The International Library of Psychology

THE PSYCHOLOGY OF EMOTION

Founded by C. K. Ogden

The International Library of Psychology

ABNORMAL AND CLINICAL PSYCHOLOGY
In 19 Volumes

THE PSYCHOLOGY OF EMOTION

Morbid and Normal

JOHN T MacCURDY

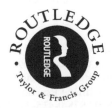

First published in 1925 by
Routledge, Trench, Trubner & Co., Ltd.

Reprinted 1999, 2000, 2001, 2002 by
Routledge
2 Park Square, Milton Park, Abingdon, Oxfordshire OX14 4RN
711 Third Avenue, New York, NY 10017
First issued in paperback 2014

Transferred to Digital Printing 2005

Routledge is an imprint of the Taylor and Francis Group, an informa company

© 1925 John T MacCurdy

The publishers have made every effort to contact authors/copyright holders
of the works reprinted in the *International Library of Psychology*.
This has not been possible in every case, however, and we would
welcome correspondence from those individuals/companies
we have been unable to trace.

These reprints are taken from original copies of each book. In many cases
the condition of these originals is not perfect. The publisher has gone to
great lengths to ensure the quality of these reprints, but wishes to point
out that certain characteristics of the original copies will, of necessity, be
apparent in reprints thereof.

British Library Cataloguing in Publication Data
A CIP catalogue record for this book
is available from the British Library

The Psychology of Emotion
ISBN 13: 978-0-415-20930-4 (hbk)
ISBN 13: 978-1-138-00738-3 (pbk)
Abnormal and Clinical Psychology: 19 Volumes
ISBN 978-0-415-21123-9
The International Library of Psychology: 204 Volumes
ISBN 978-0-415-19132-6

TO THE MEMORY OF
AUGUST HOCH

PREFACE

IN addition to its academic, or literary, *raison d'être*, every book has its human origin. The latter is generally a matter of personal interest ; yet, if the author be not wholly responsible for the material he presents, he is under an obligation to disclose as much of the history of the work as may enable the reader to apportion credit or disfavour with fairness. In this instance my duty is unusually urgent for two reasons. Many of the essential data I am now reporting were brought to light by the arduous and patient labour of others. From this standpoint I am merely the mouthpiece of a group of psychiatric investigators working with a particular method. To them, and not to me, is due whatever praise may be allotted for the originality of the observations. On the other hand, throughout the text there are a number of generalizations, theories, speculations—call them what you will—which my collaborators would not claim to have fathered and for which they would, perhaps, not care to stand sponsor. Yet even here it is impossible to discriminate accurately between ideas that I have elaborated and those which I alone originated. When one is in daily discussion with another over work that lasts for years, it is impossible to say which one first suggests that vague direction in enquiry which, months later, crystallizes out in theory. Since, in honesty, I do not know where my peculiar contribution begins, and since I am convinced that alone I could have produced very little of what follows, I am under obligation to tell something of the genesis and development of this book, if not of its tribulations.

I joined the staff of the Psychiatric Institute of the New York State Hospitals in January 1913. At that time Dr. August Hoch had been Director for three years, having succeeded Dr. Adolf Meyer in that position. Both of these pre-eminent psychiatrists had the same point of view in clinical research : that it must begin with painstaking record of what patients say and do, regardless of the pertinence of these observations for any particular theory, and, further, that descriptions of mental symptoms must be put into terms of common speech, so far as is possible, because technical labels tend to obscure individual differences of reactions. In other words that case histories should describe real people and not diseases. Every worker in the Institute was trained to follow these rules. As a result a large mass of material was available for study, equally useful in the elaboration of new theories or of old. Conspicuous among the earlier workers was Dr. George H. Kirby (now Director of the Institute) whose accuracy and thoroughness of observation, acuity of clinical judgment, breadth of experience and case memory are prodigious and, since the death of Hoch, unique in my opinion. At the same period valuable records were made by Dr. C. M. Campbell and Dr. D. K. Henderson. In my own period essential contributions were added by Dr. W. W. Wright and Dr. Glenn E. Meyers. When the present work began, there was available, as well, a considerable number of Dr. Hoch's early case histories, which were of peculiar value as control material, in as much as he made these records at a time when unimpressed by any theory of the psychological origin of mental symptoms.

In the Spring of 1913, as the result of many discussions about the applicability of psychoanalytic principles to manic-depressive insanity, Dr. Hoch and I decided to study this group with the hope of seeing whether the symptoms could be traced to unconscious mental processes in the same way as Jung had demonstrated it to be possible in dementia praecox. At the same time Dr. Hoch was anxious to effect a better classification within this huge group of psychoses, as he was far from satisfied with the existing sub-divisions. The investigations necessary for the solution of this purely clinical problem would naturally be of use in any psychological study, so it was at first planned that he and Dr. Kirby should prosecute the clinical enquiries at the same time that he and I should elaborate whatever psychological data might emerge from their work. The first material examined was made up chiefly of Dr. Kirby's observations. Preliminary conclusions were then tested out by reference to the older records and by highly detailed contemporary examinations of patients. It soon became evident that Dr. Kirby, who was now Clinical Director of the huge Manhattan State Hospital, was too much engrossed in his other work to spare time for these special researches, so Dr. Hoch and I continued alone. He did, however, collaborate with Hoch in the publication in 1919 of a paper, " A Clinical Study of Psychoses Characterized by Distressed Perplexity," a work that goes a long way towards bringing order into the chaos of manic-depressive insanity.

At the end of a year our work had progressed far enough to enable Hoch to give a preliminary, sketchy report of it (" A Study of the Benign Psychoses," *John Hopkins Hospital Bulletin*, XXVI, No. 291). Before this (May 1914) I had read a paper dealing with one aspect of our psychological investigations (" A Psychological Feature of the Precipitating Causes in the Psychoses, etc.," *Journal of Abnormal Psychology*, IX, p. 297.) Otherwise the work went on for years without publication. Nevertheless it was our chief pre-occupation all the time. Early in 1917 Dr. Hoch was forced by ill health to resign his directorship and moved to California. At the same time the War claimed me. When demobilized in the Spring of 1919, I went at once to California and spent several months working with my former chief. We then rehashed all we had done, got our general conclusions formulated and, at the same time, reviewed a large mass of his material on Involution Melancholia, working out together a classification and criteria for prognosis in this sub-group. We were now ready to begin writing and at once difficulties arose as to how the work should be divided up.

These difficulties were not merely as to how the literary task should be apportioned, for we were both equally aware that credit or discredit would inevitably be assigned to him whose name appeared on the title page of every publication. And we ourselves could not decide who was responsible for what. The best we could do was to use, as a basis for division, the preponderating contribution of each. The situation was this : Dr. Hoch had for years been engaged in clinical observation and had at his disposal a wealth of knowledge to which I could not even pretend. But, in the course of his work he had seen so many hypotheses fail in fulfilling their promise that he developed a conservative attitude, invaluable in a critic but hampering to a speculator. On the other hand I had approached the problem with only one method of attack—the psychological—and innocent of anything but the rudiments of clinical knowledge. Naturally, then, I tended to be the one who thought first of psychological explanations, while he, just as naturally tended to be the destructive critic. Countless speculations had thus an ephemeral birth and death. Yet, to say of the final theories, that I was their sole author would be grossly wrong. The first suggestion probably came most often from me but Dr. Hoch added not merely evidence but countless emendations in their elaboration. Had I been working alone I would either have published fantastic hypotheses or have delayed writing till I had acquired twenty-five years of psychiatric experience. Had Dr. Hoch been working alone he would probably have concentrated his attention on the almost purely clinical problems of classification, diagnosis and prognosis. Our mutual dependence was obvious ; yet, at the same time, each was responsible for different kinds of contribution to the joint result.

We finally escaped from the dilemma with this decision, that both accepted with equal satisfaction. Dr. Hoch had been especially interested in the stupor and involution melancholia cases, so he would write detailed clinical studies of those conditions. Having already published his work on the perplexity group, this made him responsible for the chief classificatory novelties that had emerged from our work. I, then, should expose our psychological theories about manic-depressive insanity as a whole. With this understanding we parted in June 1919 and each set about his task. He outlined his book on stupor and wrote the first five chapters. Then came his sudden and calamitous death in September, 1919.

At the end he asked that I should finish his " Benign Stupors," a small return for the incalculable debt I owe him. This I did gladly. The publication of the Involution Melancholia studies presented more of a problem. I could find in his notes no indication of how his work was to proceed beyond his records of the conclusions we had arrived at jointly. So, using the material just as it had been elaborated to date, I published it under both our names, ("The Prognosis of Involution Melancholia", *Archives of Neurology and Psychiatry*, VII, p. 1).

In the course of writing out our psychology of manic-depressive insanity extensive developments have naturally taken place. In the first place, when composition extends over a period of five years, changes in formulation naturally creep in. Therefore, although I have spent hundreds of hours in checking up these emendations against clinical records, I would not care to claim that Hoch's imprimatur—with all that it means—is to be put on every detail in the theories exposed. I alone admit responsibility for what is printed, although I do not claim credit for all the ideas. Secondly, the general objective of the book has changed, under my hands, from that of psychopathological to one of psychological conclusions.

. At this point I should explain the intolerable length of this volume. I found myself with four different ends in view. One was the exposition of clinical material ; the second was a psychological theory to explain the first ; the third were conclusions of general psychopathological import ; and the fourth was a theory of emotions as they occur either in morbid or in normal states. Different audiences would be interested in these different aspects, readers with experience in different fields. The first and second had, obviously, to go together. The third might, perhaps, be able to stand alone and I attempted to make it do so in *Problems in Dynamic Psychology* (another interruption in the production of the present book !). With the general theory of emotions I was in great doubt. If I separated it off, I would either have to indulge in a vast amount of repetition or else ask the psychologist to accept my statements about clinical facts without any evidence for him to examine. I decided, with continued misgiving, not to treat the lay reader so cavalierly. But this means a book of grotesque dimensions, likely to arouse a feeling of prospective lethargy in any but the indomitably industrious. If, however, a reader is willing to accept an argument without evidence, he may shorten his perusal of it considerably by skipping the case histories which are printed in smaller type.

The separation of Hoch's work on the Stupors and of my psychological conclusions that appeared in "Problems of Dynamic Psychology" has resulted in economy of space, but has necessarily involved the omission of pertinent material. So far is the latter true that I doubt if certain points will be fully clear to one who has not read these other books. To remedy this defect in small measure I have made extensive quotations from Hoch's book in Part III, and from my own work in Chapter 49. I wish to record my gratitude to the Macmillan Company of New York for the privilege they have generously granted me of making citations from books which they published.[1]

Although in the psychiatric portion of this study I am very largely reaping what others have sown, I have to assume responsibility for the part which has general psychological reference. Yet here again I must record a debt. If my psychological Introduction and Conclusion fall short of complete incomprehensibility, it is because of the shrewd criticisms of Mr. F. C. Bartlett of the Cambridge Psychological Laboratory. How much his suggestive criticisms may have contributed, insensibly, to my final formulations I do not dare to conjecture. Perhaps at this point I should mention that the form in which the psychological theory of emotions is presented does not at all represent the history of its development in my mind. I arrived at my conclusion—as I suppose everyone does—independently of the literature. My views grew out of the clinical studies I was making. But, in presenting an argument, it is fairer to others, and often much more logical, to elaborate the theme historically than in terms of the peculiar set of influences that shaped it in the mind of the author.

The purpose of the Glossary at the end of the book should be explained. It is hoped that readers may be drawn from among not only psychiatrists and psychologists but also from among lay men interested in psychological problems. I have tried to write in an every day vocabulary but it is inevitable that there should creep in technical terms belonging to general medicine, psychiatry and psychology. All such I have gathered, I hope, into the Glossary. But it has—or may have, I hope—another service to perform. Both psychiatry and psychology are young and growing sciences, their advances are made by workers with great variation in point of view. Consequently their technical terms are given different meanings by different schools and even by different writers in the same general school. Before the critic abandons hope for my salvation I would ask him to consult the Glossary in order to learn in what sense *I* am using any given term.

For the convenience of the reader I should add a descriptive word about the Psychiatric Institute, because many of the quoted remarks of patients may otherwise be inexplicable. The Institute

[1] Specifically these quotations are as follows :

From Hoch's " Benign Stupors," page 6 line 24 to page 11 line 9

,,	35	,,	14	,,	39	,,	9
,,	72	,,	11	,,	74	,,	2
,,	82	,,	11	,,	91	,,	39
,,	104	,,	17	,,	122	,,	last
,,	186	,,	2	,,	204	,,	last
,,	234	,,	11	,,	240	,,	9
,,	246	,,	17	,,	248	,,	last

and from my " Problems in Dynamic Psychology " :

page	101	line	13	to page	109	line	29
,,	111	,,	1	,,	111	,,	25
,,	113	,,	4	,,	115	,,	last.

has two wards, a male and a female, for clinical investigations, that are set apart from the general wards of the Manhattan State Hospital, situated on Ward's Island in East River, New York City. On one side lies Hell Gate and, on the other, across the western division of East River, Manhattan is to be seen. All the patients arrive by ferry boat, having had a preliminary examination in a special ward of Bellevue Hospital, which is referred to here as the " Observation Pavillion." They are all patients in Manhattan State Hospital, technically, and only the more curious among them ever learn that they are being studied by members of the Institute staff. The Hospital is, by all, referred to indifferently as Manhattan State Hospital or as " Ward's Island ".

J. T. M.

Corpus Christi College, Cambridge, May 1924.

CONTENTS

xvi   CONTENTS

PART I

PSYCHIATRICAL INTRODUCTION

CHAPTER I

THE MANIC-DEPRESSIVE GROUP

A CONVENTIONAL opening to psychiatrical monographs is a tedious discussion of the literature pertinent to the field in which explorations are to be described. The reader will be spared this for the following reasons. It is expected that he will be a technical psychiatrist, a professional psychologist, or a layman interested in psychological problems. In the first case he will have ready access to, or be already familiar with, digests laboriously compiled by experts, whose pens turn with greater facility to such tasks than does mine. If, however, he be either an "academic" or a lay psychologist, his interest will be confined to the text with its clinical material and argument ; he will be indifferent to the question of the relative or absolute originality of what he reads. Nevertheless, since psychiatrical and psychological discussions cannot be utterly divorced, since the classificatory and diagnostic problems with which we are to be concerned have important psychological implications—and would otherwise be out of place in this book—for these reasons the non-medical reader must be put *au courant* with some matters of psychiatrical debate. It is mainly for him that this chapter is written.

Older than medicine and older than recorded history is the observation that madness may be temporary. Of almost equal antiquity is the knowledge that such attacks tend to recur in the same individual and to be of roughly the same type when they do reappear. But it was probably not until psychiatry was sufficiently advanced to be called a specialty, that recognition came of the fact that temporary insanity was apt to be characterized by marked

I   B

changes in mood, that is, that the patients were morbidly sad, happy,
fearful and so on.

Recoverability, recurrence, and emotional disturbance, fundamental generalizations as they are, are still features too vague and
too general on which to base a satisfactory classification. Modern
efforts have been aimed at the establishment of groups in which a
reasonable internal consistency could be found. The first important
one of these was in France. Forty-five years ago Falret and Bail-
larger described what the former termed " Folie Circulaire ", a
psychosis[1] in which oscillations occur between elation, or maniacal
excitement, and a depressive condition. Such phenomena have
since then been observed with such regularity that there can be no
doubt that striking alternations of emotional reaction are characteristic of many recoverable psychoses. This is so well recognized
that, for " Circular Insanity ", the more pompous term of " Cyclothymia " has become current, while the adjective " cyclothymic "
is applied even to personality. One who is given to marked mood
swings is spoken of as cyclothymic.

The occurrence during one attack of apparently antithetic emotions
would seem to indicate some, if only a pathological, relationship
between them. Naturally it was not long before psychiatrists
began to say that it was accidental whether the mania and
depression occurred in one attack or were separated by a period
of normality, or of apparent normality. This extension of
the term made it possible to include under this heading all
recurrent attacks of emotional insanity : if a severe depression
terminated with a short, mild elation, the attack could be
called cyclothymic ; if the elation were not present at all, it
might appear in the next breakdown. Nay, further, an isolated
psychosis could be similarly labelled, because with all recurrent
disease the first attack is necessarily an isolated one and, in this
instance, if the aberration was of an emotional order, one could
expect other attacks to appear, justifying the diagnosis. This
elasticity robbed circular insanity of its specific meaning, which lay
in its implication of alternation, the latter being generalized into
mere recurrence. The next phase was a reaction against this loose-
ness. In the last decade of the last century strenuous efforts were
made to keep cyclothymia a clinical entity, and clinical research aimed
at finding criteria, which might be used effectively to differentiate
between true circular insanity and other disturbances that might or
might not be periodic, let alone alternating. These were attempts
to erect and maintain landmarks on shifting sands.

About the turn of the century Kraepelin began to unravel this
Gordian knot by grouping together under the title of " Manic-
Depressive Insanity " all periodic, emotional insanities, regardless of
whether they were circular or merely recurrent. In 1904, in the

[1] See the Glossary.

seventh edition of his text book, he cut the knot by including simple mania[1]. Still later[2] he brought in most melancholias as well. (These are conditions of anxious depression, often with much hypochondria, occurring mainly in the advancing years of life.) His present standpoint, which is almost universally accepted, may be given most fairly by quoting his own words of introduction to this section in the last edition of his text book.

" Manic-depressive insanity . . . includes, on the one hand, the whole domain of the so-called periodic and circular insanities and, on the other, simple mania, the majority of the clinical pictures labelled ' Melancholia ' and also a not inconsiderable number of cases of amentia[3]. Finally we reckon here certain mild, even very mild, mood nuances, sometimes periodic, sometimes permanent, that are to be viewed on the one hand as preliminary to more severe disturbances, and on the other glide over into the domain of personality make-up. In the course of years I have become more and more convinced that all these phenomena are manifestations of only one pathological process. I grant that a series of subsidiary forms may possibly be built up later, or that individual little groups be entirely split off again ; but, if this happens, then according to my view, it is quite certain that those symptoms should not be used as criteria, which up to that time were customarily placed in the foreground."

At this point a comment may be made parenthetically, which is, I believe, pertinent. The essence of Kraepelinian psychiatry is displayed in this quotation. He begins by formulating a classification of great practical value. Then comes a theoretic generalization that seems sound, namely that all the symptoms are manifestations of one pathological process. But at once a vigilant proprietorship forces an inconsistency. If there be one pathological process it must be the central fact or theory, the ultimate justification of the classification, for which the symptoms are of secondary importance. He proceeds, however, to claim that the classification rests on the presence of certain symptoms that derive their importance from a point of view. Since it is his imprimatur that dignifies these symptoms, he is, in effect, making an appeal to his authority rather than to clinical experience or to the demonstrability of a fundamental pathological process. The significance of this criticism will appear more clearly as we proceed.

The arguments he adduces for the unity of the manic-depressive group are excellent. We find a certain small constellation of aberrations in all forms of manic-depressive insanity, appearing in

[1] Simple mania is an isolated excitement, nor recurrent and not turning into any other abnormal emotional state.

[2] Kraepelin, *Lehrbuch der Psychiatrie*, 8te Auflage, Leipzig, 1910.

[3] " Amentia " is " a dreamy confusion with perception falsified through illusions and hallucinations and accompanied by bodily unrest ". In its purest form it often follows infections : hence in America it is usually known as " Toxio-Exhaustive Psychosis ".

manifold expressions and combinations, it is true, but persisting side by side with shifting, transitory symptoms. These give a stamp of unity to all cases, although not necessarily pathognomic in any given case. If one is familiar with the type picture he can recognize it in the majority of cases, even at one interview, in spite of the variety of disguises it may assume. Of still greater importance is the experience that all the different syndromes, which are grouped together in manic-depressive insanity, melt off into each other imperceptibly, or may replace each other even during one attack. In the same patient we see changing places, not merely mania and depression, but also states of deepest confusion and irrationality, striking delusional fabrications and, lastly, mild mood variations. Again, there is usually a prolonged, monotonous, emotional background against which is developed a full-blown, circumscribed attack. A further bond between the different clinical pictures is their common prognosis ; fast or slowly all the patients recover, and dementia does not appear even after many repeated attacks. Hereditarily too, a close relationship between the different types is to be discovered. One member of a family may have periodic and another circular attacks, or one manic, another depressive and a third confusional episodes, and so on.

In making his sub-divisions of manic-depressive insanity Kraepelin disregards the older groups of " periodic " or " circular ", etc., and proposes three broad types. These are : mania with its symptoms of flight of ideas, feeling of elation and over-activity ; depression characterized by sadness or anxiety, with retardation of thought and action ; and the mixed conditions where some manic and some depressive symptoms appear side by side, producing a state that can be called neither mania nor depression. We shall have a good deal to say about this classification, for the principles involved transcend the technical problems of psychiatry. It is not merely a matter of hospital expedience but of fundamental, psycho-pathological theory. Before entering into this discussion, however, we must see what Kraepelin concludes as to the basic pathology of these psychoses.

" Manic-depressive insanity occurs in attacks, the appearance of which is, in general, independent of external influence. This fact points to the view that the essential and fundamental cause of the disease is to be sought in a permanent morbid condition, that must also exist during the times when no attacks are present. We assume this most readily when frequent illnesses recur at approximately equal intervals. But when the disease appears only a few times or even once in a life time, its roots have already been growing for a long time or are to be sought in a perversion of psychic life established since youth."

He admits that in some cases there seems to be an exception to this generalization. They are the psychoses that look as if they were precipitated by exogenous factors. Such accidents are due to alcoholism, syphilis, injuries to the brain, bodily diseases (particularly infections), pregnancy and child-birth. But only a small proportion of the patients show a history of such intercurrent factors, and the same patient, who now seems to have broken down after one of these physical insults, may have had previous attacks in which no external agency was discoverable. A statistically more important group is that in which some mental cause seems to operate. Deaths of relatives and friends are particularly prominent ; then there are quarrels, frights, lawsuits, betrothals, threats, housemoving and so on. But here again he finds that many patients seem to have causeless attacks, and that in the same way one psychosis may seem to be precipitated by mental stress, but another come out of the blue. (It may be marked here that our experience fails to confirm this last claim. We always find that *something* untoward has occurred with which the breakdown is connected, although careful and extensive inquiry may be needed in order to discover what it is. Of course we regard such events as pregnancy and child-birth as having psychological significance, whereas Kraepelin looks on them merely from the physical standpoint.)

So Kraepelin comes to the conclusion that exogenous influences play an inconstant and therefore negligible rôle ; a basic predisposition must exist. Statistical demonstration of this appeared in 377 of nearly 1,000 cases in the Munich clinic, such cases showing a history of peculiarities in their free intervals. Sometimes these abnormalities seemed merely to be exaggerated when a definite psychosis appeared, but in others the symptoms of the attack were apparently opposite in nature to the characteristics of the normal life of the patients. A further interesting observation is that other members of the patient's family might also show these oddities, although these others never broke down.

He does not say how often such temperamental abnormalities appear in families where no psychoses intervened.

His conclusion therefore is that " there are certain predispositions that may be regarded as early stages of manic-depressive insanity. They can exist throughout the entire life as peculiar formations of the psychic personality without further development ; but they may also under special circumstances become the point of departure for pathological developments occurring in separate attacks." He calls these predispositions the " fundamental conditions " (Grundzustände) of manic-depressive insanity. The principal forms that the fundamental conditions assume are a depressive (or anxious) predisposition, a manic, one of emotional excitability, or a cyclothymic tendency. The manic personalities are characterized by flightiness, buoyancy, overconfidence, and superficial judgment. The depressive people worry much, take everything hard, have a pessimistic outlook and have to force themselves into activity. Those with emotional instability over-react to circumstances that are in the slightest degree out of the ordinary : they have hasty tempers, facile tears, and " take on " about anything. The layman would call many of them " hysterical ". The cyclothymics are always either on the crest of the wave or wallowing in the depths.

When Kraepelin comes to discuss the etiology of magic-depressive insanity he says, " The causes of the disease we must look for essentially, so it seems, in the pathological predisposition ". He then proceeds to enumerate the customary factors of heredity, age, sex, chronic physical disease, etc. that may be at the back of this predisposition.

The most impressive evidence he offers is of heredity. A number of authors, agreeing with Kraepelin's experience, have found hereditary taint in 4-5ths of manic-depressive cases ; abnormality was discoverable in the parents of 1-3rd of their patients.

Age seems to be a factor of no small moment. 16.4% of 903 cases showed the first attack between 15 and 20 years of age ; 15.3% and 15.4% initiated psychoses between 20 to 25, and 25 to 30 respectively. From then on the frequency of onset declines steadily up to 85 years, with the exception of a slight rise of the curve between 45 and 50. A full 50% begin their psychotic careers before the age of 30. With the exception of the rise between the ages of 45 and 50, the curve follows, roughly, that of the number of survivors in a given population at the different age periods. So, if these were the only attacks from which the patients suffered, there would be nothing very remarkable about these figures. There are a decreasing number of people living from the age of 20 on who may develop manic-depressive insanity. But it is a matter of common psychiatric observation that the younger the patient at the time of the first attack, the greater is the liability to recurrence and the greater is the proportion of subsequent life to be spent in an institution. A man who first breaks down in his teens is liable to many more psychoses, whereas if he is, let us say, 35 years old when the first break comes he has a fair chance of never having another. These impressions receive confirmation from a study of the statistics collected by Pollock[1] from the data gathered in the New York State Hospitals. One is forced to the conclusion that some kind of a constitutional defect exists in manic-depressive insanity, which tends to be checked by the greater elasticity and adaptibility of youth, or comes to expression with the gradual increase of stress and strain as life advances. If one succumbs in spite of the relative freedom from responsibility in youth and of its greater resilience, then it must be assumed that this constitutional weakness is unusually pronounced.

Another interesting point which Kraepelin discusses in connexion with the age factor is the change in proportion of the different types of illness as the years go on. There is a tendency for reduction in the relative number of manias and mixed conditions with a corresponding increase in the proportion of depressions. At the extremes

[1] Not yet published.

the contrast is striking ; up to the age of 20 years, there are approximately an equal number of manias and depressions, but after 60 years there are 4.3 times as many of the latter. Kraepelin, quite rightly, I think, ascribes this both to the effect of physical regression which tends to limit activity, and also to the change of outlook incidental to increasing age.

As to the influence of sex, he points out that women are regularly more affected than men. The slight proportionate differences between the two sexes at different ages and with different types of psychosis are not so striking as the figures just discussed.

Temperamental peculiarities influence the type of psychosis that developes, particularly in the case of depressive personalities which tend to produce a large number of depressions and very few manic states. Manic predispositions are followed by more manias, but, strangely enough, by still more depressions. As Kraepelin points out, however, one may regard these predispositions, not as causal factors, but as symptoms of an existing disease.

These factors all have to do with the manic-depressive constitution, whatever it may be. In addition there are the exogenous factors of alcohol, syphilis, head injuries, bodily disease, pregnancy and child-birth. They all seem to play a subordinate rôle, as Kraepelin says. As to physical basis of the actual attacks, he has to admit that we are completely in obscurity. He discusses the hypotheses that have been advanced in favour of vasomotor or metabolic changes, auto-intoxication and endocrine disturbances. Speculation outweighs evidence heavily in this field.

Now where does all this argument get us to in the end ? The inexpedience of trying to maintain, as unrelated psychoses, simple manias, simple depressions, " periodic ", recurrent, and cyclothymic attacks seems fully proved. His proof of the existence of a common thread running through all of these seems convincing, and his claim of there being some common constitution lying back of it all seems to be justified. But, when we come to examine the meaning and implications of his constitutional predisposition, difficulties arise. There are two problems here : is this predisposition a tendency or an already existing disease ; and in what terms is the predisposition to be described ?

As to the first problem, Kraepelin says explicitly that the anomalies of these patients represent not merely abnormality but symptoms of manic-depressive insanity itself. If all his patients showed such temperamental peculiarities as he describes, this would be a strong argument in his favour. But he claims this history in only 37% of his cases. One might get around this difficulty by supposing that only the more severe cases displayed these " symptoms " in the free intervals. But this is notoriously contrary to the facts. Everyone knows people who go through life with a manic or depressive tendency and never have any attacks—or only one very mild one. We are familiar, too, with the emotionally labile personality that may never develop anything worse than a psychoneurosis. On the other hand, psychiatrists see severe manic-depressive attacks occurring in patients who seem in their intervals, superficially at least, to be possessed of equable temperaments. Again, the argument as to the existence of these characteristics in other members of the family of a manic-depressive patient is futile because such observations are not controlled by statistics of the occurrence of " moods " in persons unrelated to manic-depressive patients. Everyone knows emotionally unstable individuals into whose family history one must delve a long way before discoverng a case of manic-depressive insanity, although other mental diseases may be quickly discovered.   In short, he cannot prove the existence in the " normal " periods of a definite disease, although all his arguments are cogent, if this claim be merely for the existence of a pathological *tendency*.

The insistence on this discrimination is not a bit of academic hair-splitting.   It affects one's psychiatrical outlook practically and profoundly.   If one views the constitutional something as an established disease, this tends towards the notion of a specific (it undiscoverable) physical pathology and towards a pessimistic attitude as regards treatment.   If the disease be due essentially to an unknown physical cause, we cannot hope to affect its course materially until the bodily vice be demonstrated.   On the other hand, if one regards the predisposition merely as a tendency towards what is, psychologically, morbid, one can study its relationship to other abnormalities, thus enlarging our knowledge of psycho-pathology and may reasonably hope to modify the exhibitions of the disease by mental influence.

The second problem is, at bottom, another version of the first. Are we to discuss the constitutional something in terms of psychology or of abnormal bodily processes ?   Are we to regard the disease process as one in which one morbid mental reaction leads to another, the whole story being told in psychological terms, or are we to presume that a physically altered brain produces mental symptoms all or most of which are *direct* expressions of diseased tissue ?   If the latter view prevail, we could hope to trace continuity only in a series of physiologically related processes, which produced symptoms unrelated except at the physiological level where they originated. If, on the other hand, the symptoms are integrally connected as psychic entities, one might hope to discover the psychological laws which were responsible for their appearance and constellation.   In other words, this view would make of manic-depressive insanity a field for study like that of normal behaviour.

CHAPTER II

SOMATIC AND PSYCHOLOGICAL PATHOLOGY

NO one denies that, somehow, mental processes are based on physiological processes, but the physiology is unknown, so the phenomena must be discussed in psychological terms. If a man sees a bottle, draws its cork and pours himself out a drink, we can only talk about his actions in terms of ideas, their associations, etc. If enough of his brain were destroyed we know he could not associate the ideas of wine, corkscrew, etc., with sufficient accuracy to govern successful behaviour. We therefore conclude that some brain processes are essential, but as to what they are we have no glimmering. No one can translate the idea "corkscrew" in terms of physiology without being guilty of the grossest tautology. In fact, a little reflection shows a neurologist[1] that our knowledge would have to advance prodigiously before a real translation would be possible. In quite the same way no one can describe the development of a fertilized ovum in terms of physical and chemical reactions, although it is manifest to the biologist that physical and chemical changes are in progress, and that inorganic factors are essential to development. In such cases we are forced to formulate our laws in the language of the science to which the phenomena belong. There are laws of development that are expressed in biological terms ; there are laws as to the association of ideas, for instance, that we can put in none but psychological terms.

Now it should not be thought that such a method of approach eliminates all consideration of physical pathology. It merely postpones it. If we study different forms of mental disease with the ambition of establishing different psychological reaction types, we may hope to reach a point when our analysis of each reaction reveals the initial psychological abnormality which either produces the symptoms (through the operation of normal psychological laws), or is the simple morbid psychological process constituting the disease. If, at this point, a constant brain lesion is demonstrable, it may be correlated with the specific psychological error. Thus, if one reduced the symptoms of paresis to their simplest psychological terms (which no one has ever bothered to do, by the way) and did the same for arteriosclerotic dementia, some correlation between brain tissue disturbance and mental perversion might be discovered, because we are not altogether ignorant of the morbid anatomy of

[1] See, for instance, Loeb's argument in his book *Comparative Physiology of the Brain and Psychology*, Chapter XVII.

these diseases. But to find what cell changes correspond to the delusion of having a ship full of rubies is much more of a task than that of looking for a needle in a haystack. This delusion, however, might be reduced to a comparatively simple psychological error, simple enough to be the basis of some rough correlation.

An analogy from the field of general medicine may make this point clear. A patient may have a stricture at the lower end of the stomach. The direct and immediate effects of this are mechanical, and may be described in mechanical terms. But digestion is affected, the functions of the whole alimentary canal disturbed and, ultimately, serious changes in body chemistry may ensue. All these later developments cannot be described in any but physiological terms, nor can any one of them be correlated with the first mechanical cause until analysis has resolved the symptoms down to the first and simplest physiological abnormality. Among other effects acidosis may be produced. To correlate acidosis directly with a mechanical defect in the gut is absurd ; acidosis may spring from a great variety of causes and no such specific connexion could be sanely alleged. But if one proceeds : acidosis arises from disproportionate use of body tissues for fuel ; too much fat and protein is being burnt and too little carbohydrate ; insufficient carbohydrate is being absorbed ; it is not reaching the intestine ; the passage of food is obstructed :—at this point one reaches a simple physiological defect that can be described, and described adequately, in mechanical terms.

Whatever may be their differences over minor points all psychiatrists the world around seem, to-day, to belong to one or the other of these schools : those who seek a psychological explanation for mental symptoms, and those who seek a physical. To the latter school Kraepelin not only belongs but might even be said to be the head master. Only in America do the leading psychiatrists belong preponderately to the first group, although there are still many who prefer Kraepelin's dicta to any other teaching or to independent observation and judgment. In general, his word carries more authority than that of any other psychiatrist, hence the space consumed in this *Introduction* by the discussion of his views.

I have searched in vain for any unequivocal statement Kraepelin might have made as to whether the symptoms of manic-depressive insanity are to be regarded as psychologically determined or not. It is true that he says, as quoted above, that the roots of the disease " have been growing for a long time or are to be sought in a perversion of psychic life established since youth ". This might lead one to suppose that he leaned towards the psychological view, but wherever else we turn the implications of his opinions seem to tend in the opposite direction. Five examples may be cited : his failure to classify manic-depressive insanity with the psychogenic[1] disorders ;

---

[1] See Chapter 4 for the meaning of this term.

his denial of the importance of precipitating mental causes ; his insistence on heredity ; his expressed views about the psychological interdependence of symptoms, and, finally, the principle involved in his sub-divisions of manic-depressive insanity.

Psychogenic disorders are those in which the symptoms appear as psychological reactions to mental events.   The symptoms may be direct expression of the mental causes or they may represent them indirectly through the mediation of morbid psychological processes— the diseased personality.   In this group, Kraepelin includes various psychoneuroses such as those precipitated by accident, trying occupations, etc., hysteria, psychoses induced by imprisonment, the delusions of persecution in deaf people and so on.   But he does not include manic-depressive insanity.   In fact, as we have seen, he explicitly denies any but a minor rôle to precipitating mental causes, saying that they are inconstant, even in one case.   The reader may judge as to the wisdom of this pronouncement, when he has perused the succeeding chapters.   (Not a single one of our cases was chosen to prove psychogensis but merely to illustrate special clinical features.)

It is usually assumed that hereditary influence is transmitted through some structural alteration, although the latter may be occult.   Demonstration of a heredity factor is therefore usually attempted by those who incline to the dogma of the physical causation of mental symptoms.   They do not seem to consider seriously the possibility that with faulty germ-plasm there may go faulty environment, producing or accentuating mental abnormality. Kraepelin's statements, backed by statistics from other psychiatrists, as to the prevalence in manic-depressive patients of bad heredity are unquestionably striking.   But what do they prove ?

There are, I believe, only two possible ways in which hereditary factors may operate in the production of mental disease.   That which is transmitted may be a general tendency towards poor adaptation and therefore abnormality—in other words the *Anlage* of any constitutional psychosis—or there may be a special inheritance of one form of insanity.   These two possibilities may be discussed separately and we shall see that here again satisfaction with either of the alternatives depends on preference for the psychological or the physical standpoint.

The psychiatrists, who believe that symptoms of constitutional psychoses can only be understood by studying their psychological inter-relations, are not shocked by the information that patients suffering from manic-depressive insanity are burdened with bad heredity.   This is to be expected.   If their mental processes are faulty, that bespeaks an organism relatively ill-adapted to its environment.   The mental abnormality may be due simply to bad education (taking that term in its widest sense) and a consequent establishment of bad habits of reaction ; but it is much more likely, in the majority of cases, to be the product of ill-health from whatever cause, or of innate defect that renders continuous, normal adaptation impossible. Naturally both factors may, and usually would, co-operate. This is particularly likely to occur with ill-health or "nervousness" in early childhood, when the psychic organism is plastic. Effectual discipline is made impossible by the first ; or, in the second case, the symptoms of the child are beyond the capacity of the parent to circumvent. Faulty habits of mind may thus be established.

On the other hand those who hold the psychogenic doctrines are apt to be startled by figures which would indicate a very high proportion of heredity in cases of manic-depressive insanity. The mental processes which give rise to symptoms are either similar to those of normal life or they are different. If different, the symptoms should always show a contrast with normal phenomena. But it is notorious that mania glides imperceptibly over into normal happiness or that depression seems like an exaggeration of normal sadness or remorse. To be free from anything that was analogous to the symptoms of manic-depressive sanity one would have to be free of emotion. We have no foot-rule to measure degrees of emotion. If a girl loses her mother we expect her to be bowed down with grief for a short time at least. Unless she be utterly incapacitated her immediate reaction is not held to be pathological. If she broods over her mother's death for a year, however, refuses to be comforted and refuses to undertake any usual activity, we begin to speak of a depression. But there are neither laws nor conventions which tell us that grief should last just a week, or a month, or six months. The supernormal young woman will force herself from the outset to be active and cheerful, the normal one will do so in a week or so. But in how many weeks ? The girl who takes two weeks for this change is more " normal " than the one who takes a month, while the one who mopes for a month is certainly not so abnormal as the one who sits glum for a year or more. In short we have to admit grades of normality, of adaptability, or whatever you wish to call it. Theoretically, then, there should also be grades of hereditary defect. But we never hear of this ; we read of the percentage of mental disease found in the family histories of those who require (or receive) medical care, but we find no record of how frequent psychopathies may be among the ascendants of those who never seek treatment. So we have no standards of comparison against which to equate statistics of heredity for any given psychoses. All we can do is to conjecture their validity from a knowledge of the general rate of mental abnormality in the community, from comparison with the figures obtained for other mental diseases, and from methods used in compiling them.

I know of only one survey of mental abnormality in the general population that has been made sufficiently extensive and intensive to furnish anything like adequate figures. This was made in Nassau County, Long Island, New York, by a special committee financed by the Rockfeller Foundation.[1] " The staff consisted of physicians of psychiatric experience, a psychologist, and field workers of at least collegiate education and special training and expe rience." Amongst other work, " Four special districts with a total poulation of 4,668 were selected for intensive investigation, *i.e.*, a house to house canvass to collect information concerning every resident of these districts.'' As a result of this intensive investigation it was judged that 3.6 per cent. of the population in these districts was mentally abnormal.

This high proportion may surprise those who have been accustomed to accept institutional figures as representing the rate of mental disease in any community. But every psychiatrist knows such a rate is a measure merely of institutional capacity, which, in turn, reflects the enlightenment of the community. As far as my own experience goes, I have never had extensive knowledge of any family, either socially or professionally, without discovering some mental disease in it. And I do not use this term figuratively. I count only such cases as any group of psychiatrists would include. My conclusion is that, to-day, there are few, if any perfect families from a psychiatric standpoint, and that the only histories which have real significance are those in which are recorded in generation after generation cases of feeble-mindedness, epilepsy, alcoholism and flagrant insanity.

As an example of how " good " families may be demonstrated to be " bad ", I may cite the following figures compiled by two psychiatrists of my acquaintance. They considered such of the ascendants and collaterals of their own children, as were personally known to them. One of them included only two generation of ascendants (and collaterals) and the other three. Among 53 individuals only 31, or 59% were judged to be normal ; 15, or 28%, were psychoneurotic or of abnormal make-up ; 7, or 13%, had had definite psychoses ! Of the eight grandparents only one came of a family concerning which there was any tradition of mental abnormality. This line did not furnish more cases than any of the others and no one would have dreamed of questioning, from a eugenic standpoint, the soundness of the other seven stocks. It is true that not one of the seven psychotics was ever legally detained in a hospital, but in all the cases committment would have been indicated had the social and economic status of the families been different. In one case—a man of national reputation—this possibility was seriously discussed ; but even close family friends were ignorant of that.

Heredity unquestionably does play a rôle in the production of insanity but, on the other hand, its influence is apt to be slight or negligible in such psychoses as are induced specifically by demonstrable brain disease. Yet *all* cases are included, as a rule, in making up insanity rates. As we have seen there is no way of measuring latent abnormality so we can never say just how much of a given rate is due to heredity. But, if we assume for the moment that it plays no rôle at all (which is unfair), and that various diseases, faulty environment, bad education, etc., produce all the abnormality discoverable in a given group, then the effect of these chance factors on statistics of alleged heredity may be worked out on the theory of probability. A mathematician friend of mine has been kind enough to do this for me.

In Nassau County an intensive survey indicated that 3.6% of the general population suffered from some form of mental abnormality. This survey was conducted, probably, with about the same zeal as is displayed by psychiatrists who are interested in establishing heredity as a factor in the production of the insanity from which their patients suffer. The intelligence of the families of the latter is likely better, if anything, than that of the groups in Nassau County chosen for special duty. We can therefore assume, for our present argument, that the 3.6% is applicable to the families of the pschiatrists' patients. That is, if enquiry be made concerning some thousands of

[1] " Survey of Mental Disorders in Nassau County, New York, July-October, 1916." *Psychiatric Bulletin of the New York State Hospitals*, Utica, N.Y., Vol. II., No. 2, April, 1917.

releatives, 3.6% of them will show abnormality, regardless of the presence of any taint peculiar to the family.

If information be secured about 10 relatives in the case of each patient the probability is that at least one case of mental abnormality will be discovered in :

$$100\left\{1-\left(\frac{96.4}{100}\right)^{10}\right\}=31\% \text{ of the groups.}$$

If the family groups include 15 members the chances would indicate :

$$100\left\{1-\left(\frac{96.4}{100}\right)^{15}\right\}=42\%$$

If the groups be of 20 people :

$$100\left\{1-\left(\frac{96.4}{100}\right)^{20}\right\}=52\%$$

If only the parents be considered, the chances of one of them having some form of mental disease is in

$$100\left\{1-\left(\frac{96.4}{100}\right)^{2}\right\}=7.1\% \text{ of cases.}$$

From these figures we can see that before heredity statistics have absolute value one must know the number of people examined and then take their probable mental disease rate as a base line. We can see, for instance, that a 30% rate for relatives is almost certain to be meaningless, while a 30% rate for parents would have significance, unless the series were small.

If heredity be an important factor in establishing a tendency to constitutional mental disease, the frequency of mental abnormalities should vary, roughly, with gravity of the psychosis (This should be true unless there were a specific heredity, a possibility to be discussed shortly.) Dementia praecox, then, a constitutional psychosis which results in permanent incapacity, ought to show a higher proportion of mental abnormality in the families of the patients than does manic-depressive insanity, where the attacks are isolated and the patient may, indeed, have only one. But Kraepelin claims only 53.8% of heredity among 1054 of his cases of dementia praecox as against his 80% in manic depressive insanity. On the other hand he reports 50% in his cases of paresis, a disease admittedly caused by syphilis in which heredity can only be a contributory factor ! So heredity, it appears, is as important practically, in paresis as in dementia praecox, while the disease whose affliction is the lightest of the three shows a much higher rate. How can these discrepancies be accounted for ? The answer is probably to be found in the zeal for enquiry and in the methods by which information is gained.

Paresis is a condition of which the specific causation has not long been known, although long suspected. When the etiology of a disease is uncertain every reasonable lead is followed up with energy. Granted that mental abnormality is commoner in the general population than is usually supposed, a thorough-going enquiry into the mental health of any group of families arbitrarily chosen will reveal a surprisingly high percentage of morbidity. For this reason I have no hesitation in predicting that the statistics of heredity in paresis will show a relative decline during the next twenty years, although I would by no means eliminate heredity as a possible contributory cause.

As to the discrepancy between the figures for dementia praecox and manic-depressive insanity, a principle of methodological importance comes in. The people whose illnesses are reported are not observed by experts (if they were all the rates would be higher) but are called to mind by questions put to relatives who have no psychiatric experience. Now, for the layman, insanity means either demoniac fury or else the one psychosis that the layman has chanced to observe. Hence the first question, " Are there any in the patient's family who were mentally afflicted ? " is answered in the negative or else it is admitted that so and so was " put away ". Further questions have to do with the presence or absence of minor abnormalities in the family. Now, if psychiatrists like Kraepelin cannot distinguish between characteristics and symptoms, how can a layman be expected to ? Inevitably he thinks of those whose characteristics, slight or marked, were like those of the patient. This leads to the report of a relatively small number of people who resembled dementia praecox and of a large number who resembled the manic-depressive patient. In the first instance only definite psychoses and markedly psychopathic personalities are spoken of, while, in the second, characteristics that are universal and grade over imperceptibly into symptoms are brought to the informant's mind.

The other possibility as to the influence of heredity is that it does not operate to produce a tendency towards abnormality of any constitutional type but that it mediates one form of insanity specifically. A number of authors have claimed specific inheritance for both dementia praecox and manic-depressive insanity and Kraepelin seems to be in sympathy with them. But their claims would appear to be refuted by their own figures. A disease may have one specific and several contributory factors. The latter may or may not appear in any given case, but the former must always be present or the alleged cause is not specific. If heredity be specific for these insanities it ought to be found in over 90% of cases (allowing for inevitable gaps in information). Instead of that Kraepelin says that among the 80% of cases showing heredity of any kind " I found a disproportionate frequency of illness from manic-depressive insanity among parents and siblings." He also quotes Rehm who investigated the children of manic-depressive patients. Among 44 children in 19 families there were signs of mental degeneration in 52% ; this took the form in 29% of abnormal emotional predispositions, especially of depressive tendencies." If inheritance be specific, when it is discovered it should be invariably of the disease in question. In Rehm's series, then, the 52% of afflicted children should have been 100% manic-depressive, instead of only 57% of them showing that disease even in a dilute form. Kraepelin in various places mentions that manic-depressive patients tend to have offspring with dementia praecox. All these figures are excellent evidence in substantiation of a claim for general psychopathic taint being inheritable, but as a proof of specificity they are hopelessly inadequate. They are suggestive of specificity existing, however, if one makes a large assumption. This is that every form of mental disease and peculiarity has its specific inheritance, some dominant, some recessive, according to Mendelian principles. Then the 45% of Rehm's cases, who were abnormal but had no manic-depressive symptoms, did not manifest symptoms that appeared in their manic-depressive parents, but were exhibiting the psychoses of remoter ancestors.

At first blush this looks like a pretty idea but a moment's reflection shows it to be attended by insuperable difficulties. The first is that it would be humanly impossible to prove it. A second, and theoretic, objection, is that in many individuals two or more diseases would coincide. New clinical pictures would thus result. These could not be transmitted as such (except by coincidence) but only some of their elements would reappear in the descendants of these patients. Who could say which of the psychiatric syndromes we recognize are Mendelian units and which are composite ? Here again we reach a conclusion like that arrived at in discussing the problem of the correlation of the physical and the mental. It is only when the latter has been analysed into its simplest, basic processes that correlation is thinkable—that is by those who work critically. The psychological analysis of mental symptoms must proceed much further than it shows promise of doing to-day, before specific inheritance of psychopathies can be demonstrated.

A third objection is that endeavours like this lead to illogical, if not dishonest, argument. Statistics should be made up of actual data not of conjectures. Most of the symptoms in manic-depressive insanity and some in dementia praecox are analogous to reactions of every-day life. A person whose mental reactions are at all striking is showing characteristics that ally his personality with either dementia praecox or manic depressive insanity. One may make his choice and, unfortunately, one has to do so, if he is working on problems of heredity, because the inheritance chart is incomplete without all manifestations of the disease being filled in. Hence we find Kraepelin saying when arguing in favour of the specific inheritance of manic-depressive insanity, that among the parents and siblings of manic-depressive patients there were many cases of psychopathic personalities, " among which so many are to be counted in the field of the disease we are discussing." That is, we may take the presence of psychopathic personalities in a family as evidence for a manic-depressive taint. But if we turn to his consideration of this identical problem in connexion with dementia praecox, we read that, in the families of patients with this disease, there are many with eccentric personalities. " These are properly to be conceived of as mostly ' Latent Schizophrenia ' and therefore of the same nature as [dementia praecox]." He does not enlighten us as to the proportion of " psychopathic personalities " who are " eccentric " merely, and how many are really fledgling manic-depressives. And this is in a field where proof rests essentially on data of arithmetic definiteness ! In one place he speaks of emotional instability being a fore-runner of manic-depressive insanity. In another it is a precursor of dementia praecox, representing the symptom of impulsiveness in the latter disease. One would be happier (and our psychiatric literature less extensive) if this type of argument were confined to the land where it chiefly flourishes !

From this lengthy discussion of Kraepelin's views on heredity, which has assumed the character of a digression, it is hoped that the reader may conclude that Kraepelin is anxious to bolster up a belief in the physical determination of symptoms in manic-depressive insanity, but that, in the end, he has proved no more than that a tendency to abnormal mental functioning is present in the families of his patients.

His antagonism to the theory of psychogenesis in constitutional mental disease appears plainly in his discussion of psychoanalytic interpretations of the symptoms of dementia praecox. He makes no mention of any psychological theories in manic-depressive insanity[1], but his objection to our working hypothesis is explicitly stated : " If one means by ' complexes ' nothing else than the delusional ideas, in which the fears and wishes of the patients are mirrored, then this would be, in my opinion, only a new expression

[1] There is one exception. In discussing depression he mentions one of his cases who had as a symptom compulsive stealing. He goes on to say that Gross studied this case psycho-analytically and came to the conclusion that the stealing was a substitute for a repressed sexual impulse. Kraepelin's comment on this is : " We may well regard these compulsive fears and impulses as the expression of a certain relationship of manic-depressive insanity with degeneracy insanity (meaning moral degeneracy), which is supported on other grounds." When one thinks of how many great men have suffered from depressions, for instance, this statement is rather startling. Abraham Lincoln, or John Bunyan, is a good example. Are we to regard their psychoses as related to the insanity of moral degeneracy ? The two clinical groups are connected by Kraepelin in only one other place. He says that manic-depressive patients with longstanding symptoms, particularly manic ones, may be mistaken (by laymen) for swindlers and rascals. He then gives the points for differential diagnosis. If he has grounds for alleging this relationship why does he not give them in a discussion of manic-depressive insanity running over more than 200 pages ?

for an old thing and one that is not exactly worthy of recommenda-
tion.   Its danger lies in the psychological attitude of which it is a
product.   The idea of independent, parasitic structures, which,
on the one hand, are totally withdrawn from the influence of the ego,
and on the other are able to transform and almost annihilate it,
would upset such a mass of commonplace and thoroughly secure
psychological experiences, that its foundations must be based on
quite other means of proof than have appeared as yet." He thus
takes his stand with that stout-hearted little band of survivors from
the period when psychology took no account of unconscious mental
processes.   It is, of course, difficult to trace the psychological
history of many mental phenomena—particularly when they are
pathological—if one confines oneself to the obvious data of consciousness.   The theory of unconscious mentation requires imagination
of those who hold it.   But surely one who can be happy with a
physical cause for mental symptoms, a phantasm which is now in
germ cells, again in brain cells and flits anon to the thyroid gland—
such a man is surely not guiltless of imagination !

CHAPTER III

THE MIXED CONDITIONS

THE most important evidence and product of Kraepelin's point of view appear, if one examines his sub-division of the manic-depressive group. As we have seen, he recognizes mania with its elation and overproductivity of words and movements, depression with sadness, or anxiety and reduction in speech and activity and the "mixed conditions". The latter must now claim our attention. In order to understand his argument it will be necessary first to digest briefly his account of the symptoms of mania and depression.

Mania he divides into four sub-types. The first of these is *hypomania*, in which the patients are talkative, over-active, happy, full of pranks, but often fault-finding, particularly when in the family circle. They try to attract attention to themselves and show a loss of sense of propriety and proportion in their speech and conduct. Hence they are boastful, arrogant, get into fights and are apt to indulge in sexual excesses. In *florid mania* there are often strikingly queer actions which lead to legal detention. These patients are then found to be oriented but distractible and flighty in their train of thought. That is, the associations between consecutive, expressed ideas tend to be illogical, depending on sound associations, irrelevant stimuli from the environment, or irrelevant memories. They have transient delusions and even hallucinations, which usually have a religious, sexual, or expansive colouring. As to their mood, they are generally elated but may be irritable and scold. They show great over-activity, which is often silly or queer ; they decorate themselves, play pranks, and are often erotic in their behaviour. Speech, which is usually flighty, may become fragmentary, if excitement is intense. Some cases have more persistent delusions, which they may stoutly defend in argument. These belong to the *delusion form*. Patients in this group are apt to be less excited and have a poorer grasp of the environment, being particularly liable to misidentification of those about them. Finally, there are the *delirious states*. In these there is a deep dream-like clouding of consciousness, with fantastic, confused delusions and hallucinations. Such patients are living in an imaginary world, talking to people who are not present, and so on. The mood varies from an anxious whining to frank elation, ecstasy, or erotic excitement ; again they may be irritable or apathetic. Their verbal productions are often inarticulate sounds or senseless talk with repeated phrases and sound associations. In behaviour they show mild restlessness, sudden cries, yelling and smiling. Marked variations are common in this state, for the patient may become typically manic or stuporous.

(Although a considerable variety of symptoms is thus represented, a certain unity is discernible, particularly in the way in which each type succeeds to the former by the accentuation of some symptoms and the attenuation of others. Unity in the depressive conditions may be less easy of discovery.)

Simple melancholia, which corresponds to what we call " retarded depression ", is characterized by a subjectively felt difficulty of thinking that may become objectively demonstrable. With this there often goes a feeling of unreality, neither the patient's body nor the surroundings feeling real. There is a great loss of spirits, hopelessness, feeling of wickedness or the patient may be governed by vague anxiety and unrest. Ideas of sin or uncleanness are common. These melancholics struggle with a feeling of incapacity to do anything, which may proceed to such a point that complete inactivity results. They usually remain well oriented in spite of the difficulty in thinking. The inactivity may lead to the point of actual *stupor*. The patients then lose contact with the environment and become disoriented, although the intellectual loss may be less marked than the incapacity for physical activity. Their emotional reactions may fade, so that complete apathy results. In such cases catalepsy may intervene or senseless resistiveness. Another type develops out of simple melancholia by the addition of delusions and hallucinations of a painful or accusatory character. This is *severe melancholia*. Sometimes their ideas become quite queer. Delusions of punishment may be prominent and accompanied by melodramatic hallucinations. Again, there may be a strong hypochondriacal trend. If ideas of persecution are sufficiently pronounced we may have a *paranoid melancholia*. If the fearful aspect of these predominate, unrest may triumph over the tendency to inactivity, so that great agitation results. In *fantastical melancholia* the ideas become bizarre and ridiculous and are associated with many hallucinations. Most of these are concerned with punishment, torture, or hypochondriacal fancies. The *délire de negation* appears frequently in this type, that is a state wherein the patients assert that nothing exists, including their own bodies. Consciousness is often clouded, although the train of thought remain normal. The mood varies : sometimes they are dull, again fearful and agitated, again assaultive. Not infrequently an ironic humour appears with self-depreciation. There may be stupor or sullen inactivity alternating with outbreaks of anxious restlessness. Habits of monotonous, whining, repetitious complaining may develope. From this fantastic type there is an easy transition over into the *delirious group of depressions*. These patients are in a dreamy state, living with hallucinations. They may lie staring in front of them, not answering questions, or wander vacantly around. Sometimes they cry out suddenly. Their utterances are fragments of delusions or excerpts from hallucinatory experience. Naturally in such states disorientation is complete. The ideas one gathers to be similar to the last group.

Having thus described the two great types of mania and depression, Kraepelin proceeds to argue as follows : when one observes a large series of cases it becomes evident that there are many transition forms between typical mania and depression, and that many individual patients do not remain consistently manic or depressed in any one attack. In either of these cases what we see is a mixture of symptoms. This appears most plainly in the transition period between definite mania and depression. Certain symptoms have given place to those of the opposing type, while others belonging to the picture of the earlier phase persist. A great many queer symptom complexes may thus result. These atypical psychoses can be understood by assuming that there are a number of fundamental disturbances in manic depressive insanity, which do not necessarily have to appear in any given constellation. Grouped in the conventional way, they constitute classical mania or depression, but, thrown together irregularly, a mixed condition results.

A number of the symptoms of mania are the psychological opposites of those of depression. For instance, distractability, flight of ideas, expansive delusions, elation and bodily activity are the opposites of slowness in attention and thinking, ideas of wickedness and persecution, sadness or anxiety and inhibition of activity. On the other hand, there are no such antitheses in the spheres of understanding, intellectual capacity and judgment ; so these latter symptoms are not significant for mixed conditions. To simplify the problem, he considers only disturbances of the train of thought, of mood, and of activity, assuming that each one of these is a unitary, homogeneous, mental function, and that in every psychosis each is modified as a homogeneous whole. In classical mania or depression all of the three are modified in one direction, roughly speaking, either towards excitement or inhibition. If excitement operates in one field, while inhibition affects the other two, then a mixed condition results. The possible combinations constitute his " mixed conditions ". For instance, if a patient be typically manic, but, in swinging over into a depression, becomes anxious with inhibition of thought but remains physically overactive, a mixed condition exists until such time as activity is also inhibited when typical depression is established. Not many patients show consistently, from onset to recovery, absolutely typical mania or depression ; a considerable number are never typical of either of these states. Hence the wide statistical importance of the mixed conditions.

Kraepelin has formulated six groups by following the method first outlined and describes the clinical pictures associated with the different combinations. These he calls Depressive or Anxious Mania, Excited Depression, Unproductive Mania, Manic Stupor, Depression with Flight and Inhibited Mania. As he says, if one took into consideration other entities such as attention, apprehension, intellectual capacity or judgment[1], many more combinations could be fabricated. Undoubtedly they could. One might almost fancy that he looks forward to the day when psychiatric diagnosis can be made by a clerk with an elaborate cash register. Press the keys labelled " distractibility ", " good apprehension ", " bad judgment ", " over-activity ", " sadness ", " flight of ideas ", and " good attention ", and the diagnosis " Flight Melancholia "—or some such title—will appear. How many of these new groups there will be is a problem for a mathematician. It would be better to postpone discussion, from a clinical standpoint, of the mixed conditions he has so far fabricated till the reader has more acquaintance with clinical material. I shall then endeavour to show that Kraepelin has made of his manic-depressive ward a dormitory of Procrustean beds.

Criticism may now be made of his method, however, on purely theoretic grounds. He has followed what may justly be called the algebraic procedure. There are three elements which he considers in their plus or minus aspects. a is activity, b is the mood disturbance, c is the disturbance of thinking. There are eight combinations of these[2]; $\overset{+\,+\,+}{a\ b\ c}$ (mania), $\overset{-\,-\,-}{a\ b\ c}$ (depression), $\overset{+\,-\,+}{a\ b\ c}$ (depressive or anxious mania), $\overset{+\,-\,-}{a\ b\ c}$ (excited depression), $\overset{+\,+\,-}{a\ b\ c}$ (unproductive mania) $\overset{-\,+\,-}{a\ b\ c}$ (manic stupor), $\overset{-\,-\,+}{a\ b\ c}$ (depression with flight), $\overset{-\,+\,+}{a\ b\ c}$ (inhibited mania). This type of argument is seductive, because, once fairly embarked on it, its logic is unassailable. But is it applicable at all ; are the primary assumptions justifiable ? If the assumptions are justifiable, the method is surely sound.

Two chief assumptions are made and each is an example of psychological audacity. The first is explicity stated : that physical activity, train of thought and mood are psychological units. If they are units, they must be incapable of further analysis, they must represent themselves and not latent factors, in their clinical behaviour. But a score of objections to this assumption spring to one's mind at once, objections, at least, to the application of this view to ordinary life. Bodily activity, for instance, is held to be significant in virtue of its quality, not of its presence or absence ; it is an expression of something else. A boxer who dances about

[1] It should be noted that he does not say, " 21 other clinical syndromes te discovered." The point of departure for his classification is not clinical observation but psychological theory.
[2] See his diagram on page 1287 of the *Lehrbuch*.

the ring, continuously waving his arms is not held to be more active than his opponent, who may make a tithe of the movements, but each one with accuracy and speed. The inactivity of a cat asleep, and of a cat about to spring, are not to be taken as equivalents.

Anomalies in the sphere of thinking Kraepelin judges of by examining the verbal productions (although he assumes an internal train of thought when it suits his scheme, but does not do so in other instances, where the evidence is as good). The quietness of " the strong, silent man " and the speechlessness of embarrassment are not at all the same thing, although both are silence. The kind of thinking disorder, to which Kraepelin confines himself, has to do with attention to the environment and the richness or poverty of ideas in the train of thought. Either these are both expressions of the same principle, or they are simply related elements. In mania a heightened kind of attention leads to distractibility which is correlated with the richness of successive ideas in manic flight. This fits Kraepelin's concept of a homogeneous unit. But, when we come to his excited depression group, we meet with a certain dissociation. Ideation has become pathologically poor, but attention is, apparently, normal, for he describes the patients as being clear as to their surroundings, having normal apprehension and being always anxious to talk to someone. Again he says that in the unproductive manics there is slow and uncertain perception, no attention to questions, failure to understand quite simple things. So attention is morbidly diminished. But at once he goes on to say that they laugh with or without stimulus and rejoice over every little thing. Trifles (and *every* trifle) cannot produce joy, unless attention is given to them. We are forced to conclude that attention itself is capable of dissociation. Of course, this is no novelty. We all know that attention is constantly selective and hence cannot be an independently functioning mental unit.

I shall not now anticipate the discussion of Part II by mentioning more than one argument against the concept of the mood in manic-depressive insanity representing a single entity. According to Kraepelin this unit changes its nature by moving in one dimension, moving up or down, becoming greater or less—one can express the change in a variety of terms. As a matter of fact more than three emotions do appear in manic-depressive insanity, but he does speak of three, elation, sadness, and anxiety. According to him, when elation moves in the minus direction[1], it becomes either sadness or anxiety. No unitary element can have two different opposites.

Still more important than the criticisms of Kraepelin's units is the assumption that they operate independently. He does not make this assumption in so many words, but it is implicit in his whole argument. General pathology has liberated itself from the notion that the functions of any one organ can be studied alone,

[1] See again his diagram on page 1287.

as if that organ existed *in vitro*. Much less should we expect mental faculties to be isolated, since the mental is, essentially the integrated functions of the organism as a whole. There are, of course, various parts of the mental structure just as there are different parts of an engine, but in neither do we see one part ever working alone. One might imagine, of course—and this may, perhaps, be Kraepelin's view—that, when the mind is deranged, its various functions do operate independently. In fact his theory of the mixed conditions does look as if he regarded mental functions to be as separable as the cards in a pack, from which many different hands may be dealt. The presence or absence of a given card in any one hand does not influence the presence of another. There is no integration here, merely a mixture. But when integration does exist, as in an engine, each part does actuate or control others and, indirectly, all others. When an engine behaves badly it is due not to the rearrangement of parts but the excessive or diminished function of some part. If one rearranged the parts the engine would not run at all ; that is, would " die ". So with the mind. If integration of mental functions exists in health, it is highly unlikely that a rearrangement of its parts could lead to anything except cessation of all mental function. What probably does happen is the accentuation of one or more functions, producing a new type of integration.

It is true that Kraepelin does, at times, admit a psychological relationship between symptoms. For instance, he says that in mania a poor grasp of the environment may be due more to defective attention than to any essential loss of apprehension. This, of course, is, on most superficial reflection, na obvious conclusion. But he does not go further than this. To him the notion that attention or apprehension were psychologically related to the kind of ideas and emotions present would probably seem idle, if not pernicious, speculation. His problem is to find permutations and combinations of basic symptoms which may coincide with puzzling clinical pictures. If this is a good method, then his mixed conditions are psychiatrically useful. If, however, the method is unsound, his classification is a useless encumbrance. The question turns on the relative validity of the physical and psychological attitude. What, therefore, seems at the first glance to be a technical psychiatric problem turns out to be a matter involving a fundamental principle, as important for psychology as for psychiatry. . If all the reactions of the normal man were easily explicable in the light of current psychological knowledge, psychologists might not be interested in this problem. But, since perversions of disease may explain anomalies in normal life, no psychologist can afford to remain in ignorance of psychiatric issues involving basic theory.

CHAPTER IV

THE THEORY OF PSYCHOGENESIS

AGAINST the Kraepelinian attitude in psychiatry, with its grudging admission of psychology to explain the obvious, its explicit denial of the mental determination of symptoms as a whole, and its insistent emphasis on non-mental factors, protests have been appearing with increasing frequency. The chief of these have been in Switzerland and America and both owe their genesis and development mainly to the teachings of Freud.

Psychogenesis, as applied to the psychoses, and in its modern sense, begins definitely with a brief analysis[1] of a case of what Freud then called " Chronic Paranoia ", but which he would doubtless diagnose to-day as dementia praecox. In this he demonstrated the origin of hallucinations, queer behaviour and false ideas from early experiences, some of them going back to childhood and some of them forgotten before treatment. In studying this case he arrived at the opinion that the psychological mechanisms in such psychoses were analogous to those he claimed to exist in some of the neuroses. Further than this he did not go. This publication does not seem to have met with much recognition.

In 1904 Tilling published a highly important work[2], in which he made unequivocal generalizations about the genesis of symptoms in the constitutional psychoses, specifically dementia praecox and manic-depressive insanity. He claimed that the origin of the psychosis was to be found in the weakness or disproportion of the personality before actual disease was manifest. " In general it becomes evident that the illness exaggerates an already existent disharmony of the elements and factors of the mental organism of the personality. Certain predisposed parts are developed more strongly, feeding on others, so that a caricature appears, in which certain features are accentuated." The clinical pictures and course of the disease are caused by individual factors and are only to be understood psychologically. In fact, he went so far as to say that psychiatry was, properly speaking, only a branch of psychology. The fundamental inferiority of the predisposed personality, he traced

---

[1] Freud, S., " Analyse eines Falles von chronischer Paranoia," *Neurologisches Zentralblatt*, 1896, No 10. Reprinted in *Sammlung Kleiner Schriften zur Neurosenlehre*, 1893-1906, Zweite Auflage, Deuticke.
[2] Tilling, *Individuelle Geistesartung v. Geistesstörung*, Wiesbaden, Bergmann, 1904.

to some organic cause, but denied the specificity of the latter for these forms of mental trouble. The break-down, he said, was a product of inner incapacity and environmental stress, so that chance might decide whether a man had merely a neurosis, or manic-depressive insanity, or crossed the Rubicon and became a sufferer from dementia praecox. Anticipating the obvious criticism to the effect that disease could not be a product of a personality, when the former was the opposite of the latter, he mentioned his observations in the Baltic Russian Provinces, where he witnessed the effects of revolution on sedate, dull people. Whole communities, under the excitement, became typically manic and indulged in behaviour that was a complete reversal of their normal reactions. This showed that purely psychological influences could turn a personality upside down by freeing certain impulses, as Tilling said, that had been in the background, while those of an opposite nature were repressed.

Needless to say, German psychiatrists received this theory with the enthusiasm of hounds for a fox. The pack was led by Neisser, who instituted a polemic the details of which are irrelevant. Boiled down, Neisser's arguments amounted to this : he did not like Tilling's views because they upset one's preconceptions and he was not going to change his opinions till he was forced to by more weight of evidence. A typical criticism came from Reiss, who disposed of Tilling's analogy of the Russian revolutionists by saying that, of course, these phenomena were hysterical—as if such a label could annihilate the fact that the mechanism *was* psychological !

Two years later (1906) appeared publications, which may safely be said to be the foundations of modern psychiatry. In Switzerland Bleuler[1] claimed that Freudian mechanisms were applicable for the understanding of psychotic symptoms, particularly in paranoia. The next year his associate Jung published his classical study of dementia praecox[2]. In this he demonstrated the origin of many symptoms from conflicts of pre-psychotic life and illustrated many Freudian mechanisms in the development of symptoms. This latter contribution especially has been the inspiration for innumerable studies of the kind, so that now, whether they sympathize with psychoanalysis or not, psychiatrists are all familiar with the application of Freud's principles to the understanding of dementia praecox. The kind of work which Jung started going has been essentially mechanistic and analytic ; that is, it has been concerned with the development of specific symptoms rather than with an explanation of the disease as a whole.

At the same period in America interest in psychogenesis took

---

[1] Bleuler, " Freud'sche Mechanismen in der Symptomatologie von Psychosen," *Psychiatrisch-Neurologische Wochenschrift*, 1906, VIII., Nos. 34, 35, and 36.
[2] Jung, *Ueber die Psychologie der Dementia praecox*. Halle, Carl Marhold, 1907.

a form that has been, I think, still more fruitful. In 1906 Adolf Meyer published a paper[1] in which he spoke not merely of mechanisms and specific symptom determination, but emphasized the rôle of the personality as a whole in the production of the disease as a whole. That is, the early conflicts were given their significance in virtue of a defective personality, a personality that was poorly adapted to its mental (and particularly emotional) environment, and so could not handle the problems of life in an adequate manner. Given this poor adaptation, conflicts become more serious, these produce further faulty reactions, until the last finally become symptoms. The next year August Hoch embodied the same views in a discussion of the principles of psychogenesis[2].

These two men, who were successive Directors of the Psychiatric Institute at Ward's Island, New York, became the founders of what is sometimes called the " Ward's Island School ", but would more accurately now be termed the " American School of Psychiatry ". The fundamental position assumed by it is that mental disease (of the constitutional order) is to be understood as a reaction of an organism functioning inadequately, that is, inadequately in reference to the demands actually made upon it. The task, which the organism has to meet, is determined by two major factors, the nature of the environment and the nature of the individual. Success in this task depends on the environmental obstacles that are approached, not being beyond the intellectual, instinctive or physical capacity of the subject. (This leaves plenty of scope for the operation of intercurrent or chronic physical disability, no matter where it may be situated anatomically.) Whether an obstacle is approached or not depends on its ubiquity or rarity (an environmental factor) and on the instinctive organization of the individual. The latter is determined by a *reaction type*, and this term may be said to be the watchword of American Psychiatry.

A normal reaction type is a personality. In general it may be said that any two men in any community are dowered with the same instinctive tendencies. We all tend to seek food and comforts, both physical and mental, to protect ourselves from harm, reproduce our kind, nurture our young and run with the herd. But differences in intellectual equipment and innumerable environmental influences tend to accentuate some of these propensities (all of which are not compatible of equal development) and to diminish others. Habit appears greatly to reinforce certain of our inborn propensities. Men differ then in the relative prominence of some tendencies. A situation, that may be met in different ways, produces, therefore, different responses in different people. Because there is a con-

[1] Meyer, " Fundamental Conceptions of Dementia Praecox ", *British Medical Journal*, September 29th, 1906, and *Journal of Nervous and Mental Diseases*, May, 1907.
[2] Hoch, " The Psychogenic Factors in the Development of Psychoses ", *Psychological Bulletin*, vol. IV., No. 6, 1907.

sistency in the reactions of any individual, he is said to have a personality. But it must not be thought that this personality is a fixed, immutable thing. Every time a given act is repeated, the tendency to behave in this manner is strengthened. On the other hand every change in environment elicits new reactions. From birth to death personality is gradually changing, although violent changes are almost always material for psychiatric study. Another important point to bear in mind is that personal characteristics appear only when the tendency to some special type of behaviour is more marked than in the normal man. Anyone who acted in all situations as his fellows did would have no distinguishing characteristics beyond those attaching to his legal identity ; he would have no personality in the proper sense of the term, but merely a name, age, house address, finger-prints, and characteristic set of physical features.

Now it is a matter of common observation that the mental functions do not operate singly and independently of all others. Where one's mood changes, not only is the subjective feeling tone altered but behaviour is different as well. Intellectual processes will also be affected. In a panic one's judgment is apt to be faulty, we think more quickly when happy, more slowly when sad. There are a wealth of proverbs illustrating this, of which " Love is blind " is a good example. When the emotion of love is activated, judgment is impaired pretty much in proportion to the strength of the passion. This co-operation of various functions is " integration ". The characteristics, then, which go to make up personality, appear in virtue of integration of different mental functions. It is this integration which involves the whole organism in its various reactions.

It has just been remarked that a special type of behaviour must be marked before it can be called an individual characteristic. This implies that it is peculiar, and peculiarity is the special field of the psychiatrist. If one wishes to study anomalies of any kind he turns first to those which are most pronounced. The natural material with which to begin a study of characteristics is the mind in disease rather than in health. A man may have a mild tendency to take life hard, to worry over trifles. This is one of the elements in his personality. Since his preoccupation with any given trouble is disproportionate to its cause, it is a safe assumption that the excess of worry is not a response to the external situation, but to something internal. But what is the latter ? He cannot tell us, and it does not appear in his behaviour. We presume, therefore, that it is unconscious. If, however, this worrying tendency increases in severity until it becomes pathological, its inner cause must be increasing its intensity. If the aggravation proceed far enough it is reasonable to suppose that this inner cause would eventually appear in the light of day. And this is just what we see when we come to examine manic-depressive insanity from the psychological point of view. From the mild worries of the normal man to the more chronic cares of the subject predisposed to manic-depressive insanity the transition is so gradual as to be recognizable only in its extremes. The same imperceptible gradations lead from predisposition to actual symptoms. We may indulge the hope that the study of the last may reveal the principle that has been operating with increasing strength from the beginning of this sequence.

A corollary of this proposition is immediately evident. Taking thought over a problem is allied to worry. The normal man does not puzzle himself over a situation that is not present. A perplexing environment furnishes a stimulus for this response. Similarly one who is merely inclined to worry does not do so without some occasion. It is only in the pathological field that we find the occasion for worry manufactured. Except in flagrantly morbid conditions, a stimulus is present in the external world. To be in terror of a tiger that has broken its bonds is only natural, but to have the same terror in the presence of a domestic cat is a symptom. This means that the reaction itself is not pathological, it is its irrelevance to the stimulus which gives it the stamp of disease. The predisposed subject is one who tends to react disproportionately to common stimuli. Granted an absence of these stimuli, predisposition would occasion no breakdown. Theoretically, then, it ought to be possible to prevent manic-depressive attacks by isolation in a sheltered environment. Practically this is often difficult or wholly impossible. Nevertheless, t his principle can probably be invoked to account for the otherwise inexplicable fact that of two persons who seem to have the same predisposition, one breaks down and the other does not. The latter leads, for some reason or other, a more sheltered life.

This leads us to one clue in detecting the unconscious factor which lies back of the predisposition. Everyday problems do not produce manic-depressive attacks, otherwise every predisposed subject would be in a continuous psychosis. The unknown, unconscious, factor which leads to abnormal reactions must be stimulated by some unusual event. This event must have some connexion with, some meaning for, the unconscious factor. Study the precipitating causes of the attacks and we may discover something about the latent psychological cause.

So much for the conjectures as to the initiation of manic-depressive psychoses. There remain the problems of symptomatology. If our psycholological principles hold, the changes that occur when a psychosis appears, are not due to a sudden appearance out of the blue of disconnected mental functions. New reactions appear in virtue of new integrations. A tendency to react in a given way that has been latent, becomes more prominent ; this affects a variety of mental functions, which are interrelated to form a new, and pathological, reaction type. If this hypothesis be sound, we ought to be able to demonstrate connexions between the pathological elements in the clinical picture that are identical with the connexions observed in every-day life. In other words, we should not expect to find new elements but only new constellations, that are new in virtue of unusual predominance being given to one or more tendencies.

These constellations are reaction types. Every personality is a reaction—or an alternation of—reaction types, for any man may behave differently to the same stimulus under different general conditions. For instance, the average citizen responds differently to the idea of bloodshed in peace time and during war. In an analogous way a psychosis represents one new reaction type or a series of them. The ordinary delirium is a single reaction type induced, as a rule, by toxaemia. On the other hand manic-depressive insanity shows a series of reaction types. Kraepelin gives three : mania, depression and mixed conditions. We find that this group is more easily understood if mixed conditions are eliminated and a number of other distinct reaction types added to the list. These others are : stupor, involution melancholia, anxiety and perplexity. The adoption of these six types is urged, not by à priori theory, but by expedience. We find that we cannot understand our cases when they are forced into Kraepelin's pigeon holes, while, on the other hand, a number of riddles seem to be solved if our classification be used. The reader must judge of the value or uselessness of our procedure, when he has perused the clinical argument.

At this point, however, one difficulty must be met. It is true that under such dramatically different conditions as peace and war a normal man may show radically different behaviour. But such upheavals do not come often in any man's life. There *is* a consistency in his personality. On the other hand a manic-depressive patient may show great inconsistency in his reactions from day to day, when he is living in an environment (the hospital) much more unchanging than that of the work-a-day world. Is there a psychological explanation for this or must we fall back on the facile theory of diseased brain tissue turning out a disorganized, disconnected product ?

There is a hypothesis which would account for the inconsistency, if sufficient data could be secured to support it. Let us consider the minor inconsistencies of normal life. A man wakes in the morning, feels sluggish, does not want to get up, and succeeds in doing so only with effort. He forces himself to go through his toilet ritual and dresses, although every minute sees a diminution in the effort he is called upon to make. This is like a miniature depression. He goes down to breakfast and is irritable because his coffee is cold ; he scolds his wife and discovers some naughtiness in his children ; after commenting harshly on this he retires huffily behind his newspaper. This mood accompanies him to· his office, where he complains of the inefficiency of his staff. But soon a man comes in with whom he concludes an important bit of business. Elation sets in and he makes mildly erotic advances to his stenographer.

He lunches with some friends at his club, drinks a little, and becomes jovial, laughs boisterously at his own jokes. In the afternoon, it seems that the deal he thought was consummated may not be securely settled. He begins to worry over this and other transactions as well. But soon he finds that his venture is going to go through and he returns home in a cheerful frame of mind. Here he repairs to the nursery, and runs around on his hands and knees with his children, uses baby talk and, in general, indulges in behaviour that in any other environment would stamp him as insane.

This picture is slightly, if at all, overdrawn. We do show variations in our reactions in the course of even a single day that are like those of manic-depressive insanity, although none of the changes are extreme as in the psychosis. In the main we see that these alterations are produced by variations in the environment. In manic-depressive insanity quite dramatic shifts occur without any discernible external causation. Now if we suppose that the stimuli, when a man is insane, come from within rather than without, a possible explanation is forthcoming. We know that the greater the intensity of a psychosis, the less is the contact with the surrounding world, the more, therefore, must the patient be living in an inner world of his own creation. Many factors, both social and physical, conspire to check marked changes in the outer world, but there is no check to be put on imaginings, except a subjective judgment. If that be defective, the inner world may suffer momentous changes, producing responses that would be normal, if the fancied environment were real. If a man sees himself in Hell about to be attacked by a sulphurous Devil, panic is quite natural. If the vision changes to one of Heaven and a benignant God, awe and ecstasy are just as natural. Moreover, since the vision contributes the entire world for the time being, it is natural that the emotional response should be melodramatic. In our normal lives our emotions are dilute because attention is being constantly distracted by other than the specific stimulus, we keep thinking about the effect we are producing on others and so on. It is only when we "lose ourselves" in any situation that our emotions approach the intensity of those witnessed in manic-depressive insanity.

To justify the hypothesis it is necessary to determine three things. Are the "mixed conditions" of Kraepelin really alternations of reactions, the contrasting reactions appearing as a mixture because of a cross-section being taken of a day, a week, or a month? If one described the reactions of the normal man detailed above as if they occurred at the same time, we would get a queer, mixed personality! He would be showing depression, irritability, gaiety, tenderness and playfulness all at once. (As a matter of fact the reactions of a manic-depressive patient show, as a rule, more consistency than those of normal life. The reason presumably being that his inner environment has less change in it than the outer world affords in the course of normal existence). Secondly, can we discover what the data of his inner experiences are? Thirdly, can we learn what the mechanism is whereby those experiences change? These last two are the main problems of the psychiatric study which follows.

CHAPTER V

PROBLEMS OF DIAGNOSIS

IN this *Introduction* no mention has been made as yet of the problems connected with diagnosis. Since this study—so far as it is psychiatrical—has not the purpose of text-book discussion in view, many important nosological points will be omitted. Only such psychiatrical features of manic-depressive insanity will be included as have psychological interest and pertinence, moreover, for our special theme. Among these, however, is the problem of differentiation of dementia praecox from the psychoses, that are the object of our intensive research. To confuse a typical case of dementia praecox with a typical mania or depression would be a psychiatrical crime. But both are constitutional psychoses, both seem to arise on analogous backgrounds, so it is not surprising that many cases appear which resemble both diseases. These furnish, probably, the largest group of diagnostic puzzles in institutional practice. In New York State official cognizance has been granted to this difficulty by the establishment in the lists of psychoses of the divisions " Allied to Manic-Depressive Insanity " and " Allied to Dementia Praecox ". These diagnoses have been copied elsewhere. If the essence of either dementia praecox or mania-depressive insanity lies in a peculiar reaction type, the analysis of the symptom picture, betraying the specific reaction type, should facilitate diagnosis. It will appear that some progress has been made along this line.

But this is not merely a psychiatrical problem solved (or partially solved) by psychological means, the solution inevitably involves psychological theory. One example may make this clear. In a typical case of dementia praecox emotional reactions are inappropriate or inadequate. This is a matter of prime significance for diagnosis. On the other hand, the emotional reactions in manic-depressive insanity are appropriate and adequate as a rule (we need not discuss exceptions at this point.) One sees, therefore, the same idea associated in the one case with a normal kind of emotional response, and in the other with a queer or insufficient response. The different reaction types must be responsible for this, and no theory of emotions can therefore afford to neglect these phenomena.

The material of this book may throw light on one question that is of rather grave psychiatrical importance. So far the *raison d'être* of the manic-depressive group has rested on the appearance in all the constituent psychoses of periodicity and prominent emotional reactions as well as the presence of gradations between the various types. Since gradations also exist between dementia praecox and manic-depressive insanity, that criterion can hardly be used to maintain the classification. Periodicity is frequently absent and marked emotions may fail to appear. Against the validity of his group, as Kraepelin describes it, some argument might be directed. If the various reaction types show fundamental similarities this would argue in favour of the maintenance of the diagnostic group. If they are found to differ fundamentally, some of them should perhaps be split off as isolated and unrelated recoverable psychoses.

PART II

PSYCHOLOGICAL INTRODUCTION

CHAPTER VI

DEFINITIONS

THE logical beginning of a discussion of the psychology of emotion would seem to be a definition of emotion. Unfortunately we are not dealing with an exercise in logic, so we cannot lay down a definition and then deduce further meaning from the terms of the definition. This is what used to be done in the study known as psychology ; it may have sharpened men's wits ; it taught them much about the products of the mind but little about how the mind worked. This was a tolerable method when biology was a primitive science concerned only with living creatures other than man. But, as the view developed (culminating in the evolutionary doctrine) that man was a specialized animal, the purpose of psychology began to change. Students began to look on " mind " as a general term covering a group of functions having to do with the adaptation of the organism to its environment. This makes it an instrument, its phenomena data expressible in terms of functions of the instrument. A philosopher might object that this definition is too narrow, that the mind mediates influences more extensive and subtle than the stimuli from any " biological " environment. To this the modern psychologist would reply, if he were an honest man, that he is not pretending to solve the riddle of the universe ; that he is deliberately narrowing the scope of his science and that the only bearing which psychology has on metaphysics is to provide knowledge as to the capacity and range of mind. An analogy may make this clearer. A biologist may be studying minute structures with a microscope. Only the science of optics can tell him what range his lenses will have and how much of what he sees will be a product of imperfections in the instrument—as, for instance, chromatic aberrations.

Every science must begin by observation ; the data thus secured must then be classified.   Classification involves hypothesis, for it implies some inter-relation between the phenomena grouped together.   Hypothesis is then further elaborated and stimulates further observation in an effort to establish or to destroy the validity of the theory advanced.   Once a theory is accepted a classification to which it refers has more than a tentative value.   We have no hesitancy, for instance, in regarding fishes and birds as belonging to different phyla.   A discussion on birds could begin properly with a definition that anyone would accept.   But this was not always so. The savage at an animistic stage is not at all sure that the bird is not his father.   Even in our own civilization it is only a recent theory that denies the possibility of geese developing from barnacles.   To the savage the fish may be part of the water.   These comparisons are invaluable in showing how primitive a science psychology is. It is only at the uncivilized level of preliminary classification, so that one psychologist may say that a given mental act is emotional, another that it is instinctive, a third that it is intellectual.   If our knowledge of our own minds were as accurate as our knowledge of the animal world there would be no more confusion in our descriptive psychological terms than in our differentiation of horses and cows.   The situation is not hopeless, however, for we are beginning to be sceptical of the validity of our classifications.   The faculty psychologists were not ; they were happy in the belief that their divisions of mental phenomena correspond to true differences and separable functions.

When we know more we shall probably abolish our present terminology altogether, but in the meantime we must have some classification with which to work.   So, recognizing its tentative character, we may use the word emotion, even though we expect to give it up long before we are in a position to define it accurately. This implies that our use will be adjectival rather than substantive. We are not assuming that there is any such thing as an emotion ; we are simply going to study the phenomena that have an emotional colouring.   To what kind of mental operations may we apply this adjective ?   What added significance appears if we say a thought or deed is emotional ?   To what functions of the mind may the use of this term be irrelevant ?   In this indirect way we may frame our tentative definition.

It is perhaps easiest to begin by answering the last question. Neither the layman nor the psychologist describe as emotional the behaviour of a bank clerk adding up figures or that of a policeman directing traffic.   Each knows what he is doing and the reason for each operation that he makes.   We should say that he was using his intelligence rather than his instincts or emotions and by intelligence we imply exercise of memory, reasoning, and so forth.   We feel that the man is voluntarily and consciously controlling his thoughts and actions.   We would not be so sure that emotion was absent in the small boy adding figures or in the country-bred woman crossing a crowded city street. In these latter cases conscious knowledge does not seem to be so exclusively responsible for the behaviour, nor so adequate to guide it. There is, then, some lack of voluntary control about emotional phenomena.

In daily speech we are apt to describe conduct that is not thought out beforehand, conduct that is automatic, as instinctive. When danger impends, one cowers or runs ; when insulted, one strikes blindly ; one picks up a child who has fallen without hesitation. Such actions are commonly ascribed to instincts of self-preservation, of aggression, of protection, or, equally often to fear, anger or sympathy. The latter are emotions. So frequently do instincts and emotions appear together that both the layman and the psychologist are apt to label behaviour with either term indifferently. It would therefore seem that instincts and emotions—whatever they may be—are closely related. A little reflection, however, shows that they are not identical, nor invariably associated. For instance, one steps out of the way of an on-coming motor in a purely automatic way but (ordinarily) betrays fear neither objectively nor subjectively. A fly alights on my cheek and I brush it off. My action is instinctive, but, if the fly does not return I neither feel nor show anger. If, however, the insect keeps buzzing around my head, irritation will surely appear. On the other hand, if a man be insulted and strike a blow, it is practically certain that anger as well as the instinct of aggression will be called forth. From these examples we may conclude that the unreflective, immediate action we call instinctive is not an inevitable accompaniment of emotion, although we would demand that any theory of emotions should show why it is that the association is so intimate.

There is another criterion often employed for the demonstration of emotion. This is what is known as emotional expression. It appears in changed attitude of the body, distortion of the face, modulations of the voice and in various gestures. There is no need to describe them further for everyone knows them. At first glance one would be apt to say that when they are present emotions must also be. But an actor may assume them ; he may show all the objective manifestations of fear, yet tell us he is not frightened and we believe him. Or, on the other hand, with sufficient self-control one may hide signs of fear and yet be frightened.

Now Darwin, whose book *Expression of the Emotions in Man and Animals*, was the starting point for objective study of this field, showed that many, if not all, emotional expressions in man are relics of adaptive behaviour in the lower animals. The dog, which walks growling, stiff-legged and with bristling hair around its opponent, is prepared for instant movement in any direction and has assumed an appearance likely to induce a reaction of retreat in the other dog. Is this dog angry or not ? If we say that he is we have assumed that his state of mind is identical with that of a human being behaving in a similar way (and not acting). That is, we are ascribing self-consciousness to the dog. At this stage we are not in a position either to affirm or deny the validity of this assumption. But presuming consciousness to be present, might we not with equal justice allege the actions to be calculated ? They are adaptive ; if the dog be conscious, why should he not be thinking to himself, " I am going to frighten this fellow, but I must stay on my guard lest he turn on me ". Such an attitude is hardly emotional. On the other hand, a dog without cerebral hemispheres may perform somewhat similar actions. It is true that we do not know with finality that consciousness is necessarily a function of the cerebrum alone, but it would be a bold man who would insist that a dog with only a spinal cord and brain stem could have the same sort of consciousness which we enjoy. For these reasons it would seem preferable to regard the dog's " angry " expression as part of its combative instinct and not regard the accessory details of its fighting behaviour as conclusive evidences of emotion. But it would be idle to pretend that this is a solution of the problem of emotional expression ; it is merely restating it in terms of instinct, which is equivalent to saying once more that emotions and instincts constitute a single problem.

Modern writers on emotion are now apt to include with emotional expression some accompanying physiological phenomena of an involuntary nature. Gestures, facial movements and body attitudes depend on the contraction of voluntary muscles and these, in turn, are controlled by the voluntary nervous system. But there is as well, an involuntary, or, as it is sometimes called a visceral or vegetative, nervous system. This latter has to do with the regulation of movements and secretions in the digestive canal, variations in the calibre of blood vessels sweating, erection of hairs, dilatation or contraction of the pupils and so on. It is, of course, notorious that emotions include bodily changes apart from voluntary muscular movements. Everyone knows the blushing of shame, the pallor of anger or fear (dilatation or contraction of the small vessels in the skin), the sweating or even passage of urine and faeces in panic.

Cannon[1] and his co-workers have recently enlarged our knowledge of these phenomena. They have shown that when emotions are aroused, that are usual accompaniments of violent exertion, that part of the involuntary nervous system which is known as the " sympathetic " is predominantly active. This results in a relative paralysis of movement in the digestive canal, heightened blood-pressure and increased pulse rate, dilatation of the pupil, sweating and certain changes in body chemistry. The last are mediated by the excessive secretion of a substance, adrenalin, which is produced by one of the glands of internal secretion, the suprarenal bodies.

[1] W. B. Cannon, *Bodily Changes in Pain, Hunger, Fear, and Rage.* New York, 1915.

When the amount of adrenalin in the blood is increased, glycogen, a starchy, fuel substance stored in the liver, is transported rapidly to the muscles, where, in the form of dextrose, a simpler starchy substance, it provides the fuel for muscular contraction. In some curious way, as well, adrenalin assists in the rebuilding of chemical compounds broken down in muscular work, so that it reduces fatigue.

All these changes can be easily understood as helpful accompaniments to violent physical exertion. Heightened blood pressure and more rapid beating of the heart mean better circulation of blood ; paralysis of the digestive organs leaves more of the total bodily energy free for use in the muscles ; dilatation of the pupil allows more light to enter the eye and so lowers the threshold for visual stimuli ; while the adrenalin supersecretion obviously facilitates prolonged muscular work. All the bodily changes can thus be regarded as natural expressions of instincts involving great exertion. This would seem again to make emotion really only an instinctive phenomenon. But, were the case as simple as this, one would expect the visceral changes to appear only when violent action had begun. All these chances may be demonstrated, however, when the animal is motionless, except, perhaps, for some tremors. One would be tempted then to suspect that an emotion was a preliminary phase of an instinctive reaction.

So far we have considered all the emotional phenomena, which are open to objective observation, and all of them seem capable of being treated as instinctive. Why have they not been so treated either by the layman or the psychologist ? The answer is that we have not yet considered that which is most central and vital in emotion, an element not open to the gaze of the dispassionate observer but infinitely and eternally subjective. This is the feeling-tone accompanying the emotion, or, to use the harsh but inevitable term of the modern psychologist, the *affect*. The central mystery of emotions is the affect ; without it there would probably be no problem that was not just a problem of instinct and so described. The movements of my body are open to the scrutiny of any man, and the working of my inward parts to the vision of the physiologist, but what I feel belongs to me alone. So much is it mine that I cannot even share it. It is true that a companion understands when I say I feel angry or afraid, but such crude emotions as fear and anger play a minor rôle in normal civilized life. What I feel in the presence of a sunset, a power plant or a little child, I might in a series of word pictures communicate inaccurately and incompletely.[1] But could I describe how a Bach fugue makes me

---

[1] One of the major functions of art is to produce in the reader, auditor or observer, a subtle emotional reaction. This is done by portraying a situation with which the subject identifies himself unwittingly. I cannot feel tenderness on demand but let me become interested in the sorrow of some imaginary creature in need of protection and that peculiar feeling may arise. Browning

feel ? People live and die for the sake of experiences that yield these subtle affects. If a man tells me that he loves his wife or his work, that means little more to me than the obvious fact that he prefers this woman to another or this profession to that ; but to him it means a feeling that is all his own and more precious than any material thing the world might give him.

Some of the coarser affects, like those of fear and anger, are so common that we have not only all experienced them, in what we presume to be a similar way, but we have even named them. Such affects are usually the accompaniment of action, or at least external expression. Consequently we assume that a person who acts aggressively and destructively is angry. We believe ourselves justified in this assumption because the subject will so often confess to having felt something stirring within him that he has been taught to call anger. We even go further and assume that a dog feels anger and a rabbit fear, in spite of the difficulties we land ourselves in with the implied assumption of consciousness in these animals. In ourselves we never confuse the affect and the expression of emotion, but as to others we always do. If I tremble and turn pale in a motor accident, observers may say I was frightened and scoff at me when I protest that I was not. It is an idle dispute because we are speaking of different things. The observer is speaking of what I did and how I looked ; I am speaking of how I felt, and I may *know* that I felt no fear, because I was surprised that I did not. I am the only one who is entitled to an opinion as to my affect, indeed, this is probably the only subject in which dogmatism is both justified and inevitable. Yet psychologists have almost to a man assumed that affect is open to objective observation and have framed nearly all their hypotheses on this assumption. Turn to almost any text-book of psychology and you will see a problem stated in terms of many different emotions, but the answer given in terms of only one—fear —or, perhaps, two, when anger is included. The behaviour and feeling of fear are so often found together that expression and affect are assumed to have an inevitable association, and one is explained in terms of the other.

has well expressed the insufficiency of art relative to actual experience in arousing feeling :

> " What does it all mean, poet ? Well,
> Your brains beat into rhythm, you tell
> What we felt only ; you expressed
> You hold things beautiful the best,
> And place them in rhyme so, side by side.
> 'Tis something, nay, 'tis much : but then,
> Have you yourself what's best for men ?
> Are you—poor, sick, old ere your time—
> Nearer one whit your own sublime
> Than we who have never turned a rhyme ?
> Sing, riding's a joy ! For me, I ride."

This is a particularly good example of what I mean, because the whole of " The Last Ride Together " is an effort to paint an affect and the picture produces quite different responses in different readers.

The same error has crept into psychopathology. Here again we read only of fear and of conclusions even more ridiculous. For instance, there are theories about " repressed " or " unconscious " affects. This is, of course, a contradiction in terms. An affect as such has not and cannot have any existence until it is conscious, because it is something that a person feels ; whatever may be its cause it does not exist as an affect until it be felt. But it is easy to see how the error arises. Fear, the affect, is confused with fear, the behaviour. The latter can be repressed and have a more or less demonstrable existence as unconscious ideas of escape, etc. But if the affect of fear be put out of mind it cannot have any existence. One can no more harbour a feeling of fear of which one is unaware than a pain of which one is unaware. A physical injury may or may not be present in the body but pain does not exist until it is felt. And similarly a pain can be felt when injury is not demonstrable. Sapient physicians tell patients their pains are imaginary but the patients know better ; they do feel them, so they know they exist.

Now when we try to ally affect with instincts serious difficulties are encountered. It seems reasonable to connect fear with danger instincts ; it is not unreasonable to see in the feelings of love some expression of breeding, parental or herd instincts. With love or fear some behaviour is observable and may be conceived as being in abeyance. But what behaviour is appropriate to a sunset ? What instinct is aroused by a Bach fugue ? One can avoid this problem— as many psychologists do—by inventing an instinct that would produce the puzzling affect. But this is mere tautology ; it is running in a circle. The question of definition of instincts is one that will occupy us shortly, but I may anticipate this discussion by saying that—whatever else it may or may not be—an instinct must express itself in behaviour or be capable of so doing. There cannot be a specific instinct for enjoying a sunset that is not merely the affect induced by seeing one. It is, of course, quite conceivable, that various instinctive tendencies might be activated, any one of which could, when operating alone, result in behaviour. But this view is incompatible with a theory of specific relationship of instinct and affect. Affect, too, shows a curious tendency to be dissociated from behaviour. Our most poignant feelings are stirred in dreams as a rule, in sleep during which not a muscle may move to betray to the onlooker the ecstasy or torment in which the dreamer lies. Further than this, affect may exist without recognizable stimulus. We have all of us had the experience of being sad, and sometimes of being happy, without discoverable cause for our feeling. Such isolation of affect is commonest in morbid conditions, when it is most frequently seen as a " free floating anxiety ", a fear without ground in either outward stimulus or inward thought that the patient knows about. If, then, instincts are manifested in affect, they must be operating in some unusual way.

If affect be the element in emotion that leads us to separate emotions from instincts, it must be its most characteristic component. Solve the problem of affect, and one has solved the problem of emotion, it is tempting to say. For instance if affect could be demonstrated to be a derivative of instinct, the latter only need be studied further. But, unfortunately, things are not so simple, as this affect is a peculiarly personal feeling. It belongs to the subject and to no one else. The colouring, then, of pleasure or pain that accompanies certain sensory experiences would have to be an affect. If the prick of a pin hurts me, my pain is an affect—according to our definition. Similarly, if touching a piece of velvet or hearing the note of bell seems pleasant, this pleasure is an affect. Are we then to include simple, primitive pleasure and pain as emotion ? If so, we would be explaining the simple in terms of the complex.

Most psychologists have avoided this dilemma by boldly separating pleasure and pain from affect and emotion. This was not difficult because traditional psychology, engaged in labelling mental phenomena rather than explaining them, had long ago invented two pigeon-holes into one of which any behaviour could be stuffed. In their simple view we did things because we liked them and ran away from things which hurt. The logical juggling and writhing they went through before facts could be made to fit now afford amusing reading.[1] Since emotions seemed also to determine behaviour, they naturally, in so far as they dealt with emotions at all, classified them into pleasure and pain groups. Of this William James said :

" The essence of emotion is pleasure and pain ? This is a hackneyed psychological doctrine, but on any theory of the seat of emotions it seems to me one of the most artificial and scholastic of the untruths that disfigure our science. One might as well say that the essence of prismatic colour is pleasure and pain. There are infinite shades and tones in various emotional excitements which are distinct as sensations of colour are, and of which one is quite at a loss to predicate either pleasant or painful quality."

As to the existence of pain with quite simple sensations there can be no dispute, and the relationship of it to other affects is an alluring topic for speculation. But I cannot see that, theoretically, it is possible to admit the existence of pleasure with simple sensations. If we are to be accurate in our terminology, we must admit that a simple sensation is something possible only to a new-born babe. Once experience has begun, sensation gives way to perception, an

---

[1] That is to the modern psychologist. But the doctrine of hedonism is far from dead. It still operates openly or implicitly in economics, which consequently has to produce a new theory every year. This ludicrous sight, equalled only by the spectacle many omniscient psychologists make, might be avoided if the economist frankly admitted that people only tended to do what it paid them to do, if they adopted the view that economics was a branch of the study of human behaviour, *i.e.*, man's conduct in business affairs. The laws of his behaviour would then be deduced from " economics ", history, and psychology—a prodigious task !

interpretation of sensation in the light of experience, a blending of present sensations with those of the past. Except in infancy, therefore, we can have only perception and, as perception implies associations, it cannot be simple. The pleasurable affect must therefore be attached to the complicated series of mental processes which even the most primitive perception implies. It is easy to see how, in the same way, a dilute affect of comfort or discomfort can be attached to most complicated intellectual operations.

It seems to me that this is one of the problems in which the behavourist attitude is helpful. A stimulus—afferent impulses—produce a response that implies attraction to, or repulsion from, the source of the stimulus. As conscious and, we hope, rational beings we detest the notion of our being blindly impelled one way or another. So, when our instincts drive us to or fro we rationalize our conduct and invent a motive. We pretend that we like that towards which we find ourselves going, because, as a rule, we do feel pleasure in the anticipation of instinctive outlet. Similarly, because we associate pain with withdrawal, we say we don't like that which we avoid. Roughly speaking the classification holds, but it holds only when it is so obvious as to be superfluous. The bashful girl, who treats her lover frigidly when she is consciously hoping he will advance, or the man who is attracted willy-nilly to a scene of horror, are hardly following the pleasure-pain principle.

The hedonists meet such objections as this by making impulse-towards equivalent to pleasure, and repulsion the same as pain. They thus give new meanings to pleasure and pain. How helpful this torturing of common speech may be is seen in the theorizing of J. Mark Baldwin[1] who makes "pleasure" responsible for the establishment of adaptive reactions in the beginning of such evolution. If "pleasure" means impulse, this is pure tautology. If it means what any one, man or boy not a psychologist, means by it, it implies consciousness, an awareness of something pleasant, which seems a precocious development for an organism at the tropistic level. This is an excellent example of a form of bad logic which is peculiarly apt to arise in studies of emotions, and which might be termed alternate anthropomorphism and theriomorphism. The conscious mental functions of man are assumed to exist in an animal at a time when certain physiological events are demonstrable. The investigator then turns around and says that, when this mental state is present in man, the animal's physiological processes are going on in the man and are the cause of what he experiences !

Fundamentally, I think, the basis of hedonism is the passion for simplification which governs most theorizers. There are workers in every field trying to reduce most complicated problems to two opposing factors. The moralist says every action is good or bad ; politeness forces us to say we are either well or ill ; one is held to be

[1] *Psychological Review*, 1894.

sane or insane ; behaviour is instinctive or voluntary ; matter is living or dead ; functions are physiologic or psychic and so on. Even such a bold thinker as Freud has fallen into the temptation of dichotomizing and has adopted the pleasure-pain principle. As a result he is forced to talk of painful wishes. But he is, at least, in respectable company !

For these reasons I am inclined to the view that the pleasure aspect of " pleasure-pain " need not give us pause in studying affect. It may be regarded as a mild feeling tone accompanying certain behaviour or experience. But pain is not so easily disposed of. If we are to group it with other affects we must find some formula which will cover its phenomena as well as those of complicated emotional states.

In order to avoid any misconception I shall now state exactly the sense in which I shall use the terms emotion and affect in this book. *Affect is any subjective experience that, when examined introspectively, is considered to originate in or belong to the subject's individual organism. It may be felt to be either mental or physical, to be stimulated by sense perception, by a thought, or to be causeless. But in no case is it thought to be a quality of the stimulus, except in relation to the subject.* For instance a pin may prick me : I think the pin has a point, but I regard the pain as something produced in me. I see a bear and am frightened : I think the bear has teeth and claws but the fear is the effect of the bear on *me*. I think of winning a prize and feel happy : the thought " prize " I do not consider as an inevitably happy one ; it must be *my* prize before happiness can appear.

Emotional expressions are objective phenomena which may qualify instinctive behaviour or betray an attitude. They consist of gestures, postures, movements of parts of the face, vocal expressions, modulations of the voice and many visceral changes.

In self-conscious man affect is usually associated with emotional expression. *A complete emotion is a combination of affect and emotional expression.* When, therefore, I speak of " emotion " in a man I assume that he is feeling as well as behaving in an emotional manner, unless the statement be qualified. But, if I speak of emotion in an animal, I refer only to emotional expression with no implication whatever of affect being present. The same meaning will be given to emotion in an infant before consciousness is developed, as is given to an animal's emotion. If I speak of affect, I mean only subjective experience. The adjective " affective " may be used to qualify behaviour of a conscious being : in this case it will be synonymous with " emotional ", but the implication is that the behaviour in question is presumably accompanied by affect.

If the term emotion is used to cover a number of related but often dissociated phenomena the same can be said of instincts. The layman uses the word to label inherited behaviour, habit, unthinking conduct, and a driving force, much like interest or desire directing programmes of activity. For each of these usages some psychologist can be found to do battle. It is impossble to give a specific meaning to a popular term used in a general sense ; inevitably the writer is misunderstood because the reader has his own usage firmly established and, with all the will in the world, is certain to apply *his* meaning of the term in all his spontaneous thought. If, for the sake of argument, I agree to call a horse a cow, whenever my opponent mentions the word, I visualize " cow " as something with horns, unless I keep my attention so firmly fixed on the definition as to be incapable of other mental exertions. In other words I agree to do something beyond my capacity ; I cannot think of horse by any other name and, if I try to use the word " cow ", I begin to think of the creature that gives milk. This is, of course, an extreme example, but I believe it exhibits in striking form a principle that is much neglected. If one has used the term instinct in a general sense since childhood, it will be extremely difficult to give it a specific meaning and stick to the narrowed significance.

One often finds that popular expression is more accurate than scientific terminology because the former leaves vague and fluid what is not yet sufficiently known to be made specific. " Instinct " is a good example. For instance, let us take one of the broadest definitions given to instinct, that adopted by William James. " Instinct is usually defined as the faculty of acting in such a way as to produce certain ends, without foresight of the ends, and without previous education in the performance." It is true that any animal without consciousness acts without foresight and, to this extent, the definition might be applicable to many animals, if not all. But a wealth of experimentation has shown that practically every instinct is modified by experience, so that education has taken place. Consequently this definition would cover only the behaviour of new born animals and that which occurs only once in the life time of the individual, such as that of an insect laying eggs in the body of a special caterpillar. The definition is totally inapplicable to man, because he sees, or can see, the ends towards which his conduct is shaping, even though his behaviour be involuntary. Any definition of instinct, I believe, which makes of it an entity, can be shown to have a ridiculously narrow range, unless it be stated that this entity operates only in conjunction with other factors in the production of such behaviour as we actually observe. In other words, instinct as an entity is a hypothetical factor in, not a type of, behaviour.

I think it would therefore be wise for psychologists to follow the lead of common speech and use " instinct " in an adjectival rather than a substantive sense. Our task would then be to describe the nature of these mental events, to which the term instinctive is applicable. I have elsewhere[1] discussed this question

---

[1] *Problems in Dynamic Psychology* 1922 ; The Cambridge University Press, 1923 ; Macmillan Company, New York.

but that we are sad because we weep. This statement was unfortunate ; literal-minded critics held orgies of excommunication over it, till James was finally forced to explain that by " tears " he meant the sum total of bodily response, a meaning which would have been clear to any mind not " debauched by learning ".

This, then, is the theory in a nutshell. Its application James limited to the " coarser emotions ", *i.e.*, those like fear, rage, or sexual passion. He also discussed " subtler emotions " : " These are the moral, intellectual and æsthetic feelings. Concords of sounds, of colours, of lines, logical consistencies, teleological fitnesses, affect us with a pleasure that seems ingrained in the very form of the presentation itself, and to borrow nothing from any reverberation surging up from the parts below the brain." With such presentations he admitted that there might be a secondary emotional admixture, which gives them more colour and glow. The difference between the romantic or classical taste he traced to the presence or absence of this secondary affect. When it is present, reminiscence brings up visceral sensations, he claimed. The primary subtle emotion he concluded is really a cognitive function, whereas, when the æsthetic excites us, there is a secondary emotion.

Under fire of his critics James had to elaborate his views. The most important extension had to do with the psychological mechanism of production of emotion. He made it clear that the " object " of an emotional reaction is the total situation which calls it forth. " ' Objects ' are certainly the primitive arousers of instinctive reflex movements. But they take their place, as experience goes on, as elements in total ' situations ', the other suggestions of which may prompt to movements of an entirely different sort. As soon as an object has become thus familiar and suggestive, its emotional consequences, *on any theory of emotion*, must start rather from the total situation which it suggests than from its own naked presence. But whatever be our reaction on the situation, in the last resort it is an instinctive reaction on that one of its elements which strikes us at the time being as most vitally important. The same bear may truly enough excite us to either fight or flight, according as he suggests an overpowering ' idea ' of his killing us or one of our killing him."

I have quoted James at length here because he makes it clear that he grasped an important point which many psychologists have missed. A subject does not produce a given emotion automatically and inevitably when confronted with a given stimulus. A process of association is first set up which gives a *meaning* to the situation. This meaning is derived from the man's conscious thoughts, his actions and his affect. It is this meaning which determines the type of emotion that appears ; or, indeed, whether there will be any at all. So the nature of the associations ensuing on presentation of the stimulus is an even more important object of study than the discovery of what is the immediate excitant of the feeling.

Since the James-Lange hypothesis is stated in physiological terms, clinical and laboratory findings may be used in testing it. The work of Cannon seemed at first blush to confirm it, as he showed how visceral changes under emotional excitation could be even more extensive than James and Lange knew. On the other hand it seemed to destroy the idea of differences in visceral discharge accounting for differences in feeling tone because different emotional states in his animals produced the same internal phenomena. (It must be borne in mind that in all experimental work there is only the emotional expression present from which the emotion is deduced. We have no knowledge as to whether the animal feels or not.)

One can imagine James's answer to this criticism because a similar one was made to which he replied : " Dr. Worcester acutely remarks that the actions accompanying all emotions tend to become alike in proportion to their intensity. People weep from an excess of joy ; pallor and trembling accompany extremes of hope as well as fear, etc. But, I answer, do not the subject's feelings also then tend to become alike, if considered in themselves apart from all their differing intellectual contexts ? My theory maintains that they should do so ; and such reminiscences of extreme emotion as I possess rather seem to confirm than to invalidate such a view."

This is probably another way of saying that coarser emotions (those studied by Cannon) tend to become mere excitement. As excitement increases, the attention of the subject to his own feelings diminishes, action becomes automatic, he is " beside himself ", loses that shade of subjective feeling that ordinarily serves to accelerate, inhibit or direct his thoughts and actions. In short the affect goes as excitement increases. Naturally, then, all emotions tend to become alike with excitement, the feeling is degraded to mere inner tension or may be quite absent, as in reckless action. The organism is then just behaving, the guidance of consciousness (self-awareness) is removed. As we shall see later there is evidence for this in psychopathological material : we meet with cases in which no trace of any affect can be discovered nor inferred. The patient is simply in tense excitement.

This would correspond with Cannon's findings, and indicate that the visceral effects he studied were the accompaniment of excitement rather than of affect. The biological purpose of such visceral reactions is to prepare for violent exertion or to perpetuate it—that is for action of any kind. James would say that with milder grades of emotion there are differing visceral discharges. Experimental and clinical observations ought to furnish evidence as to the validity of this view.

Sherrington[1] cut the spinal cord and the vagus nerves in a dog given to emotional display. This destroyed all skin sensibility

[1] *Integrative Action of the Nervous System*, York University Press, New Haven, 1911, p. 259.

back of the shoulders and all visceral sensibility.. The dog continued its normal emotional behaviour except for an absence of bristling hair on the back when enraged. This, said Sherrington, eliminates the James-Lange hypothesis because, he claimed, the dog did feel ! This, however, involves the assumption of the dog having a consciousness which is the *sine qua non* of affect. So this experiment shows only that visceral and peripheral sensibility are not necessary for a display of emotional *expression*. Sherrington goes on to quote the experiment of Goltz, who removed the cerebral hemispheres of a dog and kept it alive for months. The animal showed signs of anger but of no other emotion. He concludes from this and his own experiments that emotion is a cerebral function[1] merely reinforced by sensations from the viscera, the latter tending always to have an affective tone. The reason of this is that : " All sensations referred *to the body itself rather than interpreted as qualities of objects in the external world,* tend to be tinged with feeling." He goes on to explain this in words that enunciate what seem to me to be fundamental principles :

" Sense organs which initiate sensations tinged with feeling [are those which] tend to excite motor centres directly and imperatively. Hence in animals reduced to merely spinal condition stimuli calculated to produce pain (although, of course, unable to do so in a spinal animal) evoke movements appropriate for escape from or removal of the stimulus applied. Now, ' feeling ' is implicit in the emotional state ; the state is an ' affective state '. In the evolution of emotion the revival of ' feelings ' pleasurable and painful must have played a large part. Hence the close relation of emotion with sense-organs that can initiate bodily pain or pleasure, and hence its connection with impulsive or instinctive movement. There is no wide interval between the reflex movement of the spinal dog whose foot attempts to scratch away an irritant applied to its back—both leg and back absolutely detached from consciousness—and the reactions of the decerebrate dog that turns and growls and bites at fingers holding his hind foot too roughly. In the former case the motor reaction occurs, although the mind is not even aware of the stimulus, far less percipient of it as an irritant. The action occurs, and plays the pantomime of feeling ; but no feeling comes to pass. In the latter case the motor reaction occurs and is expressive of emotion ; but it is probably the reaction of an organic machine which can be started working, though the mutilation precludes the psychosis [mental state]."

Even in the dog with an intact nervous system we can have no

---

[1] Lloyd Morgan suggested that in Sherrington's experiments the after-effects of earlier emotions might be re-awakened, although direct effect from visceral disturbances could no longer take place. Sherrington adopts this view and even goes so far as to speak of " memories and associations " of visceral and organic sensations contributing to primitive emotions. (*Integrative Action*, pp. 267-8.)

proof of emotional expressions being more than "the pantomime of feeling" until we can prove that the dog has a consciousness like ours. More compelling evidence comes from cases of injury to the nervous system in man. When the spinal cord is divided in man, although the body is completely paralysed and insensitive, affect may be fully retained and show no abnormalities. For instance I have seen a man, whose paralysis was complete from the level of the sixth cervical segment down, in full possession of his normal emotional feelings. It is true that, in such a case, the vagus nerves are intact, although the entire sympathetic system is disconnected from the brain. The upper part of the alimentary canal might then be furnishing afferent stimuli, but this would surely, according to the James-Lange hypothesis, result in a distorted affect. It would give just that kind of predominance of one kind of visceral impression which should result in a peculiar feeling tone. Such patients have, of course, no awareness of their genital organs. But they are still susceptible to the charms of the other sex and often fall in love with their nurses. Further, it is well known that removal of the gonads in adult life may not affect sexual feeling in the slightest degree.

On the other hand, isolated, or even co-ordinated, visceral discharges may take place without any affect whatever. For instance there is hiccoughing, shivering sweating, projectile vomiting [without nausea or disgust], rapid heart action, flushing with high temperatures, or all the visceral changes consequent on muscular exertion. In some brain diseases (often in arteriosclerosis) we see "labile emotions"; the patients laugh or cry on the slightest provocation. Some of these will complain of it as a particularly irritating symptom because, with their laughter or tears, there is no mirth or grief. It is as if their bodies were emotional and not themselves. James met some of these objections by assuming that other visceral discharges were or were not present but, at such a point an hypothesis becomes pure tautology. The more clinical and experimental evidence accumulates the less basis does there seem to be for the James-Lange hypothesis in its literal form.

Another criticism of a more general nature may be directed against James's theories. Why should only the coarser emotions be explained and not others? To say that moral, æsthetic and intellectual feelings are a part of the concepts incorporating them is to avoid a problem with tautology. An adequate theory of affect should cover all affects. The remarks made above in connection with the pleasure attaching to "pure sensations" are pertinent here, I believe. James admits the importance of associations in the establishment of the coarser emotions. When the subtler emotions are generated, why should we not assume that a "total situation" exists which owes its pleasurable quality to the suggested reminiscences of pleasant experience? A good example of affects, seemingly intrinsic in the perceptions themselves, and therefore of the "cognitive" type of which James speaks, is seen in different kinds of quietness.   There is the stillness of a city street at three a.m., the stillness of a Sunday, the startling quietness of the country after alighting from a train, or the muffling of sounds with a fall of snow. In each of these the stimulus is the same, a contrast, a lack of noise. Each feels quite different and the differences are plainly to be traced to the associations which each situation calls up instantaneously.

A final inadequacy may be mentioned.   James explained that " We are afraid because we run " is a shorthand expression, for " run " means visceral as well as voluntary movements.   But we know that when voluntary movements are complete and effective— as in avoiding an on-coming motor—no fear is present.   He tells us nothing of the mechanism which, in this case, prevents a visceral overflow, or what causes the internal discharge when affect is present. Dewey, as we shall see in a moment, met this objection.

So, in the end, we must abandon the James-Lange hypothesis. But we do so regretfully because, having annihilated it, it seems still to contain a large measure of truth.   Sherrington following Lloyd Morgan, suggests that visceral changes may have some kind of representations in the brain and that these, when activated, produce the feeling.   Such an idea is attractive.   But I believe the truth that is hidden in James's words lies even deeper than this.   It seems to me that his hypothesis is struggling to say that what is felt is occult and obscure for normal consciousness.   It is the vague perception of something not, or not fully, conscious.   In the language of the late nineteenth century this was put into terms of physiological processes.   Were James alive and working to-day, I suspect that he would formulate his views in terms of unconscious mental processes, of which more is now known.

In his 1894 article James made it clear that he included three elements or sources of emotional consciousness.   These are : (1) The " object " with which much past experience may be associated ; (2) A feeling-tone that goes with the primary perception, that is the subtler emotional element; and (3) The back-wash of peripheral particularly visceral, commotions.   John Dewey[1] took up the argument from this point, elaborating James's views in pregnant fashion.   It is strange that little attention has been paid to Dewey's work but this may be due, I fancy, to a confusion of psychological and physiological categories that makes his writing incomprehensible at first glance.   Yet I suspect that, if his formulations were translated into purely psychological language they would gain recognition, because the germ of a competent   theory of emotions is in them.

Dewey's elaboration has to do with the train of events resulting in emotion, an analysis of what James's " total situation " consists. He also takes account of a phenomenon which had previously been neglected, namely that, when instinctive behaviour is immediate

[1] " The Theory of Emotions ", *Psychological Review*, 1894 and 1895.

and complete, no affect appears. His fundamental claim is that the total situation includes the response of the subject as well as the reception of the original stimulus. The "meaning" of the percept is something not established until reaction to it is generated. " . . . the mode of behaviour is the primary thing and . . the [conative] idea and the emotional excitation are constituted at one end and the same time ; . . . indeed they represent the tension of stimulus and response within the co-ordination which makes up the mode of behaviour." Further quotations may make clear what he means by this "co-ordination". "The idea or object, which precedes and stimulates the bodily discharge, is in no sense the idea or object (the intellectual content the ' at ' or ' on account of ') of the emotion itself. The particular idea, the specific quality or object to which seizure [affect] attaches, is just as much due to the discharge as is the seizure itself. More accurately and definitely, the idea or the object is an abstraction from the activity just as much as is the ' feel ' or seizure. We have certain organic activities initiated, say in the eye, stimulating, through the organized paths of association in the brain, certain activities of hands, legs, &c., and (through the co-ordination of these motor activities with the vegetative functions necessary to maintain them) of lungs, heart, vaso-motor system, digestive organs, &c. The ' bear ', is, psychologically, just as much a discrimination of certain values, within the total pulse or co-ordination of action, as is the feeling of ' fear '. The ' bear ' is constituted by the excitation of eye and co-ordinated touch centres, just as the ' terror ' is by the disturbances of muscular and glandular systems. The reality, the co-ordination of these partial activities, is that whole activity, which may be described equally well as ' that terrible bear ' or ' Oh, how frightened I am ! "

His view therefore is that the automatic response to a stimulus enters into consciousness with the awareness of the stimulus. Outer and inner afferent impulses are integrated together to give the meaning of the percept. When attention is directed towards the "object" one thinks of the integration as the occasion of the behaviour ; when attention is directed towards the inner impulses one thinks of the emotion. But in both instances the content is really the same ; it is the co-ordination of all the impulses reaching consciousness.

The next problem is, why is attention often directed so forcibly towards the inner impulses ? He points out that this does not always occur, that when we respond immediately and adequately to the stimulus presented, we are not aware of emotion. When there is hesitation in performance of an instinctive act, emotion appears. This hesitation is occasioned by the presence in the mind of alternative plans of action, prevision of the effects of action, recognition of the incompatibility of the instinctive action with moral standards and so on. Dewey speaks of, as tendency, or attitude, an instinctive reaction which once was the regular response to a given situation but is now held in check pending the adoption of the final co-ordinated activity. Whenever an instinctive response is controlled, there is *inhibition* and an attitude is produced. Until such time as the instinctive response may be co-ordinated with the ideas of action, inhibition exists. The resultant " tendency " or " attitude " overflows into the viscera and this we feel as affect. So, whenever there is inhibition of instinctive response, overflow into viscera takes place. When there is no inhibition there is no overflow and no affect. " The attitude stands for a recapitulation of thousands of acts formerly done, ends formerly reached ; the perception or idea stands for multitudes of acts which may be done, ends which may be acted upon. But the immediate and pressing need is to get this attitude of anger [for instance] which reflects the former act of seizing into some connection with the act of getting even, or of moral control, or whatever the idea may be. The conflict and competition, with incidental inhibition and deflection, is the disturbance of the emotional seizure [affect]."

It is easy to criticize Dewey destructively because he has given us a theory that is, as it stands, very largely meaningless. He seems to be one of those psychologists who fancy mental phenomena are explained when once they have been described in physiological terms, no matter how impossible of demonstration the alleged physiologic processes may be. So he speaks of activated eye and touch centre, association paths in the brain, efferent discharges to viscera and muscles and reflected afferent impulses from the latter. Some of these are conscious, some, like the efferent discharges of the " tendency " or " attitude " are, he says, not at all conscious. If, having framed his problem in terms of physiology, he continued to discuss these elements in physiological terms, all would be well. But what he really does is to discuss their inter-relation in psychological terms. Hence, with his tautology he introduces only confusion. It is difficult to understand why he should insist on this " physiologizing ", yet he does so with vehemence, even when his statements controvert facts of general knowledge.

For instance, in the following quotation he makes a hypothetical " peripheral excitation " first a contributory, and then the essential, element of an idea of movement. " The idea of running away must certainly involve, as part of its content, an excitation of the ' motor-centres ' actually involved in running [tautology for motor images !] ; it would seem as if this excitation must involve some, however slight, innervation of the peripheral apparatus involved in the act. What ground is there for supposing that the idea comes to consciousness save through the sensorial return of this peripheral excitation ? Is there any conceivable statement, either in terms of introspection or of nervous structure, of an idea of movement coming to consciousness absolutely unmediated peripherally ? " Has he never heard of a man with an amputated leg imagining himself walking or wiggling his toes ? Does he not know that a man with total paralysis of his body can imagine himself making any kind of movement and may even dream of running races ?

From the purely psychological standpoint a criticism may also be made. His point about the meaning of the situation depending on the reaction is an excellent one, but he presses it too far. Dewey says that this view is an extension of hints given by William James, but the latter claimed explicitly that emotional reaction is to some special feature of the situation ; that is, James made a specific concept, resulting from the total situation, the essential stimulus. The fact is that—whatever be the mechanism involved—some " meaning " is given to the stimulus *before* affectful reaction takes place. For instance one meets a bear in the woods. There is fear. One sees a bear in a cage, there is no trace of fear but only curiosity. Again, one is hunting and sees a bear, pleasurable excitement appears. Now, if one does not see the bars of the cage, or thinks exclusively of the bear, fear may develop. Or, if the hunter be inexperienced, forget his rifle, or have no confidence in it, he may experience fear. In each one of these cases, a concept has been generated on sight of the bear and the emotional reaction appears as a consequence of the concept. It is quite possible that some of the associations involved in establishing the concept are potentially capable of giving rise to an affect ; but the fact is that detectable emotion appears only after the concept is elaborated. It is idle and even pernicious to talk of potential emotions because that robs emotion of any specific meaning. It makes it so universal as to be synonymous with mental activity. My own opinion is that it is practically impossible to think without utilizing processes that are potentially capable of arousing affect ; but that is quite another matter from invoking, in the explanation of a phenomenon, its hypothetical pre-existence.

On the other hand I am sure that Dewey's theories contain buried in tautological verbiage some useful truths. If one accepted Sherrington's suggestion that peripheral processes may have some kind of representation in the brain, called these images (either conscious or unconscious or both) and then translated Dewey's theories into purely psychological language one would arrive at some such formulation as this :

A situation arouses by associations a concept which would naturally lead to some action. If this action takes place completely and with dispatch no affect appears. But before the action takes place physically it is rehearsed mentally. The thought of this action, stirs up further associations as to its effects. At the same time the situation has called up alternative plans of action and thoughts of desirable ends. If the end of the first reaction be incompatible with the desirable end, there is conflict. Either one end or the other must be abandoned and the action tending toward it inhibited. Until such inhibition is effective in suppressing the action utterly, the image of the action exists as a " tendency " or

" attitude ".   In spite of the inhibition some overflow takes place, images of visceral action are particularly prominent and often lead to actual visceral discharges.   Then these images of voluntary movement, images of visceral response, or actual visceral changes, somehow or other, filter through to consciousness as the " affect ".

Such a theory takes account of more phenomena than does the James-Lange hypothesis and it does no violence to clinical facts. Moreover it is expressed only in psychological terms, involving no undemonstrable physiological processes.   On the other hand it makes a large assumption—that there are " images " of visceral processes—and it has some gaps.   The most important of these is the failure to account for inhibition affecting voluntary rather than involuntary discharges.

CHAPTER VIII

MCDOUGALL'S THEORIES

SHAND[1] is one who has contributed largely to our knowledge and theories of emotional life. But, from the standpoint of the psychology of emotions *qua* emotions, his work has been synthetic rather than analytic. He has shown how emotions or emotional processes are united with ideas to form sentiments and how these latter become units of construction in character building. Not being primarily interested in discovering the origin of emotions he has not gone into this problem with the accuracy and imagination characteristic of the major part of his work. To me, at least, his use of the terms impulse, instinct and emotion is confusing, and I believe that in some passages he interchanges these terms. At any rate he offers no definite theory as to the ultimate nature of emotions, so his work will be dismissed—regretfully—with this mere mention.

More space must be accorded to the writings of William McDougall.[2] This is not because I have been able to discern much of value for our present purposes in his theories but because his sententious dogmatism has popularized interest in the psychology of emotions, which, a few years ago, needed advertisement badly. I have no hesitation in criticizing him freely for his polemical utterances invite it.

In his earlier writing he adopted a truth tacitly accepted by previous workers, such as William James. This is, that instincts and emotions are closely inter-related, and that, when an emotion emerges, somewhere an instinct is in operation. This generally recognized principle he elevated into a theory, viz., that every instinct has its peculiar emotion and vice versa, and that whenever an instinctive reaction is liberated an emotion appears. This view has attracted many people on account of its simplicity and originality. It goes without saying that the simpler the theory, the better ; but it does not follow that the greater the simplicity the greater its truth. The originality of McDougall's doctrine lay in its affront to common experience. It is clever to show that things are not what they seem. Regardless of the validity of any theory it appeals to people if it circumvents the obvious ; that is getting the better of

---

[1] A. F. Shand, *Foundations of Character*, Methuen.
[2] *Social Psychology*, and *An Outline of Psychology*, Methuen, 1923.

Nature, which is the object of science. So his claims have been accepted with avidity and one can find in many books his comfortable list of instincts each with its appropriate emotion, and those who use them do not seem disquieted by the fact that sometimes the emotion is named after the instinct and sometimes the instinct after the emotion. Other less simple-minded folk have wondered why, in some cases, instincts and emotions should have the same names and in others that the names should be different. They have wondered whether, perhaps, certain clear-cut and easily recognizable emotions are naturally associated with certain clear-cut and easily recognizable types of behaviour, and these have separate names ; whereas there may be much more complicated and fluid instincts and emotions that do not naturally fall into pairs but might be made to do so, were they first academically baptized.

In his " Social Psychology ", McDougall recognized two types of emotions. These were the primary ones, which were the affective aspects of instinctive reaction, and the complex emotions, which appeared when more than one instinct was in operation, the affect being a combination of the two. In this second group one can see the unwitting admission of the principle of conflict appearing for the first time. Now it runs through all his psychology of emotions, although he stoutly and constantly protests against it. If two instincts are aroused together, it seems plain that neither can reach full expression, for full expression involves the undivided energies of the whole of the organism. Blending of two processes not identical must, therefore, involve curtailment of expression in both. Each is thus to some extent inhibiting the other.

McDougall has, of course, been much criticized. The effects of this have been to draw from him expostulations of invulnerability and, possibly, to induce the present modifications of his theory that go much further, in effect, than he probably realizes. These changes may all be summed up by saying that he has greatly extended the operation of the principle of conflict or inhibition. This principle appears, I believe, in his introduction of sense of effort (experience of conation) as part of a primary emotion ; in the formulation of a third group, the derived emotions, and his now arguing only about impulses to action instead of instinctive reactions, using the latter term only when he gives definite formulations. We shall consider these points presently.

But first it must be made clear that I am alleging the introduction or extension of a principle which McDougall vehemently denies. The following passage will demonstrate this, a passage typical of his best polemical style :

" There is a curious dogma which crops up from time to time in the discussions of emotion and which requires a remark in passing. It asserts that emotions are experienced only when our natural tendencies to action are obstructed or in some way suspended. I have recognized that this is true of angry emotion ; that such obstruction is the specific condition of excitement of the combative instinct ; and that the impulse of this instinct serves to re-inforce all other impulses, when they are obstructed. But as regards other emotions, I can see no jot of valid evidence that supports this doctrine. It would seem to be a distortion of the simple truth that we do not become explicitly aware of our emotions, so long as we give ourselves wholly to action. We become self-consciously aware of the quality of our emotion only when we are not wholly absorbed in action, in the pursuit of our goal, and in the choice of means towards it. But that is not to say that the emotional quality is not there, qualifying all our experience while we strive."

Two comments may be made on this quotation. In the first place it seems to me that he contradicts himself. First he says that we are explicitly aware of our emotions, when wholly given to action, and then at once states that at such times we are unaware of the quality of our emotions. Now, as I have said before, and I believe it to be in harmony with McDougall's views,[1] the subjective aspect of an emotion is the affect. If the affect is not quality of feeling, what is it ? If it be quality of action, that is part of the objective behaviour. If affect be not quality, it must be pure excitement, and then all affects become alike.

But this is mere debate. The question at issue is not one of logic but of fact. McDougall says a given statement is " a distortion of the simple truth ". The reality or fancifulness of alleged phenomena is not to be settled by argument from an easy chair nor by the introspection of one author. We all of us introspect to the advantage of our pet theories and it is a rash man who will claim that what he finds in his psyche will be duplicated in others—particularly if they be psychologists who hold opposing views. The most valid material is to be derived from the experience of those who are not trained introspectionists. It is natural to think of fear, for instance, appearing with retreat or with an avoiding reaction, so, if one does not feel fear, his testimony is all the more striking, unless the investigator assumes with McDougall that the informant lies. Has he never heard the phrase, " I hadn't time to be frightened " ?

Being interested in this matter, I have, during recent years, questioned many people who have been in situations of danger, probably some hundreds in all. Except for the psychoneurotics, all soldiers have given me the same account. Once familiarity with dangers was established (the learning of adaptive actions and attitudes) fear was never present when any action was possible.

[1] In this I am perhaps wrong. McDougall uses the term affect (so far as I can discover) only in connection with pleasure-pain feeling-tones. If he used the term as I do for the purely subjective experience in emotion, he might, perhaps, divide this affect into " quality " and " experience of conation ". These are both subjective elements. But, as we shall see presently, he makes the same admission about " experience of conation ", namely that one is not aware of it till, activity being suspended, attention is turned to the impulse that is working within one.

A shell was heard coming, its destination was judged by the sound it made ; if coming close the soldier threw himself on the ground ; if passing overhead he gave no more thought to it. So long as attention was given to behaviour there was no fear. But, with very few exceptions, fear was universal in the contemplation of danger when no appropriate action could change the mental situation. Decorations were won by men who acted and did not think (self-consciously at least). I have frequently been told that a real stand-up bayonet fight was practically unknown. One antagonist or the other became frightened and immediately was killed. That is, with fear there was relative paralysis of his adaptive actions.

In the neurotics, of course, conflict was omnipresent, and it is interesting that one of the early symptoms was an invariable loss of the capacity to guage the direction of a shell by the sound it was making. An adaptive reaction was inhibited and fear emerged. Rock climbers have given me the same sort of story. When they have slipped in a dangerous climb, all attention was given to scrambling or planning for safety, and not a trace of fear was present. It would appear in retrospect. Some of these were surprised at the complete lack of anxiety when the danger was most acute. One inexperienced climber added that when he was making his way up a perpendicular face of rock his head gave him no trouble, but that giddiness was apt to appear if he gained a broad, safe ledge on which he could stand and rest. He spontaneously ascribed this to his attention being no longer directed to action, so that it was free to contemplate the possible danger.

In introducing his latest discussion of emotions, McDougall begins, as I have done, by rejecting the concept of their having substantive value and states that he means the term in an adjec-tival sense. The problem is, then, he says, not " What is an emotion ", but " What emotional experiences are there, what is their occasion and what services do they perform ? " He divides the phenomena into three groups : " quality " (subjective), bodily expression and " experience of conation ". The last is derived from a sense of effort, a feeling of striving, that is present whenever an emotion is. One becomes aware of it because it has variations in intensity and is thus not a constant with emotional behaviour. He defines it in the following paragraph :

" Conative experience is the felt impulse to action ; and it is felt, or is prominent in experience, in proportion to the strength of the working of the impulse. *It takes the forms of mere craving for some undefined goal, of definitely directed desire, of conflict of desires, of resolving, choosing, willing*[1] ; and, when we are actively occupied in working toward our goal, either by thinking or by bodily activity, this conative experience is complicated and obscured for introspec-tion by the kinæsthetic sensory qualities set up by muscular strains.

---

[1] My italics.

Now such felt impulse is present in all emotional experience.[1] When we are afraid, we feel the impulse to retreat or escape from the object that frightens us ; when we are angry, we feel the impulse to attack the object that angers us ; when we are curious, we feel the impulse to draw nearer and examine the object that excites our curiosity. It is true that we become introspectively aware of the the impulse to draw nearer and examine the object that excites our curiosity. It is true that we become introspectively aware of the impulse, only when we do not give ourselves up to it, but, arresting or suspending it, turn our attention from the object to ourselves ; but that is the peculiarity of all introspective awareness."

I cannot find any reference to this aspect of emotional experience in his " Social Psychology ", so I conclude that this addition to his formulations—and the most significant of them—is the product of his experience since that book was written. As he reports no new observations, it is safe to assume that enlargement of his views comes from further reflection, a reflection perhaps not uninfluenced by the remarks of his critics. At any rate, there seems to be here an admission of the principle of conflict, of inhibition of action, an admission made almost in so many words. In the last sentence quoted, he says that experience of conation does not exist till the impulse is checked. Now, when we give ourselves up to an impulse, personality (or consciousness, or whatever one terms the directing agency) is for the time being concentrated on the action or thought ; it is not felt to be an impulse but a willed act. In this case there is no conflict ; we do not feel that a " something " is impelling us, as we always do when an affect is present. In fact, the feeling of the " something " stirring in us often is the affect. An example he gives of experience of conation is one in which conflict is the most prominent characteristic. This is of the feeling of effort accompanying an attempt to perform two different kinds of movement with the two hands. Indeed it is—to me at least—impossible to conceive of unimpeded action giving any sense of effort whatever.

In reading the paragraph quoted above, and particularly the last sentence, one cannot keep from wondering in what sense McDougall uses the term " introspection ". Does he mean by it simple awareness of what is going on within one's self, either mentally or physically, or does he mean a willed turning of attention to the inner events. The latter is surely its usual meaning, yet, if that be the sense in which he is using it, he is apparently implying that all affect (*i.e.*, both " quality " and " experience of conation ") is not in full consciousness until introspection is employed. But he could hardly claim that, for it is a notorious characteristic of strong affects that they arise and smite us. We do not look for them. On the other hand, if he means simple awareness, I doubt much if any but a sedulous introspectionist is ever aware of conation except in volun-

[1] Author's Italics.

tary and difficult activities. And simple instinctive behaviour— the kind his theories are built upon—is involuntary or it is nothing. But it seems that in reality he is no longer talking about simple instincts. He has enlarged his classification and in a new one has added a category in which experience of conation would not be inappropriate. In his earlier work he speaks of primary and secondary emotions. He now adds a third, the derived emotions. In order to understand this classification it may be well to give his lists. The primary emotions are these : where the corresponding instinct is not obvious, I have added it in brackets : fear, anger, disgust, tender emotion (parental instinct), distress (appeal) lust (sex), curiosity, feeling of subjection of inferiority (self-abasement), elation (self display), loneliness (gregarious instinct), appetite (food-seeking), feeling of ownership (acquisition), feeling of creativeness (construction), amusement (laughter). As to the validity and relevance of these lists, one could argue till doomsday, but it would be unprofitable debate, for the court of last resort is individual preference, not objective experience. Facts are not the basis of this classification but interpretation thereof. But one cannot refrain from asking why he stops with only fourteen. Why, for instance, are cruelty, swimming (or bathing), climbing, dancing, or sleeping omitted from the list of instincts ? They are occupations followed with equal zest and irrationality as many on his list and they are as untaught as construction is.

The secondary or blended emotions occur when more than one instinct is stimulated at once. Some instincts are directly opposed in reaction and in these cases one dominates. But others may fuse in the behaviour elicited and then the blended emotions appear. These are peculiarly liable to development in man on account of his organization of sentiments. These combinations may present infinite gradations in the proportion of one element to another. Such emotions are : Scorn, a mixture of anger and disgust to which positive self feeling may be added ; horror, that is fear and disgust ; admiration is a compound of wonder (curiosity) and negative self feeling, although pleasure may be added ; when admiration is combined with fear, awe is the product ; while awe with gratitude gives reverence. Gratitude is tenderness mixed with negative self-feeling and pity is tender feeling plus distress (via sympathy). Reproach results from the addition of tenderness to anger.

The derived emotions are the new ones. These McDougall lists as joy, sorrow, chagrin, disappointment, surprise, regret, remorse, confidence, hope, anxiety, despondency and despair. They are neither primary emotions (because they are coincident with no specific instincts), nor are they blends : " The word derived is here used to denote the fact that one emotion of this class is not constantly correlated with any one impulse or tendency, but rather may arise in the course of the operation of any strong impulse or tendency ; the emotion being dependent upon or derived from the working of

the impulse under certain conditions which we have now to specify."
It soon appears that the "certain conditions" are intellectual
judgments which qualify desire, the latter being the formulation
that impulse has taken. For instance, the "prospective emotions
of desire" are confidence, hope, anxiety, despondency and despair.
In each of these conditions an impulse has been consciously recognized as desire and an intellectual judgment is added as to the
probability or improbability of its function. Then, too, there are
the "retrospective emotions of desire". When one has not obtained
his wish there is regret. If to this he added self-reproach, remorse
appears ; while if tender feeling is united with regret, the result is
sorrow. Similarly joy is a progressive satisfaction of desires
connected with love, and, if this be self-love, the combination gives
elation. [He has previously classed elation with the primary
emotions]. All the derived emotions are epiphenomena ; they have
no force in themselves, for the energy comes from the impulse. On
the other hand, he thinks, the primary emotions are so bound up
with impulse that they can be spoken of as having energy.

It is plain that in this last group of derived emotions McDougall
is no longer dealing with instinctive reactions appearing in simple
and direct form. In fact he confesses as much when he says the
impulse is expressed in desire. When one wishes for anything,
one is obviously not reacting to its immediate presence. If instinct
there be, therefore, it must be in abeyance, it is stimulated but not
in direct operation. This is the phenomena which Dewey alleged
as the *sine qua non* of emotion. In such cases experience of conation
would be a natural enough detail to be added to the picture.

But we may not go farther and claim that every impulse—in the
sense in which McDougall uses that term—involves an instinct in
abeyance ? If we examine his quoted language in defining experience
of conation (in the words which I have italicized), we see that he is
speaking not of an impulse that is actuating behaviour at the moment
but of an impulse that is going to determine : "mere craving for
some undefined goal, of definitely directed desire . . . of resolving,
choosing and willing". He even includes "conflict of desires" !
Not one of these refers to a simple instinct in operation, expressing
itself freely in action. By what perversion of logic can "resolving,
choosing and willing" be regarded as simple instinctive reactions ?

In all this I quite agree with McDougall. The terms he now
uses in his argument—impulse, craving, tendency and so forth—all
refer to the preliminaries of instinctive response, to the effect which
stimulated instincts have on consciousness before they emerge as
actual behaviour. These are some of the conditions in which affect
appears. If, having used these concepts in his argument, he then
went on to modify his earlier formulation of emotion being an
inevitable component of every simple and direct instinctive action,
I would have no quarrel with him.

As a matter of fact he comes perilously close at times to a denial of his original theory. For instance, when discussing the James-Lange hypothesis, as it might be applied in the case of a man whose body was totally anaesthetic, he says : " . . . the experience would remain strongly conative as well as cognitive : that is to say, the subject would continue to be aware of a strong impulse to action of some kind. This conative factor in emotional experience is perhaps its most essential mark. If this could be subtracted, leaving the specific emotional quality, we should perhaps recognize the emotion, but it would seem as though all the life and strength and all that constitutes its urgency and vital significance were gone out of it."

In these sentences he is surely talking about prospective action, not of action in being. And it is the felt urge to do something that he now says gives emotion its vividness. An impulse is a cause of action, not the action itself, so McDougall is saying, in effect, that the essential factor in affect is the recognition of an instinct that wants to be operating, so to speak. If we were to follow the logical implication of these words, we would have to think that an emotional reaction begins to lose its subjective warmth when the prospective character of the instinct begins to wane. An impulse, desire or plan is a cause not an effect. When its effects begin to appear it is being translated into something else, that is, action. Therefore he is now allying emotion with the stirring up of instincts, not with their direct operation. If their activation be momentary, the emotional by-product would be brief or escape notice altogether. On the other hand, if the activation were prolonged it could only be so in virtue of something standing in the way of immediate motor expression of the instinct. In other words, McDougall's arguments lead one to the conclusion that felt conflict is an essential feature in emotional experience. Since he explicitly rejects this view, his arguments and his theories seem to me to be in opposition.

A final word must be added about his views as to purpose of emotions. He has an excellent suggestion to make, which, did he leave it as a suggestion, would be admirable. Unfortunately he gives it as a dogma, as a theory having, apparently universal reference After having stated that he includes emotions of animals and believes them to enjoy affective experience of some kind, he says : " The primary ' emotion ' is then an indicator of the instinctive impulse at work ; its bodily expressions serve to indicate the nature of the impulse to our fellows and to evoke in them the same instinctive impulse, attitude, and emotional excitement ; and the emotional quality serves also to indicate, to the subject himself, the nature of his excitement and the kind of action to which he is impelled."

I am inclined to think that these ideas, properly elaborated, would be helpful in understanding some matters which are now obscure. For instance, if emotional expression belongs to prospective instinct reaction, it may well be that the occult means of communication between herd animals may be subtle emotional expressions. These expressions would not be evidences of instincts *per se*, of activities that animals imitate from one to the other in the group, but they would be by-products of incubating instincts, evidences of the hatching of instinctive action, which could be communicated throughout the group so that the actual behaviour could appear in all members at once. It is striking, for instance, to observe with what instantaneity a whole flock of birds will suddenly change the direction or mode of their flight. It occurs with such suddenness and unanimity that imitation of changed movement seems inconceivable. In man speech may, perhaps, have developed as an elaboration of emotional cries, that originally produced analogous instinctive impulses among the neighbouring anthropoids in a purely automatic way. This kind of process we still know, of course, as intuition of another person's emotional state.

The value to the individual of affect is also, I am inclined to believe, much as McDougall has stated it. The knowledge, " I am getting angry ", may be quite useful. But what he forgets, or neglects to mention, is that emotion is often not merely useless but baneful. Of what possible value could fear be (either in its objective or subjective manifestations) to a solitary animal. Then, too, it is a commonplace of experience that emotional behaviour is apt to be less skilful than coldly-planned conduct. The vigour of the instinctive action is often offset by its recklessness. A man's opponent may be pleased to see his adversary becoming angry : the angrier he is the less judgment will he use. McDougall should have guarded his statements ; had he said that emotions were potentially useful, little criticism could have been directed against this claim.

If, then, we sum up what McDougall has contributed in the same way that we did the work of Dewey, that is, neglecting his actual formulations but deriving what we can from his arguments, we would say : emotion is apt to appear, both objectively and subjectively, when instinct is aroused but not in operation as such. The function of emotion is to warn oneself or others of the nature of the behaviour that is likely to develop.

CHAPTER IX

THE VIEWS OF FREUD AND JANET

WHENEVER one examines one's own emotional reactions, a prominent element seems often to be the mysterious way in which the feeling seems to come from nowhere. One feels possessed, some immaterial influence seems to have seized the body and mind and to be directing both behaviour and thought. This phenomenon, of the cause seeming to lie outside of consciousness, is naturally suggestive of unconscious mental activity. Such being the case, it might be expected that psychopathologists, who are more familiar with the psychology of the unconscious mind, would have furnished us with some theories of emotion more interesting or more adequate than those of the academic psychologists. When we turn to psychopathological literature, however, the search is rather disappointing. No satisfactory theories are found there, although interesting data and pertinent suggestions do appear.

The one who has written most about the unconscious is Freud. He has given only one generalization about emotions. This is that they represent dramatic re-living of earlier experiences, just as the symptoms of hysteria do. In the latter case the earlier experience was individual; in the former it may be racial. This might seem to be repeating McDougall's view that the emotion is part of an instinctive reaction; but it goes beyond this, because it introduces, with the suggestion of reminiscence, the idea of the emotional reaction not belonging purely to the immediate situation. The emotional person is not merely indulging in an automatic response to the actual environment, but is, unconsciously, reliving earlier experiences as well. Most of Freud's discussion of emotion is found in connection with fear. As to this he has some theories about libido turning into anxiety which are partly physiological and partly psychological. They do not seem to have much direct bearing on the problems of emotion as a whole, and, since I have criticized them elsewhere[1], shall not pause to consider them further.

Freud and Janet began their psychopathology in the same school, that of Charcot, and they also worked at this period mainly with hysteria. It is therefore not unnatural that Janet's conclusions are

---

[1] *Problems in Dynamic Psychology*, Chapter IX, Cambridge University Press ; The Macmillan Company, New York.

much like Freud's—or vice versa. Since the former has put his views with admirable conciseness a quotation may be justified.[1] With his clinical material he showed that in hysterics stimuli do not arouse appropriate reactions but tend rather to stir up old systematized emotions, which appear automatically. The personality of the patient is not strong enough to develop sufficiently accurate perceptions for the guidance of behaviour, that is, these automatic emotions are not inhibited. In concluding his discussion of emotions in hysterics he offers a tentative theory of emotions in general. He has spoken of the hysterical emotion being exhibited in disturbances of ideas, in internal and external bodily phenomena and so on. He then proceeds :

" . . . But the principle thing, the thing that governs all these disturbances, is the lowering of the mental level, the reduction of all the higher functions of will, of attention, of personal assimilation. The disturbing emotion behaves here—and I am disposed to believe it a general rule—like exhaustion or fatigue. It belongs to the general class of all the phenomena half normal, half pathological, which comprises conditions of fatigue, sleep, intoxication, the neuroses which are always characterized by a lowering of the higher functions of adaptation, and by an over-reaction due to the operation of lower functions in a more or less automatic way.

" In order to understand emotion it is necessary to adopt the point of view of objective psychology and observe the individual from without at the same time taking cognizance of the group of circumstances in which he is placed, rather than to give all one's attention to the feelings, more or less incomplete, that one experiences himself in emotion. The phenomena of emotion are produced when a being, living and conscious, is suddenly exposed to a change of physical environment, particularly of the social environment in which he is immersed, when he is not prepared by previous education for automatic adjustment to the change and when he has not the necessary vital force or sufficient time to adapt himself to it at the moment. There then occurs an inco-ordinate, useless, nervous discharge, which has all the characteristics of a state of exhaustion and which takes place in just the same way as in conditions of exhaustion, fatigue, sleep or intoxications. Emotion is distinguished from these other states by the suddenness of the phenomena and by the external conditions which determine it."

What Janet is saying is, then, something like this : In mental behaviour we see two contrasting groups of phenomena. On the one hand there is thought or conduct determined by personality, by intelligence, by accurate observation of the environment and reasoned response to the situation. On the other hand there is automatic, ill-adapted, over-reacting and, perhaps, irrational conduct and thinking. The latter type occurs in mental and nervous

[1] *Pierre Janet, L'état Mental des hystériques,* Paris, 1911, p. 543-4.

disease, but it also appears when we are tired, when we sleep or when we are emotional. The emotion is not an adaptive reaction to the immediate situation, based on conscious recognition of the needs of the situation, but is a low level response merely precipitated by present circumstances. It has its origin in the past, but the subject is not aware of the situation—or situations—to which it refers.

Janet thus leaves us with the theory that emotions come from non-conscious levels of the mind. They are the products of unconscious mental activity ; but he says nothing as to the mechanism by which the unconscious elements are activated, nor has he mapped out that vague region, the unconscious, so that he could tell us what kind of processes are involved. " Unconscious " as here used is a purely negative term : it includes everything of which we are not at the moment aware, providing a deceptively facile explanation for anything inexplicable in terms of introspection. Another deficiency in Janet's formulations is manifest. He says nothing about what it is we feel, when affect is experienced. (He is not antagonistic to the James-Lange hypothesis but regards it as limited.)

The reader may be slightly shocked by the casual way in which Janet classes emotions with morbid phenomena, so a passing comment on this topic may be justified. The psychopathologist who is constantly examining and analysing symptoms is perpetually impressed by the close relationship in kind of the symptom to the mental operations of normal people. So close is this relationship that practically every psychopathologist regards the nature of the two as identical. In other words the symptom, as a kind of thinking is not morbid, it is its relative prominence that makes it a symptom. Any type of mental operation is normal if it be adaptive, *i.e.*, integrated with the personality, but abnormal if it is functioning independently or dominating consciousness. The consequence of symptoms is a distorted personality, which is abnormal. It is the final product—the irrational patient—which the layman sees. The psychopathologist, however, when he analyses symptoms, finds (as a rule) nothing that is not found in normal life. To take a simple example. The dissociated behaviour of a fugue seems pathological. So it is, because the dissociated mental processes are governing behaviour in a way incompatible with the personality. But, *qua* dissociation, there is nothing morbid. A woman who knits, counting her stitches automatically, while she reads a book or talks, is exhibiting dissociation. The psychopathologist has the best material for studying dissociation, but that does not mean that the process is necessarily morbid. There is an important corollary to be added. The psychopathologist, being familiar with dissociations, takes their existence for granted ; they feel real to him. The layman, or lay psychologist, less familiar with it, feels of it as something abnormal and unreal. He may admit the expedience of including psychopathological data in psychology, but they do not have for him the same nutritious taste as the data of introspection and experiment.

CHAPTER X

THE CONTRIBUTIONS OF MORTON PRINCE

THE work of Morton Prince carries us a bit further, for he has made an intensive study in many patients of the unconscious mental processes actually coincident with conscious emotion, as revealed by hypnotic and similar technical methods. The value of his work on the unconscious lies not in his demonstration of it by inevitable inference (the psychoanalytic method), but in his demonstration of the thinking that goes on parallel with conscious mental operations, although totally beyond the reach of the subject's introspection. Whatever one may think of his theories, Prince's data cannot be neglected by anyone who wishes to formulate broad psychological principles. I should state at this point that, in addition to some familiarity with his writings, I have had the frequent privilege of discussing the phenomena of emotion with him both in person and by correspondence.

Before discussing the material which Prince has reported, it may be well to mention briefly the nature of his views on emotions, lest confusion arise as to what I am borrowing from his theories and what conclusions I am drawing from the material he has published. In the bulk of his writings[1] he treats instincts and emotions as if they were the same, using the terms synonymously and interchanging them in consecutive sentences. He has not, then, made any effort to separate off the problem of emotions from that of instincts. He has, however, made observations of value in discriminating the two groups of phenomena. His theories of instinct-emotion are borrowed from the division of these processes into cognitive, affective and conative elements. The first represent perception of stimuli ; the last the efferent side, the expression, instinctive or emotional ; while the affective component gives the power, the drive, to the whole mechanism. He claims that in this analysis he is following McDougall, but I have not been able to confirm him in this. So far as I can discover from the latter's publications, the urge of the instinct process is always held to be the impulse, the conative

---

[1] The publications of which I have made use are : *The Dissociation of a Personality*, 1908 ; *The Unconscious*, 1914 ; " Co-Conscious Images ", *Journal of Abnormal Psychology*, XII, 5, Dec., 1917 ; " Miss Beauchamp, The Theory of the Psychogenesis of Multiple Personality ", *Journal of Abnormal Psychology*, XV, 2 and 3, June, 1920.

element, the affect being regarded as a secondary effect, which may contribute to the direction of the impulse but does not actuate it.

It is possible that, in ascribing dynamic influence to the affect, Prince had dimly in mind its separation from the purely instinctive reaction, for he eventually comes to this view. In January, 1921, he wrote me : " . . . I have been reading over some manuscript written about a year ago, from which I quote the following passage, which seems to me to bear upon the point we were discussing.

" ' Now, while such innate emotional dispositions may properly of themselves be regarded as instincts because of their inherited innate organization and behaviour, nevertheless to identify them with the particular biological instincts that he does raises contentious problems which, for our purposes, as we are not dealing with biology as a whole, but only with human psychology, are unnecessary and are bound to land us in a sea of troubled waters. For instance, the innate mechanism of fear, or "instinct" of fear, if you prefer to so name it, though it induces impulses to flight, may not be the whole instinct of flight, as Mr. Shand maintains. Thus in insects and animals the disposition to flight and concealment may very well function as far as we know and as there is reason to believe, without any conscious emotional quality taking part. In such cases the fear disposition would play the part of an auxiliary force, a reserve power to be called upon in emergencies to reinforce the instinct. It seems to me that Mr. Shand may be quite right in this view. Indeed it seems difficult to imagine that the constantly manifested flight of birds and wild animals reminding us of mere habits should always be motivated by fear, however faintly.' " The same remark might, quite properly, be made about the " fear " reactions of human infants.

In human psychology, Prince thinks, emotions or instincts, owe their wide influence to their union with ideas. This union, following McDougall[1], he calls a sentiment. He quotes McDougall's definition, " A sentiment is an organized system of emotional dispositions centred about the idea of some object " and adds this comment : " . . . But when we say that an emotion becomes linked to, *i.e.*, organized with, that composite called an idea, *we really mean (according to this theory of emotion) that it is the whole instinct, the emotional innate disposition of which the emotion is only a part that is so linked*.[2] The instinct has also afferent and efferent activities. The latter is an impulsive or conative force discharged by the emotion. Thus the affective element of an instinctive process—a process which is a biological reaction—provides the driving force, makes the idea a dynamic factor moves us to carry the idea to fulfilment."

All Prince's theories centre around the activity of the conative

---

[1] But not Shand, who does not so define a sentiment, although Prince implies that he does !

[2] Italics in the original.

aspect of the instinct linked to the idea. He says there are three exhibitions of conation : overt conduct and thoughts, internal visceral discharges, and the inhibition of other impulses belonging to other instincts, other sentiments. The last of these is responsible for the repression which makes some sentiments unconscious, and thus leads to psychopathological phenomena. If two instincts tend to be activated at the same time, the impulse of one is stronger and represses the other ; *i.e.*, it represses the sentiment. (The dominance of one sentiment over another is due to its " setting ", that is, its development in the life history of the individual, but this is not germane to our present problem.) When repressed, the sentiment is, or may be, still active and may produce various phenomena. These are all kinds of automatic behaviour of which the subject is not aware, or becomes so only retrospectively, or, perhaps, is aware of but cannot prevent. The last class includes compulsions and phobias of many varieties. The automatic behaviour may, of course, lead to somnambulisms, fugues, and even dissociation of the personality, if the sentiments split off from consciousness are sufficiently extensive and integrated to form a new personality. In normal people all behaviour that is analogous to these symptoms is similarly determined. Prince claims that the activity of unconscious sentiments is experimentally demonstrated by the " psychogalvanic phenomenon ". If, in the course of a word-association test, the subject be given a stimulus word that touches a buried sentiment, a visceral discharge will take place, of which the subject is unaware, but which is responsible for a change in the electric conductivity of the body.

This, with unfair brevity, represents Prince's theory. His great contribution is the experimental study of the activity of the unconscious sentiments. When such a complex is not conscious but is active, he calls it *co-conscious*. Many of his patients, when under hypnosis, described the thoughts actuating automatic behaviour as having been accompanied by co-conscious images. In others a record of co-conscious thought was obtained from automatic writing, and so on. Frequently the phenomena being investigated were emotional reactions which the subject could not account for ; hence the importance of his observations for our present problem.

His results bear on one important question. Are pathological emotions independently excited entities as William James claimed, and as Freud has, at times, suggested ? Prince has in many instances showed that an affect, or mood, apparently unrelated to anything in the environment or to anything in the patient's consciousness, may be correlated with co-conscious thoughts. I have asked him whether his experience justifies him in believing that moods can exist without ideas occasioning them, or whether he considers that it is possible artificially to produce an emotion by suggestion, without somehow suggesting a cause (idea) for the reaction. In reply he stated that he did not think a mood was a mood unless it was an emotion organized with ideas, and that he was sceptical of the possibility of effecting a true emotional reaction without ideas. The only exception to human emotions being associated with ideas he thought might be seen in the behaviour of an infant confronted with a moving situation. (But this could well be viewed as a purely instinctive reaction, like the " fear " reactions of animals mentioned above, in which it is unnecessary to assume the presence of affect.)

We may now consider some of the many examples Prince gives of emotional reactions, inexplicable to the subject, being correlated with co-conscious processes. The first of these has to do with a submerged personality. In his " Miss Beauchamp " article, he speaks of how B IV had a realistic outlook on life and, sincerely, thought she was a sceptic in religious matters, whereas B I was given to religious observance and preoccupation. B I continued her mental life co-consciously at such times as B IV had control of the consciousness of Miss Beauchamp. Hence B IV would be moved by stimuli significant only for the co-conscious personality of B I. " B IV had an aversion, as already stated, to religious services, including the music, and yet she was emotionally stirred by them. This is easily accounted for on a well-known psychological principle. The emotions emerged from the religious complexes of B I, which, though dissociated and dormant, were technically, of course, sub-conscious. Vibrant with emotion they sent their thrills of feeling through her whole being. (Numerous and varied examples of this principle were observed in this case. It is the same as that governing some types of phobias in which the emotion derives from the conserved dispositions of long-forgotten experiences)[1]."

In his paper on " Co-conscious Images ", Prince gives some beautiful examples of moods being correlated with specific co-conscious images. The subject referred to in the following quotation described, under hypnosis, certain images, vividly recalled when in this state, as having been present co-consciously at times concerning which she was questioned[2]. The " observer ", so to speak, of these co-conscious images, was spoken of as " C 2 ".

[1] *Journal of Abnormal Psychology*, XV, 2 and 3, p. 125.

[2] We may regard the process of hypnosis in such cases as operating by extending the range of consciousness beyond its usual limits. In fact, one can sum up all the phenomena of hypnotism by saying that the functions of consciousness are directed by the hypnotist instead of by the subject, and that the range of this vicarious control is much widened. Hence there results, conatively, an activation of bodily processes or of ideas which is normally impossible, while on the cognitive side there is a recognition of afferent stimuli and production of memories such as cannot be brought into consciousness voluntarily. In the resuscitation of memories of co-conscious images such as Prince reports, we have a process very like the normal one, that of recalling by effort or as a result of chance association, the images of a dream that has been forgotten. When aroused these images may seem vivid and to have been very " real " ; yet, like the co-conscious images they were not betrayed by any conduct while the dream was in progress. The co-conscious images are like a dream going on in the unconscious while the subject is, apparently, awake, and attending to other thoughts.

" Not infrequently these visualizations were manifestly allegorical representations of ideas entertained by the subject, and specifically were expressive of her outlook towards life and the particular problems it presented to her, or of her relation to the environment, etc. These allegories took different shape according to her emotional mood, varying as she was elated or depressed. Evidently there was a close correlation between these co-conscious phenomena and the contemporary mood, *i.e.*, the affective colouring of co-consciousness the former appearing to determine, or at least reflect the latter, or vice versa ; or as may be more probable, both being determined by deeper sub-conscious processes from which the affect emerged. A few examples, out of many that might be given, will make clear what I mean.

" 1. Often when the subject felt full of courage but not really happy, according to the introspective statement given by the hypnotic personality, there would be in C2 the picture of a man toiling up a steep mountain side, with a heavy pack on his back. If she felt hopeful the mountain looked bright at the top, but if she felt doubtful about accomplishing whatever she wanted to do the mountain top was in the clouds.

" Sometimes the road up the mountain seemed very rough, and at others it was smooth, according as she felt. On one occasion, for instance, the subject ' was more depressed than she had been for a long time. She felt as if she could not bear a disappointment that had come to her. There was not one bright or hopeful thought in her mind. She felt that she had come to the end of her endurance and was ready to give up the fight.'

" Now the correlated co-conscious picture was of a road ' so rough as to be almost impassable ; the man was bent under the weight of his load and the top of the mountain was hidden by black clouds '. After a psychotherapeutic talk ' the picture was still there but changed. The clouds had lifted from the top of the mountain and the atmosphere had cleared. The man was still toiling up the mountain side but he stood up straight and the road was not so rough. The man in the picture looked a little like Pilgrim in " Pilgrim's Progress ". He had on a sort of frock, belted at the waist and reaching to his knees and heavy laced boots, quite high. His hair was long and he had no hat. His bundle was slung over his shoulder on a stick.' *With the change in this picture there came a change in the subject's thoughts and feeling*[1] : ' She felt some hope and courage, some strength to meet the demand made upon her. She felt she had exaggerated the importance of the matter which had disturbed her and that she ought to be very thankful that it was no worse, but still felt depressed and sad, though stronger.'

" It will be agreed, I think, that if the subject had wanted to picture, allegorically, her conception of the road of life which she

[1] Italics in original.

had to travel and its final goal, she could not voluntarily have done it better. But this allegory cannot be construed as a wholly new subconscious fabrication of the moment. She had previously often consciously thought of the road of life which she had to travel in similar allegorical terms and this rough rocky road had appeared in her dreams. Such thoughts therefore were conserved when out of mind in the subconscious, and we are permitted to infer, from all we know of the subconscious, that they took on functional activity and by some mechanism manifested themselves through these co-conscious pictures. They had, however, in the allegory, undergone much secondary elaboration. The colouring of the conscious content of the mind by the affect belonging to a subconscious process is a phenomenon which has been frequently demonstrated[1]. Although in a given instance the subconscious source of the affect may not be clear, in other instances there seems no room for doubt.

" 2. Another set of cinematographic pictures appeared about this time. The scene was my office. I was ' blowing bubbles— gorgeous great bubbles—and there were pictures of herself holding out her hands to catch the bubbles. And then the bubbles burst. When the bubble was there she felt elated, and when it burst she felt depressed.'

" These pictures can be rationally interpreted as an allegorical representation of actual psychotherapeutic experiences. I was in the habit of encouraging her with roseate plans for her future, of what she could do in the way of literary and other work to solve the problem of her life. But these plans almost always " burst " and for one reason or another came to nought. This, too, was her point of view and caused considerable unhappiness. With the acceptance of the plans, however, she was always highly elated, but when they finally ' burst ' she became correspondingly depressed."

We may interrupt the quotation for a moment to comment on a possible implication of this second example. The visions described are of an essentially childish occupation. Everyone is familiar with the liveliness of emotional expression observable in a child who is playing a game. Such dramatic expressions are infrequent in the adult, but, if we assume them to be represented co-consciously, we can understand how a vivid affect may be their conscious product. This principle will be elaborated presently. To resume :

" 3. There were certain lines upon courage which had appealed to her and which appeared at times as visualized words in C 2, but without coming into the conscious content of her mind. These lines began :

" ' Of wounds and sore defeat
I made my battle stay,
Winged sandals for my feet
I wove of my delay.'

[1] See Prince, *The Unconscious*, Chapters XII, XIII, XXVI.

When these words appeared she felt more courageous and had more endurance.

"4. Again, it was observed that at times in the C 2 part of her mind there was a curious religious connection with her mood.

"Thus when she felt very depressed and rebellious there was a picture of Christ on the Cross. Correlated with this picture, of which, of course, there was no awareness, her conscious thoughts at the moment were of undeserved suffering. She realized that suffering is not always a punishment for sin (as Christ's was not), or happiness the reward of virtue. When, on the other hand, she felt peaceful and her mind was more or less at rest, the picture became that of Christ calming the waters. He stood with His Hands outstretched. Sometimes there were words there like 'Let not your heart be troubled', 'Yea, though I walk through the valley of the shadow', etc.

"5. It was noted that after a therapeutic talk, when she felt 'hopeful and sometimes exalted, there would be in C 2 coming and going, pictures of meadows with lambs frisking about, children dancing around the maypole, flowers and music, beautiful landscapes with the sun bright and shining; everything gay and light. When', the testimony ran, 'there is music in C 2 or sound, it is a perception, not a visual picture'.

"The subject volunteered the suggestion that it seemed to her 'that in this C 2 part of her mind could be found the explanation of many seemingly strange things. Certain perceptions may be registered in C 2 of which the personality is unconscious, and those perceptions may work themselves out in various ways. This may account, sometimes, for the moods of depression or gaiety for which we know no reason.'"

Janet has occasionally quoted phenomena of the same nature as these last; that is, the explanation of a mood in which the emotion present in consciousness seems to be determining the ideas that find entrance there but where hypnotic investigation shows the activity of unconscious ideas that are the more probable determinants of the mood. One of these examples is quoted in the discussion of depression. (See p. 351).

In the cases so far cited the emotion present in consciousness has been the natural one, when the co-conscious image has been detected. This is because the co-conscious image has been of a simple kind (representing physical exertion, play, etc.), or, if of a complicated nature (as with a religious presentation), is at least one for which the emotional reaction is predictable. No matter how intricate the organization of instincts may be in such a complex as constitutes religion, it tends to function as a unit. But some stimuli, some ideas, may easily be associated with instincts calling up unexpected emotional reactions. In the following examples the co-conscious images seem to suggest sexual implications, although the conscious thoughts did not, which makes the conscious feeling of embarrassment or shame quite understandable. These examples are taken from Prince's article on " Co-conscious Images " and on observations made in the same case as above. The first has to do with an emotional disturbance interfering with complete obedience to suggestions for post hypnotic behaviour.

" . . . The suggestion was given to the subject in hypnosis that after waking, on the entrance of Dr. Waterman into the room, she was to go to the book-case, take down a book, take it to the table and place it by the telephone instrument. She was then to take a cigarette from the box and put it in her mouth. The latter suggestion she refused to accept saying that she ' would not do it ', that ' I could not make her do it ', etc. Nevertheless I insisted.

" This suggestion after waking, was accurately carried out up to the point of putting the cigarette in her mouth. Instead of doing this she laughed [a cover for embarrassment as later appeared] and, after some hesitation, offered a cigarette to me and then to Dr. Waterman.

" The subject was then put into three different hypnotic states and the following memories elicited of what occurred subconsciously during the suggested post-hypnotic action. I will give substantially the exact words used in one of these states. In this state, not in the others, the subject speaks of herself in the third person as ' C.'

" ' You know after you woke her up and you went into the other room to summon Dr. Waterman, there began to be pictures in the subconscious portion of her mind. There was a picture of the book case, then one of Dr. P.—very bright, much brighter than that of the book case—and then there was a picture of a woman walking across the room, taking a book out of the book case and then coming back and putting it down by the telephone. (The picture was not of the subject.) She was in black, tall, had gray hair. A picture of you alternated with all the pictures. . . . These pictures first came after awaking, before getting up from the sofa (perhaps a minute). C did not see them but she thought of a book case alone and nothing more. Afterwards she got up and as she proceeded to carry out the act the pictures kept coming and going, subconsciously. When she took down the book, a picture of the woman taking down a book came into C's mind and each picture alternated with a picture of you. After she laid the book down she turned to the table where the cigarettes were when there came a very bright picture of a ballet or chorus girl. The girl had short red skirts of tulle and she was sitting at a table with her feet crossed. A three-cornered hat was on her head and she was *smoking a cigarette!* She looked very gay. This was when C picked up the box of cigarettes, and as she did so there came the thought that she would put a cigarette in her mouth, and then she felt shocked at the idea. It was with the picture of the ballet girl that the *thought*[1] came to put a cigarette in her mouth and

---

[1] Italics in original.

then she felt shocked at the idea of doing such a thing. No pictures came into her conscious mind, only two thoughts, one of the book case, the other of putting a cigarette in her mouth. The pictures were subconscious (C2).'

"The picture of the ballet girl had an interesting history. It transpired that the picture was a replica of a real picture which she had seen elsewhere and which previously had brought to her mind, much to her disapproval, the kind of people who smoke cigarettes. This general aversion, without any specific memory of the picture, was why she had been consciously unwilling to accept the suggestion to smoke them. But smoking cigarettes had been actually associated in her mind with the ballet girl type of person, and apparently this strongly associated idea, symbolized in the form of a previously experienced picture, arose subconsciously at the moment when the suggested act was to be performed. When she felt shocked that she should have the idea of smoking a cigarette this subconscious fiction of a ballet girl appeared."

The suggestion of putting a cigarette into her mouth (she was not even told to smoke it) seems to have produced co-conscious images with a double implication. The first, like the picture of the woman with the book, was a signal for performance of the action required. The second implication was in the elaboration of the picture to include details which she could *not* carry out without running counter to deep-seated prejudices of a moral kind. It is surely not straining interpretation to suggest that the behaviour of a ballet girl may be more than merely undignified, or, at least, is supposed by people like this patient to include sexual laxity. Grant this and the reaction is comprehensible. No emotion is reported in connection with getting the book. But there *all* details of the image could be copied in overt behaviour. The second command touched an idea that was associated with sentiments involving sexual (and perhaps other) instincts. These latter led to an elaboration of the co-conscious images, intruding details not included in Dr. Prince's suggestions at all. It was these accessory elements that aroused conflict and produced the affect.

In the next example the sexual element appears much more plainly. The story, memory of which was excited co-consciously, is about sexual transgression.

"At one time she had the habit of putting her hand unconsciously to her left breast, particularly if a stranger was present or if a number of people were in the room. I had noticed her doing this several times. On investigation it transpired that when she made this gesture there developed, co-consciously, pictures of her initials embroidered in red, quite large, fanciful, corresponding to the description of the 'scarlet letter' in Hawthorne's novel of that name. It will be remembered that the letter as there described is an embroidered capital letter.

"The history of the development of this phenomenon is as follows:

"I had made use of the subject, incognito, on one occasion, to demonstrate hypnotic phenomena before the medical students at the school. Later, on reading an article of mine on the " Unconscious ", she came across a reference to her own case. She did not recognize at the time that this, in connection with the school demonstration, would discover her identity, but nevertheless, at the moment, there occurred the co-conscious thought of which she was not aware : ' Now she is branded '. *And right after that, within a few moments, the co-conscious picture of her initials came*[1]. It should be explained that for a long time she had been dominated by the idea that if it should be known that she exhibited subconscious phenomena a social stigma would be fastened upon her and would affect her socially. This formed a sort of complex which troubled her.

"Now it so happened that a day or two *still later* she attended a lecture of mine at the hospital and she noticed that some women students looked at her and whispered among themselves. At the time she thought it was because she had been exhibited at the medical school and was slightly annoyed. When she got home, for some reason or other, it flashed into her mind (emergence of the previous co-conscious knowledge ?) that I had described in the published article the vision which she had produced for me at the school. The thought at once came to her, ' Now they will know me'. She felt ' terrible ', ' torn ', etc., and wrote me a letter in which she said, ' I feel as if I bore three scarlet letters on my breast ' (emergence from the co-conscious). And when she wrote these words a co-conscious picture of Arthur Dimmesdale developed, and it was after this that she made the gesture of putting her hand to her breast.

"For a time the initials and the picture of Arthur Dimmesdale constantly kept coming and going accompanied by the gesture. To take a specific instance : when I first noticed the gesture I had just asked her about her repressed thoughts, and then the gesture occurred. This question had brought to her mind the thought of her illness, and then, according to the hypnotic personality, the co-conscious initials came. It was as though the subconscious ' stigma ' complex was awakened by thoughts of illness, etc. ' After the letters came a picture of Arthur Dimmesdale, and then she put her hand to her breast. The picture of Arthur Dimmesdale resembled that of the description in the book, tall, slender, clerical dress, pale, *with his hands on his breast.*[1]'

"When examining this statement it will be noted that the co-conscious initials first followed immediately after a co-conscious thought—' Now she is branded '—without conscious awareness thereof. Second, that it was not until a day or two after that the co-conscious knowledge flashed into her mind that her identity would be known and she felt that she bore three scarlet letters on

[1] Italics in original.

her breast (branded) *coincidentally with the co-conscious picture of Arthur Dimmesdale*[1] (and the initials ?). Third : The behaviour of the whole was *as if*[1] an associated subconscious ' stigma ' complex was awakened in which the initials and the picture of Arthur Dimmesdale were incorporated as elements. Fourth : It is also worth noting that this subconscious complex, apparently, induced the somatic phenomena, the gesture, which was performed automatically (involuntarily) and almost, if not wholly, unconsciously."

In this example Prince has exposed the mechanisms of a painful emotion with great clarity. But the point in which we are for the moment interested—the question of the instinctive processes involved—he does not discuss. It is, of course, quite possible that one, in whom thoughts of purely social approval or disapprobation were potent influences, might react violently to the thought of having mental peculiarities emerge from concealment. Rightly or wrongly society does discriminate against the mentally diseased—once this abnormality is labelled as such. But if this were the only factor, we should expect to find co-conscious images of her being scorned, pictures of people pointing fingers at her, avoiding her and so on. Instead of this a special kind of social error is indicated, one for which no logical, conscious justification could be found. In the co-conscious she is not being treated as insane but branded with the sign of a sex delinquent. Somehow or other the idea of exposure of what had been secret was associated with loss of modesty. The latter is a sexual affair, that is, it evokes a powerful instinct which produces co-conscious images and automatic behaviour. The affect it produces is not inappropriate to the consciously conceived situation (social stigma is the essence of either situation), hence the patient feels that her exposure in the clinic is a terrible thing. The really terrible thing is the Scarlet Letter.

The mechanism is the same as that of a phobia : an affect engendered elsewhere is attached to a conscious percept or concept. When the affect is inappropriate to the latter, the emotion is felt to be a symptom ; when appropriate, the conscious content is given a special meaning by the emotion and the whole reaction is regarded as normal. Psychoanalytic investigations are persistently indicating that strong emotional bias is apt to depend on unconscious associations. It is only when the affect is grossly inappropriate that we interpret it as anything but the natural and proper expression of the " meaning " of the conscious content.

From data such as these we may conclude, tentatively, that the nature of an affect is determined in part at least by the nature of unconscious associations. May we go further than this and suggest that the strength or vividness of the affect may be correlated with the extent to which the processes involved are *un*conscious rather than conscious. Theoretically we might expect this to be true.

---

[1] Italics in original.

If an instinctive reaction be immediately and completely carried out, the mental processes involved should all be of a conscious order. That is to say, they should be all available for introspection, whether the subject's attention be directed to them or not. We would expect associations to reverberate off into the unconscious only when the reaction is inadequate. In fact, if there be unconscious associations, that is equivalent to saying that the reaction as a rule is incomplete : the unconscious expresses itself only in two ways, by affecting consciousness indirectly (the kind of reactions we are studying), or in automatic movements.

An automatic movement, in turn (if we are to give that term its proper meaning), must have its mental initiation, its " purpose ", hidden from awareness. If the subject's attention be turned to the movement, he will regard it as something produced by an unknown influence, as something uncanny. Some kind of an affect will then be present. On the other hand, if no attention whatever be paid to the movement, there may be no affect. This is probably the only case in which an instinctive process can succeed in arousing unconscious associations that have no effect on consciousness whatever. (We must bear in mind that, normally, some affect is present constantly during waking hours, even though it may be quite mild. This is proved by the subjective state when apathy develops.) But the unrecognized voluntary movement may impress an outsider as an emotional expression. In fact this is the form that involuntary movements usually take ; when not of this order it is a frankly hysterical phenomenon, whether it occurs in an otherwise normal person or in a patient. We may conclude, therefore, that, if instinctive processes are not directly and adequately expressed in action, some affect will appear.

The corollary of this would be that the impression the affect makes on consciousness would be proportionate to the degree in which the unconscious associations are mediating the energy of the organism. If, for instance, a dominating instinct, like that of self-preservation or of sex, be aroused but gain no overt expression, and few of the instinctively inspired ideas penetrate consciousness, then the subject would feel overwhelmed by an affect. The whole of the theory of " catharsis " in psychoanalytic treatment rests on this principle, and the theory receives support from common as well as technical experience. When a subject succeeds in getting a disturbing thought fully into consciousness the emotional reaction it subsequently produces is greatly reduced. The process of getting it into awareness will be a painful one. In fact, it must be so because it involves the stimulation of the unconscious idea to such a degree of activity as will force its entrance into consciousness. Until it succeeds in reaching the light of day the conditions we have assumed to be necessary for the development of emotion are ideally present. This is the reason for the psychoanalyst's opinion that it does a patient little good to recount the thoughts it is easy for him to express. A psychoanalysis which costs the patient no effort is not an analysis at all ; it is merely a field day for symptoms.

Such a theory as this is not an integral part of Prince's system. He has not, therefore, been at any pains to record experiences in support of such a view, yet a number of examples bearing directly on our contention can be found. Some of these are worthy of citation. The first occurs in his description of the famous " Church bell phobia ". He tells how the patient was thrown into a violent and painful emotional state whenever she saw a church steeple or tower, or often when one was spoken of. It soon appeared that the anguish was really associated with the ringing of church bells and an effort was made by the free association method to recover the memories on which the reaction was founded. This was unsuccessful. Then Prince tried another method[1] :

" . . . While she was in hypnosis I put a pencil in her hand with the object of obtaining the desired information through automatic writing. *While she was narrating some irrelevant memories of her mother*[2], the hand wrote rapidly as follows : ' G . . . M . . . church and my father took my mother to Bi . . . where she died and we went to Br . . . and they cut my mother. I prayed and cried all the time that she would live and the church bells were always ringing and I hated them.'

" When she began to write the latter part of this script she became depressed, sad, indeed anguished ; tears flowed down her cheeks and she seemed to be almost heart-broken. In other words it appeared as if she were subconsciously living over again the period described in the script. I say subconsciously for she did not know what the hand had written or why she was anguished. During the writing of the first part of the script, she was verbally describing other memories ; during the latter part she ceased speaking.

" After awakening from hypnosis and when she had become composed in her mind, she narrated, at my request, the events referred to in the script. She remembered them clearly as they happened when she was about fifteen years of age. It appeared that she was staying at that time in G . . . M . . ., a town in England. Her mother, who was seriously ill, was taken to a great surgeon to be operated upon. She herself suffered great anxiety and anguish lest her mother should not recover. She went twice a day to the church to pray for her mother's recovery and in her anguish declared that if her mother did not recover she would no longer believe in God. The chimes of the tower of the church, which was close to her hotel, sounded every quarter hour ; they got on her nerves ; she hated them ; she could not bear to hear them, and while she was praying they added to her anguish. Ever since this time the ringing of bells has continued to cause a feeling of anguish. *This*

---

[1] *The Unconscious*, pp. 391-2.
[2] Italics in original.

narrative was not accompanied by emotion as was the automatic script[1]*."*

There are several points of importance in this example. The first is that no emotion accompanies the recital of a memory which is in full consciousness, whereas the activation of the same memory in the co-conscious (as evidenced from the automatic script) was the apparent occasion of a violent reaction.

The second point is of considerable interest either to the psy-- chologist or the psychopathologist. No strong repression was in operation keeping the memory from awareness, else it would not have appeared so easily, and in such detail, and with no comment from the patient that this recollection was a sudden acquisition. She felt that she had not forgotten the incidents at all. Whatever repression there may have been must have been directed against associated thoughts of which she did not speak. If no repression were overcome, no fundamental change in her mental processes was accomplished, and no cure could be expected. And, indeed, this was so. We learn in reading further that the phobia continued for eighteen months and disappeared only with a thorough discussion of other thoughts the patient had at the time of her mother's death, a discussion which changed the meaning of the incident for the patient. It was of these other thoughts that she hated to think ; it was these other thoughts that kept the associated memory from appearing as such when church steeples were seen ; and it was these other thoughts, we assume, which mediated the energy appearing in the emotion, for it was these that were connected with powerful instinctive processes ramifying off into the unconscious.

The third point to note is one that will have some importance when we come to study the nature of unconscious associational processes. This patient was not an hysteric with highly organized dissociated systems comparable to those of a multiple personality. The automatic writing was therefore reproducing ordinary co-con- scious thoughts as they came, not the thinking of a separate con- sciousness with its orderly arrangement. Hence the elements do not appear in logical order (*e.g.*, the mother dies before she is operated on) and the vocabulary and sentence structure is childish. There are *free associations*, as they have been called by psychoanalysts.

Incidentally the principle we are now discussing is exemplified in experiments on the psycho-galvanic reaction. What the phy- siological nature of the electrical changes produced with emotion is, nobody knows, but they must represent some kind of discharges which the subject does not cognize directly. The extent of the swing in the galvanometer may, in some instances at least, be correlated with the *un*consciousness of the stimulated thought. This was shown by Prince and Peterson[2]. Their subject was BCA;

---

[1] My italics.
[2] " Experiments in Psycho-Galvanic Reactions from Co-Conscious Ideas in a Case of Multiple Personality ", *Journal of Abnormal Psychology*, vol. III, 2, p. 122.

C was the " normal " personality who was aware of herself in both A and B. A had no knowledge of C or B. But B was co-conscious with both A and C and therefore remembered their experiences ; she also knew the co-conscious thoughts of C of which C was not aware. Each personality was susceptible to hypnosis, the resulting states being known as a, b and c. The experiments I am going to quote were performed in the hypnotic states.

" To test the relative reactions of the different hypnotic states a, b and c, to the subconscious and conscious memories, the test words ' Smith ' and ' ring ' were used. . . . of the test words, ' Smith ' referred to an experience in B's life of which the corresponding hypnotic state b only (of the hypnotic states) had a memory. Of this experience B *now felt ashamed.* It appeared that B, pretending to be A, had disclosed to a Mr. Smith the secret of her psychological disintegration into personalities. A and C[1] knew nothing of this and therefore a and c had also complete amnesia for it.

" The word ring referred to a past experience in the life of B when there was a disintegration of character without amnesia, so that both A and C knew of it. It therefore was part of a common *conscious* memory in all three personalities, A. B and C. B had enjoyed the experience ; A, owing to the peculiarity of her character had suffered intense remorse and anguish to a morbid degree. She had, emotionally, almost torn herself to pieces over it, wearing sack-cloth and ashes, and the memory of the experience awakened similar feelings. C, however, now remembering the experience, is sorry but philosophical. While regretting it, she in no way suffers.

" Examining the tracings, . . . we find rises corresponding to both these words . . . With ' Smith ' the greatest disturbance occurred with the hypnotic state c, who had no knowledge whatsoever of the experience connected with the name. The reaction must have been, therefore, due to a *subconscious* memory (belonging to B). [The reaction was as violent as any shown in all the series of experiments. It is important to note that ' Smith ' was not merely an unconscious idea for C ; it must have been actively repressed because amnesia for it was a specific symptom in a personality with few, and only localized, amnesias. The strength of the reaction is here correlated, apparently, with the strength of the repression.]

" With a, with whom the memory was also subconscious, there was a rise, but much less marked, and approximately the same as that obtained with b, with whom the memory was *conscious*. c, it should be said, was first tested and, therefore, the surprise element may have been a factor in the height of the curve obtained in this

---

[1] " This was one of the few hiatuses in C's memory and has since been filled."

state ; and yet this explanation will not hold good with the word ' ring ' which gave curves with each of the hypnotic states, *corresponding to the intensity of the feeling which each experienced* in remembering the episode[1]. . . . "

Another example of the *un*consciousness of an emotional stimulus being correlated with the strength of the affect has been mentioned earlier. In his " Miss Beauchamp " article, Prince discusses the reaction of B IV—the non-religious personality—to religious situations. She was moved by them and of this Prince remarks : " Of the two probably the feelings of B IV were the more intense." That is, B I, who revelled in religious exercises, was not so stirred by them as was B IV, who fought against all such activities and interests as " sentimental ". When, therefore, B I as a submerged personality reacted to a religious service, the affect that penetrated to B IV's consciousness was all the stronger for the conflict which the latter's " reaction " engendered.

Prince generalises about these symptoms of Miss Beauchamp as follows[2] : " An emotion, apparently paradoxical, would be aroused in B IV in connection with a strange person or place, or in consequence of a reference by someone to an unknown event. B IV, without apparent reason, would feel an *intense*[3] emotion in connection with something or other which she did not remember to have ever heard or seen before. A face, a name, a particular locality where she happened to find herself would arouse a *strong*[3] emotional effect without her knowing the reason. The memories of the experiences to which these emotions belonged were a part of B I's life and could easily be recalled by her when the personalities again alternated and B I came into existence. When B IV came again these experiences, of course, would be forgotten, and become dormant, but the emotions associated with the visual, auditory, and other images of a given person or place, or whatever it might be, would be liable to be aroused in her by the perception, in spite of the amnesia, whenever the given person or place, as it might be, came into her daily life."

Reading these sentences led me to ask Dr. Prince two questions. He very kindly answered them and even took the trouble to discuss

---

[1] I cannot refrain from pointing out one highly suggestive feature of these psycho-galvanic experiments. A, B and C shared a common body, and, at bottom, a common mental machine. The difference between them were in psychic systems essentially conscious. Marked emotional reactions were produced by activation of unconscious memories (fundamentally common property) when these memories were subjected to repression. Now this repression was a function of a special, largely conscious integration, the personality. From this it might be deduced that factors belonging to a conscious (or mainly conscious) system may contribute to an emotion, even though the subject be unaware of the disturbing idea. Unfortunately, Peterson and Prince did not perform the crucial experiments which might have demonstrated this conclusively.

[2] *The Unconscious*, pp. 387-8.

[3] My italics.

his theory of the point involved. The first question was : " When B I reported the affective experiences did she show the same degree of *emotion* as did B IV when confronted with reminders of these experiences ? " To this he replied. " No ". The second was a general question : " Is the emotional reaction inversely proportional to the conscious grasp of the idea or memory arousing the emotion " ? Prince's reply was, " Substantially, Yes ". He then went on :

" The fundamental principle involved I conceive to be as follows : Emotion emerging into B IV's consciousness came from dissociated memories, or dispositions, or ' complexes ' (used in my sense). Now any *dissociated* system when *functioning* outside of awareness is necessarily more autonomous, independent, uninhibited and uncontrolled than a system within the field of awareness. Its emotion is therefore more intense. There is no conflicting or controlling point of view to modify it. We do, however, as I have seen again and again, get the same intensity when we reduce the total consciousness to this ' complex ', a mere extract of personality. This is reducing the total consciousness to what was before subconscious. The subconscious complex becomes now not only *the* ' conscious ' but, substantially, the whole of it. It is now therefore just as much free, independent, and uncontrolled as it was before when subconscious (*co*-conscious). Hence the same intensity. This reduction can be done by hypnosis or suggestion, and often occurs ' spontaneously ' as result of autosuggestion and associated ideas, etc. Of course, the word ' proportional ' can only be used in a figurative sense, as we have no measurements for such things."

Before agreeing or disagreeing with these generalizations one has to be certain of just what elements of emotion are referred to. If Prince is speaking of what may be observed by an outsider, I would certainly agree with him. As we shall see the essence of many manic depressive psychoses (*e.g.*, hypomanic and florid manic states) seems to be just this restriction of consciousness to certain ideas and the emotional display observed in them can be nicely explained by this formula. But I would not agree that this mechanism heightened affect. I suspect that it is more likely to reduce its intensity.

CHAPTER XI

A TENTATIVE THEORY OF EMOTION

FOLLOWING the suggestions derivable from Prince's observations, we are now in a position to formulate with greater exactness a tentative theory of affect. Dewey's theories leave one a little cold because his " conflict " is described so much in intellectualistic terms that one feels such conflict to be dispassionate in its nature, of a different order from the kind of thing one would expect to find as the central factor in a dynamic situation. Furthermore his views demand the operation of unconscious thinking without his giving any demonstration of it. Now, however, we are in a position to fill in these gaps, although several of our terms involve assumptions the validity of which is still to be proved. Our new formulation, then, would be :

A given stimulus, if it be productive of emotion, does not merely arouse conscious perceptions and overt behaviour but activates unconscious mental processes as well. These are associated instinctive tendencies incorporated with what can be spoken of for the time being as ideas. These instinctively impelled ideas or " complexes " tend to come into consciousness but are blocked by an inhibition, not engendered for the first time in this situation, but pre-existent. In fact, it is the same inhibition as that which has made and kept these complexes unconscious. Being activated the complexes are now co-conscious, that is, they constitute mental reactions in many respects like those of consciousness in nature but different in content. There are thus two different systems of thinking going on, a conscious system with one content and a co-conscious with another content. Repression prevents the co-conscious series from emerging as such but the latter does reach expression in two ways, as emotional expression and as affect, *i.e.*, objectively and subjectively. The subject then regards the affect as a product of his conscious mental state ; in his ignorance of the co-conscious mental activities, he regards his conscious percepts, concepts and judgments as producing the peculiar feeling with which they are accompanied.

The quality of the affect is determined by the sum total of unconscious complexes that are activated, and may therefore have an infinite variety. The strength of the affect depends on the dominance over other instincts, in the unconscious at the moment, of the instinctive tendencies aroused. For instance, if self preservative tendencies, which always tend to monopolize the energies of the organism, are activated but are prevented of adequate expression, a feeling of fear is experienced so poignant as to be called " paralysing ". As a matter of fact the paralysis is a result of the inhibition which is preventing movement on the one hand and the entrance of co-conscious ideas into consciousness on the other. Similarly, a situation may tend to evoke sexual complexes that do not reach consciousness ; the sexual is bound up with so much experience that its associations with other instinctive processes are extensive. The conscious perception is then echoed by innumerable unconscious reactions, which, according to the nature of the dominating co-conscious image or thought, will colour the perception with an affect of love, hate, ecstacy or shyness, etc., and this affect will be as powerful as the unconscious ramifications are extensive.

This formula, although designed to account for the more dramatic emotions, would cover the more trivial affective states that we experience continuously. One has only to assume in these a narrow range of unconscious elaboration. The theory as stated, however, is probably inaccurate as regards one type of situation in which poignant feelings may arise. If a man be trapped in some perilous position whence he cannot escape, the impulse to escape may be inhibited by a purely intellectual judgment of the complete futility of any effort to avoid his fate. In such a case one would be justified in assuming that the escape reactions go on reverberating in the unconscious, but one does not need to assume that their inhibition is a product of long-established repression. As a matter of fact, in normal civilized life, such experiences are probably rare ; they are even uncommon in warfare, it would seem, for a little examination of the mental reactions of the soldier shows that a good deal of repression is used in establishing the military adaptations and that this repression contributes largely to the development of fear, if the soldier fall a victim to it. It should be admitted as well, of course, that our formula does not cover " emotions " in animals or human infants. Emotional expressions must be viewed as secondary manifestations of instincts which appear when the primary behaviour of the instinct is inhibited from any cause. According to our present theory affect will appear in such cases if the subject have self-conscious awareness, but if this awareness be absent the emotion will be limited to objectively observable expressions.

If this view be sound three stages in the development of instincts into emotion should be expected. If the organism responds to a stimulus immediately and adequately with instinctive behaviour no emotion whatever is engendered. If the instinctive reaction be held up, emotional expression and, if the subject be self-conscious, some affect as well, will appear. The latter represents the activity which is not expressed overtly in any way. Therefore, if the inner tendency to activity be regarded as a constant, the urgency of the affect will be reduced not merely by instinctive behaviour but also by emotional expression. The third stage is, then, one in which affect alone appears, which is as poignant as the emotion is purely subjective.

This hypothesis has been built up by argument from the data, mainly introspective, that have provided psychologists with material for their speculations and also from the data reported by psychopathologists, particularly Morton Prince. Before the hypothesis can be established it should be buttressed with a greater weight of evidence. The bulk of this book will be devoted to a description of phenomena observed in manic depressive insanity, from which, it is hoped, some of the principles of our hypothesis may be derived with a reasonable degree of confidence. There are three general headings under which the data may be subsumed.

Some writers on emotion, both among psychologists and psychopathologists, have assumed that emotions can have some kind of independent existence, dissociated from other mental processes and have considered that abnormal emotions have this nature. Our first enquiry must be directed towards the confirmation or refutation of this claim. Morton Prince has, with the comparatively exact technique of hypnosis, demonstrated the existence of images or thoughts below the threshold of consciousness that seem to be correlated with subjective states of feeling otherwise inexplicable. Now it is characteristic of psychotic conditions that unconscious ideas and types of thinking tend to come more directly into consciousness than they do in normal life. So we might reasonably expect in the psychoses, where emotional symptoms are most prominent, to find something akin to Prince's discoveries, that is, a correlation of the unusual emotion with ideas not referable directly to the environment nor to normal consciousness. This expectation, will, I hope, be justified.

The second subject of enquiry will be relationship of repression or inhibition to emotion. Since a psychosis is apt to be an exhibition of unconscious mentation, acting more or less autonomously, changes in inhibition must be present on any theory which assumes that repression is concerned in the establishment or maintenance of the unconscious. Our material should, therefore, teach us something about the co-incidence of repression and emotion.

The third division of our study will be the nature of the unconscious mental processes that lead to one emotion or another being produced. Is there rhyme or reason in the unconscious ? Is it pure chance which determines what of the myriad possible instinct complexes will be activated to a co-conscious level and thus determine a given affect ?

With any considerable amount of such data most of the principles involved in our hypothesis might be established. But at one point —it may as well be admitted in advance—our evidence is bound to be lacking. The last claim made above is that affect will seem strongest to the subject when not only instinctive behaviour but emotional expression as well is at a minimum. No truly objective data as to affect can ever be secured because the phenomena are inevitably patent only to introspection. The psychotic patient is no better than the normal man as an introspectionist, in fact, he is worse. Of course one can go a certain distance on inference from objective observation coupled with introspective account. For instance, if a patient report that he is or has been suffering acutely, intolerably, yet give little evidence of any kind of externalized activity, one has a right to conclude that the affect was strong, particularly when there seems no reason to doubt that the affect in question has so thoroughly absorbed the attention of consciousness that nothing, or little, else would intrude upon it.

The best material we have from which to study the quality of affects is the writing of literary artists whose material is essentially introspective. (I shall return later to this theme, but at the moment should remark that all affects not belonging to the cruder emotions are invariably described in metaphors or similes ; and for this an excellent reason can be found.) Now in reading accounts of actual or imaginary subjective emotional experience I have been struck by the phenomenon that, when the feeling is described as most intense, the externalized activity is reduced or absent. The subject feels as if in contact with or in sympathy with the whole universe, but *does* nothing. For instance, the ecstasy of a mystic is accompanied by immobility, so complete, perhaps, as to constitute a trance. Or a lover in a passive embrace may feel that he holds the world in thrall. For instance, take these lines of Browning :

> " Hush, if you saw some western cloud
> All billowy-bosomed, over-bowed
> By many benedictions—sun's
> And moon's and evening-star's at once—
> And so, you, looking and loving best,
> Conscious grew, your passion drew
> Cloud, sunset, moon-rise, star-shine too,
> Down on you, near and yet more near,
> Till flesh must fade for heaven was here !—
> Thus leant she and lingered—joy and fear !
> Thus lay she a moment on my breast."

Goethe describes something quite similar in his famous " Gefühl ist Alles ", lines in which he makes of this feeling the essence and proof of religion. Faust has been reproached by Margaret with lack of belief in God ; to this he replies that man cannot know God by reason but that his feeling convinces him of the existence of an All-Embracing and All-Sustaining spirit. Turning to Margaret he assures her that their love *is* this Divinity : " Do my eyes not gaze into yours and does not all that throbs into your heart and head weave beside you the eternal secret, invisible, visible ? Fill your heart with this, so great it is, and, when you are quite beatified with this feeling, then give whatever name you wish to it, call it Happiness, Heart, Love or God! I have no labels for it! Feeling is everything; the name is sound and smoke, obscuring Heaven's glow." In this situation all that an observer could have seen would be a man and woman looking at each other; he might have inferred a feeling of joyous affection but could he have guessed that the participants felt themselves possessed of the secret of the universe, sharing the glory of God?

Some epileptics are prone to have as warning of their attacks a brief experience of this kind in which they stand, as a rule, motionless. It is, perhaps, these experiences which have led some of them to found new religions or sects, like Mohamed or Joseph Smith. Dostoievsky[1] knew these inspired moments and has described them, both to his biographers, and in the course of his novels, most of which contain an epileptic. Perhaps the best of these descriptions comes in *The Devil*, concerning the character Kiriloff : " . . . His contemplations are religious-mystic, which are rooted in his illusions and hallucinations. He has no convulsions but psychic equivalents. He says of these, ' For seconds, not over five or six in all, in which there is a sudden feeling of infinite harmony which fills the whole of existence.' This feeling is not earthly nor is it necessarily heavenly. But an earthly being cannot tolerate it, and must be physically transformed or perish. It is as one suddenly felt within him the whole of Nature and said, ' Yes, that is Truth '. So the Creator might have spoken as he finished the world. Here is no commotion, only simple joy. The feeling is not only that but something higher. Terrible it is that these feelings are so clear, this joy so powerful. If this mood should last over five seconds the soul could not endure it and must perish. During these seconds one lives through an entire life. Of what need is posterity, when the entire goal of life has been attained ? "

After all, many of us know that we have experienced keener feeling in dreams than in any adventures of waking life—in sleep during which we lie motionless, betraying absolutely nothing of our thoughts, as a rule, to an onlooker. One thinks at once of nightmares. A characteristic of these is that the subject not merely is relatively or absolutely motionless in bed, but that a most painful element in the dreamed situation is his paralysis. Very often one feels that, if movement were possible, the torture would not be so extreme. Those unfortunates who suffered from states of anxiety in the War, reported that the fear in their dreams was more terrible than that in the field. But dreams may give us pleasant affects as well. Some people occasionally experience true ecstasy while asleep that far exceeds that known in the work-a-day world. The rare flavour of such dreams is beautifully described in Du Maurier's *Peter Ibbetson*.

---

[1] L. Pierce Clark, " A Study of the Epilepsy of Dostojewsky ", *Boston Medical and Surgical Journal*, January 14th, 1915.

CHAPTER XII

THE OEDIPUS COMPLEX AND INFANTILE SEXUALITY

THE reader may, perhaps, be better oriented for the understanding of the clinical material which follows, if an introductory word be given as to our psychological method of approach in studying manic-depressive insanity. The old psychology took for its data the phenomena revealed by introspection, that is, what one could observe about one's own conscious thoughts. Such data were then elaborated into systems, which, to the modern *intransigeant* psychologist, seem rather futile exercises in logic. Objective study of the mind appeared with Wundt's application of the methods of the physiological laboratory ; but, since the mental phenomena available for examination by this technique are relatively simple, the gain from experimental psychology has been largely an exploration of the psycho-physiology of the special senses and muscular co-ordinations. It has also frunished us with some information about more elaborate mental processes but the value of such data has been more suggestive than extensive. Probably influenced indirectly by the researches of psychopathologists on unconscious mental activity, a new group of psychologists has arisen in recent years, the behaviourists. It is their doctrine that the " facts " of introspection are an illusion and that what the organism is about can best be learned by watching it, rather than by listening to what it says about itself. In spite of the affront which a practical denial of consciousness gives, one is bound to admit that psychology has been broadened by the writings of the behaviourists, narrow though their view may be. The marked discrepancy between the estimate a man places on his motives and ideals and the judgment his neighbour may give about them is a phenomenon that academic psychology had previous neglected. Moreover the method of behaviourism seems to be the only possible one to use in studying animals and human infants.

The psychopathologist, on the other hand, approaches his problems by all these routes, in particular, he combines the method of the introspectionist with that of the behaviourist. The two chief schools in psychopathology are those employing psychoanalysis and hypnotism. The advantages and disadvantages of these do not concern us now[1], and I need only mention the general principle that has

[1] If the reader be interested in a discussion of this topic he may read my *Problems in Dynamic Psychology*, Part II.

guided work at the Psychiatric Institute. In a word, it is the method of psychoanalysis adapted to psychotic material. The data of consciousness are not held to have any fore-ordained or incontestable validity, but they are viewed as part of the behaviour of the organism and so studied objectively. If the thoughts and actions of a person seem adequately accounted for by the mental processes which he describes, these conscious data are held valid. But if introspection cannot account, or account adequately, for the thoughts or actions of a patient, the assumption is made of unconscious processes having produced the anomalous phenomena. As large a collection of the latter as is possible is made and these are studied with a view to discovering some system in them, analogous to the system in conscious thinking which the introspectionist constructs. If a workable system can be constructed, the validity of the unconscious is held to be established. It must be admitted that the unconscious cannot be " proved " with any greater finality than this ; it is only an hypothesis. But cannot the same objection be made to any generalization in psychology ?

In collating the data, anomalous from the standpoint of consciousness, some system of classification, some pattern must be in mind. It is to the genius of Freud that we owe the discovery of a theme which will rationalize much, and frequently all, of the apparently lawless productions of the mind diseased. This theme is the *Oedipus complex*. To the psychoanalyst it is the ark of the covenant, to the neophyte it seems incredible, while the inexpert critics seize on it with joyous abhorrence as evidence of the folly or vice of Freud and his perverted followers. Where there is so much smoke there must be some fire and, since the Oedipus complex will constantly be invoked to explain the ideational content of the psychoses described in this book, some preliminary remarks should be made as to what I think to be smoke and what fire.

It is many years since I have been able to summon any enthusiasm for the polemics of this question, that is for discussion as to whether the thing exists or not, as to whether it is universal or not. "Evidence " has obtruded itself with such persistence that I cannot escape it. The nature of this evidence will be seen by the reader in the following pages, for the cases cited represent a fair average of institutional material. They have not been selected to " prove " the Oedipus complex. If that were the object of this work it could easily have been made much more impressive. The problem is, in my opinion, a discovery or formulation of what is to be deduced from the evidence. A thoroughly satisfactory answer to this question will be given only when psychological, psychopathological, criminological and anthropological research has gone much further than it has to-day, but a tentative formulation may be put forward now, one that does no violence to facts so far elicited. This and allied problems I have elsewhere[1] discussed at greater length than is now

[1] *Problems in Dynamic Psychology*, Chapter XX,

expedient in this book, so that the topic must be dealt with here in very few words.

The Oedipus complex is often defined as an unconscious wish for incestuous relations with the parent of the opposite sex, coupled with unconscious hostility toward the parent of the same sex. Conscious love and tenderness for the mother (or father) is held to be paralleled by, or based upon, an unconscious lust for sexual satisfaction in the literal sense of the term, while the antagonism for the parent of the same sex is presumed to take the form of a definitely murderous wish in the unconscious. Without an interpretation that modifies the meaning of several of these words, such a definition implies something so monstrous as to be silly. And, indeed, in actual practice, the psychoanalysts who accept such a definition with literalness belong to that class of unthinking people who cluster around any new banner and whose cries are apt to drown out the words of the real readers.

The first stumbling block in this definition is the phrase " unconscious wish ". A wish is a voluntary and, therefore, a conscious thing. It implies a wisher and so no wish can be unconscious except in the case of a patient who has a submerged personality, existing unconsciously with its own system of self-awareness. Since the Oedipus complex is unconscious it must be repressed and be repressed because of its incompatibility with the standards of the conscious personality. If it appeared in consciousness as such it would be regarded as a hideous, compulsive thought. not as a wish. Frank *incest* does appear now-a-days in three forms. As an act, it is performed more frequently than is often supposed in the uncultured levels of civilized people. So far as I know no competent psychiatric investigation has ever been undertaken of actually incestuous people to determine what their mental organization is or what their mental state at the moment when the crime is performed. As an idea, it appears rarely in dreams, which, as remembered, excite violent revulsion of feeling. Thirdly, in dementia praecox delusions of incest are not uncommon, but these occur only when the personality of the patient is grossly disintegrated.

If our evidence for the existence of the Oedipus complex rested merely on these data, its occurrence would be held to be an anomaly. There is, however, a large accumulation of evidence pointing towards the existence in the unconscious of a *tendency* in this direction. Now no-one is ever directly conscious of a tendency either in himself or others. A tendency is deduced from observation of behaviour or thought ; it is an hypothesis which correlates and explains phenomena of conduct. Whether, then, a tendency be held to have any existence or not is a problem for philosophers. If one believes that a tendency can exist then one can believe in the existence of the Oedipus complex—provided he be satisfied that this hypothesis is a suitable one to explain the large range of phenomena which it is held to correlate.

These phenomena are to be grouped under several headings. In the first place there is much in the behaviour of normal people that can be thus explained. Many features of the relationships between parents and children seem more understandable if the relationship be presumed to contain a sexual element. Again many peculiarities of sexual selection in adult life can be explained on the assumption of predeliction for certain types based on the attachments of the nursery period[1]. Allied with the latter are peculiarities of social adaptation, antagonism or undue subservience to authority, insensate devotion to unusual political and religious creeds and so on. Secondly the symptoms of many neurotics seem to be a direct or indirect expression of the Oedipus tendency. Thirdly in dream analysis a simple and understandable latent content can often only be arrived at by reduction of the dream thoughts to an Oedipus situation. Lastly in the delusions and hallucinations of the insane a relevance and coherence can often be given to their apparently incoherent utterances by assuming that they are producing variations of this same fundamental theme. Of such wide application is this principle that I cannot conceive of anyone, who has once found it of use, who has ever understood it, abandoning it.

On the other hand one may very well doubt whether it ever existed in many cases as a conscious idea, perpetuated in the mind as an unconscious memory. Children who have never known their parents have it. Adults whose childhood was cursed by parental neglect and cruelty, in whom filial affection seems unthinkable, will also give evidence of these unconscious tendencies. Finally the unconscious ideal, as derived from observation of adult sexual selection may be radically different from any actual parent. The ideal may seem to be derived from association with a sister, aunt or nurse; it may even seem to be a product of childish fantasy. For these reasons it seems best to consider the object of unconscious interest to be an *Imago*, *i.e.*, an idealized imagined parent, rather than the real one. Again, if one is to assume that memory is responsible for the unconscious Oedipus ambition, the period of formation of this complex must be that of very early childhood, at the time when inhibitions are not yet developed or still very weak. But at this stage sexual impulses are of a primitive order, genital cravings being still rudimentary. Without physiological capacity for coitus, full consciousness of genital satisfaction cannot exist. The ambition of this period could then be only for perverse forms of sexual gratification. (This is indeed the form in which the Oedipus tendency is most often expressed in dementia praecox).

[°] Recent psychoanalytic literature is so full of discussions of these points that reference to it would be superfluous. I may mention three classical papers, however. Freud, " Beiträge zur Psychologie des Liebeslebens ", *Jahrb. f. Psychoanal. v. Psychopath. Forschungen*, Bd. II, s. 389, and Bd. IV, s. 40 ; Jung, " Die Bedeutung des Vaters für das Schicksal des Einzelnen ", *Jahrb. f. Psychoanal. v. Psychopath. Forschungen*, Bd. I, s. 155.

Only with true sexual sophistication could a desire for actual incest arise and so this could not appear until physiological puberty had been established. But, long before this, repression has taken place. So, on these grounds, we are forced to conclude that the Oedipus complex is not an unconscious memory but an unconscious fabrication.

If an unconscious fabrication, how can it be said to exist? No mental process is directly known until it is conscious. This one is known in incomplete form in early life and in indirect expression when the subject is grown. If it be known in literal detail in adult life, it may fairly be said to be a product of an abnormal personality. Normally, then, one might say it was known only by its effects. That which is recognized by its effects alone is a tendency. So we may safely conclude that the Oedipus complex, viewed as a definite formulation such as the word " wish " implies, has no existence, but that viewed as a tendency the concept may have great usefulness.

A materialistically-minded reader may be shocked by the suggestion that anything can be held to exist, which is recognized simply as an hypothesis to explain certain phenomena. But an analogy may make this clearer. The embryologist says that a gill stage exists in the development of the human body. What is observed is that, at a certain stage, ridges appear in what is going to be the neck of the foetus, ridges that look like those from which gills of fish develop. In and about these ridges various organs appear that owe their subsequent relations (particularly nerve supply) to their formation in this situation. But these " gill arches " have no functioning respiratory circulation ; they are therefore not gills. The nerve supply to muscles in the mouth, ear, chest and abdomen of the adult is not a supply to gills. To this the embryologist would reply that an overwhelming weight of evidence shows that the mammalian body has evolved from that of fish ancestors and that a *tendency* for the development of gills still remains. This is shown in the actual gill-like ridges that appear in the embryo, in the existence of the arch of the aorta, in the nerve relationships of adult organs and even in the situation in which certain tumours may develop in adult life. " Gill " is the only possible term he can use to correlate these and other phenomena, so he does not worry over the fact that the human body never has and never will have real gills. But ask him therefore to deny the pertinence of the term gill and he will doubt the sanity of his questioner. I venture to state that the evidence for the Oedipus complex as a tendency is more easily demonstrable than that for the existence of the gill tendency in the human body.

In the following pages the word " infantile " will often be used to characterize certain symptoms or tendencies ; so it may be well to discuss this term briefly. It means, of course, primitive or un-developed, but psychoanalytic usage has given it a somewhat more specific significance. I shall employ it to denote a definite type of interest, type of activity and type of thinking, or the tendency towards any one of these three. Elements of an unconscious order are spoken of as infantile because they are characteristic of the mental life of little children as opposed to that of adults. Sometimes the phenomena are of a kind universally recognized in the nursery, or they may be noted there only when observation is directed by a scheme of developmental reconstruction.

The infantile type of interest is the beginning of love, the first sign of attachment to other people, which later in life will take on a more altruistic colouring. The suckling is a pure egoist, a kind of parasite who depends for his maintenance and comfort on the maternal host (or nurse). Mere trial and error will lead him so to behave towards those who tend him most lovingly as to attract the maximum of attention. The primitive adaptations of affection are thus fostered in him. Demonstrations which later in life would be the unequivocal sign of love or sexual passion are thus developed. At some point truly objective interest appears, at first sporadic, later permanent, but in general the infantile attachment is essentially selfish. On this soil is grown the Oedipus complex, or, to put it in a more accurate metaphor, from this clay is modelled the *Imago* which becomes the unconscious object. It cannot be urged too often or too strongly, that the object is not the real parent but the Imago and the type of attachment is selfish rather than altruistic. Many parents are actively hated or feared by their children so far as conscious reactions of the latter are concerned, and the influence of the former is confined to stirring up unconscious tendencies in the offspring. On the other hand a parent may be really—that is, consciously and altruistically—loved by the child but, when a neurotic or psychotic reaction appears, the infantile potentialities of the relationship are crystalized and the patient becomes exigent and selfish.

The type of activity which we describe as infantile is the indulgence of practices essentially *autoerotic*. Applying the introspective criteria of later life, we say the infant derives pleasure from stimulation of the mouth and other areas of the body, particularly the breasts, genital and anal regions. Whether pleasure is actually enjoyed or not we cannot say but we do know that the indulgence of impulses gives us adults pleasure. Eating, drinking and copulation are banal examples of such impulses. We say we do these things because they please us. It might be more accurate to say that we are impelled, instinctively, to do them, and that the pleasure is a by-product. The pleasure or discomfort consequent on yielding to impulse certainly favour repetition or inhibition of the impulse. These impulses have obvious biological values and are classified according to their biological purpose, as different appetites.

Any organ or part of the body may be used in the indulgence of more than one appetite. The mouth may serve for eating or speaking, the male genital organ for excretion or copulation, whereas the utility of the hand is manifold. An activity which finally results in behaviour of a specific biological type is labelled in terms of the final act. Biting is part of a nutritional cycle, but it may also be an exhibition of pugnacity. If this principle of nomenclature is sound, we have a right to call any stimulation of the body, which may be an excitant to an unequivocally sexual act, an erotic procedure, provided such stimulation is not part of a cycle of behaviour belonging to some other instinct. It is reasoning of this order which led Freud (as well as some non-psychoanalytic writers) to label many impulsive habits of children as autoerotic. Thus finger-sucking, which not only does not lead to taking of food but may actually be a substitute for it, is, according to Freud, an autoerotic practice. He claims that originally many parts of the body are capable of giving " sexual pleasure ", and that it is only as puberty is approaching that such pleasure is concentrated in the genital region.

This diffuse body pleasure is " infantile ". Not only is it auto-erotic, but the same bodily areas may give satisfaction when stimulated by another person. Hence the Oedipus complex is apt to be expressed in terms of perverse, rather than normal, sexual contacts. It is not difficult to see how childish theories of reproduction may be focussed about parts of the body yielding an unusual amount of " pleasure ". For instance, if the sensations of defecation are considerable and come to be cultivated for their own sake, it is not unnatural that theories should be built up as to impregnation and birth taking place *per anum*. Many such infantile fantasies are reproduced in the delusions of dementia praecox. It is important to note one point of difference between infantilism in object and infantilism in practice. The relationship to another person, although it may be preponderantly selfish at the outset, is always capable of developing altruistically. Stimulation of the body, however, must always remain an indulgence of something selfish. For this reason the attachment represented in the Oedipus complex can be developed, *qua* attachment, without implication of anything antisocial. It is only when it is portrayed as a specifically sexual union that it falls under a tabu. Body stimulation, on the other hand, apart from its genital component, can only develop into perversions, and these, with exception of a few like kissing, are socially discountenanced. Love for a parent is not decried by the community. But autoerotism must be outgrown ; this means conflict and repression of these improprieties to the unconscious with re-appearance in symbolic behaviour or ideas, or in symptoms.

It has just been mentioned that many delusions echo childish sexual and birth theories. These are constructed by mental processes of a primitive order which we call " *infantile thinking* ". Its prime characteristic is not so much that it is imaginative, but that the imagination has the value of " reality " for the child. " Primitive " would probably be a better term than " infantile "

H

because mythology and folk-lore are full of examples of the same kind of mental processes. There is probably not a single infantile sexual theory that cannot be duplicated in myth or savage belief[1]. With the advance of culture, either racial or individual, adaptation to the material environment becomes more and more accurate. Without ideas, an animal's adaptations are confined to a few set modes of behaviour, so thoughts are a first essential in human development. All men can think more or less. We are, however, still learning to distinguish between thoughts and things, between thoughts that are pure imaginations and thoughts that duplicate actual or potential experience. The child or savage has progressed but a little way on this latter road. Hence the behaviour of either towards a pure imagination may be identical with his behaviour towards the material environment. For instance, observe a child playing " train " with a row of chairs. We call it a game and say he pretends that they are railway carriages. But kick one of the series out of line and a torrent of tears results. He behaves much as we might—*ceteris paribus*—if some of our property were destroyed. For the time being it is, to the infantile mind, a " real " train. Thus do we think when we dream, and so do many of the insane.

This leads to our last introductory principle—regression. It is a fundamental principle of all pathology that adaptations or specializations of recent evolution are more unstable than ones of longer standing. This means that if the health of an organism be in any way affected the first functions to be altered will be those of most recent acquisition and that the alteration will be in the direction of reinstatement of more primitive functions. This principle was elaborated for the nervous system by *Hughlings Jackson* in theories that have inspired the best modern work in neurology. He called the tendency " devolution " as it was an undoing, a reversal, of evolution. The corner-stone of psychoanalytic theory is just this principle applied to mental functions, here called " regression ".

Just as infantilism has three general exhibitions, so regression may be, artificially, considered under three heads. When the type of thought developed in adaptation to the social and material environment is rendered difficult, the innate tendency towards fantastic rather than " directed "[2] thinking becomes stronger. By easy gradations this regression may run from mere idle wishing to day dreaming or actual delusions. Whenever imaginations are not utilized in planning but become an end in themselves, regression has taken place.

Physical activities as well may show a regressive tendency. The satisfactions of normal adult life all represent highly complicated acts having a long individual developmental history. The primary instincts of the suckling are expressed in sucking, blinking, crying,

---

[1] See, for instance, E. S. Hartland, *Primitive Paternity*, as well as the wealth of material in Frazer's *Golden Bough*.

[2] An excellent term used by Jung.

execretion and (when some co-ordination has been acquired) autoerotic acts Compared to these even the simplest behaviour of the adult is complicated and pleasure is attained—if we are to speak hedonistically—by round-about means. A tendency to indulge impulses directly, rather than as they have been modified by moral and physical expedience, is regressive. To strike blindly, or to shrink and cry out in danger, may be regressive behaviour. Similarly autoerotic practices are invariably regressions and often furnish obvious proof of this tendency in the mentally diseased.

The third heading under which regression may be discussed is type of interest. The play of the nursery leads to the games of the school boy, these in turn merge into contests of adolescence and the business of the grown up. Similarly the people we are fond of are, progressively : nursery companions, school fellows, chums, partners in flirtation and lovers. Each stage represents a higher development of interest, which yields a richer satisfaction but involves a more intricate, and therefore more unstable, mental organization. If the task of maintaining the more highly developed interest prove too much for the organism, regression takes place to earlier interests, earlier objects of affection. When weary, when bored with our work, we turn to the simpler pleasures of games, out-of-door activities, vicarious adventures in novel-reading and so on. All vacations represent interests that are regressive in type, although their indulgence is healthful simply because permanent adaptation on a high level is impossible, and the attempt to achieve it therefore unwise. Similarly the tired husband or wife finds temporary pleasure in reminiscence of early love affairs. Such regressions fall within normal limits and their phenomena are common-place experience. But the process may be more extensive. Then the dissatisfaction with responsibilities is more or less complete and the reversion is regarded by the subject—now a patient—as natural and permanent. The former activity or object of affection is looked on as preferable to the present one, thanks to a kind of retrospective falsification ; memory fails to reproduce the incompleteness of the youthful interest which in fantasy is held to be as capable of yielding pleasure as anything elaborated at a more mature period. In still more serious regressions quite primitive impulses are given full play without any hedonistic rationalizations. Then consciousness is flooded with delusions of the Oedipus type.

No professional psychologist has ever described regression in better terms than did George Meredith in his novel, " Evan Harrington " :—" We return to our first ambitions as to our first loves : not that they are dearer to us—quit that delusion : our ripened loves and mature ambitions are probably closest to our hearts, as they deserve to be—but we return to them because our youth has a hold on us which it asserts whenever a disappointment knocks us down."

This statement is incomplete from a psychiatric standpoint only in the last clause. Regression is occasioned by two other general factors in addition to that of failure in the mature adaptation. As has been mentioned above, final products of evolution are intricate and therefore unstable. So whenever the organism is weakened or embarrassed from any cause, such as physical disease or old age, regression is apt to take place. Another factor is the occurrence of something which stimulates an unconscious tendency directly ; such an event is spoken of as an infantile wish-fulfilment. It is not necessary to elaborate these statements further. All the precipitating causes for mental breakdown in the ensuing pages will be found to fall into one or more of these categories : an internal change reduces the capacity of the organism to function at its highest level, or an environmental change either renders the maintenance of an adaptation difficult or, on the other hand, lures the unconscious directly to retrograde infidelity.

PART III

THE STUPOR REACTION

Not to be born is, past all prizing, best ; but, when a man hath
seen the light, this is next best by far, that with all speed he should
go thither, whence he came.

Oedipus Coloneus (Jebb's Translation).

CHAPTER XIII

DESCRIPTION OF THE STUPOR REACTION

MOST stupors have generally been looked on as catatonic in
nature and therefore as a form of dementia praecox.
Psychiatrists were often puzzled by the fact that some
cases recovered, a problem that was first studied seriously
by *Kirby*[1] in 1913. He pointed out that many stupors, showing
symptoms considered to be definitely catatonic, not only recovered,
but that stupor psychoses could replace depressions in circular
insanity, behaving exactly like the ordinary clinical states universally
recognized as phases of manic-depressive insanity. Research with
stupors continued at the Psychiatric Institute, the fruits of this
labour appearing finally as a posthumous volume on the stupor
reaction[2]. Since these psychoses are little understood, and have
never before been accurately delineated, it may be well to describe
them here, following Hoch's text, often in literal quotation, in order
that the reader may be oriented as to the nature of the material
discussed. Some case summaries from Hoch's book will also be
included as illustrations.

We may begin with typical cases of deep stupor. In these we
found the clinical picture composed of the following symptoms. In
the foreground stands emotional poverty. The patients are almost

---

[1] Kirby, George H., " The Catatonic Syndrome and Its Relation to Manic-
Depressive Insanity ", *Journal of Nervous and Mental Disease*, vol. 40, No. 11,
1913.
[2] Hoch, August, *Benign Stupors : a Study of a New Manic-Depressive
Reaction Type.* The Macmillan Co., New York, 1921.

unbelievably apathetic, giving no evidence by speech or action of interest in themselves or their environment, unmoved even by painful stimuli. Their faces are wooden masks ; their voices as colourless when words are uttered. In some cases sudden mood reactions break through at rare intervals. The second cardinal symptom is inactivity. As a rule there is a complete cessation of both spontaneous and reactive movements and of speech. So profound may this inhibition be that swallowing and blinking of the eyes are often absent. The trouble is not a paralysis, however, for reflexes without psychic components are unaffected. Possibly related to the inactivity is the maintenance of artificial positions, which is called catalepsy, a fairly frequent phenomenon. A tendency opposite to the inactivity is seen in negativism. This perversity is present in all gradations from outbursts of anger, with blows and vituperation, to sullen, or even affectless, muscular rigidity. This last occurs most often when the patient is approached, but may be seen when observations are made at a distance. Frequently *wetting* and *soiling* is due to negativism, when the patient has been led to the toilet but relaxes the sphincters so soon as he leaves it. A constant feature is a thinking disorder. On recovery, memory is largely a blank, even for striking experiences during the psychosis, and, when the patient is accessible during the stupor to any questioning, intellectual inefficiency is apparent. An *ideational content* may be gathered, while the stupor is incubating, during interruptions, or from the recollections of recovered patients. Its peculiarity is a preoccupation with the theme of *death*, which is not merely a dominant topic but, often, an exclusive interest. Probably to be related to this is a tendency, present in some cases, to sudden *suicidal impulses*, that are as apparently planless and unexpected, as the conduct of many catatonics. Finally the disease is prone to exhibit certain *physical* peculiarities. A low fever is common and so are skin and circulatory anomalies. A loss of weight is the rule, and *menstruation* is almost always suppressed.

CASE 1. *Anna G.* Age : 15. Admitted to the Psychiatric Institute July 25, 1907.

F.H. The mother and two brothers were living and said to be normal. The father died of apoplexy when the patient was seven.

P.H. The patent was sickly up to the age of seven, but stronger after that. It is stated that she got on well at school, though she was somewhat slow in her work. She was inclined to be rather quiet, even when a child, a bit shy, but she had friends and was well liked by others. After recovery she made a frank, natural impression. She was always rather sensitive about her red hair. She began to work a year before admission and had two positions. The last one she did not like very well, because, she alleged, the girls were " too tough ".

Three weeks before admission she came home from work and said a girl in the shop had made remarks about her red hair. She wanted to change her position, but she kept on working until six days before admission. At that time her mother kept her at home as she seemed so quiet, and when taken out for a walk she wanted to return, because " everybody was looking " at her. For the next two days she cried at times and repeatedly said, " Oh, I wish I were dead—nobody likes me—I wish I were dead and with my father " (dead). She also called to various members of the family, saying she wanted to tell them something, but, when they came ; she would only stare blankly.   For a day she followed her mother around, clung to her, said once she wanted to say something to her, but then only stared and said nothing.

Four days before admission she became quite immobile, lay in bed, did not speak, eat or drink.   She also had some fever.

The patient herself, when well, described the onset of her psychosis as follows : She knew of no cause except that her brother, some time before the onset (not clear how long), was run over by an automobile and had his foot hurt.   She claimed that while still working she lost her ambition, lost her appetite, did not feel like talking to any one ; that when she went out with her mother it merely seemed to her that people stared at her.   The day before she went to the Observation Pavilion, her cousin came to see her, and she thought she saw, standing beside this cousin, the latter's dead mother.   She also thought there was a fire, and that her sister was sweeping little babies out of the room.   Then, she claimed, she felt afraid (this still on the day before going to the Observation Pavilion) because she had repeated visions of an old woman, a witch,   This woman said, " I am your mother, and I gave you to this woman (*i.e.*, patient's real mother) when you were a baby."   She also was afraid her mother was " going away".

At the *Observation Pavilion* she was described as constrained, staring fixedly into space, mute, requiring to be dressed and fed.

Under Observation : (1) For five months the patient presented a marked stupor.   She was for the most part very inactive, totally mute, staring vacantly, often not even blinking, so that for a time the conjunctivae were dry.   She did not swallow, but held her saliva ; did not react to pin pricks or feinting motions before her eyes.   Sometimes she retained her urine, again wet and soiled the bed.   Often there was marked catalepsy, and the retention of very awkward positions.   As a rule she was quite stiff, offering passive resistance towards any interference.   She had to be tube-fed at first.   Later she was spoon-fed, and then would swallow, in spite of the fact that during the interval between her feedings she would let her saliva collect in the mouth. For a time she had a tendency to hold one leg out of bed, and when it was put back would stick the other out.   Sometimes she walked of her own accord to the toilet chair, but on one occasion wet the floor before she got there.

During the first month after admission, this stupor was interrupted for two short periods by a little freer action : she walked to a chair, sat down, smiled a little, fanned herself very naturally, when a fan was given to her, though even then did not speak.

There was, as a rule, no emotional reaction, but after some moments she several times wept when her mother came, still without speaking.   Once when taken to the tub she yelled.

Her *physical condition* during this stupor was as follows : She menstruated freely on admission, then not again until she was well.   Several times she had rises of temperature to 102° or 103° with a high pulse and respiration ; again a respiration of 40, with but a slight rise of temperature, though the pulse had a tendency to go to 130 and over.   She was apt to show marked flushing of the skin wherever touched.   With the fever there was found a leucocytosis of 11,900 to 15,000, with marked increase of polynuclear leucocytes (89%). She got very emaciated, so that four months after admission she weighed 68 lbs. (height 5' 2").

(2).   About five months after admission she was often seen smiling, and again weeping, and she began to talk a little to the nurses, though not to the doctors. She also began to eat excessively of her own accord, and rapidly gained weight, so that by January she weighed 98½ lbs., a gain of 30 lbs. in two months.   Yet she continued to be sluggish.

(3.)   For two more months she was apathetic and appeared disinterested, often would not reply, again, at the same interview, she would do so promptly and with natural voice. This condition may be illustrated by the summary of a note made on January 29, 1908, which is representative of that period. It is stated that she sat about apathetically all day, appeared sluggish, but was fairly neat about her appearance and cleanly in her habits. There was at no time any evidence of emotion, except when asked by the examiner to put out her tongue, so that he could stick a pin in it. She blushed and hid her face. When asked whether she worried about anything, she denied this. When questions were asked, she sometimes answered promptly and in normal voice, again simply remained silent in spite of repeated urging. On the whole, it seemed that simple, impersonal questions were answered promptly ; whereas difficult, impersonal questions, or questions which referred to her condition, were not answered at all. She proved to be oriented. Thus she gave the day of the week, month, year, the name of the hospital, names of the doctors and nurses promptly. She also counted readily and did a few simple multiplications quickly. But she was silent when asked where the hospital was situated, how long she had been here, whether she was here one or six months, how she felt. Questions in regard to the condition she had passed through, or involving difficult calculations, she did not answer. However, some questions regarding her condition, asked in such a way that they could be answered " yes " or " no ", were again answered quite promptly. Thus when asked whether her head felt all right she said, " Yes, sir ". (Is your memory good ?) " Yes." (Have you been sick ?) " No, sir." (Are you worried ?) " No ".

(4.) This apathy cleared up too, so that by the middle of March she was bright, active and smiled freely. With the nurses she was rather talkative and pleased, though with reserve. Towards the physician only was she natural and free. She then gave the *retrospective account* of the onset detailed above. When questioned about her condition, she claimed not to remember the Observation Pavilion, although recalling vaguely going there in a carriage. She was was almost completely amnesic for a considerable part of her stay in the Institute. She claimed it was only in November or December that she began to know where she was (five months after admission). In harmony with this is the fact that she did not recall the tube-and spoon-feeding, which had to be resorted to for about four months of this period. No ideas or visions were remembered. As to her mutism she said, " I don't think I could speak ", " I made no effort ", again, " I did not care to speak ". She claimed that she remembered being pricked with a pin but that she did not feel it. She remembered yelling when taken to the tub (towards end of the marked stupor) and claimed she had thought she was to be drowned.

When she went home (March 24, 1908) some elation developed. She was talkative, conversed with strangers on the street, and told her mother that she was now sixteen years old and wanted " a fellow". When the latter would not allow her to go out, she said it would be better if they both would jump out of the window and kill themselves. She then was sent back to the hospital. In the first part of this period after her return, she was somewhat elated and overtalkative, though she did not present a flight of ideas, and was well behaved. She soon got well, however, and was discharged, four months after her re-admission, fully recovered.

After that, it is claimed, she was perfectly well and worked successfully most of the time with the exception of a short period in the spring of 1909, when she was slightly elated.

In 1910 she had a subsequent attack, during which she was treated at another hospital. From the description this again seems to have been a typical stupor (immobility, mutism, tendency to catalepsy, rigidity). According to the account of the onset sent by that hospital (it was obtained from the mother), this attack began some months before admission, with complaints of being out of sorts, not being able to concentrate and fearing that another attack would come on. Finally the stupor was said to have been immediately preceded by a seizure in which the whole body jerked. She made again an excellent recovery.

The patient was seen about two years after this attack, and described the development of the psychosis as follows : She claimed she began to feel " queer ", " nervous ", " depressed ", and got sleepless. Then (this was given spontaneously) she suddenly thought she was dying and that her father's picture was talking to her and calling her. " Then I lost my speech." As after the first attack, she claimed not to have any recollection of what went on during a considerable part of the stupor, but recalled that she began to talk after her brother visited her.   It is not clear how she was during the period immediately following the stupor.

She made a very natural impression, came willingly to the hospital in response to a letter and was quite open about giving information.

As to the frequency of stupor no figures are available, for the simple reason that the diagnosis in large clinics has not been made with sufficient accuracy to justify any statistics.   Most of these cases are usually called catatonia, depression, " allied to manic-depressive insanity " or " allied to dementia praecox ".   The majority of the stupors reported by Dr. Hoch were in women, but this is merely the result of chance, since it has been easier in the Psychiatric Institute to study functional psychoses in the female division, while the male ward has been reserved largely for organic psychoses.   The majority of the patients seem to be between 15 and 25 years of age, so that it is, presumably, a reaction of youthful years.   In our experience most cases occur among the lower classes, which agrees with the opinion of Wilmanns, who found this tendency among prisoners.

This gives a brief description of the deep stupor.   But even our typical cases did not present this picture during the entire psychosis. They showed phases when, superficially viewed, they were not in stupor but suffered from the above symptoms as tendencies rather than states.   There are also many psychoses where complete stupor is never developed.   This gives us our justification for speaking of the *stupor reaction*, which consists of these symptoms (or most of them) no matter in how slight a degree they may be present.   The analogy to mania and hypomania is compelling.   The latter is merely a dilution of the former.   Both are forms of the manic reaction. We consequently regard stupor and partial stupor as different degrees of the same psychotic process, which we term the stupor reaction.

To illustrate a " partial stupor " the following case may be cited.

CASE 2. *Rose Sch.* Age : 30. Admitted to the Psychiatric Institute, August 22, 1907.

F.H. Both parents were living (father 74, mother 68), as were two brothers and two sisters.   All were said to be normal.

P.H. Nothing was known of the patient's early characteristics, expect that she herself said she was slow at learning in school and did not have much of an education.   But when well she made by no means the impression of a weak-minded person.   The husband had known her for ten years.   He married her eight years before admission, by civil process, keeping this from his own family because he was a Jew and she a Christian.   He said that this undoubtedly worried the patient at times and that she often asked him when he would take her to his family.   The patient herself later also said that this used to worry her.   Finally one and a half years before admission she agreed, on account of the children, to accept the Hebrew faith, and they were then married in the synagogue. But he still did not take her to his family.

There were four pregnancies : the first child died ; of the survivors, one was 8, and another 5 years old. Finally, a year before admission she became again pregnant. During the pregnancy one of the children had whooping cough and she herself was thought to have caught it. The baby was born three months before admission. It was a blue baby, which died two days after birth. The patient flowed heavily for three weeks and was taken to a hospital, where she continued to flow intermittently for some weeks more.

Finally, three weeks before admission, a hysterectomy was performed. Several days after this, when the sister-in-law visited her, the patient begged her to take her home, said the doctor wished to shoot her and to give her poison. Later the patient confirmed this, saying that she thought they wanted to give her saltpetre, and that she heard them say they wanted to shoot her.

When taken home she refused food ; gazed about, was absorbed, seemed obstinate, and several times tried to jump out of the window. Retrospectively the patient stated that she heard children on the street call " Katie ". She thought they meant her child and heard that it was to be taken away from her. A similar idea came out later in her psychosis, namely, that somebody was going to harm her children.

At the *Observation Pavilion* she appeared stupid, rather immobile ; her attention was difficult to attract.

Under Observation : On admission the patient appeared sober, impassive, moved very little, was markedly cataleptic, though not resistive. On the other hand, her eyes were wide open and she looked about freely, following the movements of those around her not unnaturally. When questioned, she looked at the questioner rather intently, was apt to breathe a little more rapidly, and made some ineffectual lip motions, but no reply. To simple commands her responses were slow and inadequate. She flinched when pricked with a pin, but made no attempt at protecting herself. She had to be spoon-fed. The catalepsy persisted only for two days.

After this she continued to show a marked reduction of activity, moved a very little, said nothing spontaneously and had at first to be spoon-fed (later she ate naturally enough). But she never soiled herself and went to the closet of her own accord.

Emotionally she seemed dormant for the most part, though for the first few days she appeared somewhat puzzled, and one night when a patient screamed she seemed afraid and did not sleep, whereas other nights she slept well. She replied only to repeated questions and in a low tone. Very often, though her attention was attracted easily enough, her answers were remarkably shallow and also showed a striking, off-hand profession of incapacity or lack of knowledge. This often occurred without any admission of depression or concern about her incapacity. She would usually say, " What ? " or " Hm ? " or repeat the question, but most often would say, " I don't know "—this even to very simple questions. For instance, when asked, " What is your name ? " she answered, " My name ? I don't know myself " (but she did give her husband's name), or when asked to write her name, she said, " I don't know how to write ", or " Call Annie, she will write my name ". When requested to read or write (even when asked for single letters), she would make such statements as " I can't read ". However, she finally named some objects in pictures. This condition was characteristic of her first two weeks.

Then her psychosis changed a little. She spoke a little more freely but was similarly vague. The following interview of September 9, is characteristic : When asked how she was, she said, " Belle ". (Are you sick ?) " No ". (Is your head all right ?) " Yes ". (Is your memory all right ?) " Yes ". (Do you know everything ?) " Yes ". (Understand everything ?) " Yes ". (Are you mixed up ?) " No ". (Do you feel sick ?) " No ". But when asked where she was, how long she had been there, what the name of the place was, what was the occupation of those about her, she said, " I don't know ". (How did you come here ?) " I couldn't tell how I came up here ". (What are you here for ?) " I am walking around and sitting on benches ", but finally, when again asked what she was here for, she said, " To get cured ". She now gave and wrote her name and address correctly when requested, also gave the name of her children. Yet when asked about the age of the girl, said " I don't know, my head is upside down ". When an attempt was made to force her to repeat the name of the hospital, or the date, or the name of the examiner, she did so all right ; but, even if this was done repeatedly, and she was asked a few minutes later, she would say, " I couldn't say ", or " I forget things ", or " I have a short memory ", or she would give it very imperfectly, as " Manhattan Island ", or " Rhode Island " for " Manhattan State Hospital, Ward's Island ". (How is your memory ?) " All right ". But when at this point the difficulty was pointed out, she cried. (Why ?) " Because I forget so easily ". All this was while her general activity was much reduced, and she seemed to take very little interest in her surroundings.

Then she improved somewhat, asked her husband some questions about home, andon one occasion cried much and clung to him and implored him not to leave without taking her. She also began to work quite well, but still said very little spontaneously. During this period when asked questions, she spoke freely enough, but seemed somewhat embarrassed. What was quite marked still were striking discrepancies in giving dates, and her utter inability to straighten them out, when attention was called to them, as well as her inability to supply such simple data as the ages of her children. Her capacity later was not gone into fully but it was certainly less defective on recovery than at this time. She was rather shallow in giving a retrospective account during this period. Even later, when she had developed a clear insight and made, in respect to her activity and behaviour, a natural impression, she was not able to give much information about her psychosis, although she apparently tried to do so.

She was discharged recovered four months after admission, her weight having risen from 93 lbs. on admission to 133 lbs. on discharges. For the first two weeks of her stay in the hospital, her temperature varied between 99° and 100°.

Retrospectively : She said, in reply to question about her inactivity and difficulty in answering, that she did not feel like talking, felt mixed up, could not remember well, did not want to write.

Before she was quite well she knew of her entrance to the Observation Pavilion and her transfer to Ward's Island, of which she could give some details, but though she had been in the Observation Pavilion two weeks instead of three days, and in the admission ward one month instead of a few hours. As to the precipitating cause of the attack, she spoke of her flowing so much after childbirth and after operation.

She was seen again in March, 1913, when she seemed quite normal mentally and claimed that she had been well ever since leaving the hospital.

To understand the reaction represented in both deep and partial stupors, the symptoms should be separately analysed and then correlated.

The most fundamental characteristic of the stupor symptoms is the change in affect, which can be summed up in one word— apathy. It is fundamental because it seems as if the symptoms built around apathy constitute the stupor reaction. The emotional poverty is evidenced by a lack of feeling, loss of energy and an absence of the normal urge of living. This is quite different from the emotional blocking of the retarded depression, for in the latter the patient shows either by speech or facial expression a definite suffering. The tendency to reduction of affect produces two effects on any emotions, such as internal ideas or environmental events may stimulate. Exhibitions of emotion are either reduced or dissociated. For instance, anxiety is frequently diminished to an expression of dazed bewilderment ; or, isolated and partial exhibitions of mood occur, as when laughter, tears or blushing are seen as quite isolated symptoms. This latter—the " dissociation of affect "—seems to occur only in stupor and dementia praecox. It should be noted, however, that inappropriateness of affect is never observed in a true benign stupor. A final peculiarity is the tendency to interruption of the apathetic habit, when the patient may return to life, as it were, for a few moments, and then relapse.

Closely related to the apathy, and probably merely an expression of it, is the inactivity which is both muscular and mental. It exists in all gradations from that of flaccidity of voluntary muscles, with relaxation of the sphincters, and from states, where there is complete absence of any evidence of mentation, to conditions of mere physical and psychic slowness. After recovery the stupor patient frequently speaks of having felt dead, paralyzed or drugged.

By far the commonest cause of emotional expression, or interruption in the inactivity, is negativism. This is a perversity of behaviour which seems to express antagonism to the environment or to the wishes of those about the patient. In the partial stupors it is seen as active opposition and cantankerousness. In the more profound conditions it is represented by muscular resistiveness or rigidity, or refusal to swallow food placed in the mouth. Occasionally, too, the patient may, even in a deep stupor, retain urine so long that catheterization is necessary. All the explanations which one may gather from the patients' own utterances, mainly retrospective, seem to point to negativism expressing a desire to be left alone. The appearance of perverse behaviour in aimless striking or mere muscular rigidity seems to be an example of " dissociation of affect " (of emotional expression, really).

Catalepsy is an important symptom because, although it occurred in slightly less than a third of our cases, it seems to be a peculiarity of the stupor reaction found but rarely in other benign psychoses. Apparently it never occurs without there being some evidence of mental activity, and, consequently, we are forced to conclude that it is of mental rather than of physical origin. Just what it means psychologically it is impossible to state without much more extended observations. We conjecture tentatively, however, that the retention of fixed positions is in part merely a phenomenon of perseveration, and in part an acceptance of what the patient takes to be a command from the examiner, and sometimes a distorted form of muscular resistiveness.

The intellectual processes suffer more seriously in stupor than in any other form of manic-depressive insanity. Not only do the deep stupors betray no evidence of mentation during the acme of the psychosis, but retrospectively they usually speak of their minds being a blank. Incompleteness and slowness of intellectual operations are highly characteristic features of the partial stupors and of the incubation period of the more profound reactions.   The features of this defect are a difficulty in grasping the nature of the environment ; a slowness in elaborating what impressions are received, with resulting disorientation ; poor performance of any set tests ; and incomplete memory, when recovery has taken place, of external events during the psychosis.   At times the thinking disorder may develop with great suddenness or improve as quickly, and a tendency to isolated evidences of mental acuity is another example of the inconsistency which is so highly characteristic of stupor.   We should note, however, that these sporadic exhibitions of mentality are always associated with brief emotional awakening.

CHAPTER XIV

THE CASE OF CHARLOTTE W

BEFORE beginning the discussion of the psychology of the stupor reaction, it will be advisable to quote in some detail a case which illustrates, not merely different phases of stupor, but also other manic-depressive reactions.

CASE 3. *Charlotte, W.* Age : 30. Admitted to the Psychiatric Institute, October 21, 1905.

F.H. The father was alcoholic and quick-tempered ; he died when the patient was a child. The mother was alcoholic and was insane at 40 (a state of excitement from which she recovered). A brother had an attack of insanity in 1915. A maternal uncle died insane.

P.H. The patient was described as jolly, having many friends. She got on well in school and was efficient at her work.

She was married at 23 and got on well with her husband. The latter stated, however, that she masturbated during her first year of married life. The first child was born without trouble.

First Attack at 25 : Two or three days after giving birth to a second child her mother burst into the room intoxicated. The patient immediately became much frightened, nervous, and developed a depressive condition with crying, slowness, and inability to do things. During this state she spoke of being bad and told her husband that a man had tried to have intercourse with her before marriage. This attack lasted six months and ended with recovery.

When 29, a year before her admission, she had an abortion performed, and four months later another. Her husband was against this, but she persisted in her intention. Seven months before admission she went to the priest, confessed, and was reproved. It is not clear how she took this reproof, but at any rate no symptoms appeared until three weeks later, after burglars had broken into a nearby church. Then she became unduly frightened, would not stay at home, said she was afraid the burglars would come again and kill " some one in the house ". The patient herself stated later during a fault-finding period, that at that time she was afraid some body would take her honour away, and that she thought burglars had taken her " wedding dress ". " Then," she added, " I thought I would run away and lead a bad life ; but I did not want to bring disgrace to the family ".

The general condition which she presented at this time is described as one of apprehensiveness when at home. For this reason she was for five weeks (it is not clear exactly at what period) sent to her sister, where she was better. About a month before the patient was admitted the husband moved, whereupon she got depressed, complained of inability to apply herself to her work, became slow and inactive, and blamed herself for having had the abortion performed. She began to speak of suicide and was committed because she bought carbolic acid. She later said that while in the *Observation Pavilion* she imagined her children were cut up.

Under Observation the condition was as follows :

1. For the first three days the patient, though for the most part not showing any marked mood reaction, was inclined at times to cry, and at such times would complain that this was a terrible place for a person who was not insane

2. On the fourth day the condition changed, and it will be advisable to describe her state in the form of abstracts of each day.

On *Oct.* 24 the patient began to be preoccupied and to answer slowly. A few days later she became distinctly dull, walked about in an indifferent way or lay in bed immobile. Twice on *Oct.* 27 she said in a low tone and with slight distress, " Give me one more chance, let me go to him." But she would not answer questions. At times she lapsed into complete immobility, lying on her back and staring at the ceiling. When the husband came in the afternoon she clung to him and said : " Say good-bye for ever, O my God, save me." Again, very slowly with long pauses and with moaning, she said : " You are going to put me in a big hole where I will stay for the rest of my life." On *Oct.* 28 she was found with depressed expression and spoke in rather low tone, but not with decided slowness as had been the case on the day before. She pleaded about having her soul saved : " Don't kill me " ; " Make me true to my husband " ; once, " I have confessed to the wrong man the shame of my life ". Later she said she did not tell the truth about her life before marriage. Again she wanted to be saved from the electric chair. At times she showed a tendency to stare into space and to leave questions unanswered.

3. From now on a more definite stupor occurred, which is also best described in summaries of the individual notes.

Oct. 29. Lies in bed with fixed gaze, pointing upward with her finger and is very resistive towards any interference. She has to be catheterized.

Oct. 30. Can be spoon-fed but is still catheterized. During the morning she knelt by the bed and would not answer. At the visit she was found in a rather natural position, smiling as the physician approached, saying, " I don't know how long I have been here ". Then she looked out of the window fixedly. At first she did not answer, but, when the physician asked her whether she knew his name, she laughed and said, " I know your name—I know my name ". Then she would not answer any more questions but remained immobile, with fixed gaze. When her going home was mentioned, however, she flushed, and tears ran down her cheek, though no change in the fixedness of her attitude or in her facial expression was seen.

Nov. 1. Lies flat on her back with her hands elevated. She is markedly resistive.

Nov. 2. Free from muscular tension and more responsive. When asked whether she felt like talking, she said in a whining tone, " No, go away—I have to go through enough ". Then she spoke of not knowing how long the nights and days were, of not having known which way she was going. When asked who the physician was, she whimpered and said, " You came to tell me what was right ". She called him " Christ " and another physician " Jim " [husband's name]. However, later in the interview, she gave their correct names. When asked about the name of another physician, she said : " He looks like my cousin, he was here, they all came the first night. I did not take notice who it was till I went through these spirits, then I knew it was right." She paused and added : " My Godmother it was, she is here on earth, somewhere in a convent. Sister C. [who actually was in a convent] she was here too, I could see her ". She said they all came to try to save her. When asked whether she had been asleep, she said : " No, I wasn't asleep, I was mesmerized, but I am awake now—sometimes I thought I was dead ". (When ?) " The time I was going to Heaven." Again : " I went to Heaven in spirit, I came back again—the wedding ring kept me on earth—I will have to be crucified now ". (Tell me about it.) " Jim will have to pick my eyes out—I think it is him. Oh, it is my little girl." (Who told you ?) " The spirits told me." Again : " Little birds my children—I can't see them any more—I must stay here till I die ". (Why ?) " The spirits told me—till I pick every one of my eyes out and my brains too." When asked what day it was, she said, " It must be Good Friday ". (Why ?) " Because God told me I must die on the cross as He did." When asked why she had not spoken the day before, she said that " Jesus Christ in Heaven " had told her she should not tell everything " till all of you had gone, then I could go home with Him, because that is the way we came in, and it was Jim too, all the time ". Fina!ly she said crossly, " Go away now, you are all trying to keep me from Jim " (crying).

Nov. 3. Knelt by bed during night. In the morning she lay in bed staring, resistive ; again was markedly cataleptic. She had to be spoon-fed, and was totally unresponsive. In the afternoon she was found staring and resistive. Presently she said with tears : " I am waiting to be put on the cross ".

Nov. 4. Still has to be catheterized. She sits up, staring, with expressionless face, but when asked how she felt she responded and said feebly : " I don't know how I feel or how I look or how long I have been here or anything ". (What is wrong ?) " Oh, I only want to go to a convent the rest of my days ". (Why ?) " Oh, I have only said wrong things, I thought I would be better dead, I could not do anything right." Later she again began to stare.

Nov. 5. During the night she is said to have been restless and wanted to go to church. To-day she is found staring, but not resistive. When questioned she sometimes does not answer. She said to the physician, " I should have gone up to Heaven to you and not brought me down here ". She called the physician " Uncle James ". Again she said, " I want to go up to see Jim ". Sometimes she looks indifferent, again somewhat bewildered.

Nov. 6. She eats better, catheterizing is no longer necessary. She is found lying in bed, rigid, staring, resistive, does not answer at first, later appears somewhat distressed, says " I want to go and see Jim ". (Where ?) " In Heaven." She gave the name of the place and of the physician, also the date.

Nov. 8. In the forenoon, after she had presented a rather immobile expression and had answered a few orientation questions correctly, she suddenly beckoned into space, then shook her fist in a threatening manner. When later asked about this, she said : " Jim was down there and I wanted to get him in ". (And ?) " You was up here first." (And ?) " I thought we was going down, down, up, up—the boat—you came in here for—to lock Jim out so we wouldn't let him in." Later she said, when asked whether anything worried her, " Yes, you are taking Jim's place ".

Nov. 9. During the night she is reported to have varied between stiffness with mutism and a more relaxed state. Once, the nurse found her with tears, saying, " I want to go down the hall to my sister—to the river ", and a short time later, with fright : " Is that my mother ? " Again she said : " Oh dear, I wish this boat would stop—stop it—where are we going ? " In the forenoon she was quiet and unresponsive. In the afternoon she said in a somewhat perplexed way, " We were in a ship and we were 'most drowned ". (When was that ?) " Day before yesterday it must have been." Again she said in the same manner : " It was like water. I was going down. I could hear a lot of things." She claimed this happened " to-day ". " I saw all the people in here, it was all full of water." " I have been lying here a long time—do you remember the time I was under the ground and it seemed full of water and everyone got drowned and a sharp thing struck me ? " " I was out in a ship and I went down there in a coffin." When asked whether she had been frightened at such times, she said : " No, I didn't seem to be, I just lay there ". She also said " the water rushed in ", and when asked why she put up her arms, she said, " I did it to save the ship ".

Nov. 10. She is still fairly free. She said that when she was on the ship things looked changed ; " the picture over there looked like a saint, the beds looked queer ". (How do things look now ?) " All right." (The picture too ?) " The same as when I was going down into a dark hole." When asked later in the day where she was, she said, " In the Pope's house, Uncle Edward is it ? " but after a short time she added, " It is Ward's Island, isn't it ? "

Nov. 11. Inactive, inaccessible, but for the most part not rigid.

Nov. 14. Varies between mutism with resistance and more relaxed inactivity. To-day lies in a position repeatedly assumed by her, namely, on her stomach with head raised, resistive towards any interference, immobile face, totally inaccessible.

Nov. 15. Freer. She said : " One day I was in a coffin, that's the day I went to Heaven ". She also said she used to see " the crucifix hanging there " (on the ceiling)—" not now, but when I was going to Heaven ". (When was that ?) " Over in that bed " (her former bed). Later she added, " The place changed so . . . things used to be coming up and down [dreamily]—that was the day I was coming up on the ship or going down ". She is quite oriented.

Nov. 17. Usually stands about with immobile face, preoccupied, but she eats voluntarily.

Nov. 24. When the husband and sister came a few days ago she said she was glad to see them, embraced them, cried, and is said to have spoken quite freely. To-day she speaks more freely than usually. When asked why she had answered so little, she said she could not bring herself to say anything, though she added spontaneously, " I knew what was said to me ". When shown a picture of her cataleptic attitude with hands raised, she said dreamily, " I guess that must have been the day I went to Heaven, everything seemed strange, things seemed to be going up and down ". (Did you know where you were ?) " I guess that was the day I thought I was on the ship." When the sister spoke to her she seemed depressed ; said, " If only I had not done those things I might be saved ; if I had only gone to church more ".

Dec. 3. Seems depressed. She weeps some, says she is sad : " There seems to be something over my heart, so I can't see my little girls ". Again : " I should have told you about it first—I should not have bought it "— (refers to buying carbolic acid). She wrote a natural letter but very slowly.

4. There followed then a state lasting for *six months*, during which the patient was rather inactive, preoccupied, even a little tense at times. Sometimes she did not answer ; again at the same interview spoke quite promptly. For the most part the emotional reaction was reduced, at other times she appeared a little uneasy, bewildered, or again depressed. She said that sometimes a mist seemed to be over her. Now and then spoke of things looking queer, and she asked, when the room was cleaned, " Why do you move things about ? " and she added irrelevantly : " I thought the robbers broke into my house and stole my wedding dress and my children's dresses " (refers to the condition during the onset of her psychosis). In the beginning of this state, when asked about the stupor, she spoke again of the " ship " and about going " down, down," but also said that on one occasion she heard beautiful music, was waiting for the last trump and was afraid to move. Moreover, she had some ideas referring to the actual situation which were akin to those in the more marked stupor period. Although she admitted she was better, she said on Dec. 8 that she still had queer ideas at times. " I sometimes think the doctor is Uncle Jim " (long dead). She also spoke of other patients looking like dead relatives, and added, " Are all the spirits that are dead over here ? " " We never die here, the spirits are here." But after that date no such ideas recurred, in fact this whole period seems to have been remarkably barren of delusions. Exceptionally isolated ones were noted. Thus, on Jan. 28 it is mentioned that she stated she sometimes felt so lonely, and as though people were against her ; and on Feb. 13 she said she felt as though the chair knew what she was talking about. It is also mentioned in January that she wept at times, but this seems not to have been a leading feature at all. In March, when asked why she was not more active and cheerful, her lips began to quiver and she said, " Oh, I thought my children would be cut up in Bellevue. I don't know why I feel that way about them." She sometimes cried when her friends left her.

5. Then followed a week of a rather fault-finding, self-assertive state, during which she demanded to be allowed to go home, saying indignantly that she was not a wicked woman, had done nothing to be kept a prisoner here ; she wanted justice because another patient had called her crazy. But in this period also she said that, after the robbery (at home), she felt afraid that her honour would be taken away. When told that her husband had been with her, she said, " Yes, but I was afraid they would get into a fight ". (You mean you were afraid the other man would kill him ?) " No, he is not dead." She further talked of a disagreement she had at that time with her husband,

I

and that she felt then like running away and leading a bad life, but thought of the children. With tears she added : " I would not do anything that is wrong. I have my children to live for ". Quite remarkable was the fact that she then told of various erotic experiences in her life, though with a distinctly moral attitude and minimizing them.

6. On *June* 16 another state was initiated with peculiar ideas, the setting of which is not known, as she told them only to the nurses. She said that she was not Mrs. W. but the Queen of England ; again, that she was an actress ; or again, the wife of a wealthy Mr. B., and that she was going to have a baby. But at night she is said to have been agitated and afraid she was to be executed. She asked to be allowed to go to bed again, then stopped talking, and remained in this mute condition for about a week. She often left her bed and went back again ; she usually had a perplexed expression. On one occasion she put tinsel in her hair and saying it was a golden crown.

7. At the end of that time she became freer and more natural, and remained so for three weeks. She occupied herself somewhat. When asked what had happened in the condition preceding, she said she thought she was a queen, or to be a queen.

8. Towards the end of this period she had again three more absorbed days, but when examined on the third of these days, got rather talkative, drifting on superficial topics.

9. Two days later she began to sing at night, kissed everybody, said it was the anniversary of her meeting her husband, but again cried a little. On the following morning she began to sing love songs, with a rather ecstatic mood, and at times stood in an attitude of adoration with her hands raised. This passed over into a more elated state, during which she smiled a good deal, often quite coquettishly ; she sang love songs softly ; on one occasion she put a mosquito netting over her head like a bridal veil ; or she held her fingers in the shape of a ring over a flower pinned to her breast. But even during this state she said little, only once spoke of waiting for her wedding ring, and again, when asked why she had been singing, said, " I was singing to the man I love ". (Why are you so happy ?) " Because I am with you " (coquettishly).

This, however, represented the end of the psychosis. She improved rapidly. At first she smiled rather readily, but soon began to occupy herself and made a perfect recovery.

She gave a rather shallow retrospective account about the last phase at first she said it was natural for people to feel happy at times, and that she did not talk more because the inclination was not there. The only point she added later was that she held her fingers in the shape of a ring because she was thinking of her wedding ring.

She was discharged on *Oct.* 11.

The patient was seen again in *Sept.* 1915. She then stated that she had been perfectly well until 1912, when she had a breakdown after childbirth. (A childbirth in 1910 had led to no disorder.) The attack lasted six months. She slept poorly, lost weight, and felt weak, depressed, " my strength seemed all gone ". In *July*, 1915, again following a childbirth, she was for about six weeks " despondent, weak, and tired out ".

At the interview she made a very natural, frank impression, and displayed excellent insight.

CHAPTER XV

PSYCHOLOGY OF THE STUPOR REACTION

SINCE I collaborated with Dr. Hoch in the psychological analysis of his material and elaborating the resultant formulations, and, as editor of his book, wrote the chapter, "Psychological Explanation of the Stupor Reaction", I can find no better way of presenting our views than by quoting the arguments that appeared there.

The first problem—following our usual programme—is to discover what ideational content, if any, is characteristic of stupor. It is not likely that many observers have any preconceptions on this subject, because psychiatrists, as a rule, have not been in the habit of paying much attention to the classification of *what* patients are thinking about, concerning themselves rather with *how* they are thinking. One might have expected to find rather multiform ideas, and it was distinctly interesting to discover that there was a marked tendency for the content of the delusions and hallucinations to remain within a certain small compass[1]. It was possible, to state this at once, to show that in by far the majority of cases the same set of ideas returned, and that these ideas had among themselves a definite inner relationship, being concerned with thoughts of "death". In isolated instances other ideas were found as well, and they will have to be discussed later. For the present we shall take up more habitual content.

In a survey of thirty-six consecutive cases of definite stupor, literal death ideas were found in all but one case. They seem to be commonest during the period immediately preceding the stupor, as all but five of these cases spoke of death while the psychosis was incubating. From this we may deduce that the stupor re-action is consequent on ideas of death, or, to put it more guardedly, that death ideas and stupor are consecutive phenomena in the same fundamental process. Two-thirds of these patients interrupted the stupor symptoms to speak of death or attempt suicide. which would lead us to suppose that this intimate relationship still continued. One quarter gave a retrospective account of delusions of being dead, being in Heaven, and so on. From this we may suspect that in many cases there may be a thought content, although the

---

[1] Kirby, *loc. cit.*, pointed out that stupor showed resemblance to feigned death in animals, that the reaction suggested a shrinking from life, and that ideas of death were common.

patient's mind may seem to be a complete blank. It is important to note that when a retrospective account is gained, the delusions are practically always of death or something akin to it, such as being in prison, feeling paralyzed, stiff, and so on.

In the one case of the thirty-six who presented no literal death ideas, the psychosis was characterized essentially by apathy and mild confusion, a larval stupor reaction. It began with a fear of fire, smelling smoke and a conviction that her house would burn down. It is surely not straining interpretation to suggest that this phobia was analogous to a death fear. When one considers the incompleteness of anamneses not taken *ad hoc* (for these are largely old cases), and that the rule in stupor is silence, the consistence with which this content appears is striking.

To exemplify the form in which these delusional thoughts occur we may cite the following : Henrietta H. said, retrospectively, that she thought she was dead, that she saw shadows of dead friends laid out for burial, that she saw scenes from Heaven and Earth. Anna K. claimed to have had the belief that she was going to die, and to have had visions of her dead father and dead aunt, who were calling her. She also thought that all the family were dead and that she was in a cemetery. Rosie K. said she had the idea that she wanted to die and that she refused food for that purpose, and during the stupor she sometimes held her breath until she was cyanotic. Mary F., before her stupor became profound, spoke of the hereafter, of being in Calvary and in Heaven. In this case, as well as in the above-mentioned Henrietta H., we find, therefore, associated with " death " the closely related idea of Heaven. Whether Calvary merely referred to the cemetery (Mt. Calvary cemetery) or leads over to the motif of crucifixion, cannot be decided. It is, however, clear that this latter motif may be associated with that of death, as is shown in Charlotte W. [Case 3], who, during intervals when the inactivity lifted, spoke of having been dead, of spirits having told her that she must die, of having gone to Heaven, of God having told her that she must die on the cross like Christ. But this patient also showed, in a second sub-period of her stupor, another content. She said : " It is like water. I was going down ". Or again, she spoke of having gone " under the ground ", " I went down, down in a coffin." She spoke of having gone down " into a dark hole ", " down, down, up, up ", again, of having been " on a ship ". We shall see in the further course of our study that this type of content occurs not at all infrequently.

The internal relationship among the different ideas associated with stupor : Before we go any further it may be advisable to examine the meaning of such ideas when they arise in other settings than those of the psychoses. If we consider these ideas of death, Heaven, of going under ground, being in water, in a boat, etc., we are impressed with the similarity which they bear to certain mythological motifs. This is, of course, not the place to enter into this topic more than briefly. We are here concerned with a clinical study, and, therefore, among other tasks, with the inter-relationship of symptoms, but for that purpose it is necessary to point out how these ideas seen in stupor can be shown to have not only a vital connection when viewed as deep-seated human strivings, but also are closely related to, or identical with, ideas found in mythology.

To one's conscious mind death may be not only the dreaded enemy who ends life, but also the friend who brings relief from all conflict, strife, and effort. Death may, therefore, well express a shrinking from adaptation and reality, and as such may symbolize one of the most deep-seated yearnings of the human soul. But, from time immemorial, man has associated with this yearning another one, one which, without the adaptation to reality being made, yet includes a certain attempt at objectivation, the desire for rebirth. We need not enter further into possible symbols for death *per se*, but it is necessary to speak briefly of the symbolic forms in which the strving for rebirth has frequently found expression. The reader will find a large material collected in various writings on mythology, for the psychological interpretation of which reference may be made to Jung's " Wandlungen und Symbole der Libido " and Rank's " Mythos von der Geburt des Helden ". From them it appears how old are the symptoms for rebirth, and how they deal chiefly with water and earth, and the idea of being surrounded by, and enclosed in, a small space. Thus we find a sinking into the water of the sea, enclosure in something which swims on or in the water, such as a casket, or a basket, or a fish, or a boat ; again, we find descent into the earth.

The striving for rebirth might be assumed to have adopted these expressions, or symbols, on account of the concrete way in which the human mind knows birth to take place. The tendency for concrete expression of abstract notions causes the desire for another existence to appear, first as a rebirth fantasy and then as a return to the mother's body. One thinks of Job's cry, " Naked came I from my mother's womb and naked shall I return thither ", as an example of the literal comparison of death with birth. We need only refer to the myths of Moses and the older one of Osiris, and the many myths of the birth of the hero, to call to the mind of the reader the examples which mythology furnishes. There is probably not one of the ideas expressed by our patients which cannot be duplicated in myths. We have, therefore, a right to speak of these ideas as " primitive ", and to see in them, not only recurrent expressions of a fundamental human tendency, but to recognize in them an essential inner relationship. It is especially this last fact to which at this point we wish to call attention : that without any obvious connection the fantasies of our forefathers recur in the delusions of our stupor cases. We presume that in each case they represent a fulfilment of a primitive human demand. In one of our cases a vision of Heaven and a conscious longing to be there was followed by a stupor. On recovery the patient compared her condition to that of a butterfly just hatched from a cocoon. No clearer simile of mental rebirth could be given.

Brief survey of the ideas associated with the states preceding the stupor : If we now return to the study of the further occurrence of such ideas in the cases described, we find motifs, similar to those seen in the stupor, in the period which immediately precedes the more definite stupor reaction. Indeed we find the ideas there with greater regularity. In Meta S. the stupor followed upon six days, in which there was reduced activity and crying, with self-accusation, but also with entreaties to be allowed to go home and die with her father. At the very onset of her breakdown, the desire for death had also occurred. Anna G. [Case 1] expressed a wish to be with her dead father, and, at the visit of a cousin, she had a vision of the latter's dead mother. A second attack of this same patient began with the idea that the dead father was calling her. Maggie H. saw dead bodies, and during outbursts of greater anxiousness, she thought her husband was going to die. In Caroline De S. the psychosis began with a coarse excitement, with statements about being killed, with entreaties to be shot, with the idea of going to Heaven, again with frequent calling out that she loved her father (who was dead since her ninth year), while immediately before the stupor the condition passed into a muttering state in which she spoke of being killed. Mary D. began by worrying over the father's death (dead four years before), had visions of the latter beckoning, and she heard voices saying, " You will be dead ". Mary F. had a vision of a " person in white ", and thought she was going to die. In Henrietta H. the stupor was preceded by nine days of elation, with ideas of shooting and of war ; but this had commenced with hearing voices of dead friends, and with ideas that somebody wanted to kill her family. In the case of Annie K. we find, before the stupor, a stage of worry, with reduction of activity, and then a vision of the dead father coming for her. In Charlotte W. [Case 3] the stupor was preceded by a state of preoccupation, with distress and entreaties to be saved, partly from being put into a big hole, partly from the electric chair.

We see, therefore, in the introductory phrase of the stupor in almost every case ideas of death, and in one case an idea belonging to the rebirth motif, namely, of being put into a dark hole. In well observed cases, apparently, we do not find the stupor reaction without either coincident or preceding ideas of death.

Relation of death and rebirth ideas with affect : In order to investigate the relation of these ideas to the affective condition associated with them, it will be necessary to study not only the abstract ideational content but the special formulation in which the content appears. In looking over the enumeration of the ideas given above, it is very clear that these formulations differed considerably from each other. A priori we would say that it is, psychologically, a very different matter whether a person expresses a desire to die, or has the idea that he will die or is dead, or says he will be killed. We associate the first with sadness, the last with fear, while our daily experience does not give us much information about the delusion of being dead. A vivid expectation of death is usually accompanied by either fear of resignation.

In studying the ideas which we obtained from the patients by retrospective account after the psychosis, or from a retrospective account during freer intervals, it is, of course, difficult, especially in the former case, to say whether they had persisted for any length of time. Probably in most instances this was not the case, and we must remember in this connection that in a considerable number of cases the patients recalled no ideas whatever.

Of the five cases which we may consider as types, Henrietta H. and Mary F. formulated their ideas simply as *accepted facts* during the stupor. The former thought she was dead, saw dead friends laid out for burial, and scenes from Heaven and Earth. The latter spoke during the stupor, of being in " Calvary ", " The Hereafter ", or " Heaven ". We have seen that these stupors were essentially affectless reactions and we can therefore say that, so far as these two cases are concerned, the ideas thus formulated were not associated with any affect.

Annie K. was a little different. During the stupor she made a few utterances about priests and " all being dead ", and retrospectively she said that she thought she was in the cemetery, was going to die, that she had repeated visions of her dead father and once of a dead aunt calling her ; that she had thought her family were dead ; again, that her baby (who was born just before the psychosis) was dead. The formulation is therefore less one of fact than of something prospective, something which is coming—the *going to die.* Correlated, perhaps, with this anticipation were slight modifications of the usual apathy. The patient often had an expression of bewilderment. She was also more in contact with her environment than many stuporous patients are, for, not infrequently, she would look at what was going on about her. Her apathy was also broken into in a marked degree by her active resistiveness, which was sometimes accompanied by plain anger. It seems that a prospect of death may occur in other instances in a totally affectless state. We have recently seen it in a partial stupor during which the patient spoke and had this persistent idea in a setting of complete apathy. We see here also, as in one of the former cases, the idea of other members of the family being dead.

More difficult and deserving more discussion are the two remaining cases, Rosie K. and Charlotte W. [Case 3]. Rosie K. showed a peculiar condition. She said, retrospectively, that during the stupor she had the desire to die and that for this purpose she refused food. Moreover, she was repeatedly seen to hold her breath with great insistence, though without emotional expression. This is worth noting. We often say in a case like this that " there is no affect ", and yet there is evidently a considerable " push " behind the action. We shall later have to mention in detail a patient whom we regard as belonging in the group of stupor reactions, and who for a time made insistent, impulsive and most determined suicidal attempts, yet with a peculiar blank, emotionless, facial expression and with shouting which was more like that of a huckster than of one in despair. Here also then, there was a great deal of " push ", yet not associated with that which we call in psychiatry an emotion. In both instances we see acts which we are in the habit of calling for this very reason " impulsive ". Evidently this is an important psychological problem which leads directly into the psychology of emotions and deserves further study. For the present it is enough to say that, in stuporous patients who harbour a wish to die, there is not, as in other psychoses, a definite affect, such as sadness or despair, but no affect at all, apparently, through there may be a good deal of " push " or impulsiveness.

The case of Charlotte W. [Case 3] is a complicated one, for she had short stupor periods with inactivity, catalepsy, resistiveness, etc., which were interrupted with freer spells. A careful analysis of her history has been instructive and justifies a detailed and lengthy discussion. For the purpose in hand it is necessary to separate the ideas—which she expressed only in the freer periods (during which some affect was at times seen)—into those which referred retrospectively to the stupor phase, and those which referred to the freer periods themselves.

We find that the time, during which more marked stupor symptoms appeared, may be divided into two subperiods. This is not possible in regard to the manifestations belonging to the general reaction, which seem to have undergone no decided change, but only in regard to the form of the delusions. In this we find there was a first phase in which ideas of death and Heaven (and crucifixion) occurred, and a second phase in which ideas were present which belonged essentially to the motif of rebirth but which were also associated with ideas of Heaven.

About the first subperiod she said : " I was mesmerized ", or " I thought I was dead ", or " God told me I must die on the cross as he did ", or " I went to Heaven in spirit ". About the second subperiod she said retrospectively : " We were on a ship and we were 'most drowned ". " It was like water, I was going down, down." She said she saw the people of the hospital and " it was all full of water " ; or again, " I went under the ground, and it was full of water, and everyone got drowned, and a sharp thing struck me " ; or " I was out on a ship and went down in a coffin ". She claimed she put up her arms to save the ship. Again she spoke of having gone into a dark hole. She also said : " One day I was in a coffin—that was the day I went to Heaven ". " They used to be coming up and down, that was the day I was coming up in a ship or going down ". And when shown her picture in a cataleptic attitude, she said, " That must have been when I went to Heaven—everything seemed strange, things seemed to go up and down—I guess that was the day I thought I was on the ship ". Finally she also said : " Once I heard beautiful music—I was waiting for the last trump—I was afraid to move ".

We see, therefore, that most of the ideas which she thus spoke of retrospectively as having been in her mind during the stupor, and which belonged both to the death and the rebirth motifs, were formulated as facts (as in the cases of Henrietta H. and Mary F. above mentioned). It was, moreover, a condition which was accepted without protest. Here again an affect was not associated with these ideas, and when the patient was asked whether she had not been frightened, she said herself, " No, I just lay there ". The idea that God told her she would have to die on the cross like Christ, is, in the religious form, like the beckoning of the father in Henrietta H. The only exception to the claim, that the ideas were formulated as facts and accepted as inevitable, seems to be the statement that she held up her arms to save the ship. This would seem to be, in contradistinction to the rest, an intrusion of the thought, if not of the feeling of, danger. However, this was isolated and we can do no more than to determine main tendencies. We must expect, especially in such variable conditions as we see in this patient, to find occasional inconsistencies.

In summing up, therefore, that so far as the stupor itself is concerned, the ideas are formulated as a rule :—

(1) As accepted facts (being dead, being in a ship, etc.)

(2) As accepted prospects (going to die).

(3) As the wish to die.

In the first two types the ideas are not associated with affect ; in the third, though not associated with affect, they may be combined with " impulsive " suicidal attempts.

In order not to complicate the analysis of Charlotte W. [Case 3] too much, we may begin our study of the intervals and the conditions preceding the stupors with the ideas which this patient produced when the stupor lifted somewhat. We shall see that the ideas are closely related to those mentioned above but formulated differently.

It will be remembered that Charlotte W. had freer intervals when she responded and was less constrained generally, and that it was in these that the ideas above mentioned were gathered. Since they were spoken of in the past tense, we regarded them as not belonging to the actual situation but to the more stuporous period. It seems tempting now to see whether the ideas which are expressed in the present tense are different in character, the general aim being to discover whether any tendencies can be found for the association of different clinical pictures with specific types and formulations of delusions. We see that on November 2 the patient, when speaking much more freely than before, said she had felt that she was mesmerized, was dead, and that she had gone to Heaven, ideas which we have taken up above as belonging to the stupor period. In addition to speaking much more freely in these intervals she showed at times some affect. Thus to the physician whom she called Christ she said, with tears, " You came to tell me what was right ", or again, with tears, " I will have to be crucified ", or she spoke in a depressed manner about her children, " I can't see them any more ", " I must stay here till I die ", and she spoke of having to stay in the hospital till she picked her eyes and her brains out ; or she claimed her husband or her children had to pick them out. Once she exclaimed crossly and with tears, " You are trying to keep me from Jim " (husband). Another idea was not plainly associated with emotion. She said she had come back from Heaven, " The wedding ring kept me on earth ". What strikes one about these formulations is that they are, on the one hand, sometimes associated with an affect, and that, on the other hand, they refer much more to her actual life, her marriage, her husband, her children. At least this seems to be a definite tendency. A similar tendency may be seen later : On November 4, while generally stuporous, this suddenly lifted for a short time, and with feeble voice she uttered some depressive ideas. She said she wanted to go to a convent, that it would be better if she were dead, that she could not do anything right. On November 5 and 6 she said she wanted to go to Jim in Heaven (in contradistinction to the retrospective statements that she had gone to Heaven) ; and on the 8th, when she had the idea of being in a boat, she said with some anger that she wanted to get her husband into the boat, but that the doctor kept him out and took his place.

Later there were at times ideas expressed which referred to the actual situation or essentially depressive ideas in a depressive setting. Thus on December 3 she appeared sad, retarded, and spoke of not being able to see her children and that she had done wrong in buying carbolic acid (her suicidal attempt). So far as this case is concerned, therefore, we do find a distinct tendency for the ideas which refer to the more stuporous condition to differ from those which refer to the actual situation in the freer intervals, a difference which we may formulate by saying that, though primitive ideas are expressed, the tendency seems to be to connect them more with actual life, or that the primitive character is lost and the ideas take on a more depressive character with a depressive affect. A few words should be added in regard to the peculiar ideas that she or her husband or her child had to pick out her eyes (or her brain). It is probable that this idea belongs to the motif of sacrifice (the *Opfermotif* of Jung) into which we need not enter further, except to say that in this instance it was plainly connected, like some of the other ideas just spoken of, with the real situation of her life (husband, children).

It will now be necessary to examine the earlier state of Charlotte W. The condition preceding the stupor set in with preoccupation, slow talk, and slight distress. During the time she asked to be given one more chance, and said to her husband she would not see him again. Then followed a day when she was very slow, and with moaning said she was going to be put into a dark hole. Again on the next day, when speaking more freely, she begged to be saved from the electric chair, and also said, " Don't kill me ; make me true to my husband ", etc. (Again the connection with real life !) We see here the idea of death and especially an idea pertaining to the rebirth motif in a setting of distress and slowness, as an introduction to the stupor which had in it both of these motifs. We must leave it undecided whether it is accidental or not that the distress was associated with more slowness (i.e., more marked stupor traits) when she spoke of the dark hole than when she spoke of the electric chair or death. But what interests us is that distress and reduction of activity (not sadness and reduction of activity, which seems as a rule to have a different content) are here associated with ideas seen in stupor but formulated as prospective events. We know from experience that we often find associated with the fear of dying considerable freedom of action, and we see at times in involution states conditions with freedom of motion and marked anxiety, whereas the ideas seem to belong to the motif of rebirth ; e.g., the fear of being boiled in a tank[1].

In this connection, however, two other cases should be considered, which show a condition reminding one somewhat of that we have just discussed, but in which the rebirth motif appeared, not prospectively, but, as in the stupor, as an actual situation. At the same time this situation was not passively accepted but conceived as a dangerous situation. The significant phenomenon in both these conditions was that there was not anxiety with freedom of action, but a bewildered uneasiness with marked reduction of activity.

The first case is that of Johanna S. At one stage of her psychosis, she presented two days of typical stupor with the idea that she was dead. We are familiar with this. But it was followed by several days of bewildered uneasiness and slow restlesness, with ideas that she was at the bottom of " the deep, dark water," and for a time she made attempts at stepping out of the water or at swimming motions. All of this was in a general setting of reduction of activity with bewildered uneasiness. In the ideas about being at the bottom of the deep, dark water, we recognize again the rebirth motif, yet the situation is not accepted, for attempts are made by the patient to save herself, i.e., the attitude is one of avoidance. It is interesting in this connection that immediately following this state there was one day of ordinary retardation with sadness and with ideas of being bad and ill. That is, when the element of anxiety, the uneasiness,

---

[1] We may ention that since this study was made we risked a prediction of stupor, which events justified, in the case of a patient who showed expectation of death without affect. Such opportunities are rare, however, since we usually do not see these cases till the stupor symptoms are manifest. It would be unsafe to dogmatize on the basis of such meagre material.

disappeared and sadness supervened, the rebirth ideas were no longer present.

In Mary C. we have, unfortunately, not a direct observation, but we have, at any rate, a description from the Observation Pavilion, which seems so plain that we should be justified in using it here. The condition we refer to is described as a dazed uneasiness, with ideas of being shut up in a ship, of the ship being closed up so that no one could get out, of the boat having gone down, of the people turning up. We should add here that the condition was not followed by a typical stupor. Essentially it was a retardation in which only on one occasion was a complete inactivity observed. During this phase she soiled her bed. Perhaps the persistent complaint of inability to take in the environment belonged also more to the incapacity of stupor than to that of depression. We have again, therefore, in this initial phase, a similar situation, namely, ideas belonging essentially to the rebirth motif, formulated as of a threatening character, if not as actually dangerous.

We can say, therefore, that what characterizes these three cases and brings them together is the fact that all three had ideas belonging to the rebirth motif, but formulated as dangerous situations. Associated with this there was not a typical anxiety with the relative freedom of activity belonging to this state, but an anxiety, or distress, or uneasiness, with traits of stupor reaction, namely, slow movements, lack of contact with the environment, and a dazed facial expression. It would seem that these facts could scarcely be accidental but that they must have a deeper significance. However, as a discussion of this would lead us more into the theoretic part of this study, we shall defer it for the moment, and be satisfied with pointing out here the clinical facts of observation.

In brief, then, our findings as to the ideational content of the benign stupor are as follows : From the utterances during the incubation period of the psychosis, from the ideas expressed in interruptions of the deep stupor, as well as from the memories of recovered patients, we find an extraordinary paucity and uniformity of autistic thoughts. They are concerned with death, often as a plain delusion of being no longer alive, or with the closely related fancy of rebirth. The rule is a setting of apathy for these ideas, but when they are formulated so as to connect them with the real life and problems of the patient, or when rebirth is represented as a dangerous situation, some affect, usually one of distress, may appear.

It is our view that manic-depressive insanity is a disease fundamentally based on some constitutional defect, presumably physical, but that its symptoms are determined by psychological mechanisms. In accordance with this hypothesis we seek, when studying the different forms of insanity presented in this group, to differentiate between the different types of mental mechanisms observed, and by this analysis to account for the manifestations of the disease on purely psychological lines. If benign stupors belong to this group, then we should be able to find some specific psychology for this type of reaction.

All speech and all conduct, except simple reflex behaviour, are presumably determined by ideas. When an individual is not aware of the purpose governing his action, we assume, in psychological study, that an unconscious motive is present, so that in either case the first step in psychological understanding of any normal or abnormal condition is to discover, if possible, what the ideas are that lead to the actions or utterances observed. In the case of stupors the situation is fairly simple, in that the ideational content is extremely limited. As has been seen, it is confined to death and rebirth fancies, other ideas being correlated with secondary symptoms, such as belong to mechanisms of other manic-depressive psychoses. Our task is now to consider the significance of these death and rebirth delusions and their meaning for the stupor reaction.

Thoughts concerned with future and new activities require energy for their completion in action and are, therefore, naturally accompanied by a sense of effort which gives pleasure to an active mind. When the sum of energy is reduced, one observes a reverse tendency called " regression ". It is easier to go back over the way we know than to go forward, so the weakened individual tends to direct his attention to earlier actions or situations. To meet a new experience one must think logically and keep his attention on things as they are, rather than imagine things as one would like to have them.

Progressive thinking is therefore adaptive, while regressive thinking is fantastic in type, as well as concerned with the past— a past which, in fancy, takes on the lustre of the Golden Age. Sanity and insanity are, roughly speaking, states where progressive or regressive thinking rule. The essence of a functional psychosis is a flight from reality to a retreat of easeful unreality.

Carried to the extreme, regression leads one, in type of thinking and in ideas, back to childhood and earliest infancy. The final goal is a state of mental vacuity such as probably exists in the infant at the time of birth and during the first days of extrauterine life. In this state what interest there is, is directed entirely to the physical comfort of the individual himself, and contact with the environment is so undeveloped, that efforts to obtain from it the primitive wants of warmth and nutrition are confined to vague instinctive cries. Evolution to true contact with the world around implies effort, the exercise of self-control, and also self-sacrifice, since the child soon learns that some kind of *quid pro quo* must be given. Viewed from the adult standpoint, the emptiness of this early mental state must seem like the Nirvana of death. At least death is the only simple term we can use to represent such a complete loss of our habitual mental functions.

When life is difficult, we naturally tend to seek death. Were it not for the powerful instinct of self-preservation, suicide would probably be the universal mode of solving our problems. As it is, we reach a compromise, such as that of sleep, in which contact with reality is temporarily abandoned. In so far as sleep is psychically determined, it is a regressive phenomenon. It is interesting that the most frequent euphemism or metaphor for death is sleep. Sleep is a normal regression ; but it does not always give the unstable individual sufficient relaxation from the demands of adaptation and so pathological regressions may take place, one of which we believe stupor to be. It is important to note that objectively the resemblance between sleep and stupor is striking. So far as mental activity in either state can be discovered by the observer, either the sleeper, or the patient in stupor, might be dead. Briefly stated, then, our hypothesis of the psychological determination of stupor is that the abnormal individual turns to it as a release from mental anguish, just as the normal human being seeks relief in his bed from physical and mental fatigue. When this desire for refuge takes the shape of a formulated idea, there are delusions of death.

The problem of sleep is, of course, bound up with the physiology of rest, and as recuperation, in a physical sense, necessitates temporary cessation of function, so in the mental sphere we see that relaxation is necessary if our mental operations are to be carried on with continued success. This is probably the teleological meaning of sleep in its psychological aspects, for in it we abandon diurnal adaptive thinking and retire to a world of fancy, very often solving our problems by " sleeping over them ". The innate desire for rest and a fresh start is almost as fundamental a human craving as is the tendency to seek release in death. In fact the two are closely associated both in literature and in daily speech, for in many respects we correlate death with new life.

If one is to visualize or incorporate the conception of new life in one term, rebirth is the only one which will do it, just as death is the only word which epitomizes the idea of complete cessation of effort. Not unnaturally, therefore, we find in the mythology of our race, in our dreams, and in the speech of our insane patients, a frequent correlation of these two ideas, whether it come in the crude imagery of physical rebirth or prejected in fantasies of destruction and rebuilding of the world. Many of our psychotic patients achieve in fancy that for which the Persian poet yearned :

> " Ah Love ! could you and I with Him conspire
> To grasp this Sorry Scheme of Things entire,
> Would we not shatter it to bits—and then
> Re-mould it nearer to the Heart's Desire ! "

A vision of a new world is a content occurring not infrequently in manic states, but before the universe can be remoulded it must be destroyed. Before the individual can enjoy new life, a new birth, he must die ; and stupor often marks this death phase of a dominant rebirth fantasy. In this connection it is significant that stupors almost always recover by way of attenuation of the stupor symptoms, or in a hypomanic phase where there seems to be an abnormal supply of energy. Antaeus-like, they rise with fresh vigour from the earth. They do not pass into depressions or anxieties.

Rebirth fancies unquestionably, then, contain constructive and progressive elements, but, as has been stated above, any thinking which implies a lapse of contact with the environment is, in so far as that lapse is concerned, regressive, and in consequence, rebirth fancies, as dramatized by the stupor patients, are regressive, just as are the delusions of death itself.

It is obvious that an acceptance of death implies rather thorough mental disintegration. Before that takes place there may be some mental conflict. The instinct of self-preservation may prevent the individual from welcoming the notion of dissolution, so that this latter idea, though insistent, is not accepted, but reacted to with anxiety ; hence we often meet with onsets of stupor characterized by emotional distress. It has already been suggested that death may foreshadow another existence. Often in the psychoses we meet with the idea of eternal union in death with some loved one, whom the vicissitudes and restrictions of this life prevent from becoming an earthly partner. This fancy is frequently the basis for elation. Similarly, new life in a religious sense, as expressed in the delusion of translation to Heaven, is a common occasion for ecstasy. These formulations of the death idea may occur as tentative solutions of the patient's problems, leading to temporary manic episodes while the psychosis is incubating. It seems that stupor as such appears only when death and nullity is accepted.

The above are more or less priori reasons for regarding the stupor as a regressive reaction. We must now consider the clinical evidence to support this view. In the first place, we always find that stupor occurs in an individual who is unhappy and who has found no other solution than regression for the predicament in which he is. There is nothing specific in the cause of this unhappiness. At times the factors producing it are mainly environmental ; at others, the problem is essentially of the patient's own making. Of course almost any type of functional psychosis may emerge from such a state of dissatisfaction, but it is important to note that unlike manic states, for instance, stupors invariably develop from a situation of unhappiness. Quite frequently the choice of the stupor regression is determined by some definitely environmental event which suggests death. This often comes as the actual death of the patient's father (in the case of a woman) or employer, events which inflate the already existing, although perhaps unconscious, desire for mutual death. Again, the precipitating factor may be a situation which adds still another problem and makes the burden of adaptation intolerable, forcing on him the desire for death. In these cases the actual psychosis is sometimes ushered in dramatically with a vision of some dead person (often a woman's father) who beckons, or there are dream-like experiences of burial, drowning, and so on.

A few cases taken at random from our material exemplify these features of the unhappiness in which the psychosis appears as a solution with its development of the death fancy.

Alice R., at the age of 25, was much troubled by worrying over her financial difficulties and the shame of an illegitimate child. Retrospectively she stated, " I was so disgusted I went to bed . . . I just gave up hope." Shortly before admission she said she was lost and damned, and to the nurse in the Observation Pavilion she pleaded, " Don't let me murder myself and the baby ".

Caroline De S. for some time was worried over the engagement of her favourite brother to a Protestant (herself a Catholic) and the threatened change of his religion. At his engagement dinner she had a sudden excitement, crying out, " I hate her—I love you— papa, don't kill me ". This excitement lasted for three weeks, during two of which she was observed, when she spoke frequently of being killed and going to Heaven. The conflict was frankly stated in the words, " I love my father but don't want to die ". Then for two weeks she had some fever, was tube-fed, muttered about being killed or showed some elation, there being apparently interrupted stuporous, manic, and possibly, anxiety episodes. Finally she settled down to a year of deep stupor.

Laura A. had for three months poor sleep with depression over her failure to study. Another cause for worry was that her father was home and out of work. She reached a point where she did not care what happened but continued working. Ten days before admission she was not feeling well. The next morning she woke up confused, frightened, speedily became dazed, stunned, could not bring anything to her memory. This rather sudden stupor onset was not accompanied by any false ideas, at least none which the family remembered.

Mary C. was an immigrant who felt lonely in the new country. Two weeks before admission her uncle, with whom she was living, died. She thought she had brought bad luck, complained of weakness and dirziness, then suddenly felt mixed up, her " memory got bad ", and she thought she was going to die. Next she was frightened, heard voices, thought there was shooting and a fire. For a short time she was inactive and later began shouting fire. When taken to the Observation Pavilion, she was dazed, uneasy, thought she was on a boat or shut up in a boat which had gone down ; all were drowned. Then came a mild stupor.

Maggie H., while pregnant, fancied that her baby would be deformed and that she would die in childbirth. Three weeks before admission the child was born. For five days she worried about not having enough milk, about her husband losing his job (he did lose it), and thought her head was getting queer. On the 5th day she cried, said she was going to die, that there was poison in the food, that her husband was untrue to her. She became mute but continued to attend to her baby. She saw dead bodies lying around, and by the time she was taken to the Observation Pavilion was in a marked stupor.

Turning now to the symptoms of the stupor proper, we note, first, the effects of the loss of energy which regression implies. The inactivity and apathy which these patients show is too obviously evidence of this to require further comment. Another proof of the withdrawal of libido or interest is found in the thinking disorder. Directed, accurate thinking, requires effort, as we all know from the experience of our laborious mistakes when fatigued. So in stupor there is an inability to perform simple arithmetical problems, poor orientation is observed, and so on. Similarly what we remember seems to be that which we associate with the impressions received by an active consciousness. Actual events persist in memory better than those of fancy, in proof of which one thinks at once of the vanishing of dreams on waking, with the re-establishment of extroverted consciousness. This registration of impression requires interest and active attention. Without interest there is no attention and no registration. The patient in stupor presents just the memory defect which we would expect. Indifference to his environment leads to a poor memory of external events, while on recovery there may be such a divorce between consciousness of normal and abnormal states that the past delusions are wiped from the record of conscious memory. Withdrawal of energy then produces, not only inactivity and apathy, but grave defects in intellectual capacity.

The natural flow of interest in regression is to earlier types of ambition and activity. This is betrayed not merely by the thought content dealing with the youth and childhood of the patient, but also is manifested in behaviour. Excluding involution melancholia, there is probably no psychosis in which the patients exhibit such infantile reactions as in stupor. Except for the stature and obvious age of these patients, one could easily imagine that he was dealing with spoiled and fractious infants. One thinks at once of the negativism, which is so like that of a perverse child, and of the unconventional, personal habits to which these patients cling so stubbornly. Masturbation, for instance, is quite frequent, while wilful wetting and soiling is still more common. We sometimes meet with childishness, both in vocabulary and mode of expression. In one case there was evidently a delusion of a return to actual childhood, for she kept insisting that she was " in papa's house ".

The frequency with which the delusion of mutual death occurs in stupor is another evidence of its regressive psychology. The partner in the spirit marriage is rarely, if ever, the natural object of adult affection, but rather a parent or other relative to whose memory the patient has unconsciously clung for many years, reawakening in the psychosis an ambition of childhood for an exclusive possession that reaches its fulfilment in this delusion. Closely allied with this is another delusion, that of being actually dead, which the patients sometimes express in action, even when

K

not in words. The anæsthesia to pin pricks, the immobility and the refusal to recognize the existence of the world around, in patients who give evidence of some intellectual operations still persisting, are probably all part of a feigned death, with the delusion expressing itself in corpse-like behaviour.

Finally we must consider the meaning of the deep stupor where no mentation of any kind can be proven and where none but vegetative functions seem to be operating. This state is either one of organic coma, in which case it marks the appearance of a physical factor not evidenced in the milder stages, or else it is the acme of this regression by withdrawal of interest. As has been stated, back of the period of primitive childish ideas there lies a hypothetical state of mental nothingness. If we accept the principle of regression, we find an analogue, to what is apparently the mental state of deep stupor, in the earliest phases of infancy. This view receives justification from the study of the phenomenon of variations in symptoms. Mental faculties at birth are larval, and if such condition be artificially produced, mental activity must be potentially present (as it would not be if we were dealing with coma).

In discussing the memory of recovered cases, Hoch notes that isolated facts may be remembered when the rest is blank.

Anna K., for instance, while very vague about most occurrences, recalled a sudden angry outburst in detail. We can scarcely account for such phenomena in any other way than by assuming that certain influences may temporarily lift the patient out of the deepest stupor. In spite of stupors often lasting for one or two years almost without change, a fact which would argue that the stupor reaction is a remarkably set, stable state, we see in sudden episodes of elation that this is not the case, and other experiences point in the same direction. A similar observation was made on a case of typical stupor with marked reduction of activity and dullness. A rather cumbersome electrical apparatus (for the purpose of getting a good light for pupil examination) was brought to her bedside. Whereas before she had been totally unresponsive, she suddenly wakened up, asked whether " those things " would blow up the place, and whether she was to be electrocuted. During this anxious state she responded promptly to commands, but after a short time relapsed into her totally inactive condition. We have, of course, similar experiences when we try to get stuporous patients to eat, who, after much coaxing may, for a short time, be made to feed themselves, only to relapse into the state of inactivity.

Such variations are paralleled by a suddenly pronounced deepening of the thinking disorder. We have already seen that the onset may be quite sudden. All this indicates that, in sipte of a certain stability, sudden changes are not uncommon. Finally, we know that, notwithstanding the fact that stupor is an essentially affectless reaction, certain influences may produce smiles or tears, or, above all, angry outbursts, which, again, must be interpreted by assuming that such influences have temporarily produced a change in the clinical picture, in the sense of lifting the patient out of the depth of the stupor. All these facts suggest that inconsistencies in recollection are correlated with changes in the clinical picture.

One case is now of particular importance in demonstrating that an appropriate stimulus may dispel the vacuity of complete stupor by raising mental functions to a point where delusions are entertained. This patient retrospectively recalled only certain periods of her deepest stupor, occasions when she was visited by her mother. At these times, as she claimed, she thought she was to be electrocuted and told her mother so, adding, " Then it would drop out of my mind again ". Otherwise her memory for this state was a complete blank. Here we see a normal stimulus producing not normality but something on the way towards it, that is, a condition less profound than the state out of which the patient was temporarily lifted.

This case exemplifies the principle of levels in the stupor reaction which we have found to be of great value in all our study. These levels are correlated with degrees of regression, as a review of the symptoms discussed above may show. In the first place, the dissatisfaction with life, the first phase of regression, leads to the quietness—the inactivity and apathy—which is the most fundamental symptom of the stupor reaction as a whole. Initiative is lost and with this comes a tendency for the acceptance of other people's ideas. That is the probable basis for the suggestiveness which we concluded was a prominent factor in catalepsy. Indifference and stolidity may exist with those milder degrees of regression which do not conflict with one's critical sense, and hence may be present without any false ideas. The next stage in regression is that in which the idea of death appears. Although not accepted placidly by the subject, its non-acceptance is demonstrated by the idea being projected—by its appearance as a belief that the patient will be killed. This notion of death coming from without has again two phases : one with anxiety where normality is so far retained that the patient's instincts of self-preservation produces fear, and a second phase where this instinct reaction lapses and the patient so far accepts the idea of being killed as to speak of it with indifference. The next step in regression is marked by the spoiled-child conduct, interest being so self-centered as to lead to autoerotic habits and the perverse reactions which we call negativism. When death is accepted but mental function has not ceased, the latter is confined to a dramatization of death in physical symptoms or to such speech and movements as indicate a belief that the patient is dead, under the water, or in some such unreal situation. Finally, when all evidence of mentation in any form is lacking, we see clinically the condition which we know as deep stupor and which we must regard psychologically as the profoundest regression known to psychopathology, a condition almost as close to physiological unconsciousness as that of the epileptic.

Naturally we do not see individual cases in which all these stages appear successively each sharply defined from its predecessor. To expect this would be as reasonable as to look for a man whose behaviour was determined wholly by his most recent experience. Any psychologist knows that every human being behaves in accordance with influences whose history is recent or represent the habit of a life time. At any given minute our behaviour may not be simply determined by the immediate situation, but may be the product of many stages in our development. Quite similarly we should not expect in the psychoses to find evidences of regression to a given period of the individual's life appearing exclusively, but rather we should look for reactions at any given time being determined preponderantly by the type of mentation characteristic for a given stage of his development. As a matter of fact, we see in psychoses, particularly in stupor, more sharply defined regressions to different levels than we ever see a consistent domination in normal behaviour of one set of interests.

Our psychological hypothesis would be incomplete and probably unsound if it could not offer as valid explanations for the atypical features in our stupor reactions as for the typical. The unusual features which one meets in the benign stupors are ideas or mood reactions occurring apparently as interruptions to the settled quietude, or in more protracted mild mood reactions, such as vague distress, depression or incomplete manic symptoms. The interruptions are easily explained by the theory of regression. If stupor represents a complete return to the state of nothingness, then the descent to this Nirvana or the re-ascent from it should be characterized by the type of thinking with the appropriate mood, which belongs to less primitive stages of development. A review of our material seems to indicate that there is a definite relationship between the type of onset and the character of the succeeding stupor. For instance, in the cases quoted in Hoch's book, the onsets, characterized by mere worry and unhappiness and gradual withdrawal of interest, had all of them typical clinical pictures. On the other hand, of those who began with reactions of definite excitement, anxiety or psychotic depression, there were interruptions which looked like miniature manic-depressive psychoses (in all but one case). This would lead one to think that these patients retraced their steps on recovery, or, with every lifting of the stupor process, moved slightly upward on the same path which they had descended in the first regression. The case of Charlotte W. [Case 3], offers excellent examples of these principles.

The next atypical feature is the phenomenon of reduction or dissociation of affect. As the law of stupor is apathy, normal emotions should be reduced to indifference and no abnormal moods, such as elation, anxiety or depression, should occur. What often happens is that these psychotic affects appear but incompletely, often in dissociated manifestations. This looks like a combination of two psychotic tendencies, the stupor reduction process, which inhibits emotional response and the tendency to develop abnormal affects which characterize other manic-depressive psychoses.   There is no general psychological law which makes this view unlikely.   One cannot be anxious and happy at the same instant, although one can alternate in his feelings ; but one can fail to react adequately to a given stimulus when inhibited by general indifference.   In fact, it is because apathy is, properly speaking, not a mood, but an absence of it, that it can be combined with a true affect.   It is possible, therefore, to have a combination of stupor and another manic-depressive reaction, while the others tend to alternate rather than to combine.

Finally we must discuss the psychological meaning of such cases as seem superficially to resemble stupor, but prove on closer analysis not to belong to this group[1].   It seems likely that these patients are absorbed in their own thoughts, rather than in a condition of mental vacuity.   It is not difficult to explain the objective resemblance.   All evidence of emotion (apart from subjective feeling tone which the subject may or may not report) is an expression of contact with the outer world.   There must be externalization of attention to environment before a mood becomes evident.   A moment's reflection will show this to be true, for no further proof is needed than the phenomena of dreaming.   The attention being given wholly to fantasies, the subject lies motionless, mute and placid, although passing through varied autistic experiences.   Only when the dream becomes too vivid, disturbs sleep and re-directs attention to the environment—only then is emotion objectively betrayed.   There is an appearance of apathy and mental vacuity which the dreamer can soon declare to be false.   He was feeling and thinking intensely.   In any condition, therefore, such as that of perplexity or of an absorbed manic state, the patient may be objectively in the same condition as a typical stupor.   The histories of the two psychoses differentiate the two reactions, which may be indistinguishable at one interview.   The keynote of one reaction is *indifference*, while that of absorption is *distraction*, a perversion of attention to an inner, unreal world.[2]

In summary we may recapitulate our hypotheses.   Stupor represents, psychologically speaking, the simplest and completest regression.   Adaptation to the actual environment being abandoned, attention reverts to earlier interests, giving symptoms of other manic-depressive reactions in the onset or interruptions, and finally dwindles to complete indifference.   The disappearance of affective impulse leads to objective apathy and inactivity, while the intellectual functions fail for lack of emotional power to keep them going.

---

[1] A number of these will be described under the headings of absorbed mania and of perplexity states.

[2] This problem of " distraction " will be discussed at length in Chapter XXIII

The complicated mental machine lies idle for lack of steam or electricity. The typical ideational content and many of the symptoms of stupor are to be explained as expressions of death, for a regression to a Nirvana-like state can be most easily formulated in such a delusion. Other clinical conditions may temporarily and superficially resemble stupor on account of the attention being misdirected and applied to unproductive imaginations. To employ our metaphor again, in these false stupors the current is switched to another and invisible machine but not cut off as in true stupor.

So much for the technical, psychiatric aspects of the stupor problem. We have also spoken of it, however, as if it were a psychobiological reaction. If this be a sound view, similar tendencies should appear in everyday life, the psychotic phenomena being merely the exaggeration of a fundamental type of human and animal behaviour. Shamming of death in the face of danger and animal catalepsy come to mind at once, but since we know nothing of the associated affective states we should be chary of using them even as analogies. We are on safer ground in discussing problems of human psychology.

It is evident that there are psychological parallels between the stupor reaction and sleep, while future work may show physiological similarities as well. Apathy towards the environment, inactivity and a thinking disorder are common to both. But sleep reactions do not occur in bed alone. Weariness produces indifference, physical sluggishness, inattention and a mild thinking disorder such as are seen in partial stupors. The phenomena of the mid-day nap are strikingly like those of stupor. The individual who enjoys this faculty has a facility for retiring from the world psychologically, and, as a result of this psychic release, is capable of renewed activity (analogous to post-stuporous hypomania) that cannot be the result of physiological repair, since the whole affair may last for only a few minutes.

In everyday life there are more protracted states where the comparison can also be made. When life fails to yield us what we want, we tend to become bored—a condition of apathy and inactivity, forming a nice parallel to stupor inasmuch as external reminders of reality and demands for activity are apt to call out irritability. A form of what is really mental disease, although not called insanity, is permanent boredom, a deterioration of interest, energy and even intelligence by which many troubled souls solve their problems. A sudden withdrawal from the world we call stupor. When the same thing happens insidiously, the condition is labelled according to the financial and social status of the victim. He is a " bum ", a loafer, a mendicant, or, more politely, a disillusioned récluse. Frequently this undiagnosed dement has satisfied himself with a weak, cynical philosophy that life is not world while.

It is but a step from valueless life to death, and the same tendency which makes the patient fancy he is dead, leads the tired man to sleep, the poet to sigh in verse for dissolution, and the myth maker to fabricate rebirth. The religions of the world are full of this yearning, which reaches its purest expression in the belief and philosophy of Nirvana. The ideational content of stupor has also its analogue in crime. The desire for perpetuation of relationships unprosperous in this world is not seen only in the delusion of mutual death. One can hardly pick up a newspaper without reading of some unhappy man or woman who has slain a disillusioned lover and then committed suicide.

PART IV

THE INVOLUTION MELANCHOLIAS

On meurt deux fois, je le vois bien.
Cesser d'aimer et d'être aimable,
C'est une mort insupportable
Cesser de vivre, ce n'est rien.—VOLTAIRE.

Truly the desire for a long life hinder many from a happy life.
Exterminium Acediæ, FRANCIS NEUMAYR, 1755

CHAPTER XVI

SYMPTOMS AND TYPES OF INVOLUTION MELANCHOLIA

WE have seen that in the stupors unhappy situation may produce in the mentally unstable a regression with loss of energy and, as the regressive ideas are not combatted but accepted, a reaction of apathy. The mental content of the patients shows preoccupation with death, and to a less extent autoerotic practices and " spoiled-child " behaviour. Quite similar, even identical, regressions seem to take place in the Involution Melancholias. but the loss of energy seems to have, as a rule, more physical basis (senescence) than in the stupors, while the regressive ideas are not accepted and the struggle against them results in a clinical picture contrasting markedly, as a rule, with that of stupor. The essential difference is concerned with the disparity in age between the two groups. The stupor patients are the youngest of our manic depressive cases, while the melancholia reaction belongs more to the advancing years of life. A young person can play with the idea of death, but the instinct of self preservation is alert to defend the individual against what is a real and imminent danger in the later years of life. This is why essentially the same ideas may lead to quite different reactions at different age periods. So, instead of death ideas and autoeristism being accepted with apathy, reduction of mentation and onanistic practices, the melancholics usually react with dramatic fear of being killed, compensatory physical activity and hypochondria. It is our problem now to demonstate these processes and trace their evolution.

We have then two problems, a psychiatric and a psychological. The former has to do with the nosological positions of the various symptom complexes observed in the big group known as involution melancholia ; while the latter is concerned with the problem of detecting the types of regression, that may be observed, and relating them to the emotions produced and to the prognosis of each group. We may conveniently begin with discussion of the first problem.

Although involution melancholia, often spoken of merely as " melancholia " is one of the oldest of psychiatric groups, no settled opinion as to prognosis has obtained and the symptoms, pigeon-holed under this heading, are extremely diverse, often contradictory. Plainly the group is too large if it contain incompatible symptoms with variable prognosis. Some years ago the late Dr. Hoch set himself with my co-operation, to a solution of the problems thus presented. We secured data as to the final outcome in some 67 cases which he had examined about 20 years before. With this information as to the end results, we were in a position to classify symptoms in terms of prognosis and our conclusions have recently been published[1].

The clinical pictures presented in these cases (all of which were diagnosed as Involution Melancholia) are as follows :—

Most of the patients are in the sixth decade of life (the average age being 54.5 years) but do not suffer from physical disease affecting the central nervous system, except for a few among whom arterio-schlerosis advances beyond the stage normal for that age. Only one case showed symptoms, pointing unequivocally towards this process affecting the brain directly, and here, interestingly enough, convulsions were regularly followed by improvement of the melancholic symptoms.

The onset is gradual with complaints of a neurotic rather than of a psychotic nature. As a rule there is a definite precipitating cause : there is loss of money, or of a friend or member of the family. Sometimes the patient is worn out physically with some extra strain or is stricken with some acute somatic disease, not affecting the central nervous system. Worry begins, usually directed at the precipitating cause, so that the commonest topics of painful preoccupation are financial failure and loss of health. With this worry comes insomnia, adding its influence to a vicious circle. The patient gradually grows worse over a period of weeks or even months.

[1] Hoch and MacCurdy, " The Prognosis of Involution Melancholia ". *Archives of Neurology and Psychiatry*, Jan., 1922, Vol. VII., p. 1.

Then come the truly psychotic symptoms which may take a great variety of forms. There may be a marked feeling of unworthiness and sin with sadness and retardation and complaints of change in themselves and the world around. Or delusions may appear. These fall into two chief groups. The first is a belief in approaching death. The patient thinks he will be killed, cut up, hanged, burned alive and so on. Sometimes the death idea masquerades as a delusion of immortality : he can never die. Related probably with this idea of dissolution is a conviction that he will be left alone in the world, or that all his property is gone ; he and his family will be put on the street, or that he is really in a poor house, not a hospital. Again he may believe that he has been changed into an animal. Or all the world is changed, there is no more sun, nor trees, the trains run no more, etc.—the *délire de negation*. With such complaints the patient is apt to show dramatic exhibitions of fear and great rest- lessness or weep tumultuously. Sometimes the most naturally fearful ideas are spoken of quite calmly, the victim seeming to be indifferent or uttering his stereotyped plaint in a monotonous whine. The second group of delusions has to do with bodily change and disease. There are complaints of indigestion in all forms, of muscular weakness, pains and queer sensations. Frequently these ideas become extravagantly ridiculous or disgusting. The patient insists he is shrivelled up, only one foot high, that he is made of wire or porcelain, that his anus is stopped up (although his bowels move), that he cannot swallow, that his internal organs are all gone or are rotten, that his defecation is so stupendous that he has plugged up all the sewers in the country, or an odour proceeds from him that defiles the world. With this there may be shameless autoerotism, even going to the extent of pulling fæces out of the rectum, smearing the furniture and body and so on. These cases are apt also to show irritability and peevishness with kicking, scratching and foul language. They remind one inevitably of a spoiled child in a tantrum. Finally we see cases where there seems to be only a general washing out of all natural interests. There are few specific complaints, the patients just wander aimlessly around, whining, unoccupied and apathetic.

If all this welter of psychotic symptoms led invariably to recovery, or never did, we might be forced to consider them all as manifes- festations of one disease process, and pyshological interpretation of the various features would be futile. Yet this is the kind of description one finds in most text-books of psychiatry. Fortun- ately, we have found that certain symptoms are correlated with eventual recovery, while others seem rather inevitably associated with chronicity and further deterioration. This enables us to make some classification into different reaction types.

We have found that the prognosis may depend on the mood reaction, the behaviour, the type of ideas present or on combinations of these. For instance, if the thoughts of a patient are apparently dominated by ideas of violent death and yet he shows no emotional response in the form of fear or agitation, he will not recover. If he has ridiculous hypochrondriacal notions, the falsity of which is perfectly obvious, or if his attention be concentrated on his body with autoerotic indulgence, his case is hopeless. Or if he be persistently refractory, non-co-operative, spiteful, assaultive and destructive, his psychosis will endure until he dies. On the other hand, no matter how wicked a patient may feel, no matter how lurid may be his delusions of approaching murder or execution, his recovery may be expected, provided his emotional reaction is what one would expect it to be were his expectations justified and not false ideas. Similarly no matter how concerned he may be over his health the outlook is good, provided his theories of disease and complaints of symptoms do not assume an absurd form. That is, the hypochondria, except for its intensity, is like that seen in ordinary medical practice.

It is therefore possible to split the " melancholia " group into two great divisions, a recoverable and a chronic. Both can be re-divided as representing different kinds of processes. Of the chronic cases the majority show ridiculous delusions, indulgence in " infantile sexuality ", insufficient emotional reaction and antisocial conduct. All except the last are cardinal symptoms in dementia praecox, in which the last also occurs quite frequently. So it does not seem straining a point to regard these deteriorated individuals as suffering from dementia praecox, that appears late in life, and from a form of that disease, of complex and varying symptomatology, in which the symptoms are related to the age period of the patient.

The other subdivision of the non-recovering group is what Hoch used to call " Organic Insufficiency ". To quote from our paper : " A small but definite subgroup is that of patients who have what we have been accustomed to term organic insufficiency, since the whole picture seems to reflect a fundamental and general senescence rather than a localized cerebral abiotrophy with senile dementia or a largely psychogenic disturbance, such as characterizes so many of the involution melancholias. These cases usually begin with insomnia followed by a gradual loss of interest. If there are any self-accusations or paranoid or death ideas, these are in the background of the clinical picture. There are hyprochondriacal ideas, but these are usually concerned with the patients' condition in a vague, general way. Specific complaints are usually about constipation, with slight exaggeration, but they are never absurd or ridiculous. The patients usually wander aimlessly around whining, unoccupied and apathetic. Sometimes there is a mild restlessness—not accompanied by poor sleep, however, as in the benign cases. Organic insufficiency seems to have an invariably bad prognosis."

Having eliminated the chronic cases and their peculiar symptoms from the general mass of psychotic phenomena lumped together as involution melancholia, we can scrutinize the remaining symptoms.

In the first place we find many cases that have a clinical picture in no essential respect differing from that of the depressions of the manic-depressive type seen in earlier years. Such patients complain of feeling sad, hopeless, wicked, incapacitated, and of things seeming unreal to them, while objectively there are signs of physical and mental sluggishness and an appearance of dejection in attitude and facial expression. If delusions are present they are concerned with the moral failure of the patient, while hallucinations are extremely rare. Sometimes we see too in the involution period " reactive depressions " like those of youth and middle age, where the patient's attention is mainly concentrated on some unhappy event the constant memory of which excites great lamentation, the other depressive symptoms (remorse, retardation, unreality, etc.) being in the background. When such reactions occur in the later years of life, there is no reason for calling them involution melancholia. The psychological mechanisms of these typical depressions are discussed later in this book so we need not tarry longer with them now.

After this analysis and classification we are finally left with what is still numerically a large group, in which a fairly consistent symptomatology may be observed. These are the cases showing fears of impending death, often with great agitation and restlessness. These ideas may be distorted into delusions of immortality, of the judgment day having come or of the world being changed. In this class are also to be found poverty ideas. Or, on the other hand, the patient's attention may be focused more persistently on fancied bodily disease, with complaints tending to represent mere intensification of ordinary hypochondriacal symptoms, rather than to develop into grotesque and autoerotic fancies. The essentials of this, which we would call true involution melancholia, are fear of dissolution and change, or concern over physical health, or both. Intellectual operations are relatively immune ; the patients remain well oriented and so on. Judgment, however, when it would conflict with insistent false ideas, is faulty or absurd, and consequent misinterpretations of the environment are frequent. Often there are vivid hallucinations described.

We believe that this group represents a definite manic-depressive reaction type just as do mania, ordinary depression, stupor, and so on. There are four reasons for this.

In the first place the reaction is essentially psychogenic. Appearing so often in the declining years of life, when physical disease is apt to be manifest or suspected, one's first conjecture would be that these cases show symptoms in the mental field that are merely evidences of anatomic or metabolic changes. If no other pathology could be invoked the endocrine glands would be blamed. There is a wide-spread impression that among women the menopause, with its unquestional endocrine revolution, is responsible for involution melancholia, while a similar climacteric is presumed to take place among men. One cannot lightly dispose of such arguments and, in fact, one cannot frame an adequate psychological theory of the disease without presuming physical degeneration to be present in some vague way. But we are without any hint as to its specific nature. For instance, we were rather surprised to find among our female cases that the tendency was for the definite psychosis not to appear till five or ten years after the menopause. It seems more usual for the " change of life " to produce a neurosis rather than a frank mental disturbance. Indeed the cases occurring at this period were apt to show a somewhat different symptomatology.

There are, too, specific arguments in favour of its being essentially a psychological reaction. There usually is some definite, mental, precipitating cause, and specific ideas appear, with which the other symptoms seem to be related. There are, on the other hand, no physical evidences of any specific physical disease. In fact, in one of our cases, somatic disturbances produced apparently amelioration of symptoms. The patient's mental condition regularly improved after each of a series of cerebral attacks ! Finally we can rule out of consideration any morbid process affecting the cerebral cortex directly, because the intellectual functions (always disturbed in " organic " psychosis) remain unaltered.

Secondly there can be no question but that this is a form of emotional insanity with a good prognosis and that patients with such symptoms are often classified as " depressions " (for instance by Kraepelin). On the other hand such classification makes " depression " a collection of varied and inconsistent symptoms. It is true that many melancholics are frequently sad and feel they are wicked, while many depressives may have episodes of anxiety. But at the same time the extremes of these two types do not mix and show phenomena so different as to make their co-existence an impossibility. No one could be paralysed with despair, remorse, and conviction of sin and at the same time melodramatically agitated with delusions (and hallucinations) of destruction. The deeply depressed individual welcomes any thought of approaching death. We recognise reaction types by their extremes, not in their dilute forms, which may be interrupted by the exhibitions of some other kind of reaction. For instance, anyone may be laughing gaily and spontaneously one minute and be sorrowful the next, when some reminder comes of a forgotten grief. But no psychiatrist has ever seen a florid manic turn in a minute's time into a retarded depression. We can see gradations from normal happiness up to frank mania, or from normal remorse to true retarded depression, and can recognise their relationships. But we would never think of these normal phenomena as emotional reaction types did we never encounter their exaggerations. This is what justifies us in establishing the involution melancholia reaction as a separate type from depression—its complete dissimilarity in full development.

The third reason is that this syndrome appears at all ages. It is true that it occurs most frequently and in purest form in the

6th decade, yet it is not uncommon to find, in the more depressive of the manic depressive psychoses of early life, brief episodes in which the symptoms are identical with those we are now considering. Moreover, we occasionally see in a young person an entire psychosis consist of these symptoms. Such a case will be described later. In a word " Involution Melancholia " is a collection of phenomena that appears whenever a certain type of regression occurs. This regression is most apt to happen in the advanced years of life for reasons shortly to be discussed, but the setting in which it is precipitated may develop at any time.

Finally, this psychotic type may alternate with other manic depressive reactions in the same two ways that the others do. That is, a patient with recurrent insanity may have this year a typical depression or manic attack and next year an involution melancholia. Or, during the same illness, the patient may begin with involution symptoms that give way to those of mania, then of depression or of stupor. Every characteristic, therefore, by which we recognize a manic-depressive reaction type is to be found in this syndrome.

CHAPTER XVII

TYPICAL CASES

AFTER this introduction in may be well to cite the digests of some case histories, in order to show the usual forms, which the involution melancholia reaction assume. It should be borne in mind that, with one exception, these patients were examined about twenty years or more ago, at a time when " psychogenesis " was not much talked about and little effort was made to fill in the psychological picture by stimulating the patient with pertinent questions. The records, therefore, are not so complete as they might be. but, on the other hand, they represent evidence secured merely by faithful observation, undirected by any theory. The consistency, with which certain ideas reappear, is, it would seem, all the more striking.

The first case shows how, out of a mild depression, with which were associated the involution ideas oɪ poverty and bodily disease, a dramatic anxiety state appeared, when the belief in imminent death developed.

CASE 4. *George L.* was a retired business man, aged 61 and married, when he was examined twenty-five years ago.

F.H. One uncle was insane, otherwise no data were recorded.

P.H. No description of his personality is given. In his youth he suffered a syphilitic infection. At the age of 31 he had a well-marked attack of depression, during which he believed he had syphilis of the throat.

During the half-year preceding his admission he lost some money and three months before admission began to worry over trifles. Then he became depressed, although somewhat restless ; he thought he was going to be poor, disgraced, and that people on the street looked at him. A short time before admission the old idea of his having syphilis of the throat recurred. He began to sleep badly, lost weight, and was said to be suicidal.

On admission no neurological or vascular anomalies were discovered, but he had a coated tongue, and chronic pharyngitis and laryngitis. It may have been these physical troubles which determined the specific idea of syphilis of the throat.

For the first two weeks he was depressed, staying constantly in his own room. He complained of utter hopelessness and spoke of his being an outcast, of his speedy removal to a poorhouse and, most prominently, of his syphilitic throat infection. Then during the next six weeks his condition improved particularly towards the evening of each day, although he always wanted to lie abed in the mornings. Then, two months after coming under observation, restlessness took the place of lethargy and with this there was definite apprehensiveness. At first he was merely afraid that he would be left alone to die, but soon he began to think that he would be killed, burned, drowned, strangled, or cut to pieces. Any kind of chance event would be interpreted as a preparation for his distruction and he even heard the people in the ward talk about killing him. With this he was much agitated and also suicidal. Soon fluctuations in the acuteness of his symptoms began to appear and in a little more than four months after admission he was entirely well. Eight years later he reported that he had been perfectly well and cheerful ever since leaving the hospital.

In our second case we have a man who was for some time restless and apprehensive in a vague way. From his suspiciousness it seemed likely that that he feared bodily harm would come to him and that he would be murdered. At first he either refused to admit this, or else it was not fully conscious. Later, however, in a setting of great agitation, this idea came to open expression.

CASE 5. *Charles B.* was an unmarried business man, 56 years of age.

F.H. Grandparents and parents had been normal. Of nine aunts and uncles, one aunt had a " nervous, opinionated and melancholic temperament ". Of three siblings one sister had had " puerperal insanity ".

P.H. The patient's personality was described as normal. He had had two previous attacks of depression. The first was when he was 23 ; it only lasted a few weeks and he was able to keep on working. The second occurred when he was 52. He then lost considerable money, became sad, could not attend to anything, lay in bed saying nothing, thought he would never be well again, and had to be urged to eat. In three months he was quite well again. After this he took up a new business. With this he was, with labile alternations, quite enthusiastic or gloomy.

Three months before admission he began to worry again over some poor investments and quickly became depressed. He began to sit about silently. At times he would be restless and talk of his going to rack and ruin. Gradually he began to think that everybody was against him.

On admission he was found to be in fair physical condition. He had a high blood pressure and two finely granular casts were discovered in his urine, but there was no other evidences of vascular or renal disease. His pupils showed some irregularity of outline and of reaction to light.

At the first few examinations it was difficult to get much out of him on account of his restlessness, suspiciousness and reticence. It was hard to say whether there was any retardation in addition to these other factors. In spite of frequent refusal to answer questions and invariable delay in so doing, it was evident that he was quite clear as to his surroundings. The most noticeable thing was his restlessness, sometimes becoming true agitation, as when he would get up, lift his chair and set it down heavily. Often he kept on saying " Oh my God ! " with a facial expression of woe and anxiety and wringing of his hands. Again he would breathe fast as if frightened. Frequently he seemed suspicious, would taste water before drinking it, or look suspiciously at the physician's note-book. Once he said the water was poisoned and, when his watch, etc., were taken from him on admission, he thought he would never get them back. After much questioning he admitted worrying because he ought to be at home and also having an indefinite dread that something was going to happen to him. At the same time he blamed himself for not having attended to his business properly. He said he was nervous and could not apply his mind well.

Then about two weeks after admission his agitation became pronounced. He would ring his hands, shout incoherent sounds at the top of his voice, break glass, throw the furniture about. He accused the nurses of trying to poison him and struck one of them. Once he came to the physician and spoke to him in a low ·oice so that the nurses could not hear : " They are going to harm me and put me under the ground ! . . . The nurses are going to burn me ; they have stolen my money ! . . . Last night the doctor signed the certificate to have me buried ! " He could not be reassured, often reiterating, " They think I have money ; they are going to murder me and

L

make it out I have committed suicide ! " All this time he appeared alert and fearful, watching the nurses carefully. He would answer no questions.

For two months this state continued. Then he quieted down and, for the further three weeks he was in the hospital, began to occupy himself and played games. But an undercurrent of suspicion remained as, for instance, when taking his blood pressure made him apprehensive. At no time would he discuss his condition frankly, although in other respects his talk and actions were quite normal. His family reported that within a couple of months after returning home he became quite his old self again, gained weight and seemed in perfect mental and physical health.

The next case, which is more complicated, had, as its most prominent feature ideas of negation with bewilderment and apprehension. At times there were more than hints that the fancied changes in the world around were projections of a belief in the patient's own dissolution and bodily change (for he was hypochondriacal as well). When delusions about his own undoing came directly to expression, he became markedly agitated. Another interesting thing was that he was much absorbed in his thoughts and with this was mildly disoriented. Discussion of the psychology of this correlation must be postponed till consideration is reached of " distraction of thought " in absorbed manic, and in perplexity states. It will be necessary to give a fairly detailed digest of the case history in order to present the picture with accuracy.

CASE 6. *George P.* was a married clergyman aged 49.

F.H. No data were secured.

P.H. According to friends who knew him intimately, the patient was universally well-liked because of his kindness, politeness and tact. On the other hand his intellectual endowments were not great and this, added to lack of any business judgment, led to his progressive decline professionally. He was frequently shifted from one parish to another, each time gaining a smaller congregation and a smaller stipend. Both he and his wife were keenly aware of this degradation and for years he had been a disappointed man, growing gradually more dissatisfied with himself and his life. About 18 months before his admission his wife, for years an invalid, became seriously ill and required an operation. This was a great shock to him.

Ten months before admission he lost 2,000 or 3,000 dollars in poor investments and at the same time had another disappointment in connection with a change of parish. This precipitated a definitely pathological condition with insomnia, worry over his pecuniary loss and a despondent conviction that he would never get well. After a month of this depressive invalidism, he was sent to a private sanitorium when his condition improved for some time. Then six months before admission he made a determined suicidal attempt. One month before admission he became suddenly agitated with wild hypochondriacal fancies and ideas of negation. He said he was filled up and could not swallow and that his anus was stopped up ; also that all the people in the world were dead and that no more newspapers were being published, etc. [These hypochondriacal delusions are of a type we have found to be associated with a bad prognosis when they are persistent. Here, however, they appeared only in one episode of agitation and, besides, we have no evidence that they were not expressed as similies although recorded as beliefs].

On admission he was found to have no physical anomalies of any significance. It is particularly important to note that careful examination failed to reveal any localized sensory disorders, although his complaints might have led one to suspect them.

For about two weeks his condition was as follows : He lay in bed un-occupied, occasionally moaning to himself ; when spoken to he replied in a whining way not suggestive of true, deep sadness nor yet of real fear. When asked what he thought of all the time, he said : " Of the noises—you—the other men—I don't want them to hurt me ". The only other remarks ex-hibiting apprehension were his frequent statements that it hurt him when he was touched, to which he would add, " Don't touch me, don't come near me ! " Further hyprochondriacal complaints were that the nurses had destroyed his power to swallow by giving him food, and that it was impossible for him to eat. A number of hyprochondriacal notions were combined with negation ideas, the latter being the most prominent delusions, although it could be seen that they were usually a projection and extension, of his own feelings. For instance, he said it was not necessary to eat, no one in the ward ate. Or, " I used to think I had brothers and sisters like myself, but I haven't. I wished I were like them. They are like you, they come and go, they don't eat and they don't drink." The projection element in his negations was well shown in consecutive remarks beginning with complaints as to his changed sensations. He suddenly put his hand into his arm-pit and said " Put your hand here, and see how different I am ; you are not so. You would not feel it, if I did that to you ". Then he put out his tongue—" You couldn't show your tongue like that. Do you breathe ? Have you a pulse ? " Or when talking of his inability to eat, he said it was not necessary, no one did it—" Men like you don't eat." Then he pointed at another physician and said, " He lives as he is." Without any manifest connection with his hypochondria were other negation remarks. For instance, on seeing a flag outside he said : " Well, now, that's funny ; I used to think there were lots of countries and there is only one, and I used to think there were lots of people, but there are only a few—only I." When asked later if he really thought there were no countries, he replied, " I am afraid so," and to a question as to what had become of them he could anly answer, " There never were any ". These negations naturally affected his orientation as he tended to deny the existence of the hospital, but, after much urging and his giving of false names, he finally found the right one. He knew the physician for a doctor, but could not recall his name, and insisted a doctor he had known before had been changed. He was over two weeks out in his time relations, and thought he had been in the hospital for two weeks, when he had been admitted only six days before. Similarly he was slow and inaccurate in his calculations. On the other hand, he could give a fairly full and accurate account of his past life.

During the next month new ideas appeared which affected his behaviour. These were that he was going to be carried into a dark place, and that there he would fall down and break to pieces. With this he was at first agitated, pacing about the room, running his hands through his hair, screwing up his face and whining repeatedly, " Oh you mustn't carry me down to that dark place ! " Sometimes he would let himself fall on the floor, and say he was too weak to get up again. Very often he would refuse to get away from the security of his bed, fearing that he was to be taken to the dark place. He would say, " I can't see in the dark." When told that no one could see in the dark, he replied, " Yes, you can ; but you come and go. I am tangible. I have something all the time and it hurts me ".

Towards the latter end of this period he showed less agitation and more of a whining, stereotyped repetition of his apprehension. Sometimes he spoke of impulses to throw himself over the foot of his bed or on to the stone floor of a passageway to another building. He would refuse to leave his bed and room, and efforts to reassure him only led to more expression of negation. For instance, he would say : " You don't understand ; of course you don't : I am the only being in the world. You and the others are only mere shadows." Then he touched the physician and went on : " It seems real but it isn't ; you are just a shadow while I am a being with feelings and emotion. You have no feelings ; nothing can hurt you. I can't understand it. I am all at sea. You have no fear." (The last statement seems a pretty good indication of the negation ideas being connected with thoughts of the difference between others and himself, at least of a difference in feelings). At the same interview he complained of hearing nothing but voices talking of taking him down into the stone-floored passageway.

Then for two weeks he showed considerable improvement ; he began to occupy himself, did some work in the wood-carving class, and his absurd statements became less frequent. At the same time his former ideas appeared in diluted form. For instance, he said he was very delicate, and that he would suffer terribly if sent down the stairs (the trip he previously feared) with insufficient clothing. The negation delusion of his being real and other shadows persisted in the form that he would never die, but be left alone on the earth. This was to be a punishment for his misdeeds. Although this fancy could be shaken by argument, it could not be dislogded. He now gave a retrospective account of his ideas and feelings. The only additions to what had been noted from his utterances were his belief that his wife shared in the general dissolution of things, and that the nurses were spirits who could go through closed doors. (This shows that in this case the negation ideas were an expression of the death delusions projected on to the rest of the world, as they so often are).

The improvement did not endure, however. He began to be uneasy, wanting reassurance that he would not become ill again. After a week of this mere uneasiness he became quite restless, wringing his hands, crying and saying, " Oh, must that dreadful past come again, those horrible delusions I had about myself and others ? " A few days later he made a determined effort at suicide by throwing himself down the stairs, of which he had previously expressed such fear.

His restlessness gradually increased so that he would fling his arms into the air, clutch at the doctor's arm, rush about the room, throw himself on the floor or gestulate wildly. He rubbed the hair off one part of his head. Owing to his intense agitation, it was difficult to get an idea of the nature of his ideas or of his grasp on the surroundings. Usually, however, he spoke of a fear that he would injure people, and beg that it might be prevented. Once when a little quieter, he remarked, " I don't realize my condition at times ; I can't help giving away to these terrible feelings ". This state of violent agitation continued for about three months, and necessitated his being tube fed. It was also impossible to keep him properly dressed or shaved.

This dramatic distress continued for three months and then he began to recover slowly. First his excitement became episodic and appeared at longer and longer intervals. Then the interval condition improved. At the beginning he was whining and unoccupied, although he would talk. But as time went on he occupied himself more, talked more freely and gradually gained more and more insight. As soon as he became communicative, a wealth of negation ideas were recounted. Everything had been changed : the cars didn't run, time was shorter, " An hour is only ten minutes," " The seasons are so short that the fruits can't ripen " ; no one in the hospital slept ; patients did not eat, because they did not go to the dining room ; there wasn't enough to eat, there was no food in the country because the land was not cultivated as it used to be ; no more business was done ; when his relatives came to see him they never got home again, for they went out into the cold and fell down ; when his wife visited him she was not his wife because she was dead.

Many of these ideas were, quite plainly, projected expressions of his inner feelings. For instance, the delusion, that his relations went outside and fell down, was correlated with the desire that he himself might go outside and fall down because he was so worthless and ought not to be known about. This last had a trivial origin highly typical of the delusions of involution melancholics. Before coming to the hospital a doctor told him he ought not to talk about himself, should not let people know of his troubles, which he interpreted as meaning that his worthlessness should be hidden. A result of this idea was that he was constantly oscillating between an impulse to go out and an equally compulsive desire to be locked up in his room.

Then, too, a variety of apprehensions were expressed. He said he was in fear all the time but that it was more intense in his spells of agitation. He thought patients were being tortured when they were set to work ; they had teeth knocked out, some had stiff legs, others crooked toes. Such things would be done to him. He was going to be put on a paralytic's bed. When the nurse said he would cut the patient's finger nails, that meant he would cut off his fingers. When his pillow was pounded, it meant that he would be pounded. When somebody said " lobster," that meant he would be boiled alive. Once he heard some noise downstairs and enquired what it was. The nurse said it was the hopper. This was interpreted as meaning that there was a hopper in which human bodies were ground up. This, together with the strangeness of the place, made him think that the buildings, the rocks outside, the furniture and even the food was human flesh. A chair, he said, had not been in the room before, and that it must have been made out of the suffering body of someone. Moreover, he said that the colour of the furniture suggested human flesh as did the compressibility of the arm of a willow chair. Food was human flesh because a nurse once brought him his dinner and said, " Now eat her up." Even when insight was returning, he could not throw off the idea for a long time that fish was human flesh.

Another thing that troubled him was that when he thought of people they appeared. He gave several instances of this and added, " It is a strange power of thought ; I hope it isn't true."

Finally all his ideas were corrected, his natural interest in outside affairs returned and he became normal once more. His whole psychosis lasted for more than two and a quarter years.

We shall next consider some hypochondriacal cases. Hypochondria is, of course, more frequently a neurotic, than a psychotic, symptom, and at times it is difficult to draw the line between the two. It seems essentially to be a question of degree. In the psychotic patient, attention is so exclusively focused on bodily ills that all, or nearly all, sane thoughts are in abeyance. With this there is a tendency for complaints to assume an exaggerated form plainly in conflict with reality. When this tendency is so developed that the ideas are utterly ridiculous, the prognosis is apt to be bad. As intelligent laymen know, every hypochondriac regards his symptoms as being matters of social interest ; in the insane cases this self-centredness is magnified in two ways ; preoccupation with the body may be expressed in autocrotic (and often filthy) practices, while self importance leads to irritable rejection of social overtures. This may be so pronounced that the patients will object to having anything done for them by nurses or doctors.

The first case to be cited complained of many morbid sensations and showed great distress. The latter contained an element of fear, as will appear, for she fancied her illnesses might have a fatal termination.

CASE 1. *Cora O.* was a married housewife, aged 39.

F.H. One grandfather was a heavy drinker. One brother (in a large family) disappeared in the West. Otherwise there was no record of any mental abnormability in the stock.

P.H. The patients' disposition was not described. She was married sixteen years before her breakdown to a frivolous travelling salesman. He was coarse and inconsiderate, initiating many " scenes " and rendering home life most unhappy. She had had four children and two miscarriages. About a year before admission her father died and she worried over the settlement of his estate.

About four months before admission the patient began gradually to neglect her household and her own appearance, seeming to take little interest in anything. At about the same time she began to eat poorly and looked generally run-down. After a month of this dilapidation, acute symptoms began. These took the form of attacks, usually at night, when she would writhe on the bed, complain of various sensations and scream out such remarks as, " Go for help ! " " You can't hold me ! " " Kill me ! " " Oh, I'll do something ! " " Help ! " In one of these panics she tried to swallow pins apparently with suicidal intent. She often pinched herself and pulled her mouth out of shape. The day before admission she constantly thought the house was on fire and would be burned up.

On admission she was found unkempt and with many bruises, obviously undernourished, but with no other physical abnormalities that could be detected. She was always distressed and often restless. She would toss about in bed, kick off the coverings, throw her arms about. Sometimes she would even jump out of bed, run to the window, and say she would throw herself out. Irritability was also present, for she struck, scratched and kicked the nurses. Spontaneously she made many complaints and offered more in answer to questions. She protested, " I can't stay in this place ; I am vile, poisoned inside." She spoke of her insides seeming to drop out of her, of her throat being contracted, of her head feeling full and her legs cold. Frequently she put her hand to her throat and when asked how her head felt, said, " It feels as big as a bass drum, stopped up with something, and something in it boiling all the time." It was difficult to get her attention and hence impossible to guage her orientation with accuracy. She seemed to know where she was, to recognise people she had met the day before and to know roughly how long she had been in the institution. Nevertheless, she made the remark, " I am awful bad this afternoon," although she had previously said correctly that it was morning. Apparently her attention was wandering, for she said, " I don't seem to grasp thoughts quickly, I can't apply my mind to anything." But she also made this curious statement : " I have got one with me who puts answers into my mind, it comes with the suggestion," and then, when a question was asked, she replied, " You told me with your thoughts, your thoughts come to me." The following shows how this disturbance operated. She was told to subtract 3 from 22. " No, don't try to fool me. These thoughts come to me from you. I haven't been able to do anything like that for weeks and weeks—3 from 22 —3 from 22—oh, can't you relieve me, can't you relieve me ? It leaves 19, I guess. Can't you relieve that ? " (clutching at her throat). The question of 3 from 19 was then put. Continuing in restless distress she replied, " 16, now you make me do that ! " (16—3 ?) " 13, I guess. I can't put my thought to it." But when asked 13 from 3 she said at once, " You can't take 13 from 3 ".

After a couple of days she became quieter although her restlessness did not entirely disappear. There was no longer any doubt as to her orientation being perfect, and the complaint of her thoughts being suggested to her was heard no more. Still, she continued to look distressed and poured out her complaints. The chief of these was that she felt numb all over, particularly in the head, as if she were paralysed and feared she was going to die. The last would be the result of choking or suffocation. There was a constriction in her throat as if someone were pressing it tightly and squeezing her eyes out of their sockets. There were noises in her head, " as though they were pounding in it ". Then she had a variety of complaints about her gastro-intestinal tract. She felt as if her tongue were being pulled down her throat ; everything tasted bitter and there were sharp prickles in her throat ; she felt filled up ; again she felt hollow, even after eating, but her food seemed to want to come up again and choke her (she did vomit frequently). Often she complained of a fear that she would have a fit, become paralysed, lose her mind and be put in another place. Occasionally she struck the nurses, but as a rule her irritability was controlled.

This state continued for two weeks at the end of which she was so much improved as to give a retrospective account. She told of having had for some time sick headaches. These began with flitting scotomata and were followed by vomiting. Such sensations became so severe that she was obsessed with fear of paralysis and losing her mind. She assigned the carelessness at home to this preoccupation. In the hospital the fear continued and was usually accompanied by the idea that they would move her to another ward. Once she thought she was to be put into a box.

Complete recovery came only ten weeks after this, however, for there were frequent relapses to all the old symptoms, lasting sometimes for hours, days or even more than a week. They became rarer, and shorter till they finally disappeared altogether and she was perfectly normal. Even then she insisted that all her troubles began and were due to the sensations in her head and the fear of their consequences. Paralysis, of course, is an idea akin to that of death. But by translating this latter apprehension into terms of bodily disease she may have developed her hypochondria and changed fear into the milder emotion of distress.

The next case illustrates a kind of hypochondria not infrequently observed, in which the patient uses " insane ideas " as complaints as well as bodily sensations. In this particular case, as sometimes happens the patient became finally so absorbed in these fancies that they took on the " reality " of delusions, being no longer mere complaints. It is perhaps to be correlated with this that she recovered by way of a manic phase.

CASE 8. *Mary H.* was a woman of no occupation, aged 54. She had been married but her husband deserted her.

F.H. One grandmother was insane for two years at the menopause. One aunt had a depression lasting for 14 years. The patient's father deserted his family. One sister was in a mental hospital apparently with a chronic psychosis. Another sister had recently had a typical manic depressive attack.

P.H. As an infant the patient was delicate and subject to digestive troubles. Throughout her life she was never regarded as robust and had frequent illnesses ; yet, at the time of her breakdown, there was no objective evidence of her not enjoying good health physically. In disposition she was described as kind, gentle, and not at all excitable. She lived at home till she was sixteen, when she was married and then lived with her husband on a farm up to the age of 34. He turned out to be a rascal, and at that time ran off with another man's wife, never being heard of directly again. For the next twenty years the patient lived with her sister and seemed to recover from the shock of her desertion quite satisfactorily, taking an apparently normal interest in life and being moderately happy.

About three years before admission, however (when 51 years of age) she began to be introspective and hypochondriacal. She complained greatly of her stomach, " creeping nerves ", insomnia, and what not. This condition grew gradually worse, and after about nine months of it she took to her bed. She became blue, did not care to see anybody but a doctor (whom she wanted with her all the time). She said people did not understand her and that she would never get better, yet insisted that something be done for her continually. After several months of this she had to be taken to a hospital for mental diseases where she remained for two years, that is, up to the time of her admission.

From the history furnished by this hospital, it seemed that she improved for a while, but after a couple of months became excited, agitated, noisy and violent. She chewed up her eye-glasses, apparently with suicidal intent. She also complained of queer thoughts, such as that she had to chew up snakes' heads or that she would be chained up in a pit. These were not true delusions, for she retained insight. After a few weeks of this excitement she quieted down into a state of depressive restlessness and was said to be very suicidal. A year later she had pneumonia, which temporarily increased her depression and suicidal tendency, but after it she improved so much that for six months she was apparently normal. In fact she rather enjoyed the hospital life, was given some small responsibilities and was rather looked up to by other patients. About ten days before admission there was talk of her going back to live with her sister. This she did not wish to do, because she objected to life on the farm, could not get on with her sister and did like the hospital. So she immediately began to complain of weakness, took to her bed with many complaints, all of which she urged as reasons why she should not leave, this being preferable to hurting her sister's feelings by direct statement of her antipathy to her old mode of living. On the morning of admission her sister came to fetch her, whereupon she began to scream out expostulations of weakness and incapacity to move. Instead of going home she was taken to the hospital, where her case was observed.

On admission : For two weeks she lay quietly in bed talking interminably about her bodily ills in a weak languid voice, whenever she could get an auditor. She said her head ached so severely that it seemed as if it would crack open, and she had excruciating pain and a throbbing sensation all up and down her spine. When she bent her head forward all her nerves were set tingling and she was sent quivering like a jelly-fish. She felt as if her stomach and intestines had dropped down. If she made an effort to do anything, even to think, it increased all her evil sensations to an intolerable degree. Her mind was usually a blank, for she had lost her memory and power to think. She also complained of seeing things with her eyes shut after having been watching them. This she regarded as a sign of approaching insanity. When an attempt was made to reassure her as to this, she seemed to resent it. She also expressed great anxiety about her sister's mental condition. fearing that the latter was apt to have another breakdown. She did not hesitate to say, however, that one element in this worry was as to what would become of herself, if her sister did have another attack.

Then, rather suddenly, in the middle of the night an excitement appeared. She became very restless, noisy, threw her bed-clothes off so that she carelessly exposed herself, waked her arms about and moaned. Her speech was no longer languid but energetic and " agonising.". The old hypochondriacal fancies had not departed, but the focus of her attention was on a new group of symptoms. She said when examined the next day, that during the night she had had hallucinations which occurred mostly with her eyes shut, but also when they were open. She saw flames of fire and again a great sheet of flame as if the whole side of the room were ablaze ; then there were snakes with great big eyes and snakes of fire and hideous beasts with the heads of men and eyes that leered at her. She described all these as imaginations, but insisted she was a crazy woman, completely mad in a way never known before ; she feared she was going to be a mad dog. She begged to be put in restraint before she should injure herself or others. So she ran on indefinitely, invariably returning to the theme of her madness, if interrupted by questions on other topics. She had no apprehension as to anything except her condition.

During the next two weeks she achieved a good deal of what seemed to be her ambition. She became so wrought up, so engrossed in her ideas that she lost contact with the environment (as could be plainly seen) and seemed to have, occasionally at least, true delusions and hallucinations. With this, too, her abnormal thoughts became more varied and more intense, leading to genuine emotional reactions This much could be observed during her excitement. Once during this period she became quiet and occupied for a short time and, at the close of it, she was quiet and gloomy during the days, although still restless and moaning at night. Then even the nocturnal disturbance abated. The following account was gained both by direct observation and from her retrospective story.

When most wrought up she spoke of burning up, of going blind, and of worms crawling over her. Many painful thoughts passed through her mind, that seemed as if they came from without, and which she therefore sometimes thought she heard. At the same time there were occasional vivid auditory hallucinations. For instance, a voice once said, " Mary H., come here ! " which she took to be the voice of the head Devil. Again, she heard a man drive up to the door in order to take her off and murder her. The thoughts which came to her were of her sister being in a hospital for the insane, of her sister being blind, of her sister being electrocuted for murder and of people coming to murder the patient herself. In the same way she was told of a friend of hers being murdered, and she claimed to hear an explosion. Once she thought the hospital was an " opium joint ". Again, when she was asked what was in her mind, she ran on as follows : " What is the world governed by ? Why was I born ? Why was I made ? God, I have sinned ? . . . Suffered ? I can't die ; I must live ! Am I to blame ? What am I to blame for ? Where am I to be ? Where shall I go ? Who is pulling this earth to pieces ? Why was I made different from other people ? " etc. As she sat pouring out similar interrogatories to Destiny, as it were, she would sometimes speak what seemed to be answers to her questions, such as, " You will be blind ! You will be electrocuted ! " With all this she seemed to be suffering a great deal with real distress and true fears. It was evident from her statements that she was quite clouded and definitely disorientated, thinking she was in a different hospital, etc.

After a few days her conduct became normal. She went out for walks, read, occupied herself moderately and so on. But for a year she complained of fatigue and debility, of exertion bringing on the old pains and tingling. However, she was not aggressively eager to publish her woes. In fact, she presented the typical picture of a hypochondriacal neurosis rather than psychosis. A year later she again took to her bed with bodily complaints, but this time soon developed a typical manic state with elation, flight of ideas, over activity and misidentification. This lasted only a short time and then her recovery was complete. The total length of her psychosis, including remissions, was four and one half years.

The next case illustrates nicely the transition from a retarded depression to an involution melancholia type of reaction. In a later chapter it will be seen that with depression there are antisocial ideas (chiefly of injury to other people) with self blame and an instinctive effort to stifle these thoughts, that leads to an inhibition of mental activity in general. When she first came under observation this patient had such a reaction and little could be got out of her. Then self blame began to merge over into thoughts of punishment and, with the latter, fear appeared, first episodically, later as a continuous reaction. With the fear came, as always, some lifting of the inhibition, and the harassing ideas came to expression. As in all border line and ill-defined psychoses her thoughts were much in flux giving a varied picture and leaving her in much uncertainty as what she did think. When they were formulated as injury to others she was depressed, when the accent was placed on the fate in store for her she was terrified.

CASE 9. *Mary B.* was a married woman, aged 59.

F.H. There was no information about the patient's grandparents or collateral relatives. Her father became depressed and committed suicide. This, in turn, depressed her mother, who also took her own life. Two brothers and a sister were said to be normal.

P.H. She was described as energetic, but conscientious, and given to worry. A grammatical mistake in Sunday School produced a sleepless night. There had been no previous attacks. The menopause came at 48 ; her sleep was then poor and she was a bit unstable emotionally, but not much was thought of it.

Six months before admission the patient's sleep was broken owing to her nursing her sick husband. Three months later her capacity was no longer equal to attending to all her household duties and she began to worry over this inadequacy. A depression gradually developed out of this, in which she spoke of her parents' fate, and of her losing her mind. She became quite idle and cried much.

On admission she was found to be in a state of fair nutrition ; she had some tremor of her tongue and fingers but no other abnormalities were discovered. She sat about, usually unoccupied, and expressed the belief that she would not get well, because of her poor sleep and having no appetite ; she would lose her mind as did her parents. This mild depression lasted for a month.

It then became evident that the depression was deepening. She became quite unoccupied, and was retarded to the point of complete blocking when asked any personal question. Her face was not immobile and she could even be induced occasionally to smile in a conventional way. At the same time there were little spells of apprehension, sometimes with restlessness and plain fear. Occasionally the latter was evidenced mainly by rapid breathing unaccompanied by any considerable increase of the pulse rate. The nature of her speech and ideas may be gathered from the following : She was asked what she worried about, and after a long pause replied, " You mean what troubles me particularly ? " When this was affirmed she finally said, " Well, I suppose one thing that troubles me greatly is that I—— " and ceased speaking. After more prodding, she went on, " I can't seem to answer these questions, and yet I have been over it so many times to know why I am afraid ". She usually made only beginnings of answers such as the above. Again she might say, " I don't understand your question ", although it had been extremely simple. Once she said, " I ought to answer your question but I am ashamed to have you know it ". After repeated urging she was then induced to reply, " I regret my whole life ". At another interview she finally said that she was jealous of a woman friend and her husband. When she had uttered so much it seemed easier for her to speak and she explained that she thought they might be at home together. Then she blamed herself for the jealousy. On another occasion she said, " I have the greatest faith in both, but still—that's not the way to express it—please don't mix me up, [the physician was silent all the time]. Do you want me to tell you the facts about the jealousy ? " But she could get no further except to accuse herself of not being sincere in her religion, alleging that otherwise she would not have been so jealous. Ideas of an unpleasant fate began to obtrude themselves more and more. She spoke of punishment which was to come to her—" It ought to be prison ". As time went on this became more marked ; she was to be taken to a " worse place ". " This is the last time you will serve me a meal here." Occasionally she harked back to the original complaint and said she would never get well.

After about ten days, her apprehensions became crystallized into more specific ideas of a terrifying nature, and at the same time the fancied crimes were definitely formulated. She thought that she was going to be tried for the death of her husband, whom she had killed by blaming him. Seeing a box, she remarked that a box sent her by her friends was a symbol of the box she would be buried in. Again she spoke of being hanged because of doing wrong to her husband and friends. When a letter came from her husband, it did not correct her belief in his death—" It was not from him ". Sometimes she moaned out such statements as " Oh dear, oh dear, I wish I had served God," or " Think of all the innocent people who have to suffer on my account ! " Paralleling this greater productivity of ideas was more marked fear and a disappearance of her slow speech and blocked answers.

During the next month she moaned more and gradually became more restless. She often spoke in a staccato voice. She said that she constantly had terrible thoughts about various people. Someone must be reading her mind, she should not be held responsible because she did not want to have such thoughts. Yet she was going to be punished. She saw smoke one day ; again something was toasting and smoking in the bathroom. These were signs that she had to be burned or buried alive. A friend who brought some flowers said they should be put in water. This indicated that she was going to be drowned. Then the family would commit suicide. When some crows were heard she moaned, " Oh those crows ! " Asked what she meant, the reply was, " Their bodies must be exposed and they have no one to take care of them ". Again she said she felt every move she made was photographed and circulated ; much had been written and published about her.

During the eight months she remained under observation she showed almost constant exhibitions of dramatic fear. She paced up and down the floor, panting and moaning. Towards the end of the period she became irritable ; when interfered with or given directions by the nurses, she was apt to strike them. She ate little, and this, coupled with her overactivity, led to a steady loss of weight. Her " thoughts " continued. The reaction to them was explained in part by their remarks : " I put a meaning to everything ; if I look at a bed or a picture I think it means something. I accuse myself of terrible things which I know I could not do for the world, yet they come to my mind." " I can't understand why thoughts are facts." " I would never think of starving or poisoning anyone." Her false ideas regularly took two paralleling forms, injuries to others and the dreadful fate about to fall on her. Her house was broken up and her husband remarried. She had " terrible thoughts " about another patient. Once she named all the leaves on a rubber tree in her room by names of her friends. One that had notches she called by her sister's name and said the notches meant that her sister's throat had been cut. Again, hearing a church bell, she said it was tolling for her sister's death. On the other hand she was constantly referring with terror to being taken to a " cold, dark place ". She was going to hell, " Death is coming to-night ". " Punishment will be terrible ", and so on.

She was then transferred to another hospital when recovery took place very gradually over a period of two and a half years. The whole psychosis therefore lasted over three years and a half.

If we are to understand the psychological tendencies of these involution reactions it is well to examine the more complete regressions that occur in those cases where recovery does not occur. As has been stated these reactions are more of the kind one finds in dementia praecox, but the transition from the manic depressive type is gradual and, from a pychological standpoint, it is easier to see the direction of the regression, when its goal is plainly in evidence, than it is in the benign cases. There are three different kinds of symptoms which go with a grave prognosis ; the consistent presence of any one of these justifies a prediction of permanent deterioration, although as a rule when one is present the others are at least indicated. The first of these is a concentration of interest in the patient's body so intense that frank autoerotism (not necessarily, although frequently, masturbatic) occurs, as well as grotesque and often filthy hypochondriacal delusions. The second is an aggressively anti-social attitude, showing itself in negativistic irritability. The third is a reduction or loss of emotional reaction. Complaints become stereotyped in whining repetitions ; the mental horizon of the patient is more and more narrowed ; and delusions, which one would expect to excite distress or fear, are recited quite calmly. Often the only genuine emotional reaction appears as irritability, when the basis of an obviously ridiculous idea is questioned. Three cases will be cited briefly to illustrate these peculiar features.

The first case showed shallow effect, irritability, ridiculous ideas and persistent autoerotism (mouth area).

CASE 10. *Mary M.* was a married woman of 48, belonging to the leisured class.

F.H. There was no evidence of hereditary factors other than the suspicion that the patient's father had committed suicide following failure in business.

P.H. She was described as light-hearted, active, ambitious, fond of social life, and sensible. On the other hand she was apt to get " run-down " every winter, as the result of her social activities. Six years before admission she was depressed for two weeks. She had four children living and well.

Six months before admission, and one month before the onset of the menopause, she became nervous, sleepless, and downhearted, cried at times, but was able to control herself sufficiently to carry on her ordinary activities. After a month she improved, but four months before admission, the trouble recurred and she went to a sanatorium. There she expressed utter despair, although able at first to appear cheerful before strangers. Soon she became restless, uneasy, moaned, said she would never get well and tried to starve herself. Two weeks before admission she began to complain of her legs being numb and paralysed, of not being able to move her eyes and, finally, of being dead. She developed a peculiar gait, but could be made to walk normally. She slept poorly and tried to commit suicide. Nevertheless her weight rose while in this institution from 132 to 157 pounds.

On admission she was usually restless, striking her head and pounding it against the wall as she talked about her delusions. At other times she was quieter, reasonable and depressed. Once, however, she appeared moderately cheerful, got up and dressed and even did a little sewing. She complained of her legs feeling numb and of her muscles being stiff and immovable ; that she could not think except when she was speaking ; and that the moment she closed her eyes and stopped speaking, not a thought went through her mind. [A good case for one of the modern schools of psychology !] She claimed she was dead, only an image. " It is not melancholia or depression ; it is true, God has changed me. Why, I don't know. Six months ago I was well, then all in one night I was changed. All my power was taken from me. I want to die but I can't."

Within a couple of months her ideas had become more absurd and her emotional reaction shallow. Occasionally, however, when talking of her ideas, she would become excited and talk loudly. Usually her delusions were expressed in monotonous repetitions. For instance, she would repeat, " I am only a ball of wire ", or that she was all shrivelled up, that her face was drawn up and her mouth thrinking. She would put her hand into her mouth and hold it open. She said she would be nothing but an " ow-ow woman ", that is a woman who could say nothing but " ow-ow ". If she had an auditor she would continue indefinitely with such monotonous complaints. Occasionally she would say she was insane and try to frighten the nurses with affected wildness. On the other hand, she showed not the slightest insight into the ridiculousness of her beliefs.

During the next six months her ideas became quite fixed. She was changed first into an image, then into a dead body. She was, as a matter of fact, steadily losing weight. On admission she weighed 157 pounds ; in the first three months she lost 25 pounds, and after a couple of years weighed only 75 pounds. After developing the delusion that her body was dead, the next idea was that it was shrinking until she was " all dissolved ", only " a little ball ", " nothing but a rat ", " a rag-doll ", or " clothes pin ", " a spit on the end of a lip ", or " nothing but a bit of lip. " Her poor nutrition was the result of her scanty eating, and when, three months after admission, it became necessary to tube-feed her, she put up a sign over her bed which read, " Evaporated remains. Don't feed ". She would ask (without affect) that her husband be sent for to cut her head off with an axe, or that she be cut to pieces and bottled up. Sometimes she struck herself, often spoke of suicide, wanted to get out in order to find some way of killing herself. Then there were many fancies about localized changes in her body ; her brains were changed to bone, the organs of the abdomen were crowding into her chest, her breath was almost gone, her mouth was shrinking. This zone seemed to interest her chiefly, and she persistently pulled at her lips, so that her mouth finally became frightfully disfigured, drawn down on either side, and the lips hypertrophied. So great was the resulting distortion that she was barely recognisable.

At first her ideas were expressed with a good deal of loquacity, but no real affect, even when asking to be killed. Nevertheless she showed a fair degree of vivacity, even when not irritable. She said herself she was not depressed but simply knew that these things were so. When her ideas were not believed, however, she became enraged, would swear, scream and attack the nurses, hitting them with all her strength. At the end of six months she became quieter, lay in bed most of the time with a sheet drawn over her. She spoke less of her ideas, but they remained exactly the same, and she continued to get angry if they were criticised. On the other hand, she sometimes made paper flowers, and occasionally played an excellent game of chess. Once she assisted in the preparations for a little festivity, showing good taste in decorations. At another time she gave good advice on family matters. When her son died, she showed natural grief and even on one occasion cried in a natural manner in speaking of her sad fate, and of how much she would like to be with her family, and of how her life was ended by the change that had come over her. But even at this interview she reaffirmed her absurd delusions. (This demonstration of normal mental processes and emotions co-incident with the maintenance of preposterous beliefs, is highly typical of a chronic psychosis ; the " splitting " or dissociation of functions is characteristic of the dementia praecox reaction).

This condition remained absolutely unaltered till three days before her death, which occurred five years after the onset of the psychosis. She had become extremely emaciated, and one day had several slight convulsions accompanied by unconsciousness. Full consciousness never returned, breathing became more difficult until it finally ceased.

The next case illustrates the degradation of emotional reaction with a narrowing of interest down to a few hypochondriacal complaints and a delusion of poverty ; analerotism was markedly present. The case is complicated by the fact that symptoms pointing towards a mild arteriosclerotic or senile affection of the brain were present, but these were quite disproportionate in prominence to the symptoms belonging definitely to the involution melancholia picture. Moreover, the features suggestive of organic disease were present mainly on admission and largely disappeared with the better hygiene of hospital life.

CASE 11. *George S.* was a married post-office clerk, 57 years old.

F.H. All heredity was denied.

P.H. He was described as temperate, jovial, never " nervous ". He held none but subordinate positions. Some years before admission he lost all his hair, and for three years he had been fretful, although no importance was attached to it.

Seven weeks before admission he underwent an operation for " ulcerated rectum ". His fretfulness at once increased, a good deal of it being focused on a worry about proposed advancement to the postmastership of a small town. Two weeks after the operation he took oxalic acid with suicidal attempt, although he was making a good recovery physically. From then on he continued to worry about inability to fill his position properly ; he complained much of pain in his head, said he had ruined himself by taking the poison. With this he became uneasy and restless, and, by a week before admission, this symptom was so aggravated that he was constantly pacing the floor, talking in an undertone. He muttered that he was going to be taken to court because he had tried to get the post-office position, that his family and all who signed the petition for his nomination would be indicted. Sometimes he was heard swearing to himself. The informants thought he remained clear as to his surroundings, but they recalled that he said, " Now what I am talking about ? You see I forget these things ".

On admission he was found to look much older than his years would indicate. He was markedly stooped, and stood or sat in a relaxed pose. There was a definite loss of tone in his facial muscles which gave his face a washed-out expression. The arteries were thickened, but his heart was not enlarged blood pressure not measured). His bowels were fairly regular, his nutrition fair. Neurological examination betrayed no abnormality, neither sensory nor motor, except for marked increase of the knee jerks.

At first he was quite confused, almost completely disoriented, had most defective memory, and all his intellectual operations were slow. He could perform only the very simplest of arithmetic calculations. This condition improved steadily, however, so that at the end of four months he was perfectly oriented, and had no obvious defect in his intellectual functions except for his slowness. Careful examination, however, always revealed a slight but definite defect in memory.

From the outset he usually stayed alone, unoccupied, walking about and occasionally speaking to himself. Yet occasionally he would talk sensibly to the nurse about his former life. At the first interview he said he had no worry, but a few days later admitted that he had, and seemed subdued. When asked to explain his worries, however, he seemed uncertain about them. They concerned his running for office, he said, but confessed he could not bring the details to mind. Four days later, when his orientation was improving, he showed an aimless restlessness (although he would assist the attendants in dusting and polishing the furniture) and more ideas came to expression. He said it was all up. He was going to be hanged, he should have gone to the U.S. Court. " They are holding me on that case." Later, " Holding me as a criminal ". He said too that he worried about " everything," and " because I can't get away from here ". He was sleeping and eating well.

Two weeks after admission he wrote a grammatical and consecutive although poorly punctuated, letter to his son. It was entirely composed of repetitions of two ideas, that he was to be brought up for a trial that would astonish everybody, and that he was badly in need of money. After a month's residence in the hospital he had settled into a chronic, aimless restlessness ; without signs of definite apprehension or of any other emotion except a vague dispair. He was so busily engaged in walking around muttering to himself that it was difficult to get his attention on questions. While being interviewed he might take his coat off, shake it, put it on again and repeat this performance several times without the examiner being able to detect any particular motive in the actions. He seemed to be engrossed with two ideas, that his bills were not paid and that he wanted to get out. No reassurance made the slightest impression on him. He denied fearing that anything would happen to him in the hospital, but kept repeating in a vague way that everything would be all right if only he were out. Yet when he was allowed to go into the hall he walked aimlessly around, making no attempt to go further, simply muttering " Oh God ! Oh God ! " in a low voice. But when taken into another room and the door locked, he kept rattling at the handle. The only regular consistency between his ideas and his conduct was his refusal to eat on account of the expense, for the bills, he thought, were running up into the thousands. It became necessary about this time to tube-feed him.

In the course of the next month his ideas began to change, and also to some slight extent his conduct. He became less restless, as he dropped the ideas of expense and of wanting to get out, and gradually substituted, for these, analerotic fancies. He began to be untidy, because he thought he would fill up the closet if he used it ; also he believed himself to be filthy, to be covered with faeces and liable to contaminate others. Once having an attack of diarrhœa, he defecated all around his room. On another occasion he smeared his whole body. At first the desire to get out persisted, although he himself recognised its inconsequence, for he said " I want to get away from here—I hardly know where to myself ". Or he might give an equally vague statement as to his worries. They were " About the state I am in ". In six months' time his complaints had narrowed down to a few oft repeated phrases : that he was all covered with feces, that he was all gone to pieces, or such sentences as " Oh, God, oh God, it's gone, it's gone, the whole business is gone. It's awful, awful ". He also began rubbing his head and his buttocks. With all this his activity was much reduced, he still walked about muttering to himself, but not with the uneasy restlessness he had formerly shown. He had to be frequently led to the toilet in order to prevent his urinating or defecating on the floor. Often he had to be coaxed to eat, but tube-feeding was no longer necessary, when the worries over expense ceased to be insistent. With all this behaviour he seemed to pay no attention to, and be quite out of contact with, the environment. It was therefore surprising to find that he was well oriented, knew how long he had been in the hospital and so on.

There was no change in his condition till his death at 67 years of age, nine and a half years after the onset of the psychosis.

If one eliminated from the picture given above, the specifically formulated delusions one would have left a state characterized by aimless restlessness, vague unfocussed worry, and a poverty of emotional reaction. This is what we term " Organic Insufficiency ". The following case illustrates this type. Such patients give one the impression of not having sufficient mental energy even for the fabrication of delusions.

CASE 12. *Alexander C.* was a widower, a mason by occupation, and 58 years of age.

F.H. One brother was an epileptic, otherwise no evidence was secured of any family taint.

P.H. He was said to have been natural in manner and disposition, although for many years he had been given to drinking in periodical sprees. Very little alcohol would affect him, and for a month thereafter he would be nervous, have dyspeptic troubles, and so on. In his younger manhood he had worked for himself, but for 20 years had been employed by contractors. His trade naturally left him idle, as a rule, during the winter months.

Towards the end of the last off-season his home was broken up. He worried a bit about this, and when, a month later, it was time for him to return to work he did not do so. His worry, combined with sleeplessness and restlessness, grew gradually more severe. Ten days before admission he grew afraid of leaving his room, thinking he would fall. In his room he paced about complaining in a whining voice of his apprehensions, his restlessness and of his " condition " in general. He said he was doomed, there was no hope, he ought to die, but hadn't the courage ; he did not want any longer to see, hear or speak ; his condition would affect his children as well as himself. He slept only with sedatives. He ate poorly, his bowels had not moved for a week, and his weight had gone down from 120 to 100 pounds.

On admission he was found to be physically undernourished, generally of senile habitus, but without *arcus senilis*. Blood pressure was increased (not measured), and the area of cardiac dullness was slightly enlarged. There was a left hydrocele the size of a goose egg. The pupils reacted well to light, but poorly to distance accommodation. The tongue was protruded consistently to the left, but showed no tremor. When standing with closed eyes he swayed, but always caught himself before falling. The knee kicks were very active, and on the right almost produced clonus. He walked as if weak.

Mentally, the observations confirmed the history. When left alone in his room he was quiet, but if anyone entered he would begin an interminable whining complaint, walking nervously up and down. He would run on indefinitely with statements like the following : " What am I going to do ? I'm so nervous I can't sit down. I can't lie down, I can't walk, I can't sleep, I can't eat, I can't sit still and can't keep quiet. Here I have been walking, walking, walking. I shall drop. What will become of me ? " He made no complaints of any specific or localized sensory change, even when they were suggested to him by questions. His restlessness seemed always aimless in type, and never amounted to agitation. In a couple of weeks his physical condition improved considerably, but this had no effect on his mental state. He complained much about his worries, but cross questioning could bring out no fixed and permanent formulation of them. He fastened his general dissatisfaction with life on whatever came along. For instance, he complained because his bowels did not move, and, when a purgative was given, because he might suddenly have to go to the closet and not be able to hold it. He worried about going to the baths lest he might fall on the way ; he thought bathing might make him more nervous ; something was going to happen, but what he would not say; when pressed for explanation, he said he might be treated unkindly if he made a disturbance. On complaint was specific, but this had, probably, a rational basis. He suffered from sexual weakness, and spontaneously referred to absence of erections for six months. When his attention could be secured, it was manifest that he was well oriented.

Some three weeks later he was rather stirred up for several days although not noisy. This was associated, apparently with the fear that he might hurt another patient who had a lame hand. He would say with increasing vehemence : " There will be a terrible time around here in a minute. I don't want to hit a one-armed man. You don't want me to be a murderer do you ? Well then, take me away from here. Take me to the B." [ward for disturbed cases]. During this wild excitement he had to be tube-fed. Then he quieted down into his usual state and ate well, although often complaining that he felt filled up, and that it was useless to eat when his bowel movements were so scanty. It was interesting that he did not, as most of the chronic cases do, formulate this idea in a delusion of total incapacity to defecate. He would say : " I can't go on in this way eating, eating all the time and no movement of the bowels, or at least only a very small one ".

A couple of months thereafter, he often refused food and had to be tube-fed. He alleged reason was that he could only swallow a small amount of food at a time. But it was probably also determined by a perverse irritability that appeared at the same time. Not infrequently, when giving utterance to his whining complaints he would seize the physician's hand or coat and scratch or bite. He would often do this when he was being undressed or fed. Or when interfered with he would strike the attendant in a weak, petulant way, and say in excuse, " I must do it, I can't help it ". He also would sometimes become noisy, when uttering his complaints, shout them out and swear inordinately. He frequently soiled his clothes and both urinated and defecated in his bed. No matter how intractable he might be, if he were put to bed and the lights turned out he would lie there quite quietly. He claimed that he could not sleep, but observation showed that he slept about five hours a night on the average.

This condition, with mild variations, endured until his death some four years after the onset. About a week before his death he rapidly lost strength, then became unconscious, and died in a few hours without any convulsions. The general weakness reflected in the colourlessness of his whole clinical picture seemed finally to be increased to a point incompatible with life. Throughout his entire hospital stay he was well oriented, knew how long he had been in the different wards, and so on. It therefore seems improbable that either his psychosis or his death was due to cerebral arteriosclerosis.

A reduction of emotional response, particularly when painful ideas are present, implies an inconsistency in the clinical picture. What we hold to be natural relationships of thoughts to affect are characteristic of normal mental operations, and it is because, in the main, such consistency is preserved in manic-depressive insanity, that the outlook for recovery is good. When inconsistencies appear the reaction is tending towards dementia praecox. As has been pointed out by Hoch[1], reduction, and even dissociation, of affect, may occur in recoverable cases of stupor. But here again one finds a certain consistency. The expected emotional reaction is toned down as part of a general reduction of energy output, associated with thoughts of death and indifference to the environment. It is not impossible that the relative weakness in emotional response to naturally terrifying ideas, which many benign involution melancholias show, may be correlated with a certain acceptance of death. In other words such cases would be grading over into the stupor type of reaction. But for the latter to the benign it must also show consistency (so Hoch has claimed). The stupor patient is not multifariously productive and such ideas as he does produce centre closely around death.

Particularly in the melancholias of bad prognosis many of the hypochondriacal delusions are of bodily changes which imply certain death. The benign reaction to such ideas would be either distress and fear or an exclusive elaboration of the death aspect with acceptance of this implication and the development of stupor symptoms. In such a case if the ideas remain purely hypochondriacal in type but stupor symptoms appear, we have the kind of inconsistency that is characteristic of dementia praecox. The following case is cited to illustrate these two points : that the involution melancholia regression may lead to a stupor reaction and that the inconsistency of the latter is associated with a bad prognosis. (It should be mentioned that cases could be described in which a benign melancholia grades over into a benign stupor and that this one is chosen simply because it demonstrates both psychiatric principles at the same time). As the reader will observe, other symptoms—marked irritability and autoerotic behaviour—were also indicative of a malignant reaction.

[1] Benign Stupors, p. 125, seq.

M

Case 13. *Catherine H.* was a widowed housewife, aged 60, when she came under observation nearly 25 years ago.

F.H. Nothing was known of the grandparents. Her father became " demented " in his advanced years, and her mother was " an invalid for years ". A first cousin had typical circular insanity. Among 4 siblings one sister was insane.

P.H. The patient was said to have had a cheerful disposition and to have been intelligent. Her husband died 15 years before her psychosis appeared. There never had been any previous mental illnesses but for years she had suffered from " neuralgic headache ". The menopause had occurred over ten years before admission.

About a year before she was brought to the hospital she was vascillating in reaching decisions, slept poorly but had no self reproach. After some months she improved, but six months later became depressed, gradually weaker, and worried about what she should do and about her physical condition. A month before admission she was taken to a sanatorium where she rapidly became worse. Her dejection deepened, she worried over the expense, said she had no friends, that she had been living under false pretences and had committed a sin in coming to the sanatorium. She made a suicidal attempt, and then became markedly restless with the idea that she was to be put in prison. She also spoke of her brother and her son being killed.

On admission no physical anomalies were found except for mild undernourishment and signs of constipation. For the first week she showed marked agitation. Now and then she would wet herself. She talked much on a few topics : that she had no money, that she would be taken away and put in jail, that she had done an " awful deed ", and that attempts were being made to poison her. She frequently had to be tube-fed, refusing to eat by herself. Eight days after admission she was found with impacted rectum and distended bladder, passing small quantities of urine into the bed. She seemed weak and in pain, but these symptoms disappeared with evacuation, catheterization and stimulation.

During the next week the patient was often in bed, saying little spontaneously, although breaking into a moaning recital of her troubles when approached. Sometimes she got out of bed and paced restlessly up and down, talking mournfully. At times she ate a little by herself ; again she had to be tube-fed. When given questions to search her orientation, it was difficult to get her attention, since she was always reverting to her complaint. But it seemed that she was undoubtedly aware of the hospital, its name, purposes, and so on. She knew the month but could not tell how long she had been in the hospital. Doctors and nurses she recognised as such. She protested that she could not perform even the simplest arithmetic calculations. Her ideas were essentially the same as those given above without further elaboration. As to her " condition ", she was " demented ". When asked if she was afraid she said, " Afraid ! Afraid ! There is nothing I am not afraid of ! " She often refused food because she was filled up, or because it was poisoned. Even the most patient questioning elicited no explanation or correlation of her ideas ; they came spontaneously or not at all. For instance, when asked if she were afraid, she invariably answered in the affirmative, but would give no more explanation of the occasion of her fear than " that I am here ".

Fifteen days after admission she became quite upset, apparently because she had seen a nurse throw away food, which she (the patient) had not eaten. She lay in bed with increased pulse and respiration rate, disoriented and plainly quite confused. She kept repeating over and over that it was a most dreadful thing, that she should have seen to it, and so on, without ever giving any clear reason for her distress. It was presumed to be connected with her notions of poverty and some feeling of responsibility she had for the loss of the food.

During the next year there was little change in her general condition.

She usually was walking restlessly around, although sometimes lying in bed. When observed she was generally moaning out her complaints in short broken sentences such as, " Awful ! Awful ! I say—I—Oh God—up there—won't you—Oh God ! " Often she would be found peering through the panel of a door making such jerky remarks. All questioning she resented ; in fact. any attention paid to her was apt to produce violent and blind resistiveness, Frequently she gave voice to apprehensive ideas such as that she would be buried alive, cut in pieces, torn limb from limb and so on, but these thoughts were always produced without evidence of fear and with a mournful, whining intonation. Her complaints of wickedness fell into the background except perhaps for frequent statements of a queer, perplexed feeling that she was responsible for the welfare of the other patients. Worry about being in the hospital and about expenses continued, as did complaints about the way she was treated, the last even being spoken of as fiendish torture. She was not given a chance to eat (untrue), but was stuffed full of egg-nogs. With all this she seemed absorbed in her own ideas to the point of perplexity, yet when a determined effort was made to gauge her orientation it was found to be excellent. On the other hand, it was utterly impossible to get her to attempt the simplest of calculations. She would repeat the problem over and over, and finally blurt out a ridiculous answer. Towards the end of her first year in the hospital, her sentences became almost entirely broken, and little could be got out of her. For instance, she was one day found in bed with food lying beside her, saying over and over, " I can't eat such stuff ". When asked " Why not ? " she replied, " I have to be left right here for ever ". She was then asked what she meant : " I came here—oh, I am all to pieces ! " Sometimes she said she was vile and filthy or that she had lost all interest in everything.

A year after admission she developed a tendency to pinch the nurses. Once in attempting to do so she slipped on the floor and sustained a fracture of the neck of the femur. The leg was, of course, immobilized, and this seemed to inaugurate a new phase of her psychosis.

Once confined to bed she became quieter and dull. She lay with her legs bent at sharp angles and resisted efforts to straighten them out. Months afterwards, when she had been moved to a wheel chair, this persisted. At first she would occasionally straighten out her legs herself. There was also a tendency to hold her arms in a bent position. Even after her femur was well knit she claimed that she could not walk, her feet being dead. She also insisted that her throat or neck was broken as a result of being tube fed. Ordinarily she seemed dull and indifferent, but would show signs of distress when attempts were made to straighten out her limbs or when she was questioned. For a few months she occasionally repeated broken exclamations such as, " Why—you can't—my poor hands—my poor broken hands—you can't do that . . ." Later she said very little, moaned slightly or answered questions with signs. At one examination when repeatedly questioned about her health, she looked distressed and pointed to her throat. When asked if she had pain there, she was heard to whisper, " All over ". She depended entirely on the nurses for her care and gave them much trouble with wilful bed wetting, for she would be given a bed pan and would push it away from under her, then urinate and summon the nurse. During the last few months she held her hands and fingers in peculiar cramped positions and grasped anything she took hold of with her extended thumb and fore-finger. In spite of the persistent contracted positions of her extremities, no contractures nor atrophies resulted. The phalangeal joints both of the hands and feet were enlarged, the right knee kick was more active than the left, and the left Achilles jerk could not be obtained. Otherwise there were no physical anomalies.

After about 18 months of this striking inactivity, she one day got out of bed of her own accord in order to upset a pitcher full of egg-nog. The next day she left her bed, walked to the window, and sat down. From then on she remained out of bed during the day, sometimes even assisted the nurses in dressing and occasionally fed herself.   There was also a temporary improvement in her habit of excretion.   At no time, however, did she ever do anything beyond attending to these primitive needs, but would sit all day long, in or out of doors hunched up in an invalid chair.   She almost invariably hindered the nurses in anything they tried to do for her and often assumed her old muscular resistiveness when in her chair.   Rarely, when in her room alone, she would open the drawers of her bureau and look in.   She spoke very little and answered questions more rarely still.   When urged to speak she would assume a look of distressed uneasiness.   Sometimes she opened her mouth long enough to say such things as : " I cannot live," " I cannot die ", " I am rotten through and through ".   Or she said her mouth was all gone, that she had swallowed her tongue, and, quite frequently, that her neck was broken.

Her history states that there was absolutely no change in her condition till a week before death, when a gastrointestinal upset prevented her retaining nourishment.   She grew rapidly weaker and died at the age of 78, more than 18 years after the onset of her psychosis.   It was added that up to the end she would occasionally give information that was startingly correct.

The following case is included as an example of the involution melancholia reaction occurring in the early thirties.   The psychosis was typical except for the presence of paranoid ideas, which, when they were bizarre and prominent, suggested dementia praecox. It was thought at the time, however, that they were more an expression of the theories of a superstitious Italian, evolved to account for his other symptoms. than delusions of a schizophrenic order. An excellent recovery justified this view.

CASE 14.   *Vincent C.* was a married barber, aged 33.
F.H. There was no information except with regard to the patient's own generation, in which no mental nor nervous diseases were reported.
P.H. The patient was born in Italy.   He had convulsions as a child, but was subsequently healthy.   He went to school in Italy, and continued for a short time after coming to this country at the age of 13.   His progress there is not known.   He became a barber as soon as he left school and worked efficiently at that trade till a little over a year before admission.   He had been married for eleven years and had three living children.
Make-up : Nothing was known of his early life.   He was always a quiet, though sociable chap after marriage, and he had friends before marriage too.   He had never been very fond of sexual intercourse.   Whether he had any love affairs with other women is also unknown.   He was 22 and his wife 15 at the time of their marriage, which occurred after a courtship of seven months.   Unusual attachment to either parent had not been observed, although he spoke oftenest of his mother.   He had always been fidgety and nervous, and as long as his wife had known him he had had tics with his eyes, face, neck, and right hand (stretching out his fingers).   At times he was irritable, would come home angry, not telling the cause, would not eat his supper, but would scold for awhile, although he never struck either his wife or the children.   He drank beer quite moderately.
Psychosis : The first indication of any abnormalities that may have to do with his psychosis was a year before admission, when his eyes began to trouble him.   He secured glasses but would not wear them, and worked irregularly for a couple of months.   He spoke of giving up barbering on account of his eye trouble, and was so impatient with this weakness that he often would not eat for a day.   Two months later, however, he was apparently better, began to work with a barber, F., and in two months more formed a partnership with him.   A month later he had pains in his head, beginning in his left ear, so bad that he could not sleep at night.   These pains got better

spontaneously, but recurred more violently six months before admission, when he went to an eye, ear and throat hospital, where he was immediately operated on for mastoiditis. A letter from this hospital left no doubt as to the genuineness of the disorder. He came home in two weeks, but after six weeks returned to have the wound re-opened, as the pains had recommenced. This wound was kept open till one month before admission. Almost immediately on returning home after his first operation, symptoms of a fairly typical anxiety neurosis began to develop. He was very weak, and began to worry at once about his ear and said that it would never get well. It was not only the pains (which soon subsided) but the noises that developed which never left him. He worried more and more about his wife having to work, and began to think, or at least to say, that his wife was angry at his idleness. For two months prior to admission he complained that his brothers were down on him, also alleging that people turned their backs on him. At no time, however, did he hear voices or tell of any accusations being made against him. For the last five weeks at home he was very nervous, pacing up and down the house, refusing to eat or sleep. During the latter months he slept apart from his wife. He once made a feeble attempt at suicide and talked a great deal about it. He became weaker, and one week before admission went to the Observation Pavilion and reported on his return that the doctor wanted to see his wife. The next day, however, he refused to accompany her and stayed all night with his brother. Three days later he returned alone and was detained. That same night his wife went to the hospital with a friend of the family, S., and signed a paper. On the next visit she made, his whole attitude was changed, as he accused his wife of having been persuaded by S. to put him away, and averred that his brothers and his wife were glad to be rid of him.

On Admission : He was found to be rather poorly nourished, deep reflexes were over active, there was weakness of the left face and possibly of the left pharyngeal muscles with the tongue protruded to right.

He was not accessible for examination as to his intellectual status, but there was no indication of his having any organic defect symptoms and subsequent examinations confirmed that view.

He was examined daily for ten days, and during that time his mood had always a background of hopelessness with variations in his more superficial reactions. The first day he spoke in a whining, panicky voice of his troubles, but only on questioning. While in bed he lay quietly with a blank face, but on being brought to the examining room he was restless, particularly when talking, moving his hands and feet with quick back and forward motions, often apparently crying, although without tears, and again with an expression, half way between weeping and a forced laugh. Occasionally he grit his teeth. With his restlessness was an occasional evidence of distractibility. On the whole, he seemed like a nervous individual in a panic, like one exaggerating his emotions. The next day he refused to speak, sat dejectedly in his chair apparently both uninterested and depressed. Movements made on command were slow, although some spontaneous motions were quickly enough executed. The day following he presented the same picture as on the first examination, for he talked when questioned, and in the same sad but panicky way. The subsequent days it was difficult to get him to talk at first, but after some questioning he would " warm up " and begin to repeat his monotonous, lugubrious phrases, " It's a shame ", " I gotta die ", etc., as well as to talk of his paranoid ideas. He frequently spoke of his difficulty in thinking. Dejection was the keynote of his mood, though he often wore an ironical, bitter smile.

During these ten days the subject of his talk was entirely his insane ideas. All of these, he repeatedly stated, occurred to him only after they had put a thermometer with carbolic acid on it into his rectum, the first night at the Observation Pavilion. Immediately he felt his belly burn up, his guts were gone, his blood drained off from all his body and from his head, so that he could not think, and he knew he was to die, was " dead-alive ", was being kept alive by medicine, by gas, by blue medicine. He also referred to his having been killed by this operation. Immediately, too, he had realised the attitude of other people to him. His wife had been given him poison since Christmas, so had Mrs. K., a neighbour, who gave him eggs and coffee with something in it every day. The result was the noises in his head. A barber friend had put a powder in his ear and given him clams to eat which made it worse. F., his partner, had done for him with a drink. S. and his wife had put up a job on him. They got money from the Government for delivering him over to the hospital, and they were to have a good time together when he was gone. His sister-in-law had warned him against them but he had not listened. So it was his own fault, he had gone to the Observation Pavilion himself and had let himself be operated on in the first place for his mastoid. He was to be killed by poison or electrocuted (his eye falling on an electric machine) or by "electricity-poison". Again, his wife and S. were alleged to be responsible for his death. Once he said he was going to support his wife, when he had been born again.

His condition remained unchanged (except for occasional days when he cried a great deal) for a month, when, after seeing a large number of visitors, he became unusually panicky, sat in bed, trembling, and panting with raucous respirations that graded over into sobs. Spontaneously he repeated over and over again short phrases such as "My poor life", "I gotta die", "My poor children", " "Getta killed twice", interspersed with equally brief exclamations in Italian. He could be induced to answer very few questions. For some weeks he had evidenced a strong attachment to the examiner, and objected vehemently to his leaving after a talk. Then for several days he became more depressed, seemed to care little whether he was spoken to or not, and for two days would not eat. For the following two weeks he cried more, rarely used his bitter smile, and seemed more consistently depressed. Following the examiner's absence on vacation, the patient became more agitated and was transferred to the ward for excited patients for ten days. There his unrest interfered with satisfactory examination, as he would do little but repeat his stereotyped utterances of woe. This agitation calmed down and without other sign three months after admission he suddenly remarked "I want to go home". This was without any change in his general mood. A week later he brightened suddenly, and began to talk of his going home, of getting better, in place of his continual reference to imminent death. After two weeks he would talk at times for half an hour or more without making reference to his trouble, inquiring when he would be well, and frequently laughing openly at a joke. After this he was allowed up and began to work with fair efficiency in the ward, ate enormously, and in general took a new interest in his environment. For six weeks his mood was never spontaneously cheerful, and he had periods when he would give up all hope, sit in a corner and cry bitterly. It was always possible, however, to pull him out of these periods of depression by sternly ordering him to work and refusing to sympathize with him. He then became entirely normal, uniformly cheerful and had excellent insight.

The development of his various delusional ideas shows that they were all tentative and superficially determined. Sixteen days after admission he ceased to make any reference to his wife's infidelity, and two days later denied all ideas against his wife, and consistently kept this attitude. All his other ideas were shifting fancies, some of them often repeated, but many only mentioned once. They concerned first the origin of his mastoid trouble; second, his treatment as the Observation Pavilion, and third, the fate he was to suffer. For a couple of weeks references were made mostly to the incidents at the Observation Pavilion. The thermometer affair caused his guts to shrivel up, took his spine out and all the strength from his penis, so that he could no longer get an erection. They also scared him by undressing him and giving him a bath. An electric fan on the wall gave him the buzzing in his head, which he said was due to a machine put into his head. The results of these indignities may be termed loosely feelings of unreality. His skin was cold as ice and white, his blood all gone, his body turned to wood, the bones in his head loose, etc. At this period, too, he referred more to the dreadful things that were to be done to him in the hospital. He was to be castrated, his body all cut up, poisoned, electrocuted. Medicine he got was used both to keep him alive and to draw his blood out. For a day or two he talked about being turned into a monkey, interpreting movements of the examiner's hands and his stooping shoulders to be a conscious imitation of a monkey, in oder to show the patient what was to happen to him. The most persistent of all these ideas was that he was to be killed. Once on the basis of a dream he had had of all the other nations in Europe killing all the Italians, he began to talk about the Italian King being killed, his brother, himself too, and all his family. Next he referred this to hatred of the Italians in America. On another occasion he said that the rice he got was poisoned, and explained this idea thus : He knew a Mr. Reiss, who, when ill with mastoid, tried to jump out of a window. This sound association gave him the idea, and when he was told it was foolish, he replied " I think foolish, Doctor, but I feel bad ".

Persisting with his ideas of death were various explanations of his mastoid trouble. Their long duration may be accounted for by the fact that he was always conscious of the buzzing and ringing noise in his ear. For some days he had a long rigmarole about a white powder that had been put into his ear by the God-father of the child of his partner. The powder was secured from one who had been a patient once at the hospital, and was a fortune teller. The visitors, when they came to the hospital, all got stuff from the patients which, when applied to people outside, made them sick too. Then he associated fortune tellers and hypnotists together and called a patient walking past a hypnotist. The same fortune teller, who supplied the powder, wanted to cure him with hypnotism, but the patient would not allow him. Innumerable other individuals who had had social or business relations with him were at various times mentioned as the ones who caused the trouble.

Inquiries made seven years after his discharge determined that he had been unusually well for two years. Then pains in the mastoid region recurred and some discharge, this happening mainly during the summers. When he had pains he would become irritable and hypochondriacal, but he never had had to cease working.

CHAPTER XVIII

THE PSYCHOLOGY OF INVOLUTION MELANCHOLIA

WE have so far considered—in broad outline at least—the more purely psychiatric aspects of the Involution Melancholias. With these data before us, we are in a position to discuss their psychological significance. The first problem here is to determine which one of the many symptoms presented in the foregoing case histories can be regarded as peculiar to this clinical type. As the different manic depressive reactions are described, it will be seen that few patients present absolutely pure regressions, in which the ideas belong exclusively to one type. This, after all, is but natural. When we speak of a normal man as having any given kind of personality, we are not surprised to observe in him traces of other varieties of attitude or conduct. For instance, a man of sanguine temperament is capable of feeling disappointment ; we speak of him as optimistic because he is not long dejected by untoward circumstances and tends to find some ground for hope, rather than to concentrate his thoughts on distressing incidents. As a matter of fact, abnormal reaction types are much more consistent than are normal ones. Psychiatric classification is therefore a simpler matter than the recognition of normal types ; indeed, the former analysis is so much easier that it enables us to detect general psychological principles applicable to the problems of ordinary life, which is the larger task of psychiatry. We must therefore attempt to pick out from a welter of symptoms those which are present prominently and consistently—those which enable us to make a diagnosis—and subject them only to psychological analysis.

In the first place we find that the patient's interest, which has been applied to his family, business, or social activities, is withdrawn from these environmental objects and turned in on himself. He is concerned only with the insecurity of his life, the afflictions of his body or the unhealthy state of his soul. Second, this introversion is correlated with the development of various ideas, exaggerated or utterly false : he believes himself about to die by disease or violence, his property is gone, the world is strangely altered, and his soul is lost, doomed to everlasting torment. Thirdly, his mental processes suffer radical alteration in that he entertains thoughts which are patently absurd, misinterprets the intentions of those about him, and in general substitutes uncritical imagination for rational judgment. Finally his conduct alters : he abandons his former social adaptations, becoming surly, ungrateful, resentful, irritable and even brutal.   These are not mere uncontrolled impulses but reflect a true (if temporary) change of character, because, when the unkindly act is completed, there is no reaction of remorse or desire for pardon. We shall see that all these phenomena are closely inter-related psychologically.

Every abnormal reaction (at least in the psychogenic disorders) derives its characteristics from three reciprocally related factors. One is the nature of the situation from which relief is sought, the second is the occurrence of some disturbing event, which precipitates a morbid reaction, and the third is the goal towards which the resulting regression tends.

It is a matter of fairly common knowledge that most psychopathic individuals make their lives difficult by their own maladaptation. They are relatively incapable of satisfying their inner instinctive needs in the activities and emotional relationships of adult, civilized life. When something occurs to make the task of adaptation intolerable or to suggest the earlier and cruder type of outlet, regression takes place.   The histories of such people while " normal " exhibit peculiarities directly related (we can discern) to these fundamental tendencies.   So we find them shy, seclusive, prone to achieve their ambition in fancy rather than by effort, emotionally, unstable, irritable, given to blue spells, difficult to get along with and so on.   Now it will have been noted by the reader that the majority of the patients, whose histories have been cited, showed little of such defects in their past lives.   It must be borne in mind, of course, that these cases were examined long before any intelligent interest was taken in the life reactions of psychopaths, and that questions asked of relatives were probably superficial.   Nevertheless, if marked anomalies of personality were the regular precursors of involution melancholia, one would expect to find some indication thereof.   But their dispositions seem to have been, in the main, fairly normal.   If any impression is gained of abnormality, it is that they tended to have less ambition and energy than their fellows. None of them had been highly successful although relatively little handicapped with nervous or mental trouble.   From this, one is led to suspect that with this group it would be well to seek for some factor in the production of an intolerable situation that is independent of specific constitutional defect in the patient.

We may find this, perhaps, in the circumstances incidental to the age-period at which these psychoses usually occur.   If, as we have claimed, this is a reaction type, it ought (like other manic depressive psychoses) to appear any time of life.   If, on the other hand, most cases occur in the sixth decade, there must be something about the involution period, which makes adaptation peculiarly difficult, and facilitates this special type of regression.   The bodily machine is, of course, wearing out or running down, but this cannot be the only factor. If it were we would expect to find a simple dementia of the senile or arterioschlerotic type. It does not explain the peculiar changes of interest, ideas or conduct, characteristic of this psychosis. We must look rather to the problems that beset man in his declining years for a clue as to why life becomes intolerable to him.

It is possible and convenient to group instincts (or interests) under three great headings, ego-activities (self-preservation and aggrandisement), sexual proclivities (mating and parenthood) and herd or social functions. At the beginning of life biological reactions are centred around maintenance and development of the individual as such. With natural growth appear interests and activities associated with the perpetuation of the species and the welfare of the group, that is to say, sexual and social functions. The normal man expresses his individuality during the best years of his life in family and social affairs, his business, trade of profession, falling into the latter category. His life is bound up with others, his wife, his children, his social and business and political associates. At this time his primitive impulses to seek food, shelter and so on do not engross much of his attention in their primitive form, the egoism of which they are expressions finding outlet in combination with the other instincts. In fact, adaptation consists largely in the warping of ego tendencies in with sex and herd instincts. This adaptation requires more fundamental energy than is demanded for the expression of egoism in its crude form. Consequently when life force—whatever that may be—begins to abate, there is a natural tendency for these elaborate mental mechanisms to give place to simpler ones. The individual becomes more individualistic.

Other factors augment this tendency. Broadly speaking we invest our emotional interest in undertakings or human relationship that yield some return and, if such an investment fails, we become indifferent to it. The involution period of life is full of such failures. The senescent man finds he is physically and mentally unfit for the work that was easy some years before ; he realizes that he must retire from his post. What new interest can be take up ? Similar changes beset him in his family life ; his friends are dying off or have not, any more than he, the energy to maintain old social activities ; his children are growing up, establishing homes for themselves, and are independent of his assistance, hence relatively indifferent to him. What is there left to occupy his interest or utilize his intelligence ? If he retains enough of his old elasticity he can take up some hobby, game or pastime. But it is also necessary for him to realize philosophically that he is not the man he once was and cast his ambitions in a form compatible with his waning powers. No harder task comes to any man and few there are who achieve it perfectly. This is the reason why the man or woman, who grows old gracefully and contentedly, is a rarity. Almost all at some time or another exhibit characteristics distinctive of involution melancholia, although we do not call them symptoms, or the condition disease, until such changes begin to wipe out and replace the normal personality.   In other words the psychosis is merely an exaggeration of changes so universal as safely to be called normal in so far as their nature is concerned.

The break comes as a rule when some event forces on the patient a realization of something that is psychologically, if not physically, true.   For instance, a man suffers a business reverse.   He worries over this because worry is the nearest approach his enfeebled mind can make to grappling with the problem of retrieving his fortune. Soon he concludes that his life is finished.   In a physical sense this may be ridiculous, but, in so far as " life " means the maintenance of his old interests, there is considerable truth in his conclusion. Similarly a woman's children marry.   They are gone out of her life ; if her life has been her children, she must find a new career or admit that her race is run.   The inner meaning of practically all the precipitating mental causes of involution melancholia is of this kind. Sometimes it is physical disease, which at one blow reduces strength and forces what is already a tendency, introversion of attention. But no matter what may be the accident that sets off the final explosion, the mind of the senescent tends to select from its many possible meanings the more depressing ones.   One can for instance look on the marriage of a child with joy ; but, if one is becoming aware of advancing age, the festal occasion may be viewed with alarm.   This general principle of inability to develop pleasurable thoughts is illustrated in psychiatric statistics.   Depression frequently terminates in manic or hypomanic episodes.   This becomes rarer and rarer as age advances.

We have seen that there is a compelling tendency in the involution period towards the abandonment of what have been engrossing interests.   The individual becomes weary of life, because he is becoming more selfish, more egoistic.   What have been stimulants to activity become irritants.   An impulse of avoidance naturally appears ; there is an instinctive tendency to shrink away from what has become unproductive and distasteful.   Unconsciously at least we seem prone to incorporate such tendencies in definite ideas.   If one is to envisage a reaction of withdrawal from the world in a single word or concept, it is best done in the thought of death.   The weakening of sex and herd interests leads, then, to an unconscious preoccupation with death, since a naked ego finds no comfort in this world.   But the instinct of self-preservation is disproportionately strong at this period.   Hence the same factors work to produce both attraction to, and terror of, death.   In other words, an *ambivalent* attitude to death appears.   It seems that man is specialized, both biologically and in virtue of the civilization we have developed, for a social and family existence.   So far as his instincts are concerned his capacity for adaptation depends, therefore, on the strength of his herd and sex instincts.   When his ego instincts predominate, individualistic achievement is the almost exclusive source of pleasure and the successful maintenance of this achievement demands a large supply of energy. (Recent studies of the psychological mechanisms operating in idiopathic epilepsy confirm this view.) Energy is naturally reduced in the involution period. Unhappiness is therefore inevitable so soon as the sex and herd instincts become relatively weak. The isolated ego instincts, therefore, produce at this same time a tendency to withdraw from the world and an accentuation of the fear of death.

In stupor, as we have seen, shrinking from unhappiness produces a conscious longing for death, as is evidenced not merely by placid acceptance of delusions of permanent dissolution, but also by the other world appearing in fancy as a pleasant place. Resurrection follows death, the patient goes to heaven, becomes the Virgin Mary, rejoins her father and so on. In the involution group, however, the same dissatisfaction with life collides with the instinct of self-preservation, so that, when the idea of death appears, it leads to terror and, being consciously unacceptable, it is formulated as something coming from without, a death by violence and torture, while the other world is portrayed as Hell or Purgatory. It seems as if, unconsciously, instinctively, there was an overwhelming impulse to leave this world, against which the psychic organism erects such barriers as it can by picturing the event in terrifying colours. The opposition of unconscious and conscious forces is well shown by the not infrequent suicidal attempts of those who are consciously obsessed with fear of death. Any excuse seems to serve for the fabrication of delusion of a horrible fate. We see, for instance, many psychoses beginning as ordinary depressions with feelings of wickedness. In the involution period the conviction of sin is apt to develop into judgment-day delusions, with a change in the clinical picture to the melancholia type, as in the case of Mary B., which is described above.

Although many patients express death ideas in plain terms, the same tendency seems to underlie other symptoms and ideas as well. The first of these is the insomnia, so frequent at the onset and during the course of the psychosis. Some years ago I put forward the theory that many of the features of insomnia (particularly with fatigue) could be explained as a reaction to unconscious ideas of death[1]. According to this view sleep and loss of acuity of consciousness both represent a breaking of contact with the environment, and hence come to stand in consciousness for an unconscious impulse to die. The self-preservations tendencies of the organism then fight against sleep or loss of consciousness with blind activity both mental and physical, and a compulsive effort to keep attention at its highest pitch. Any hint of lapse of attention or consciousness (such as must occur in the induction of sleep) is a signal for this

---

[1] " The Psychology and Treatment of Insomnia in Fatigue and Allied States," *Journal of Abnormal Psychology*, April, 1920.

reaction to take place.   The phenomenon is analagous to, or identical with, the feverish restlessness of an epileptic trying to fight off an attack, when the aura comes over him.

If this hypothesis be sound it may explain the extreme frequency of insomnia as the first symptom of involution melancholia ; the death idea is incubating in the unconscious, is active but has not yet emerged as a conscious delusion.   The restlessness which is such a common symptom throughout the course of the psychosis may be similarly explained.   It is part of the protective reaction of the organism against death, which is a loss of consciousness.   To explain this behaviour in conscious terms, one might say that the patient feared that, if he relaxed his activity for one moment, the inactivity might become the immobility of death.   Paralleling insomnia is the worry over the things which have gone wrong. This is psychologically analogous.   Interest in normal friendships and undertakings is diminishing.   A frenzied effort to maintain it is made by filling the mind with obsessive thoughts of what the organism is becoming instinctively indifferent to.   It is an effort to substitute conscious for innate and automatic interest.

Foremost among such worries we find anxiety about money and property.   Just as sexual potency becomes symbolic of vitality in general, so money is a symbol for social power.   It is prized therefore, not merely for its intrinsic and buying value, but also because its possession attracts respect ·and establishes prestige. The reverse is also true :   poverty entails social degradation, social extinction.   In this way loss of property means loss of social life. Hence delusions of poverty are closely allied psychologically with delusions of death ;   the former are milder expressions of the latter. This is why fear of financial ruin is such a common symptom during the onset of involution melancholia and so often proceeds, as the psychosis advances, to a conviction that the ruin is an accomplished fact.   When the death idea reaches clear expression, however, the delusion of poverty usually sinks into the background of the clinical picture or completely disappears.

The feeling of unreality is a frequent symptom in all depressive reactions and occurs prominently in involution melancholia.   This, too, may be an exhibition of the death motif ;   or, to put it more accurately, it is probably another evidence of those tendencies of which death is the most dramatic expression.   This problem will be discussed more fully in connection with depression so the argument may now be merely indicated.   Things feel " real " to us in proportion to the amount of interest we take in them, they lose their meaning when we become indifferent to them.   If our indifference be great the whole world gets to be a shadowy place.   It no longer appeals to us.   Even our bodily sensations lack their normal feeling tone.   Hence in these patients we meet with complaints of the sun not shining properly, of the grass not seeming green, or of their legs feeling as if they were wood or stone, and so on.   In its more extreme development this tendency leads to definite delusions. When the unreality affects to body, delusions of such physical change contribute to the hypochondriacal half of the picture.

The representation of inner longing for death, as something that is being forced on the patient from without, shows, as we have seen, a tendency to allocate responsibility to any but the correct origin. A similar mechanism may determine the *délire de negation* and the psychologically allied delusion of immortality. According to our view death is not a primary idea but merely the commonest expression for a more fundamental tendency of shrinking from the world. The essential motif is divorce from an unsatisfactory reality[1]. This can produce a change of feeling towards the environment, *i.e.*, loss of interest or actual delusions of personal change ; it may be incorporated in ideas of leaving the earth (death) ; or, finally, the changed relationships of self and outer world may be pictured as affecting the latter alone. In the last instance the mechanism of projection appears ; responsibility for altered feelings is thrown on to the environment. Hence the patient denies the existence of material objects and doubts the capacity of other people to think or feel. This psychopathic process was prettily illustrated in the case of George P., cited above. The determination of the delusion of immortality is probably quite similar. If death is projected, it is not the patient who dies but those around him. He is then moving in a dead world. The contrast establishes the patient as immortal. Hence, not infrequently, we hear involution melancholics speak of all their friends and relations being killed, or dead, or of the nurses all being spirits, and so on. The normal emotional bonds (which give the feeling of reality to human relationships) being broken, the friendships, and therefore the friends, are dead.

A current, one might almost say conventional, view in psychological circles is that fear is part of an instinctive reaction of flight, which, when the latter is once established, may cause the production of fearful ideas. These exist then essentially as rationalizations. According to such a theory involution melancholia would be primarily an anxiety state in which the ideas of imminent death appeared as the incorporation of a fundamental and primary reaction of fear. Our view is directly opposed to this, for we think that the thought

---

[1] " Our revels now are ended.   These our actors,
     As I forefold you, were all spirits, and
     Are melted into air, into thin air.
     And, like the baseless fabric of this vision,
     The cloud-capp'd towers, the gorgeous palaces,
     The solemn temples, the great globe itself,
     Yea, all which it inherit, shall dissolve,
     And, like this insubstantial pageant faded,
     Leave not a rack behind.   We are such stuff
     As dreams are made on ; and out little life
     Is rounded with a sleep.   Sir, I am vex'd ;
     Bear with my weakness ; my old brain is troubled . . . ."

of death is the primary stimulus, to which the organism responds with the emotion of fear.   There are three reasons for believing that there is, in these cases, an independent death impulse apart from the *a priori* evidence for its existence, which we have just been considering.   In the first place suicide is not uncommon, and it may occur with patients who demonstrate most dramatic fear of death. This, surely, can only be understood as a failure of the protecting reaction to prevent the operation of a powerful impulse against which it has been struggling.   Secondly, in the chronic cases the idea of dissolution persists after emotional reactions are wiped out, so that we have delusions of imminent destruction present without any fear at all.   Finally the stupor type of reaction—that is, the acceptance of death—may, in benign cases, be evidenced in episodes where the patients seem resigned to their fate, or in the brief appearance of limp spells, a dramatization, as it were, of physical death.

Translation of the patient to another world or changes in this, constitute the theme of which half the symptoms of involution melancholia are an expression.   Indifference towards people and things result from the preponderance of ego instincts over those of the sex and herd group.   The other half may be traced to more positive exhibitions of egoism.   The patient is not merely asocial ; he is aggressively interested in self and anti-social.   The plainest evidence of this appears in irritability and negativism, tendencies that are frequently present in the recovering cases and developed to a grotesque degree in chronic ones.   Such patients kick, scratch and bite when they are approached with kindliest intent.   They are publishing a wish to be left alone.

Positive interest in self is expressed in hypochondria.   Two factors co-operate in the production of this symptom.   The first is merely an incorporation of the tendency towards exclusive self-centredness.   When social and sex instincts are intact, egoism finds vent in egotism, that is, a false idea of one's importance in the world of affairs.   When the lust for activity is gone, however, one's body, rather than one's personality, becomes the matter of supreme importance.   The former represents a narcissistic trend, the latter autoerotism.   Once interest is focussed on the body, the second factor appears, which is the derivation of pleasure from bodily sensations.   This makes the indulgence of autoerotic practices (best seen in the chronic cases) easily understood as the complete and final development of the tendencies we are discussing.   But the autoerotic root for hypochondria is not immediately obvious.   We might logically expect these patients to exhibit their autoerotism in gluttony and in the delight of muscular activity, as well as in onanistic practices ; but we find them complaining of indigestion and weakness.   The reason for this is probably to be found in the fundamental energy defect of this time of life, and also in a pre-existent habit of exploiting physical disease as a means of gaining attention.   Physical exercise is plainly incapable of yielding much pleasure to the senescent individual. Similarly the physiological effect of over eating is to produce an active loathing for food. Under these circumstances it is easier to capitalize abnormal visceral sensations for their autoerotic value. than it is to find the energy necessary for the production of normally pleasurable sensations. That this autoerotic element is present in hypochondria is shown in the many chronic cases where " disease " is inextricably mixed up with the most obvious autoerotic fantasies and practices. This is seen most frequently with analerotism.

These symptoms exhibit, of course, a break away from social custom. It is not conventional to wet and soil one's clothes, masturbate, or discuss one's excretions in public. But convention, although we do not realize it, ordinarily goes further than this. Our interpretations of natural phenomena, including bodily sensations, are based on current interpretations. For instance the theory was once held that depression was due to a disturbance of liver function. But people no longer think that, when they are dejected and morose, black bile is coursing through their veins. " Melancholy " now has a different meaning. When the involution case feels an unusual sensation, however, he interprets it according to his own whim, regardless of the knowledge or theory of his society. Hence the patient with a benign psychosis evolves a simile, and the chronic melancholic a delusion, to account for some queer bodily sensation. The former may say his throat feels as if it were closed up so that he cannot breathe, while the latter declares his windpipe is totally blocked and that he no longer breathes. Or one says he feels as if only a small part of his feces were passed, while the other insists that his bowels never move. The patient with a recoverable condition feels as if he were shrivelling up, whereas his more unfortunate fellow asserts he is only one foot high. Examples could be repeated indefinitely all pointing in the same direction, of a personally elaborated explanation having more weight than conventional beliefs.

It is abundantly manifest that involution melancholia, even in its benign form, is a regressive process. But, as it has been so far described, one might imagine it to be really two psychoses, one characterised by fear of death, and the other by hypochondria. Not only do these regressions seem to be separate, but they also stand in contrast psychologically, for death is essentially a negative thing, being a denial of life, while hypochondria with its autoerotic implications suggests actual outlet. On the other hand these opposing symptoms often co-exist or replace one another, which suggests some unconscious connection between them. The solution of the problem may lie in the coincidence of development of these two tendencies at a period of infancy to which the patient regresses.

Analytic psychologists have made little use of the theories put forward by Ferenczi and Burrow as to the psychological peculiarities of infants in the early suckling period—the " Primary Subjective

Phase ", as the latter has called it. I have recently discussed at considerable length the implications for psychopathology of the mental characteristics claimed by these authors to be peculiar to this phase[1], so only a resumé need now be given. The new-born child has sensations but not perceptions, that is, he has not had the experience necessary for the correlation of memories of past sensations with those of the present, which is essential for interpretation of current impressions. His reactions are, therefore, more physiologic than psychologic. He cannot even distinguish between himself and the environment. So rudimentary are his mental processes as to approach non-existence, and, in retrospect, this period must seem like that of death from the standpoint of adult psychic capacity. On the other hand mental effort is at a minimum and life is maintained by the labour of others : the infant's needs are satisfied without his even taking thought about them. The gradual acquisition of a capacity for self-help is accomplished in virtue of the development and exercise of more and more energy and effort. Consequently when the child or, later, the man, is weary of the struggle for existence, he naturally tends to regress in fancy and mental habit to this early stage. It is the historical origin of the death motif.

The acquisition of independent consciousness is not a sudden affair but a slow and often arduous development. At first all is subjective, for the infant does not discriminate between himself and the environment. Gradually he recognises his body as being something separate and at this time bodily sensations make up the whole of his budding consciousness. His first sensations come from sucking and excretion, but, with the growth of voluntary control of his muscles, he learns to stimulate other parts of his body. The biological importance of autoerotism is apparent to any observer who watches a baby training himself in the movements necessary for getting his thumb or toe into his mouth. The same force, which facilitates co-ordination, is at the same time leading to the correlation of sensations (perceptions) and the growth of consciousness. Preoccupation with the body is therefore necessary and useful in mental development. In psychoanalytic terms, autoerotism is an inevitable and integral part of the primary subjective phase. If one were to incorporate in words or ideas the mental state and interest of this period, it would best be expressed as " death " for the former and pre-occupation with the body for the latter. The coincidence of death ideas and hypochondria in involution melancholia are thus explained.

There are, however, other implications of this regression. The attitude towards the environment of the infant engrossed with his body is indifferent and passive, because it really has little meaning for him. But when the adult degenerates to this level he is wilfully

[1] *Problems in Dynamic Psychology*, New York, Macmillan Co., 1922, Part III, *The Preconscious Phase.*

abandoning interests that have been essential to his personality. He does not fail to include the environment in his survey of the world, he actively excludes it.   He wishes to be allowed to restrict his interest not merely to his personality but to his body alone. Hence he resents interference from those about him, even though their intentions are helpful.   He does not want that kind of help because he is no longer of this world.   This is what determines the symptoms of negativism and of irritability ; it is an inevitable accompaniment of marked autoerotism.

A second corollary has to do with an altered sense of reality.   It stands to reason that, in the primary phase, there can be no grasp of reality in the ordinary sense of the term.   Whenever we meet with a new phenomenon, we at once compare it with the huge body of our experience, a large part of which is the result of definite education, that is, of knowledge acquired from others rather than elaborated for ourselves.   The infant who has not learned speech has only one method of interpretating new impressions.   He can correlate them only with what exists already in his nascent mind. The involution melancholic falls back into this mental habit, deriving only such meaning, from what he sees or hears, as may be assimilated with the themes that preoccupy his attention.   In this way he elaborates delusions with a ridiculousness we meet with otherwise only in paresis.   For instance, if a normal man hears someone say " lobster " he thinks at once of something to eat.   The melancholic, however, engrossed with thoughts of death, jumps to the conclusion that this is a reference to a threat of boiling him alive.   The extreme development of superficial associations as determinants for most genuine delusions is characteristic of this psychotic group.

A third corollary has important psychiatric significance.   We are, in general, satisfied with such positions or situations in life as give us an opportunity for outlet.   If a man can express himself, he remains contentedly with the occupation that gives him that satisfaction.   Otherwise he becomes unhappy and tries to change his environment or his work.   The same principle holds true for the permanence or impermanence of psychotic regressions.   If a patient returns in fancy or mental habit to a more positive type of thought and establishes an outlet on that level, he becomes satisfied with it, and has no longer any tendency to exercise his more highly integrated functions.   Now death, being essentially a negation of life, is a protest rather than an outlet, and is, therefore, to be related with the psychological and physiological principle of rest.   This is why death ideas do not involve a bad prognosis, unless the accompanying behaviour and emotional reactions betray the fact that the patient is satisfied with Nirvana as a form of existence.   On the other hand autoerotism implies an outlet, so that if the psychosis shows truly autoerotic hypochondria, or autoerotic practice, a regression with outlet on the lower level is established and the prognosis is bad. Similarly marked irritability implies not merely satisfaction with the regression but an aggressive desire to maintain it, which explains the chronicity of psychoses with prominent tantrum behaviour. But terrifying delusions of imminent destruction make manifest a fight against regression as well as the regression itself. In the same way, if a patient betrays an autoerotic tendency in distressing hypochondriacal fancies, but does not incorporate them in ridiculous ideas (implying an adoption of the most primitive type of thinking), nor in delusions that are transparently autoerotic, there is again proof of the organism failing to accept the regression and recovery ensues[1].

In concluding this chapter some general applications may be suggested of the psychological principles demonstrated in this clinical material.

The first has to do with the psychology of advancing age, with those features of senescence which are to be regarded as characteristics rather than symptoms. A most prominent one of these is *conservatism*. In so far as this is connected with judgment, which is the one great asset of age, it is unquestionably valuable. Conservatism facilitates the dispassionate weighing of evidence essential to judgment and difficult for enthusiastic youth. On the other hand it inhibits action and the instigation of new ideas. At least three factors demonstrable in psychopathological studies contribute to the establishment and maintenance of this tendency. The first is an indirect effect of the slowing up of the mental machine, which always occurs to a greater or less extent as one grows older. This is, of course, a purely physical matter primarily, but it has results that ensue from its psychological effects. At any period of life it is more difficult to reason quickly and cogently about new problems than to exercise judgment that is habitual. This difference becomes more marked when physical regression begins to affect the functions of the central nervous system. We all have a fundamental tendency to concentrate our interest and attention on activities, in which we may excel, and to avoil tasks wherein we may prove incompetent. As senility approaches (and its advance is insidious) a man automatically restricts his interest to the familiar and shuns either new ideas or occupations. He becomes conservative and rationalizes this tendency in a thousand ways rather than admit to himself the truth that he is growing incompetent.

The second factor is the fear of death, which, as we have seen, is an inevitable development of the involution period. The greatest change which any of us can experience is translation to another world, hence any change becomes a painful reminder of the supreme

---

[1] The prognosis of involution melancholia is affected by the nature of the regression in a purely physical way. The hygiene of an individual who resents attention to his bodily needs and who indulges in autoerotic (particularly anal) practices is of necessity bad. Consequently the health of the chronic cases is apt to suffer quickly and they are prone to die much earlier than those with recoverable psychoses.

one in prospect. It is always an old man who says, " Things are not what they used to be " ; as the hymnist sings,
" Change and decay in all around I see,
O Thou Who changest not, Abide with me ! "
The young man sees change as does the old one, but the sight is not painful to the former ; for him it spells growth and development, not death.

The third factor involves a rather subtle psychological point. The personality of each of us—apart from such physical and material data of identification as would have weight in a law court—is a complex of reactions between the unit organism and the environment. A consistency in reaction establishes a definite personality in the psychological sense. This is the personality, which loves or is loved, hate or is hated ; it is also that which one instinctively hopes or believes will survive after death. Since it exists in virtue of interaction between self and environment the latter is essential to it. Alter the surroundings of an individual in any radical way, and his personality inevitably changes, because his opinions and habit of thought are dependent on the repetition of stimuli to which they are a response. Hence when life is beginning to peter out, there is a horror of changing one's views, as that implies changing the personality. In a certain sense immortality is achieved if opinions and attitudes are not modified. When an old man " changes his mind", he is admitting his mortality.

A second characteristic of old age is *opinionativeness*. This results from the influences just discussed and is augmented by the tendency to irritability, the origin of which has been shown in involution melancholia.

A third feature is *penuriousness* and fear of loss of property. Conservatism is nowhere better exhibited than in the investments of an old man ; and the petty economies of the aged, even when wealthy, would be ludicrous were they not pathetic. The psychology of this characteristic is, of course, identical with that of the delusion of poverty, which has been detailed above.

A fourth is the habit of *restlessness*. This is far from universal and, if well marked, is usually coincident with other changes that are definitely pathological. It is when the fear of death is coming close to conscious formulation that restlessness appears, as has been already explained. Mental restlessness is a more frequent phenomenon in old age. The desire to maintain contact with the world leads to pottering activity or an ineffective intrusion into the affairs of others.

Finally we come to a most serious tendency. Conservatism is often a grave defect in a man holding important office ; in the home and in all personal intimacies *selfishness* is prone to appear. No one who has studied the psychological mechanism of involution melancholia can fail to see how natural this development is. Among normal people it is exhibited in less crude form than in psychotic individuals. For this reason its real nature is not unmasked and infinite harm may ensue. Old people demand affection from others, whom they earlier loved to serve. Hence the aged parent insists on receiving not merely physical, but moral, support from his or her children. It is the moral support which may be harmful or disastrous. If the parent is to be kept happy his opinions and prejudices must be held sacred. His views may have been adaptive a generation back, but they have limited value in the present. Hence many a grandchild's education and happiness is sacrificed to keep peace with a mental derelict. Examples are too notorious to need citation. If selfishness appears in no other form it comes to light in the attitude of grandparents to discipline. It is easier to spoil children and win their regard (for the moment at least), than to keep their ultimate welfare in mind. Hence the grandparent, hungry for attention and affection, uses his authority to relax discipline, thereby making himself more popular with the third generation than are the children's parents. This is the easiest form for selfishness to assume because it is so easily rationalized as kindness and true sympathy.

Certain deductions of interest from the standpoint of psychoanalytic theory can be drawn from the clinical material discussed in this chapter. Freud and his followers have claimed that a number of character traits are specifically related to repressed anal erotism. These include stinginess, stubborness, irritability, conceit, untidiness, as well as opposing tendencies that are held to develop as " reaction formations ". Evidence drawn from involution melancholia— where anal erotism so often appears in crude form—would seem to indicate that these are mainly associated with autoerotism in general rather than related with anal erotism specifically. This problem has, however, been discussed at length elsewhere[1], so need not demand further attention now.

Finally a word should be said as to the findings in involution melancholia relative to the psychology of emotions. We do not see affective reactions existing independent of ideas but rather as responses to the latter and sequential to superficial associations. We cannot therefore regard this psychosis as a condition in which emotions are primarily disturbed. The primary abnormalities seem rather to lie in the false ideas. If these were real events occurring in the lives of normal people the emotional reaction would be regarded as normal. The only anomaly, from this standpoint, is found where the affect is less than what a normal person would produce. This is explicable as degeneration with loss of repression in the chronic cases, as the influence of the stupor process, or as a result of the general running down of the machine, the last being merely one expression of approaching senility. Argument on these points must be postponed, however, to the concluding part of this book.

[1] *Problems in Dynamic Psychology*, Chapter XV.

PART V

MANIC STATES

" Then, from the caverns of my dreamy youth
I sprang, as one sandalled with plumes of fire,
And towards the lodestar of my one desire,
I flitted like a dizzy moth . . . "
Epipsychidion, Shelley.

" I am convinced, too, that happiness is much such a kind of
thing as you describe, or rather such a nothing. For there
is no one thing can properly be called so, but everyone is
left to create it to themselves in something which they either
have or would have ; and so far it's well enough. But I do
not like that one's happiness should depend upon a per-
suasion that this is happiness, because nobody knows how
long they shall continue in a belief built upon no grounds,
only to bring it to what you say, and make it of absolutely
the same nature with faith. We must conclude that
nobody can either create or continue such a belief in themselves ; but, where it is, there is happiness."
To William Temple, Dorothy Osborne.
June 13th, 1654.

CHAPTER XIX

INTRODUCTORY : SUBLIMATIONS

THERE are probably no conditions to be met with among
the benign psychoses, which represent such a multiplicity
of symptoms as those grouped together under the heading
of " Manic States ". We see murderous rages and diplomacy, infectious gaiety and irritability, volubility and silence. It
is our task to show that these, and all typical symptoms, are related
etiologically and, that no matter how great may be the superficial
variations, all manic states possess in common the same type of

ideas, pathognomonic of the group. Further, we shall try to show that elation, flight of ideas,[1] distractibility and over-activity—the cardinal symptoms—are an accompaniment of a definite *motif*, furnished by the dominant ideas of the psychosis.

We cannot gain much assistance from the literature, for such studies as have been made of manic states[2] are concerned with small groups, that showed symptoms suitable for the hypotheses advanced, but not common, in our experience, to all cases. *Abraham* says that in depression the patients are cast down by certain complexes, which in manic phases come into consciousness. These are love and hate ideas. He sees a regression to early childhood, to a stage where repression had not begun to operate, so that they frequently say they feel " new-born ". Elation comes from the lifting of inhibition, he thinks, like the pleasure of wit according to Freud's[3] theory. This saved energy goes into a happiness, which also comes from deeper sources of pleasure now freed from repression. A third factor is the freedom from normal compulsion to logical thinking. Such freedom is seen in plays upon words, and constitutes a return to a childish mental state. He claims that flight of ideas makes possible the avoidance of painful topics and the substitution of pleasant thoughts, the incursion of repressed pleasure-giving thoughts as jokes. Essentially, then, he finds a flight from reality to infantilism and a prominence of the hate motive. The latter is certainly far from universal, while the former never occurs, in our experience, in the sense that definitely infantile ideas are present as such, although it is easy to infer their existence below the level of consciousness.

Freud has put forward the suggestion, in a purely tentative way, that mania may result from a freeing of energy, when libido is detached from an intolerable object and thus set free for expression. He does not support this with any evidence, and there does not seem to be any clinical justification for such a view.

Campbell follows Abraham's lead with a hypothesis of flight from conflict. In all of his cases this conflict was a conscious one, the patients being aware that they were ceasing to struggle and giving way to tendencies, which had been consciously controlled, rather than repressed. He concludes that the difficulty of adjustment is much less deeply seated than in dementia praecox. It was probably coincidence that brought such a group of cases to his attention. There are certainly many manics who have no consciousness of the pathogenic conflict. We can always infer its existence, of course, but if we do so, why should we not look on all functional psychoses as a

---

[1] See Glossary.

[2] *Abraham,* " Ansätze zur psychoanalytischen Erforschung und Behandlung des manisch-depressives Irreseins und verwandter Zuztände ", *Zentralblatt für Psychoanalyse,* IIter Jahrgang, s. 302. *C. M. Campbell,* " On the Mechanism of Some Cases of Manic-Depressive Excitement ", *Review of Neurology and Psychiatry,* May, 1914. *Freud,* " Trauer und Melancholie," *Sammlung Kleiner Schriften zur Neurosenlehre,* IVte Folge, 1918.

[3] *Der Witz und seine Beziehung zum Unbewussten,* Vienna, 1905.

flight from reality—a conception valuable from a general standpoint, but of no assistance in solving the problem of specific factors ? Campbell has done us a service, however, in pointing out the value of noting the patient's productions, as a guide to the study of his conflicts. Both authors lay stress on the unhampered expression of ideas. What are these ideas ? Are they peculiar to manic states ?

We may, perhaps, obtain a clue by studying the normal content of elation, which is undoubtedly the leading affect of the manic states. In our daily lives the greatest happiness seems to come from the prospect of achievement of cherished ambitions, whether these be concerned with one's career or with one's love affairs. When we analyse such emotions we see that contentment with actual achievement is a less violent affair. Further, we must recognize that situations which produce the purest joy are never purely altruistic. They come nearest to this in the case of parents elated over the progress of their children, or of lovers similarly overjoyed with the triumph of fiancé or partner. The egoistic component of this situation is discernible in the identification which characterizes genuine love. Even in religious fervour one does not meet with ecstasy over the salvation of the ninety and nine ; it is the hundredth sinner who rejoices when *his* soul is saved. On the other hand the altruistic element is always present, inasmuch as in all normal elation we find the pleasure giving thought to be one related to achievement in some activity, which is essentially social in its implications. We must conclude, therefore, that happiness comes from the vision of success in some undertaking which will indirectly benefit others. It might be objected that many a business is predatory, which must be admitted, but the profits from all legal trade are allowed by society as a return for some *quid pro quo* direct or indirect. Hence even the most grasping of merchants is free from the uncomfortable feeling of engaging in a criminal enterprise ; he feels instuitively that he is working with society, not against it.

The above takes no account of the apparently baseless elation, which, like depression, may colour the day for a normal man without his being able to give any explanation beyond the statement that he awoke happy. We have found such moods to depend on dreams, which are themselves forgotten, as often as not, although their affective penumbra spreads over the waking hours. This subject will be discussed in Chapter XLVIII.

To understand what ambitions mean we must study them as expressions of the personality. Few people—and they are probably abnormal—work for money alone ; the joy is in professional or business pride, or in the prospect which money opens up of a congenial activity. Each man has his particular bent, which gives an outlet to something within him calling for expression. These cravings have their history, and only by studying it can we see their significance for the individual. As indicated in Chapter XII the process of growing up is largely a question (from the emotional standpoint) of directing selfish motives into channels that lead to the general stream of social life. We may use for a rough example the case of a small boy who wants a jack-knife so immoderately that its possession seems to him to be equivalent to the *summum bonum* of life. Finally he gets one, and a new heaven and a new earth are opened up to him, as he perfects himself in the art of carving. Soon a saw and plane are essential to his existence. Next he begins to make tools for himself, and twenty years later we see him a manufacturer of cutlery. As a man he forgets this history and probably regards his business as the result of a lucky accident, which led him to seize the opportunity of an opening in this industry. We can see, however, that his choice was not free. He was blind to the possibilities of manufacturing bricks, let us say. Unconsciously he is still worshipping the jack-knife.

Psychoanalysis takes us a step further and shows the interest in the knife to be symbolic of a larger ambition—to be a man. But manliness is a complex affair and, with growing sophistication, the boy sees more of the sexual in it. There is no lawful, direct sex outlet in childhood, so such tendencies must be repressed to the unconscious, where the instinct continues to grow until it can gain outlet in adult life. Meanwhile—as the instinct is not actually suppressed—it reaches expression in symbols such as that of the knife.

The knife is a symbol while the cutlery business is a sublimation. What is the difference? This can be best discovered by analysing the factors contributing to the establishment of each. Sex is, biologically, an altruistic function, and Nature compensates, for the personal sacrifice its operation entails, by putting the premium of great physical and psychic satisfaction on the performance of copulation. Indulgence in the act for its sake alone means an incomplete development of the instinct. Now the infant is purely selfish in its motives and its bodily satisfactions are its only aims. Until real manhood is attained (which only occurs in truly normal people), the child clings to such acts as are predominantly individualistic. If the desire to be grown up takes the form of a wish to have larger and more potent sexual organs, this is a yearning for a selfish sex life.

Consequently the knife is a symbol of a selfish desire directed into the sex sphere and its hold on him is proportional to his individualism. It is selfishness speaking through sex.

In man at least the sexual object is a matter of as great importance as the act, or, perhaps, greater. As a part of all objectivity, it grows from the first instinctive recognition, which the infant makes, of people and things outside of himself. This interest is naturally given to parents and nurses and is preponderately selfish, inasmuch as it is returned a hundredfold. The task of transferring affection to others outside the home, where reciprocation is less ready and abundant, is *the* problem of psychic development. It is largely complicated by the sex instincts, for as the latter develop, they tend to follow the channels of the existing personal associations, a process which, if completed, would mean incest. As this is repressed it tends to come into consciousness in a distorted form—the sublimation. In it the potentially sexual and selfish component gains a substitutive outlet—as in the case of a woman yearning for physical contact, who devotes her life to nursing. At the same time—and this is the important point—the objective interest, primarily directed within the family, is turned to strangers or towards society as a whole. Freud has defined sublimation as . . . " A process by which outlet and application in other regions is opened to overstrung excitations from the individual sources of sexuality[1]". By analysing the " sources " as we have above, it becomes clear that Freud's definition is too narrow. Sublimation seems really to be the union of selfish and social tendencies in some activity which is a substitute for more primitive and selfish ones. Such a definition may be made to cover what one may term the " sublimation of war ", where originally repressed cruelty is allowed outlet to the soldier and applauded by society, because it now serves a social end. There is no necessity to postulate anything sexual in this " sublimation "[2]. The difference between the symbol and the sublimation is, therefore, this : the symbol stands for something physical or, at most, a circumscribed concept, something which is purely selfish ; the sublimation, on the other hand, is a substitution of a higher, more social, activity for one which originally had in it merely the elements of potential altruism.

If we look on sublimations as socialized childish objectivation, we can see how adult sex interests, culminating in marriage, are really to be grouped with them. In the adult the family attachments (so far as they are potentially sexual) have sunk into the unconscious, while a stranger comes into conscious life to gain this love. Psychological analysis demonstrates these adult objects to be surrogates for the earlier recipients of the affection, while, in the psychoses with which we are dealing, the verbal productions of the patient declare it. Two confirmations of this view appear in studying the ideational content of manic states. First the physical side of sexuality is rarely mentioned, even when the talk is much of lovers, and it is never prominent in any case. Second, we find, in contents which shift, an interchangeability of sexual and non-sexual ambitions. For instance, a woman may one day talk of some lover (whom she unwittingly identifies with her father) and the next time have a religious system of ideas when she is the Virgin Mary, Mother of Christ, the Bride of God (the Heavenly Father), or she may talk of being in Heaven with her own father.

---

[1] " Drei Abhandlungen zur Sexual theorie ", 2e Auflage, 1910, S. 83.
[2] For fuller discussion of this, see " The Psychology of War," MacCurdy London, Heinemann, 1917.

In all psychoses there is, of course, regression. Hence these sublimations are not practical ones adaptable to the real life of the patients. They are divorced from reality (*e.g.*, fantastic business schemes), or represent a less socialized form of sex interest, as in the case of a woman, unable to maintain the adaptation of marriage, who breaks down and turns to imaginary lovers, or to the sweethearts she once had. The formula might, therefore, be proposed : When adult adaptations fail, if the patient regresses to ideas of less real, or more primitive, sublimations, a manic state results.

We must direct our attention to the difference between adaptive and non-adaptive ideas, that is, sane and insane thoughts. In dreams, reveries and the fantasies of idle moments, we often dally with thoughts, whose fruition in action, might lead to disastrous results. This does not mean impracticality but, frequently, social censure. For instance, one may imagine outwitting an opponent by some shady procedure, or having an affair with another man's wife. Again we may plan impossible inventions, discoveries or philosophies, which restrained judgment would ridicule. All such ruminations may occur in sane people because they do not engross the subject's exclusive attention and normal judgment inhibits their transference into action. They belong to the general category of autistic thoughts without being psychotic. Once they are taken seriously, they are symtoms of a psychosis—usually a manic state.

But there are other ideas which normally fail to appear in consciousness, although they occur occasionally in dreams and often in certain psychoses. Psychoanalytic evidence points towards their constant presence in the normal, unconscious mind. These are expressions of crimes, for which we all have the deepest loathing, such as incest, parricide and so on. Such tendencies are so out of keeping with normal life that they are repressed to the deep levels of the unconscious. We do not repress them because they are impracticable, nor because of what Mrs. Grundy would say ; they are never subject to the restraining influences of judgment, " conscience " or fear of public scandal, because such inhibiting forces are largely conscious and so out of contact with them. Their repression is an instinctive matter. Such ideas, however, are often observed in states of profound mental disintegration like dementia praecox, epileptic deliria or paresis.

We see then that there are two groups of ideas which are usually unconscious : one remains far below the threshold of consciousness, unless there be great mental disturbance, and the other is extruded from consciousness because it is not adapted to such a life as the subject has to live. The two repressions are plainly different as well. Tendencies to incest and similar crimes are unbiological, hence their repression is instinctive. What we may term the " non-adaptive " fancies, however, are repressed on conventional grounds. The reader may be a little shocked, perhaps, by the suggestion that he abstains from sexual promiscuity, lying and thieving because of the fear of scandal. Yet he may not be so startled if he considers that polygamy has been practised in America by sects who showed no other signs of degeneracy ; that homosexuality was exalted by the Greeks, whom we admire on other grounds, as the noblest of passions ; and that " caveat emptor " is a legal maxim of the present day. As Stevenson says, " . . . we look abroad . . . and find . . . no country where some action is not honoured as a virtue and one where it is not branded as a vice ". Yet for all that our statement is a narrow one, we do not repress such thoughts merely from a logical fear of consequences. As Trotter has pointed out, we instinctively act with our herd for good or ill because we are, psychologically, herd animals. In this sense both types of repression are instinctive, but one is as basic as our biological kinship with all mankind, the other reflects the normal or expedient attitude of the society in which accident places us.

It has been necessary to dilate on these general principles, because they give a rational introduction to the study of the content of manic states. In benign psychoses the fundamental, biological repressions continue, to operate while, as part of the general failure of adaptation implied in all insanity, conventional inhibitions are lifted. Therefore, *we find in manic states ideas to be classed, broadly, as sublimations, but, often crudely unconventional.*

When we begin to group these ideas under general headings we find in our material, that men and women tend to develop their psychotic interests along different lines. The latter seem to indulge themselves either in fancies of lovers, whom they identify indirectly with the father, or else portray a union with the father, in which sex is consciously eliminated. Such a union is found in the delusion of mutual death or of joining him in Paradise, or in religious formulations where God or Christ is seen to be but an etherealized father. Men, on the other hand, seem more given to inflate themselves with fantastic ambitions, which are concerned with business or professional schemes, or with the development of philosophical, religious or pseudoscientific theories. Hence we hear them announce themselves as prophets, leaders of thought, masters of wireless electricity, hypnotism and telepathy. They remind one of the alchemists who hoped to solve ultimate moral and physical problems at one stroke. They resemble the dementia praecox patients with " constructive delusions "[1] but differ in that their theories are evanescent, less elaborate and less objectivated into definite systems of ideas. Homosexual fancies may, rarely, crop up in either sex and it is possible that, if our material contained a larger number of males, we might find inversion more commonly than we have.

As exceptions to this general differentiation between the ideas of men and women patients, we may cite the case of a woman who in a typical manic state talked constantly of her poetic and linguistic

[1] See MacCurdy and Treadway, *Journal of Abnormal Psychology*, 1915.

accomplishments, her scientific and medical capacities, etc., and the case of a man who had excitements in which his conduct and speech were erotic and coarse. In his case there was a complicating factor, inasmuch as three and one-half years before observation he had suffered from a severe head trauma with concussion symptoms and three weeks' amnesia. This was followed by a character deterioration and instability. Apparently his short attacks of hypomania were but exaggerations of his daily life.

The question may be asked, " But why these ideas or why false ideas at all ? " A complete answer would settle all problems of constitutional insanity, but some indications may be given of more general and underlying causes. Every benign functional psychosis on sufficient investigation seems to result from three psychological factors. First, there is a faulty make-up, evidenced in a continuous failure, from childhood on, to meet the more trying problems in life; second, there is a painful situation resulting from this failure and from which relief is psychotically sought ; at last comes some incident which seems to spring the mine. In a number of the cases which we shall cite the words may be found, " Apparently normal make-up " or " The patient was well when such and such happened." We feel justified, after studying many cases intensively, in claiming that such statements represent the view of relatives who observed poorly, or that lack of time or some other interference, such as a language difficulty, prevented the discovery of previous abnormality. We make this claim because we have always found the three factors, when there has been opportunity to study a case thoroughly, even after the relatives and patients themselves have vociferated and reiterated that the attack came out of a clear sky.

The most fundamental factor is undoubtedly the make-up. As in all the benign psychoses the most conspicuous defect is to be found in the sphere of affective personal relationships. There is a " seclusiveness ", a tendency to shun social contact, often evidenced by shyness, preoccupation with work and so on. The establishment of new friendships and adaptability to a new environment is more difficult than with normal people. The same faulty development is found in a more marked degree in dementia praecox. It must be confessed that the distinctions between the constitutional defects of the personalities found in the benign and malignant psychoses is a problem for the future. We can only say now that the deficiency in the latter is apt to be more obvious than in the manic depressive group. One evidence of this is in their differing abilities to meet new situations, particularly the ability to leave the home environment and live independently in the outside world. It is when this is necessary that the dementia praecox patient begins, as a rule, to break down. The manic depressive case, on the other hand, can, as a rule, make this adaptation, although he cannot maintain it.

So much for the general features common to the personalities in all the manic-depressive cases. There is, in addition, a manic make-up. These are individuals who show a chronic, very mild hypomania, or who tend to become excited and " carried away " with slight stimulus. They are inclined to derive considerable satisfaction from pleasurable fantasies and to react to distressing situations with imaginary relief into which they project themselves in fancy. An excuse for failure can always be found, or a new scheme twice as good is immediately forthcoming. These people have energy, resource and ambition, but are apt not to be practical. They waive difficulties aside or shut their ears to them. Their vivacity makes them socially attractive, so that casual acquaintances are as charmed as intimates are worried by them. This is the commonest type of manic make-up. Another is found in such a case as that of Mary S., whose case will be cited later. Her normal life was subdued, but this was the result of repression of a strong tendency to sexual promiscuity, which came to expression in her attacks accompanied with manic symptoms. In such cases the make-up may be far from hypomanic, and may even be depressive, but psychologically a unity is found between the normal personality and the psychotic ideas. This is probably the case with the circular cases who may alternate between pleasant and unpleasant formulations of the same basic unconscious trend. The essential point is that such people are limited in development ; they are so inelastic that one idea, or a circumscribed constellation of ideas, dominates their lives.

The second general factor is the intolerable situation. This may become impossible from mental weariness in maintaining an adaptation, such as the boredom of household routine—an expression of poor adaptability—or some extra burden may make the daily task unbearable. This burden may be physical, as in ill health, or it may be psychic, as loss of money, threatened failure in business, arrival of another child, and so on. These added difficulties draw attention to the weariness of the labour, hence the feeling and complaint of overwork. This is so often alleged as the primary cause of the breakdown, but is usually secondary or even the first symptom, in the sense that it is a feeling of overwork rather than true fatigue.

The third general factor is the precipitating mental cause. This is some event which stirs the patient, almost always in an inexplicable way, because it is important for him unconsciously rather than consciously. On analysis of the whole case it is seen that the latent meaning of this event has stimulated the patient's innate psychotic tendencies. The mechanism of such disintegration is best studied by citation of actual cases.

CHAPTER XX

BEFORE proceeding with our casuistic material, it may be well to state the methods of our study. We have made only one assumption in our investigations, that the productions, mood and conduct of our patients were somehow related. Our cases are not picked rarities ; they represent the routine admissions of State and private institutions and come from all walks of life. If they seem to differ from average manic cases, it is because great pains were taken to make the observations complete. It cannot be urged that these patients stated what they did as a result of suggestion, because we found the same content in cases examined a quarter of a century ago, when psychogenesis was unthought of.

Full anamneses were taken in order to discover the stresses of their lives, the stories being obtained from relatives, friends and the patients themselves, when accessible. Chance references to people or events were followed up till some explanation of their significance appeared. Some hypomanic cases were sufficiently accessible to answer questions themselves and these were allowed to talk. The flighty patients had their productions recorded and these were arranged and re-arranged until the jumble became coherent, like the solution of an algebraic equation. The working hypothesis in such instances is that ideas consecutively expressed have some other connection. If the association is absent one day, the flight of the next may give it. Such reconstructions are like the putting together of a puzzle picture, where a mass of irregular, apparently heterogeneous blocks are seen ultimately to form a definite picture with not one piece missing. Finally in the understanding of the whole history much light was thrown by the analysis of the precipitating mental causes, which showed the connection between the faulty emotional life prior to the attack and the resulting psychosis.

It is possible to separate the precipitating causes of manic states into four rough groups according as they show : first, direct opportunity for adult wish-fulfilment ; second, veiled outlet to an infantile wish ; third, plain infantile wish-fulfilment, which is quickly distorted in an adult formulation by means of autistic elaboration ; fourth, distortion of a distressing idea into a " sublimation ". These we shall consider separately.

When a poorly adapted individual, with a tendency to regress from the reality of a trying situation, finds himself committed to responsibilities which do not bind him unconsciously as they do consciously, he is in a state of mind where his unconscious interest may be easily deflected to one which pleases his inner, lower self more nearly. To such an individual the suggestion of a new type of life or activity may fire the imagination to flights of fancy that soon pass the boundaries of normal day-dreaming. The alternative offered by a new business to a man, or of promiscuity to a wife wearied with domestic dreariness, are typical of the inciting factors in the first group of precipitating causes.

An excellent example is furnished by the case of William A. W., whose history will be detailed below. During ten years he had seven hypomanic attacks, each one of which followed his abandonment of salaried employment to set up his own business. The inner psychological meaning of this change will be demonstrated later. A somewhat analogous situation existed with Alfred J., who broke down when within sight of a degree. One characteristic of his poor balance was the disproportionate importance he attached to his academic work. Hence the degree was to him symbolic of universal success. It meant a solution of all his problems and he became elated. His case, too, will be cited at greater length.

The history of Lina A. demonstrated how an erotic situation, although at first reacted to with shame, ultimately serves as the stimulus for manic fancies, which relieve the monotony of a humdrum life.

CASE 15. *Lina A.* Aged 20. Unmarried. Admitted to the Psychiatric Institute, February, 1905.

Her family claimed that she was natural, sociable and industrious ; but, as she herself admitted that she was sensitive, shy, nervous, easily embarrassed and always stayed at home at night, we can see that she was really of the seclusive type. Her father, who had been a spendthrift and alcoholic, was dead, but her mother had married again. In July, 1903, when the patient was 19, the step-father was killed. She showed considerable but not unnatural grief. In November of the same year she was offered a better position with a little more pay. Her reaction to this is typical of the difficulty in transferring interest from which such patients suffer. She hesitated, but finally took the new situation. At once she began to worry about her disloyalty to the firm she had left. The normal reaction, of course, would be to transfer her loyalty to the new employers.

Apparently her dissatisfaction with life at this time led her to seek some emotional stimulus. At any rate she so far encouraged two different men that they took decided liberties with her in December, 1903 and January, 1904. She worried over her conduct and confessed the incidents to her mother. She slept badly, talked much about the insults she had received and thought that callers at her home would talk about her. Apparently this initial reaction was highly regressive, for she refused to see visitors and made two attempts at suicide. These represent a tendency to avoid all reality ; but she also showed a trend towards infantile regression in that she had horrible dreams of her stepfather and felt her mother distrusted her (ideas suggesting attachment to the father and antagonism to the mother). Next came a progressive stage ; she built up ideas of adult love, dropped her depression, and became elated. For five months her character seemed to be changed. No longer seclusive, she went out to dances, sang loudly, accosted men, and worked poorly. She claimed she was going to have a millionaire for a husband, a central fantasy of her psychotic imaginings. By July, 1904, she had become uproarious and was sent to the Observation Pavilion, where she boasted of sexual excesses. Thence she was removed to the country and quieted down, gaining some weight.

Reaction set in and she became depressed and inactive for three months. She cried a good deal, let everything drift, did not help with household tasks, and seemed indifferent to the financial fate of her mother and herself. Then at Christmas, 1904, there was a sudden improvement, and for a few weeks she seemed normal.

For a personality such as hers this precipitating cause has a colouring of shame. Hence she could not accept it consistently and began and ended this psychotic cycle with depressions. Her spirit yearned for some autistic outlet, some relief from the narrow dullness of her life. This came in a form suggesting two fates—a sex life that struck a respondent chord in her unconscious, and a life that spelled shame to her consciousness. Hence the alternate reactions. Within two weeks, however, another incident occurred which did not include the drawback. A widower proposed marriage to her. This involved no conflict between unconscious inclination and conscience, but another struggle. Viewed as an imaginary situation marriage was alluring ; as a real bond, it had the irksomeness which all seclusive people dread. It appears from the anamnesis that for two weeks she alternated between these aspects of the problem, for it is stated that she became uncertain, wrought up, unsettled and erratic. At times she was elated and talked of what she would do when married, again said she did not want to marry.

Her condition justified commitment, and she entered the service of the Psychiatric Institute at the beginning of February, 1905. Although not funny nor mischievous, she was elated in the sense of being self-assertive or abusive with exaggerated facial movements and rolling of the eyes. She was talkative and distractible, given to an orderly flight of ideas with continuous, quite natural, and some sound, associations. In these flights she reverted to the topic of the previous attack, but had it formulated in a way more comfortable to her personality, for she scolded about men taking liberties with her, and boasted of her virtue. The sex interest appeared also in the account she gave of a pain in the groin which went to her head and nose and was followed by a delightful feeling. Occasionally she said, " You can't hypnotize me ". The infantile drama emerged as antagonism to her mother whom she repeatedly accused, with indignation, of having called her a prostitute, and in a vision of her father, to whom she said, " Papa, go away, don't talk to me ! " Again, she said that her interlocutor was God or a " religious form."

This phase lasted for six weeks, and was followed by a period of three months during which she was less flighty, but was more delusional. The evanescent ideas she expressed were almost all plain or veiled erotic fancies ; somebody is firing shots from the wall which go through her ; she has been played on all the week ; she is the hero of the bullets ; powders are shaken at her, they say, ' Don't kill me, it is like hypnotism," powders come up through her body to her nose, they make her passionate, they break her nose ; it is like hypnotism ; " I should like to see a man hypnotize me ! " ; they are knocking on the wall to try and hypnotize her ; they try to see what she can stand ; nurses put stuff in her drink ; gun powder is put with her food ; she saw saw divers come out of the river, and the nurses signalled to them ; Dr. M. (at a clinic where her case was presented) made signals to the nurses ; there are signals in the breaking of the eggs and the turning on of the water ; the doctor has people in the cellar and tom-cats crying at the window ; the stars have told her that somebody is down stairs ; her mattress and the ward are in flames ; she feels as if she would explode. That with all this symbolic eroticism, the precipitating cause was not forgotten was shown by her identifying the ward physician as the widower who proposed to her.

We consider these disjointed ideas to be essentially erotic because when they are grouped, as has been done above, associations to sex thoughts are manifest. Bullets and hypnotism are used as equivalents to powder. Powders come up through her body to her nose and make her passionate ; powder is put in food and drink also for the same effect presumably. The signal is plainly erotic. That the people in the cellar are kept there for immoral purposes is a pure assumption. This case was observed many years ago. If examined now she would be asked, " Why are these people kept in the cellar ? " If like other cases she would undoubtedly answer, " For immoral purposes," or something to that effect. The flaming mattress and feeling she would explode are unproven but possibly erotic ideas. With these exceptions, the proof lies in her productions themselves, and, by accepting this, we see a logical connection between her make-up, the setting of her psychosis, the precipitating causes and her productions.

After these three months she began to recover, and was quite well in a month, when she was discharged as recovered. She had retrospectively only superficial, perfunctory insight, and scant memory for her delusions.

Another similar precipitating cause was found in the next case.

CASE 16. *Pauline L.*, aged 49, separated. Admitted to the Psychiatric Institute, February 14th, 1914.

Her parents died when she was a child, leaving her to the mercies of a cold world and of relatives little more charitable. From her own account, it seems that she was an inferior and seclusive sort of a person. She did not learn well at school, was never lively, preferred to be alone and read, rather than to seek friends, was bashful, backward, easily offended, but with little temper. She was religious. She knew nothing of sexuality until she was 20, holding the nursery belief in storks as providers of children. She never could undress before women, and was afraid of men. When 17, a man told her to come with him, and she remained frightened for two days. When 22, she married more from weakness than love, it appears, for she merely bent to the suitor's insistence. She was afraid of sex relations, and prevented intercourse for several weeks, then submitted but without satisfaction. Later she solved this problem by telling him to go to other women. He seems not to have been much of a hero himself ; always alcoholic, he drank more and more after marriage and never got work. She became consciously bitter against him. When 16, she had worked as a domestic, and at 42, when after a psychosis she refused to live longer with her husband, she resumed this employment. She held one position for four years where her employer was very kind to her.

Always given to mood swings, she had her first manic depressive attack when 42. It seems to have been an anxiety with delirious features. It lasted for six months. After it she was fortunate enough to get the position with the kind mistress mentioned above. When she had to give up this place, she was depressed for four weeks. Later she had a second depression of a month's duration. Then her employer died. She became nervous, and, leaving the city, took a place in the country. This did not suit, and she was soon back in town. Some impulse led her to seek employment in the City Hospital, where her worries increased, and she thought the nurses had given her something. She fled this work and tried a public laundry.

Then came her psychosis. She saw two men run after a woman. She afterwards gave the following account of the affair. Two men were trying to throw a woman down some cellar steps. Perhaps one of the men was the woman's husband. If so, she resented this marital attention, and shouted loudly. At this the patient became frightened. " I thought it was cruel ; she shouted and I got frightened . . . I don't know any more. There is so much wickedness about men and women. There are very few gentlemen. The men I worked with are the same ; they were brutes . . . The men make women do things for them."

Is it surprising that from a life of such sordid dreariness this poor cramped soul should unconsciously see, even in this painful incident, a suggestion of relief ? She became immediately hypomanic with elation, excitement, flight and mischievousness. When admitted she showed a constant irritability towards the nurses, and, as the manic features subsided, remained querulous.

The precipitating causes of the group we have just discussed present to the patient, ready-made, an outlet. In the second group, the upsetting factor stirs up the unconscious infantile tendencies but suggests an adult outlet as well. The patient elaborates this suggestion himself and becomes manic.

The case of Celia C., which will later be given in more detail, illustrates this type of precipitating cause with great nicety, for she had two attacks which appeared superficially to be initiated by the same event—a quarrel. As a matter of fact, one was a quarrel with a sister and the other with a fellow worker. Each concerned essentially an alleged interference on the part of the patient with the love affairs of the opponent. This, of course, implied a desire to steal the lover. Now stealing a sister's lover lies very close to the unconscious wish to steal the mother's husband, both being family situations. On the other hand, any elaboration of the idea of interference in the love affairs of an unrelated girl would suggest the fantasy of a quite legitimate lover for herself. This difference was strikingly evident.

When 18 years of age she was working very hard in preparation for examinations and worried about passing them. This perhaps provided the general setting for her psychosis. Her sister was engaged to be married and one day while cleaning up a room ordered the patient out as she was expecting " company ". They quarrelled and the patient became at once depressed. Five years later when asked about this event, she admitted it was her lover for whose reception her sister was preparing ; then she became so upset that she could tell no more. The significance of this episode was apparent in the psychosis, for in a setting of depression and perplexity she expressed ideas of having lost her honour, being a prostitute and killing her mother with worry. All this was heavily coloured with the affect of guilt.

When 23, the patient was associated in work with a girl who was engaged to a dentist. The patient visited this dentist professionally and was plagued by her friend for information as to what he said to her at these visits. This led to a quarrel in which her co-worker called the patient a vampire. A few days later there was another quarrel, this time only about their work, and after this she went home quite upset, and in a couple of weeks had to be committed with what was essentially a manic state. In this she confused the two quarrels, insisted that she was accused of stealing the other girl's lover and developed an erotic trend, all of which will be described more fully below. At first there were symptoms suggestive of depression but the latent idea of the quarrel—gaining a lover—was acceptable, and manic features appeared with this fantasy.

The third group of precipitating causes is that of patients who react to an incident that represents an infantile wish-fulfilment by some psychotic elaboration, which adultifies the wish, as is illustrated in the following case.

CASE 17. *Sara A.* Aged 52, widowed. Admitted, January 7th, 1904.

As a girl she was nervous, sensitive and easily irritated, but on growing older learned more self-control. A feeling of inferiority persisted, however ; she felt people, even her relatives, looked down upon her ; she was now much under the domination of a brother, who belittled her. She was married for about thirty years, and had rather an uneventful life, filled with dull routine. At times she became irritable, once going so far as to throw a kettle at her husband. For six months prior to her psychosis she had several causes for worry, and made the most of them. The fiancé of her daughter had jilted her, and several law-suits were pending. She was always wondering how matters were going to turn out, and spent much time telling her fortune with cards. Apparently she did not claim great belief in this divination, for she said she did it to ease her mind ; but, that she was playing with the idea that fate would be good to her, was shown by her careful watching for the postman. She said she was looking for good news, and would never hesitate to open the letters of others in search of it. Plainly she was seeking relief in imaginations from the care and monotony of her life.

Then on December 12th, 1903 (26 days before admission) her husband died suddenly. As we shall frequently see, death of the husband or wife means the severance of a bond which is difficult for any maladapted individual to maintain. It operates, therefore, as an unconscious wish fulfilment. There was little obvious reaction to this event at first ; her worries about the future seemed merely to be accentuated. On the night of the 18th the psychosis suddenly began. She threw herself on the bed, weeping, and later told the family she had been with her father and brother (both dead), had seen them, and that they had said that all would be well. At once she was euphoric and talkative, the symptoms increasing until her treatment in a hospital was necessary. She remained there nearly eleven months, during two of which she was highly excited, elated and talkative with marked flight, misidentification and disorientation. After that she gradually quieted down to normality, making a good recovery.

It seems that following her husband's death she regressed to the infantile idea of union with her father, as evidenced by the halucination which ushered in the psychosis and also by definite identification with her mother. " I felt as if I was my mother walking up stairs." Then came a constructive reaction (corresponding with the manic phase) when she projected herself into a future that existed before marriage—an existence which her marriage had not furnished in real life.

This case was examined twenty years ago at a time when little attention was paid to a patient's production, and small effort was given to eliciting psychotic ideas. Nevertheless considerable evidence is present in the history to confirm the viewpoint expressed as to the evolution of her thoughts. The cycle was epitomized on Christmas night, one week after frank symptoms commenced. She was excited, restless and talkative, dwelling on her childhood days, once holding a cat in her arms and singing Mother Goose rhymes to it. This was apparently a little too regressive, for she would interrupt the performance with a crying spell. But getting quickly over this she would say that everything was fine, they would all be rich, there would be no more clothes to wash, no more dishes ; they would live in a fine house, have lots of company, and all she would do would be to enjoy herself and do what fancy-work she wanted to. That such statements represented a regression to a premarried period is shown by her claim that she was 20 years old and the reiteration that her name was R. (her maiden name). The uncomfortable difficulty of disposing of her husband in order to project herself into an optimistic maidenhood was smoothed away thus : " Since I have been here I have felt that my husband was alive. I never felt he was dead, and every-

body else has asked me what my name was, and I always felt I was an R."
It will be remembered that she had occupied herself for a long time prior to
her husband's death in telling her fortune with cards ; this, in her psychosis,
was taken seriously, for she announced that she could tell the future, and
assured many people that they would be rich if they followed her advice.

The precipitating cause and its implication of freedom from the domestic
yoke was not forgotten. When telling of her vision of father and brother,
she said that the moment the breath had left her husband's body a feeling
of relief came over her, and taking up his glasses she kissed them. Life up to
that time had been a nightmare, she said, now everything was bright and
beautiful ; she was going to have a new home so that people might come and
see her. (One of her trials had been her husband's lack of sociability). The
intimate connection between her psychosis and the husband's death was self-
confessed in the following production. She was asked by a hospital physician
seventeen days after the death, " When did you come here ? " She replied,
" I came here to-day when my husband died ". When surprise was expressed, she said, " Oh, oh, he's been dead two weeks ". " Why did you
come here ? " she was then asked, and responded, " Because my husband
died. Aunt Joe and Thomas have both confessed ". (" What ! ") " Oh
he has not confessed. My husband is very jealous and has red hair."

The idea of confession implies a crime, of course, and the manic state was
not complete or perfect enough for the criminal aspects of this wish for release
to be distorted. On admission she looked distressed and there were a number
of references to guilt. She identified one of the doctors as the matron of the
police court. Retrospecting she claimed to have had a feeling of guilt. She
once explained her poor sleep during the night of her excitement thus : " I
sang because I was afraid I should sleep if I didn't ; and if I slept I thought
people would think me guilty, and in the morning people always seemed
pleased to think that I stayed awake all night." Again she said that she
used to feel that she was in a terrible place, where she had been put for punishment, because she had been wicked in some way. Not unnaturally she threw
off in her psychosis other responsibilities besides that of her husband. The
children were as much of a bond. Hence she had the idea that her children
had been taken away or again that they had forsaken her, and that she had
been put into a poor-house to get rid of her—a projection of the wish to be rid
of them. In this connection it is interesting to note that whenever she
mentioned her children in her flight she always dragged in the information
that two had died of diphtheria.

In summary, then, we may say that this precipitating cause gave her a
relief from an intolerable burden, to which she responded by building castles
in the air, imagining herself going away again with another future to live.
This was the basis of her elation ; but, inexorably, the injury to others which
this implied would come to her mind, and so there ran through her psychosis
a latent tendency to depression and guilt.

Another case may be quoted to illustrate this principle of autistic
elaboration of an infantile wish-fulfilment into a more sublimated
form, which gave the patient free outlet and a manic state.

CASE 18. *Ruth B.* Aged 22, unmarried. Admitted to the Psychiatric
Institute, February 25th, 1916.

She was born in Germany, and came to the United States at the age of 17.
Her father died when she was 8 years old, her mother ten months after the
patient came to this country. Two sisters were with her. She is described
as having a jolly, happy disposition, but was a bit loose and irresponsible in
her behaviour. A pleasure loving soul, she was of the type to choose the
" Easier Way." She had never actually been a prostitute, but with her
love of being petted, fell easily into the relationship of a mistress. Her infantile tendency was evident in her preferring to accept emotional relationships, which like those of the nursery are largely selfish, rather than to assume

the responsibilities of the mutual give and take of marriage.   This tendency was strong enough to outway moral considerations.

Her abnormality may, perhaps, be traced back to the death of her mother. This occurred in Germany in November, 1911, some ten months after the patient had emigrated.   She was quite downcast over the news.   Before this she had met a man, A., of whom she became fond.   In March, 1912, three or four months after hearing of her mother's death, this friend told her that he cared more for her sister, Ella, than for herself.   She cried all night, and after that did not care what became of her, according to the story she told after recovery.   She felt that all pleasure had gone out of life, all this being made much morse by the taunts of Ella.   This depression did not interfere with her work as a nurse girl, and she soon began to crave affection again and to feel passionate.

In October, 1912, seven months after this disillusionment, she changed her place of employment, and so met a man with whom she became intimate in a couple of months.   In February, 1913, she discovered that she was pregnant, and the man promptly evaporated.   She worried, confessed to her sister, and thought of suicide.   Two months later she had an abortion performed, but was not subjectively relieved.   She felt even more gloomy.

Then in May—a month after the abortion—her sister Ella was married to the man, who had been her friend.   She was sad at the wedding, and felt that all looked down upon her.   Later, when she saw that her sister was happy, it made her feel worse.   She moved away from the neighbourhood of these associations, took lodgings down town, changed her name and worked in an ice-cream shop.

In the following spring she met a man, B., who soon became her lover.   He had some means ; got her an apartment, gave her good clothes, a riding horse, and so on.   He asked her to marry him several times, but she refused, as she thought that if she did, he would get tired of her.   Happening to meet her sister one day, she told of her life quite frankly, said she was comfortable and happy and expressed no compunctions.   In July, she again found herself pregnant, but sometime later, following a horseback ride, she miscarried. This grieved, but did not depress her.

In the following spring, 1915, she decided to leave B.   In July she met Charlie, a young man from the country.   She gradually grew to like him much, and in October became engaged to him.   A week before Christmas of the same year, when she had been engaged for two months, a girl told her that Charlie had said things about her.   She sought him out, scolded, and they had a quarrel with a sudden rupture of the engagement, and a resultant disappearance of Charlie who was heard of no more.   This initiated another depressive reaction.

On Christmas Day she visited her sister Margaret.   This sister had been there already, when the patient came to America.   She was a dissatisfied woman, prone to dwell on the disappointments of her marital life.   On this occasion she said she had ceased to care for her husband, and that her doctor had told her that " he could learn to love her and that she could learn to love him."   Apparently the patient projected herself at once into this situation, identifying herself unconsciously (we may presume) with her sister. During the recital of this confession she alwost fainted from her chair, and for six weeks was much exercised about it.   She spoke much of the doctor's wickedness, wanted to go and talk to him, or do something.   She feared something would happen between the lovers, and that, if it did, she (the patient) would jump out of the window.   Another anxiety was that her sister's husband would kill his wife, and each morning she felt that this had happened, or that her brother, who was fighting in Europe, had been killed. Having become aware of another's guilt her mind was open to recognize her own, and she began for the first time to feel some pangs of conscience about her relations with B., and to regret her loss of Charlie.

With all this she became highly irritable, particularly with her sister, and developed hypochondriacal ideas.   She thought she had a number of fatal diseases, heart disease, diabetes or dropsy, and that she would die. Early in January she had what may have been a slight attack of influenza, and, again at the end of the month, the same trouble. In the latter attack she was delirious (according to her retrospective account), and talked much of her dying and unwillingness to face death.

She was plainly in a highly morbid state, brooding over her own and her sister's misdeeds, cantankerous, rebellious, hypochondriacal, and talking much of death. This was not a healthy attack of conscience, but a psychotic unrest out of which might emerge alwost any kind of a functional psychosis. Chance led her to read a book, "The Awakening of Helena Richie." that changed her condition abruptly to a manic state. But it was not chance that caused the book to make a deep impression on her, for every vital incident in the book duplicated some event or situation in her own or in the life of her sister, with whom she identified herself, and its philosophy furnished her with a comfortable solution of her problem.

The story is a sentimental one, of which a gist can be quickly given. The characters are stock types. The heroine, Helena, is a woman who contracted an unfortunate marriage with a brutal drunkard in order to escape from an irksome home. A child dies as a result of the husband's brutality, and Helena leaves him. She soon falls in love with a selfish widower and intimate relations are established on the understanding that the lovers will be married, so soon as the wicked husband dies. Of course the latter persistently refuses to do so. Meanwhile the widower becomes more and more fond of his daughter by his deceased wife, whom be brings up in ignormnce of his illicit alliance, a child who worships her father with virginal ecstasy. When the story opens this girl is 19, and has largely weaned her father's affection away from Helena, whom he visits perfunctorily, posing as her brother, in a small village to which she has retreated. In this village is a personage with the charity of Christ, the diplomacy of Metternich, and the psychological insight of George Meredith. He is the village parson. The doctor is all the doctor of the sentimental novel should be, and is married to an efficient gossiping shrew. A third character of importance is a lovelorn country youth named Sam. The action hinges around David, an "old-fashioned" child, whom the parson presents to Helena for adoption.

Such is the background for the story. Helena, of course, falls in love with David, and would willingly adopt him. Here the plot begins. The innocent Sam, stricken with calf love, cannot keep away from Helena, who has only a mild and rather bored interest in him. Finally his grandfather, a worldly wise and eccentrically benevolent old gentleman, guesses Helena's secret past and tells it to Sam, in the hope of killing his passion. The latter asks her if it is true, and when she admits it, shoots himself. Meanwhile the doctor has been entangling himself in a high-minded, Platonic devotion for the heroine. She confesses her past to him, and he is so shocked that he makes her give back David to the parson. Just before Sam's tragedy her husband's death is announced. She looks forward to marrying her lover as an escape from all this turmoil, but the latter hesitates. Finally he gives an ultimatum ; he will marry her, if she insists, but David must be left behind. After much travail of spirit she decides to keep the child. When the decision to give up her lover is reached, she communicates it to the doctor, who still insists she is not fit to be a mother to David. In despair she turns to the parson, and tells him the whole story. He forces her to admit she it not a fit woman to bring up a child. For some days she is saddened by this renunciation ; then she leaves the village and the parson presents the child to her as she goes. The moral of this tale is announced as, "Sin does its divine work". By reaching a consciousness of guilt, Helena's soul had been saved, and she was rendered worthy of the trust of motherhood.

The parallelism to the situation of our patient (and the sister with whom she identifies herself) is really striking, and where it was incomplete the patient made good the deficiency in her subsequent psychosis. The selfish widower is her lover who kept her in luxury, whom she left but without gaining peace of mind.   Sam is Charlie in real life, who disappeared in a less dramatic way than the novelist's character, whom he learned of the patient's past. The doctor in the book stands over against the doctor who made love to the patient's sister.   David was the name of a little brother, who died in child-hood, and in the book his possession represents, not only an outlet for love, but also a sign and seal of respectability.   But the most important thing about the whole story is its shoddy philosophy.   Throughout, Helena is presented with such sympathy that one feels the respectability of the neigh-bors to be unchristian prudery.   The reader looks on her dereliction as an expression of natural human instincts.   All this would be comforting to a young woman in a somewhat similar plight.   The dénouement does much more for her.   It dignifies her transgressions.   The moral is that sin is a divine agency for salvation ; become conscious of it, and the soul finds grace it knew not before.   If we recall that the patient was suffering from remorse, we can see how much this gospel meant to her.   It was a promise of new life.

Naturally, just as her repentance was pathological so was her rebirth.   She proceeded to regress (as did our last patient) to her infancy and to build up a new fanciful world for herself.

So soon as she had read the book she felt less antagonistic, wanted to be nice and kind to everyone, or as she put it frankly after recovery, she got " sentimental ".   The first regressive step was to hunt out pictures of her early home, of her father, mother and family, and have them about her room. She also announced that she wanted to go back to Europe—a plainly irrational wish, since the war was at its height.   The manic development was then checked temporarily by the receipt of a cold letter from a sister, which worried her, because it spoke of her engagement.   Her hypochondriacal ideas con-tinued.   On the other hand she got, at about the same time, a friendly letter from another sister which made her so happy that she telephoned to her sister Ella (with whom she had broken after the marriage to A.) and wept over the telephone in her efforts to be " nice ".

But soon the novel reasserted its influence.   Helena was kept on probation by the parson for some time, before he delivered David back to her, and then she journeyed away for a new life.   The patient adopted this phase of the story by imagining that the trouble with Charlie had been brought up to test her.   Next she thought she was going to travel.   Regression began in earnest with much talk of the virtues of her father.   Increasing excitement was evidenced by sleeplessness.   Her sister thought she was abnormal, and decided she should have a change of environment, the very thing for which her psychosis was attuned.   They took her to stay with a friend in the country. On the train marked symptoms appeared.   She felt as if she were walking in a dream, everything looked queer and funny, old-fashioned yet familiar. From then on till her recovery her ideas came thick and fast.   At times she felt they were day dreams, at others she deliberately closed her eyes, because she wanted to build castles in the air and those around her interfered with it. On the train she began an extensive misidentification by recognizing in the fellow passengers, relatives and friends from Europe.   She called one man " Father ".   When she arrived at the house where she was to stay, she mis-took the friend (a woman 45 years old) for her mother, and thought the husband was her father.   The housekeeper she imagined to be her grand-mother.   It seemed as if there were ghosts around, talking and walking about outside and whispering in closets.

This was the stage setting for her regression.   She soon imagined she was a baby ; a boy in the household, Marvin, she thought was her brother.   She sang songs of her childhood, Christmas songs which she used to sing at school. This was, perhaps, the beginning of her new development.   Soon it was love songs, and with this appeared the erotic element.   At night she wanted to have Charlie in bed with her.   She felt cold, and when hot water bags were brought her, she said she wanted natural heat.   But the new life was not merely the re-possession of Charlie.   She had more ambitious fancies.   She stood before the mirror combing her hair and fancied she was turning blond.

This meant that she was a Princess of Germany. The children of her hostess, Agnes and Marvin, were her children, and they were of royal blood. She was in the country for two days, during which she was plainly hypomanic; talking interminably, singing and very happy.

She was then brought back to New York. The journey only excited her more, for she thought something great was going to happen. She became more manic, being very giddy, laughing much, singing songs which she composed at the moment, and making many rhymes. She thought she was in Germany, and saw the Crown Prince ; she was a prima donna, whose name linked with that of the Crown Prince at the time. That she also thought her father was the Kaiser, shows how the Oedipus tendency made itself known, although only by inference. She took one of her sisters for the Czarina. She assumed a variety of expensive rôles ; she was Agnes, Queen of Rumania, a saint, Ruth from the Bible or, again, her father and mother were living and she was a gypsy princess. She was sent to a general hospital, where she thought the nurses had been nursing soldiers with her sister, the Czarina. At another time the doctor was Mr. Vanderbilt and she was his daughter. This hospital, of course, quickly transferred her to the Observation Pavilion.

Up to this time those about her had rather humored her ideas, which she subsequently stated, made them worse. At the Observation Pavilion, however, the sight of other abnormal people shook her up, and she began to wonder if she too were out of her head. A few less pleasant ideas cropped up, which were, possibly, associated with some latent thought of mutual death of which no further evidence is present in the notes. She saw a boy on a stretcher, and thought it was her son, Marvin, and she cried about him. This led to the thought that they had shot her brother, and somehow she fancied he was Marvin Again, it seemed to be her little brother David, who died early. This fantasy may have been stimulated by the identity of the name with that of the little boy in the novel. Her two miscarriages may also have had something to do with these ideas of a dead child.

She was transferred to the service of the Psychiatric Institute, but by that time her ideas had largely subsided, although she continued to talk much of Charlie for a few days. She later said that the kindly criticism of one of the nurses helped her materially to come to herself. Her whole manic state lasted only for about three weeks.

To recapitulate : in this case a hypochondriacal, irritable state with a content of remorse over her own and her sister's loose living is transformed into a hypomanic psychosis, where these ideas are distorted autistically into thoughts of regeneration and a new, glorious existence. Before the expansive fancies appear a regression to childhood is dramatized.

The fourth group of precipitating cause is that where a distressing event is psychotically reacted to by viewing it from one (and a distorted) angle and building this concept into a " sublimation ". The next case is an example of this mechanism.

CASE 19. *Annie D.* A single Jewish, aged 15. Admitted, September 23rd, 1905.

She was slow of comprehension but painstaking, according to the school records. Her mother, who described her as sociable, seemed to be stupid. The father had died while the patient was a child. From the age of 13 on she worked as a nurse girl, but five months before admission took up millinery.

Three months before admission her employer shot himself and was subsequently cremated. His daughters showed the ashes to the patient. The place of business was closed, so she took another position and appeared natural. But the event had made a strong impression on her, for she began to talk a good deal about the suicide and the ashes.

If we assume that she had unconscious tendencies, such as are common property, we can see why this death meant a good deal to her. An employer is unconsciously (and often consciously) like a father. Her father was dead.

The only possible union with him, therefore, was in death.   Hence the interest in this gloomy topic.   She remained sane, however, for two and one half months.   Two weeks before admission something happened to her which suggested an abandonment of her environment, her life.   Her family moved to a new flat.   There she slept poorly.   Now insomnia may be suggestive of a latent fear of death[1] but, at any rate, after eight days she developed symptoms pointing in that direction.   While at work she slipped from her chair without losing consciousness.   She was taken home, and on her way became definitely psychotic, saying that her brother-in-law was going to be killed (a natural father substitute).   She was awake all night talking to herself and refusing food.   She was sent to the Observation Pavilion where she remained six days.   She was described there as a typical manic, being elated, talkative, rollicking, errotic and flighty.

On admission, September, 1905, she was still in this state.   Her flight was composed almost purely of erotic suggestions or references to water, a frequent death symbol.   The following is an example :

"Good luck, give me my diamond (reaching for the doctor's ring), I want to sin no more—three cheers for Theodore, go your way, I will go mine, *I want to be buried in the deepest waters*, I could fight with a will but not with a way—what did I say, good luck, I don't care who it is, I want a duck (puckering her lips as if for a kiss), Mary Lou, let me kiss you, say Lilly's Romeo." To orientation questions she gave the following : (Place ?) "Say Mount Morris, *say salt water, say the deepest water*, I want my little girl in white, I don't care who she is to-night," (Place ?) "Romeo, I want Juliet, queen of the high bounders."

The next day the motif of mutual death appeared rather plainly, and, as the promiscuous eroticism diminished, her conduct became less manic, appearing so only when she applied this tendency to the environment.   She was found whining and crying (without tears).   Her productions were as follows :

"We were kings once, I don't want anyone's photo—I haven't him two, I haven't him three, I haven't him four." (What do you mean ?)   Oh ! don't bother me, don't say what you don't mean, *I fell asleep with him* ; *I woke with him, but don't kill me*." (Are you unhappy ?)   "I am always happy—*I don't care, I didn't blow my brains out*.   *Why do you bring me in such deep water*—*I fell asleep with him, but I didn't do no harm*.   Did I play with bean stalks, hawk faces, *no death, no knife, no angels*.   Roosevelt is mine to remember" (sticking the doctor's hat on her head). . . . "My last duel is fought ; I don't want to fight, I want to see my darling to-night."

In the sentence, "I fell asleep with him, but I didn't do no harm," the keynote of her psychosis is struck.   We have the idea of mutual death which has three potentialities in it.   First there is death, a stupor content ; second, love, a manic theme ; third, sex transgression with depressive implications.

The remainder of her psychosis was a succession of these reactions, with the changes rung on these topics.   For three weeks she was mainly rather depressed, often tearful, apprehensive or appealing, sometimes, however, she lay quietly in bed and said little (a stupor tendency).   An anxiety element also appeared when the visitation of death took an aggressive form.   It was this which made her apprehensive.   She begged not to be killed.   "You will kill me, you have the battery in your pocket now."   Voices spoke to her : "You will get the electric chair.   Why should I get killed ?   I watched the eagle [an immemorial father symbol] and I watched the boats.   Lots of people watch the boats and don't get killed, why should I get killed, just because I like gay colors ? "   (An intrusion of the sex-punishment idea ?)   "I ought to be stabbed, killed, because I looked at the eagle."   At times she was highly distractible, but always twisted her observations into the trend of her thoughts.   "Why should I be killed because I watched the lead pencil ? "   (Watching the doctor write).   "Let me go, I can swim, I don't

[1] See Chapter XVIII.

care for the gold [as a watch was shown], write a little faster—Oh ! I am in
chains [as she heard money jingled], I don't care for the jingling—The candle
is waiting to burn the eyes out." (Candle seen). Next came a more stuporous
phase in which her conduct was less bizarre, but she was inactive. Once for
a week she was dull and stood about gazing at nothing apparently. This
week was followed by a day of elation with flight and a relapse to another
dull period, from which she emerged by a moderate elation without any
special flight into complete recovery. She was in the hospital five months
in all.

As another example of the distortion of a painful idea into manic
content, we may refer to the case of Mary S., which will be described
more fully later. This patient had had some seven attacks by the
time she was 29, three of which were severe enough to demand
commitment. An efficient saleswoman who could always obtain
employment, she nevertheless was continually worrying about
holding her job. When anything occurred suggestive of dependency,
intense worry would set in which soon led to excitements. In her
psychoses it became abundantly manifest that the *res angustae domi*
served as a premonition of being put on the street, while the latter
idea led inevitably to thoughts of prostitution and lovers. Once
agitated, any excuse was seized as a stimulus for erotic excitement
and manic symptoms appeared. The secret of her life, her worries
and her psychoses was simple—an unconscious trend towards sexual
promiscuity. This in her normal life was evidenced by elaborate
decorum and prudish fastidiousness ; it came to expression as a fear
of being forced into prostitution when she worried, while in her
insanity it was the keynote of her productions.

Four instances may be cited. When 19, her brother, with whom
she and a sister had been living, married suddenly. She became
at once depressed, quarrelled with her sister and speculated morosely
on a future without the brother's support. In a few months she
began talking about lovers, and was soon obviously psychotic.
When 21, she worried about not getting a raise in salary that had
been expected, and shortly after, hearing that a man acquaintance
had become engaged to be married, grew restless, visited friends and
boasted of her lovers and was soon in a marked manic state, in which
she claimed to have been married to the man whose engagement
was announced. When 28, another disappointment in not receiving
an advance in wages led to a similar cycle. In her psychosis she said
she had given up this man but was married to the examining physician. When 29, the failure of the firm for whom she worked set
her off on the same abnormal course, and this time she was again
the autistic bride of her casual acquaintance.

CHAPTER XXI

SOME TYPICAL MANIC CASES

HAVING reviewed these various etiological factors, it may be well to give a number of typical cases, which show the close relationship between what we consider to be the distinctive manic content and the excitement, productivity and elation of these patients. We shall then take up the question of the psychology of the other manifestations of the psychosis, in order to show, if possible, that there is, inherently, a close relationship between all the symptoms.

The first case to be described was observed nineteen years ago ; the records are scanty so far as notes concerning her utterances are concerned but, what there are, are illuminated by a splendid retrospective account, which she furnished on recovery.

CASE 20. *Elizabeth K.* Aged 39, married.. Admitted, March 24th, 1905.
F.H. The family history shows nothing of interest.
P.H. The patient was described as a healthy normal child, who got on well at school and graduated from college. She is said to have had a natural happy disposition. After graduation she taught school for a year. Then when 25 she was fired by an ambition to be a missionary, and was sent to Japan. On the trip over her conduct was such as to attract attention and occasion comment. On arrival her excitement increased, for she became frivolous and gadded about to parties, concerts, etc., instead of attending to her work. In a couple of months she was evidently in a typical manic state with incoherence and failure to recognize her friends. She soon quieted down, however, and then became depressed, in which unhappy condition she was shipped home again, a month after the height of her excitement. On the voyage she made suicidal attempts. After her return home she was in hospital for three and one half months with an agitated depression, and then recovered, her entire attack lasting about eight months. She was well for eight months, and then had a five months' exhilaration in which she had extravagant plans for making money, writing poetry and composing music (rather the masculine type of content). Six months later she had a hypomanic attack of only four weeks' duration, when treatment in a hospital was unnecessary. When 29, she married, and for ten years remained well. She is said to have lived a normal life but was very active. She had two children, and in addition to all her housekeeping managed to go about socially a good deal. She was popular, partly on account of her excellent singing.

Then came another attack. For two months she had been over-doing, and possibly was a trifle exhilarated. She subsequently stated that this was coincident with worry over the attentions a married man paid to her. He was a friend both of her husband and herself, who made such flattering remarks that she began to worry lest he should go too far. She thought his wife was worrying about it too. She fretted over her health, fearing that she might not be able to finish out the season. Naturally this led to thoughts of her insanity, and the idea came that her son might inherit the taint. This was probably the first hint of the unconscious idea of injuring the family, which later came to frank expression. She wished her physician to write to the hospital, and learn if her illness had really been considered insanity. Evidently her insight was beginning to fail.

The next step was definitely psychotic. She told of an incident which was, probably, precipitating cause of her first attack. On the steamer going to Japan, the next stateroom contained a man, and there was a door between the two. This suggestive situation was elaborated into a belief that she was accused of having intercourse with him. She worried and pondered over this, unable to say whether the worry was about the accusation or the fancied intercourse. She claimed that a woman medical missionary in Japan had stated that she was not a virgin. Then, suddenly, everything at home annoyed her beyond endurance ; she became highly irritable, accusing her husband of having illicit relations with the nurse, and promptly turned against the latter. She thought her two boys were being smothered in a tower like the two princes. This irritable and anxious phase passed at once into an elation in which she was excited and talkative, switching from one subject to another. She affected to be on the stage, saying she was an actress, and singing ; again she was Queen Louise ; again she was on a wedding trip with her physician. She had to be taken to a hospital at once.

Before describing her psychosis it might be well to recapitulate the events of this onset in the light of our theory. A highly superficial anamnesis reveals no trace of maladaption to her situation except over-activity, which suggests an exaggerated effort to maintain contact with her environment. The sequence of events, however, can only be understood, psychologically, by assuming that maladaption was present. A suggestion of unfaithfulness coming to her, she reacts abnormally to it with excessive worry instead of promptly snubbing the aspiring Don Juan. Next she frets over her health, which can be explained as the conscious form assumed by an unconscious wish to break with her responsibilities, as she would have to do if her health failed. Then came a projection of the wish to leave the family in a thought of injury to a child—he might become insane. Following this she revives an idea from her first attack—of an illicit sex adventure. Having thus psychotically transferred her interest to a stranger, she becomes antagonistic to all in her home, thinks her sons are being killed, and projects her own inner unfaithfulness on to her husband. This provides an excuse for liberation and her psychosis blossoms into fantasies of new activities ; she is an actress, a queen, a bride ; with the last idea she becomes manic.

For the first day or so in the hospital she was elated with contagious laughter, was under some stress of movement but not markedly so, Lying in bed she had a tendency to kick the clothes off. She made many gestures. At times she knew, apparently, that she was in a hospital, for she spoke occasionally of the nurses as such, and misidentified one doctor as another whom she had known there before. Otherwise she seemed quite disoriented. Although aware of her environment in the sense that she was distractible, it was almost impossible to get her to fix her attention sufficiently to answer questions or even to obey such a simple command as to show her tongue.

Her productions were flighty, inconsequent, but with few sound associations. It is noted that there were many repetitions in what she said, but unfortunately no record was made of the topics on which she dwelt. Apparently she made a few erotic remarks, such as saying that the doctor should put his hand on the " key of her heart " or look at her knees. In the few sentences of her talk which were written down there appear several references to Heaven and to death—" I found out how it is to die. I don't fear death any more. Fear is the greatest evil of human existence." Again, shutting her eyes and keeping quiet for a moment, she said, " How hard it is to talk when you are dead," an obviously playful, and therefore pleasant, dramatization of death. Then there were some expansive references : asked how she was, " I can express is in any language " ; another time, " I can talk as fast as any typewriter or stenographer ; I am Phillips Brooks ; I can talk as fast as he ".

The third night after admission she had a sudden, isolated attack of anxiety, the theme of which was, apparently, sudden death and descent to the infernal regions. In the midst of her excitement she screamed loudly, crying out, " Look at the picture on the wall ! See it move ! Now look it is going around the room. Oh, I am so frightened ! I am going down, down through the earth. See I am sinking ! Look at that imp coming out of my closet. Look at him ! Why am I alone here ? No light, all dark ". Then she threw herself on her knees and said, " Oh my God, what have I done that I should suffer so ? Where is my Red Cross nurse ? Oh, they have left me alone in this cell ! Won't someone come to me ? " When the nurse went in, the patient calmed down and asked her if she thought she had delusions or was it real. Later she slept, and on awaking began singing and pounding as usual. It is important to note that with this change of fomulation of the death idea to a painful form, not only is the mood changed but the thought disorder is radically altered, a phenomenon of which we shall have more to say later. In these productions there is perfect clarity without a suggestion of the flight, which usually made her remarks incomprehensible.

After her first admission note, her excitement grew steadily more pronounced. Restlessness was extreme, she pounded the wall, pulled her bed to pieces, refused to keep any clothes on, and was often untidy. She often sang and talked loudly, again, as at an interview six days after admission, she was easily kept in bed by the nurses and was unproductive, answering few questions and then irrelevantly. She kept her eyes closed a large part of the time, made some faces, laughed occasionally, and had an expression of dreamy contentment. Apparently she was completely disoriented and answered questions merely from the inner trend of her thoughts. For instance, when asked where she was, she once said, " Opera House " (her actress idea), and again, " At home, sweet home, giving the boys away " (a repetition of the wish to be rid of her family). Sometimes during this six weeks of marked disturbance she refused to speak altogether. During this period she was usually tube-fed. She became destructive towards the end of this time, tearing up sheets and pillow cases ; but with this she occasionally asked where she was. The association of these apparently opposite tendencies, she later explained herself. During this whole period she usually recognized her husband, when he called, and some times spoke rationally to him.

Then, rather suddenly, she began to improve. This was evidenced in her becoming more tractable, more comprehensible in her flight and seemingly taking more interest in her environment. She certainly commented on it freely. She was more erotic, and made frequent attempts to embrace the doctor. This improvement continued until complete recovery occurred after a month. Five days after improvement set in, she said, " I realize now that my being here is real. I thought the nurses were college friends dressed up to play some trick on me. I used to think my room went 'round and 'round, and I had all sorts of dizzy sensations. When they put me in a pack I used to think I was being done up to be thrown overboard ". In this she expresses the death idea again, and also a dramatization of return to pre-nupital life.

When she recovered, she gave an excellent account of the onset of her psychosis (which has already been quoted), and remembered the external events up to the actual entering of the door of the hospital. But from then on, for the six weeks of her marked mental disturbance, she was completely amnesic for all that went on around her. She was living in a world of her own, of which she gave an account. Her ideas may be grouped as representing different kinds of regression and a reverse process of progression by which she emerged into reality.

The first regression was one noted in the onset. She was on her wedding trip, and they had put rice and pins in her bed, which was the reason for her refusal to stay in it. Next came dramatization of her college days. The nurses were her old friends and the doctor was the brother of her husband. The whole situation was elaborated into an imagination which apparently persisted for some time. She was at a house party surrounded by her friends (her continual misidentification), who had locked her up in a room as a joke—a rather poor one, she thought. The light fixtures were a part of the joke ; if she manipulated them properly she could get out ; the scratches on the wall meant something, and a correct interpretation of them would give her the key, which would enable her to get out. (She spent much time in silently feeling the wall). This idea of the " Key " may, possibly, he regarded as the first trace of the constructive psychic processes. The incarceration fancy was also formulated as a part of larger problems. The war between Russia and Japan was raging at the time. She thought she was in a ship bound for Port Arthur (possibly an echo of her earlier manic attack), or that her room was in the fort at Port Arthur, and was the Key to the situation. Evidently she was making herself an all important personage in the struggle. The garden wall suggested the fort, and the tiling on the bath room floor made her think it was a place of refuge in the citadel, where no harm could come to anyone.

We have noted that she often referred to death in her excitement, and once was terrified by hallucinations of descending into the abyss. Now death, burial and incarceration are symbolically closely related ideas, and often preceded delusions of rebirth. The latter is a progressive tendency, just as dissolution is regressive. Hence we can see the logic of her next fantasies. The first one was closely allied to the Port Arthur imaginings. A great battle was going on outside, and all her relatives were killed. Next, quite naturally, came the end of the world. There had been a tremendous upheaval, and the earth was flat, floating on ether. She speculated much how things would be in the new world ; how could there be night and day with a flat earth ? She finally concluded that it would always be day. These delusions were apparently a projection of her personal problems. The world which she destroyed was that little world in which she moved and which had been too much for her. From its death would come a new life and better life. Hence we find that, when this imaginary destruction took place, she was the only one left alive. *All things would begin over again with her,* she thought. This isolated grandeur was properly accompanied by symbols of power. Everything was electrified ; she felt so charged that her hair stood on end, and she could feel it go from her fingers, when she touched anything. She claimed, too, that she lost ability to guage the force or her movements. Thus she was greatly surprised to find a window break when she barely touched it ; she struck the nurses when she only intended to touch them. What superhuman strength this suggests !

These last were constructive ideas, however, and naturally heralded recovery. This began with correct recognition of a doctor and nurse whom she had known in her earlier admission. Having grasped so much of her environment she built on that. Her next step in orientation was to realize that she was in hospital, but she reacted psychotically to this, for she began to tear up sheets to make bandages. Crazy though this behaviour was, it contained the germ of recovery in it, for, after all, it was an ambition to do something useful, no matter how perverted the effort was. This explains why she became " destructive " and began to ask where she was at the same time. Superficially they look like opposite tendencies, but underneath they both represent an attempt at recovery. Finally there came an illusion which illustrates exquisitely how her ideas were shaping for sanity. One day the guard on the window looked to her eyes like a cross, and the thought came to her that she should be keeping Lent. Then suddenly her feeling of rebellion, against things as they were, passed away and, immediately with this resignation, everything cleared. She looked out and saw the green grass and trees, and said to herself, " Things are not so changed as I thought, they all look as they used to ". All at once it came over her that her ideas had been imaginations, that she had been ill. From that time on, with explanations from her husband, the nurses and the doctors, she recovered rapidly and completely. Progression and sanity triumphed over regression.

The reader may have been struck by the resemblance of this account to the retrospective story of a delirium. We shall recall this when we discuss the thinking disorders of manic states.

In the cases so far described the "sublimation," which we view as the occasion of elation, has been an unreal and plainly regressive idea. The next case, however, shows how a hypomanic patient may break down when he develops the thought of going into business for himself. This is not, superficially, a regressive tendency; but repeated observation showed that this "business" was but a thread-bare cloak for distinctly regressive fancies, and that the new undertaking always implied changes in his life, which meant retreat from his struggle for adaptation. As the study of his attacks progressed it became more and more evident that his new ventures were not the product of legitimate and natural development of interest in his trade, but were prompted by psychotic ambitions.

CASE 21. *William A. W.* Aged 50, married. Admitted to the Psychiatric Institute, November 25th, 1909.

This patient is one whose case was mentioned in the discussion of precipitating causes. He was born in 1859, and was 44 at the time of his first attack. When last seen in his tenth observed attack in 1917, he was 58 years of age. He is described as being always healthy, intelligent and successful in his business as a salesman, or manager, for fashionable provision houses. Temperamentally, he was restless and eager, which qualities contributed to his business success. He earned high wages, and made a good living out of his commissions in addition. No informants were available to describe his boyhood and adolescence. Perhaps the most definite evidence we have of his inferiority is to be found in the fact that, although he had a life-long ambition to be his own master, and had had opportunity to save, he never attempted to work for himself except as a symptom of a psychosis. This is, perhaps, not unrelated to his physical cowardice. He was married twice. At 28 he wedded a woman who bore him two children; one was a boy who died in infancy, the other, a girl, was grown up and married when the patient came under our observation. This wife died in 1907, and he married again a year later. There was one child from this union, further pregnancies being prevented in the fear of transmitting the father's psychotic taint. This second wife probably had a good deal to do with the increase in frequency of his attacks, for she was hardly designed as a psychiatric nurse. Domineering, selfish and unsympathetic, she viewed the anomalies of her husband's temperament with impatience, accepted his almost servile devotion, when sane, as her natural right, but resented his individualism, so soon as his swing from the normal began.

The patient had two master passions, perhaps we should say, only one. He idolized his mother, calling her the most perfect of all women. As a daughter by his first wife grew to maturity, and his mother died, this affection was then transferred to the former and, later, in some measure to the daughter by his second wife. Apparently he was never able to carry over this love completely to either of his wives, towards whom he became antagonistic in his attacks. In fact quarrels were responsible for upsetting his balance. In one attack he epitomized his attitude very nicely when he remarked that his married daughter was a much finer woman than his wife, adding that his mother was the finest woman God ever created. He never had a cross word with her. He was her oldest son, her pet, and "took after her". With this, adaptation to wedlock was naturally difficult for him, and the situation in his second marriage was made much harder by a quarrel between the new wife

P

and daughter at the wedding. They vowed never to speak, and carried out the threat with consistency. Consequently the bridegroom was forced to make a decision and chose to be loyal to his wife, letting all associations with the daughter be broken. But this decision was conscious ; unconsciously the older loyalty remained, to be asserted with greater vehemence and plainness in each attack.

The other passion was his business—the imaginary business, which he would some day have for himself. As his career developed, however, it became ever more evident that the getting and spending of money were not primary interests, but merely a vehicle of expression for his conscious or unconscious devotion to his wife or mother. How this came about can be understood from his history. When 14, he went into his father's business ; but the latter failed after two or three years, and the patient at once assumed some responsibility for the maintainance of the home. He went to work for a man in the meat and produce business, and had only one interest, to make money for his mother. It seems that it was at this time that he developed the idea of going into business for himself in order to have more money to bring home. Up to the time of his marriage all his earnings, left over when his meagre expenses were met, went to his mother ; then it had to go to his wife.

Money was his medium for expressing devotion. So we find that he turned over all his salary, except pocket-money, to his wife, which he had her deposit in her own name at the bank. At the time we knew him, he avoided theatres and other amusements on account of the expense, and preferred to spend his leisure hours in looking after his little girl or helping with the house-work. At the same time he cherished the ambition to rear his daughters in luxury, or to leave them fortunes. Quarrels in his original home were always about money, and he remained permanently estranged from one brother with whom he differed over a financial matter. Most of his attacks were ushered in by a discussion on this subject with his wife (when a widower, with his father-in-law). Once psychotic, his habits changed completely. He would charge his wife with stinginess, say that she was rich with accumulations of his money, and that it was her parsimony which prevented their indulging in any amusements. He further would allege that she kept his money to prevent his giving it to his married daughter, an idea, it was determined, which was purely his own. He would think she interfered with his business, and ask her to go away on a visit. He would be irritable to her alone, but for years confined his accusations to a financial form. Even leading questions could induce no other complaint. Finally, however, in one of his last attacks, he broke into accusations of infidelity. Not unnatrually the dénouement of the money story also came to light at the same time. His mother sent him spiritistic advice from Heaven as to his business. The autistic partnership of his life's dream was established, and he projected his own lack of marital loyalty on his wife.

We can now proceed to a description of his attacks. Of his earlier ones we know little. The first occurred in Washington, and lasted from December, 1905, to September, 1906. As to the prodromata we have no information. He began to sell smuggled game, abusing the privilege accorded to ambassadors, of having game brought from abroad without inspection. Jubilant over his prospects, he was indiscreet enough to sell to others besides the ambassadors. The police discovered this and arrested him. At the time he spoke about Secretary Hay being involved, which made the police doubt his sanity, although he was not committed. He later explained this statement by saying that an employer in a house owned by the Secretary was implicated and arrested. During this attack he quarrelled with his first wife over some financial matter, struck her and left her for several months. The arrest ruined his business, of course, and he soon became depressed, the latter reaction being the only one of this nature he had until the last psychosis in which he was observed. During the depression he went to a sanatorium, where he is said to have made suicidal attempts.

His wife died in April, 1907. Shortly after, he quarrelled with his father-in-law and left home. He went to Atlantic City, and took up the ice-cream business. This started his second attack; he became elated, and spent a large part of the summer running around the country with a couple of girls. This is the only frankly erotic behaviour chronicled in his history, and it is interesting that he explained it later, by saying that all his other attacks had occurred while he was married, and that he had inhibited these impulses out of respect to his wives. The exact duration of this psychosis is not known, but some time in the fall he left Atlantic City, penniless, and resumed life as a salesman.

In the beginning of November, 1909, he got three hundred dollars from his new wife, and set up an independent business. He established offices in New York and Washington, making his headquarters in Atlantic City. He bought much game, and received many orders, but took no pains to determine the standing of his customers, nor to collect moneys owing to him. Consequently he went heavily in debt. Meanwhile his conduct grew more and more irrational; he put strange advertisements in the papers and so on. His ridiculous behaviour led to his arrest, commitment and subsequent admission to the service of the Psychiatric Institute. Notes made on his case at that time show that he was over-talkative, elated and expansive, expecting to be a millionaire and dilating on his intellectual and business capacity. His productions were not definitely flighty. There was no evidence of any intelligence defect, but he denied his more irrational acts. Lumbar puncture was entirely negative. He quieted down soon, and in December of the same year was paroled to re-enter the employ of the firm he had been with before the attack.

In November, 1910, a year later, he again went into business for himself, became elated as usual, and had to be put into a hospital in Washington, where he was at the time. He remained there only two months.

In the spring of 1912 he was again at Atlantic City and under similar circumstances developed another elation. His conduct in this attack was more ridiculous than in any other. He telegraphed the Republican convention to wipe out the "Beef Trust", bought a museum of stuffed birds, which he was going to establish on the Million Dollar Pier as an advertisement. He claimed to have found a child on the beach and one morning told his wife to have breakfast for three as Frank was coming, Frank being the name of the son by his first wife who died in infancy. Later he tried to make light of these irregularities by saying that the "baby" was a marble baby which he talked about for advertising purposes, and that the "three for breakfast" was a joke. This attack forced a commitment in a New Jersey State Hospital from June to September, 1912.

His sixth attack occurred two years later (1914) and, as it again led to his reception in the service of the Psychiatric Institute, the case was chosen for special investigation. It appeared a good opportunity to see whether a case of obvious hypomania, that seemed from all the records to be free from any content except business expansiveness, could be shown to have any deeper psychological mechanisms. No psychoanalytic technique was employed. He and his wife were simply asked many questions and the answers recorded and arranged.

A full account of the onset was obtained which was typical, his wife said, of all attacks she had seen. On May 15th, 1914, he was laid off for the summer by the firm which had given him winter employment. Before resuming work in another position he and his wife thought they would take a two day trip up the Hudson. It may be that this liberation from employment stirred up the unconscious wish for a different life and set the psychotic machinery a-going, far from consciousness. At any rate when his wife accidentally missed the boat, he was irritated and accused her of being late on purpose to save the money which the trip would cost. (A sudden reversal of his usual attitude in business matters.) He remained irritable for several weeks and, in spite of any obvious abnormalities, his wife was convinced that another attack was impending.

He went to work at once for a firm in Oyster Bay, with whom he had previously been employed. But he became dissatisfied—increasingly so. The shop was owned by a woman with a number of nephews and a manager above them. Apparently there was considerable jealousy on the part of all the employees of the deference paid to the patient by the owner, and he made little effort to meet them diplomatically. Knowing the unconscious tendency of the patient to work for an idealized woman, we can easily understand how this situation was an impossible one for him. Soon matters came to a crisis. He quarrelled with the manager over some trivial affair and went home in a rage. Doubtless he was assuming the airs and authority of a proprietor. His wife persuaded him to finish out his week but then he left. On Monday the owner of the shop sent for him four times, but he refused to return.

He had already rented a shop for himself, bought fixtures and put advertisements in the papers. It was only then that he became frankly excited, although his wife discovered that he had for a week or more been secretly making preparations to go into independent business. She persuaded him to come into New York and then had him committed, before he had time to do anything markedly irrational. He entered the hospital on June 22nd, a little more than five weeks after he had the quarrel with his wife, which seemed to be his first symptom.

On admission he showed a mild elation with over-productivity of speech and to a less extent of movement, but with no formal disorder of thought. He was spontaneously expansive about his business ability and prospects and, on questioning, showed considerable irritability towards his wife. He complained that she always had him committed, whenever he set up a business for himself, because she feared that if he made much money he would turn it over to his married daughter. This was his most insane idea, for it had not the slightest foundation in fact (as was determined by cross-questioning of his wife), and was plainly a projection on his wife of the latent idea of working for his daughter rather than for her. By the end of July (five weeks) he had, apparently, recovered his normal mental attitude and would admit that he had been excited. But no amount of argument could persuade him that he had at any time done anything irrational, or that he had showed any defect of judgment in any of his business dealings. His history was reviewed with him and he even defended the buying of the museum, and the talk of finding a baby at Atlantic City, as legitimate forms of advertising.

By the middle of August it was thought that his condition was sufficiently stable to justify his parole. He at once took up a position as a salesman. His wife stated that he seemed quite his old self, kind, considerate and generous towards her and the child. About the end of October, or after ten weeks of this normality, he began to have trouble with the book-keeper (a woman) of the store. This culminated in his discharge on the 31st. The next day he told his wife he was going into business for himself; but he stated later that he had been cogitating over this change for some days, which probably was the underlying basis of his disaffection at the place of his employment. He tried to get first $25.00 then $10.00 from his wife but she refused. He then went to his married daughter for money. For three days he was much upset, full of his plans but fearful of his wife's returning him to the hospital. This last was such a living apprehension that he spent all one night on the roof, for fear she would have him taken in custody, and threatened to jump off, if she interfered with him. During these days he was very irritable towards her. On the fourth day he went into business by buying (with the few dollars he had) two stalls in a public market. With borrowed money he bought fish at the piers and sold them the same day, paying back his loans in quarters and half dollars as he took in cash. After three days of this career he was so unbalanced as to give away a wagon load of fish. The market policeman thought he was drunk but not sufficiently so as to justify arrest. Two days later he was arrested on the complaint of his wife but he put up such a good story to the desk sergeant at the station, that he was liberated and the wife reproved for trying to put him away. She then appealed to the hospital authorities, who sent attendants to fetch him back to the hospital, as his parole had not expired.

On readmission (November 10th, his seventh attack) he seemed at first to have just the same kind of mental disturbance as had characterised his previous psychosis. He was again elated over his capacity and expansively voluble about his achievements. The account of his progress in five days of business sounded plausible, but cold reason made it appear highly improbable, whereas the extent of the correspondence and telegraphing he described was plainly unwarranted. Three days later, however, a change was noted. The attendants reported that he was not sociable, as he had been before, and refused to do any work. With the examining physician he was querulous and showed an over-activity in speech and manner more like that of one in anger than elation. He charged the doctor with holding up his mail and his wife with taking letters sent him by his married daughter and stealing money from them. (Again a projection of his distorted loyalty in financial guise!) With this change of mood there was an elaboration of his ideas, in much graver form, further divorced from reality, and closer to the underlying wishes. He spontaneously referred to suspicions of his wife's infidelity, claiming that he had never allowed himself to think of it before. She had always been niggardly in allowing him marital privileges, so he suspected that she might be intimate with two men living in the same house. She had probably had him returned to the hospital in order that she might have a free hand, as well as to prevent his making money to send to his daughter. A definite expansive delusion also appeared. He hinted at his possessing hidden wealth. He had always given his salary to his wife but had secreted his commissions, which, of course, to his heated imagination were huge. Then he went on to tell of his spiritistic guidance in his business, giving examples of trades he had entered into with profit as a result of influence by a medium and asserting that this assistance had increased since the death of his mother. Plainer evidence of " business " being for him a partnership with his mother could hardly be desired.

This condition of irritable assertion of delusions lasted for only four days, after which he quieted down and was superficially normal, except for once saying that he could not make out what had guided his wife's actions, unless there were some one back of her who had a lot of money. This, apparently, was a reformulation of the jealousy idea in financial terms, co-incident with the abandonment of his frank delusions. But with this improvement there was no gain of insight, he seemed particularly impervious to any suggestion that his business judgment had ever been faulty. So the experiment was tried of talking to him an hour daily in an effort to foster some self-criticism. For nine days no effect whatever was apparent and then occurred something of great significance. His wife visited him and was unusually decent in her attitude. This made him feel more kindly to her and abruptly came expressions of insight into his business difficulties. Recovery seemed to recapitulate the development of his psychosis in reverse order. Whereas he had always begun his attacks with a quarrel, and then developed fantastic schemes as a method of getting away form the domestic yoke, now, with a willingness to bow his neck again he became aware of how ridiculous his plans and behaviour had been.

This delicate relationship between marriage and employment, on the one hand and unfaithfulness and independent business on the other, was further illustrated in the next few days. Once he expressed insight, the theory of his psychosis was given him, which he accepted at least verbally. It was thought that there was a faint hope of his reformation, if he could get into business for himself, at a time when he was mentally normal, and so establish a real, rather than an autistic, sublimation. His reception of this suggestion augured well for the scheme. He accepted it with cheerfulness, but no elation. This was on the 22nd of December. He was told to write his wife asking her to come and discuss the matter with the physician on the 24th. She did not appear that day or even visit her husband on Christmas day. The following day, however, she came, but not in a co-operative mood. She stated that she was not going to pay any attention to anything the patient wrote and that the doctor should write himself, if he wished to see her. This at once produced a relapse. Naturally he became enraged at this treatment and, so soon as antagonism to his wife appeared, so did elation and he grew expansive over his prospects. This, his eighth attack, lasted for only three weeks. Its termination is also of interest. His unconscious wish for dissolution of the home received altogether too direct a fulfilment and he became depressed[1]. His wife revisited the hospital and informed him of her intention to leave him for ever. She had sold all the furniture and put their child in an orphanage His depression was somewhat relieved, when he was assured that she had no legal right to keep him in the hospital. With this his insight returned and he expressed a willingness to remain months, if necessary, in order to demonstrate his normality.

The remainder of his history is tragic. There are, of course, other ways, in which compelling unconscious trends can operate, besides the psychotic. One is, that the hidden motive may prove too strong for the moral tone of a man. We have noted already that his history showed him to be rather weak. His next débâcle was more of a lapse of probity than of sanity. After it seemed certain that his wife would do no more to aid him, he was kept one month in the hospital, while plans were laid for him to try another bout with fate. He was paroled on February 27th, 1915, and given some money as capital, with certain conditions ; he was to make no effort to see his wife or child until he should have thoroughly established himself, and he was to visit the physician or report daily to him by telephone. These promises he did not keep. His first act was to go to the orphanage where his daughter had been placed and take her out. Next he tried to secure the family furniture, which had been sold, threatening suit if it were not immediately delivered. This was with the hope of starting housekeeping with his five-year-old daughter ! Direct fulfilment of his deepest craving was more attractive than the round-about satisfaction to be gained through the sublimation of business, so he misappropriated the fund furnished him for the latter. A five-year-old child requires some attention, and this the father was not loath to give. Naturally little time and no money was left for his legitimate venture. He appealed to his brother-in-law, who gave him a room for himself and daughter temporarily, but soon wearied of him and reported his whereabouts to his wife. His return to the hospital was accomplished only five days after his liberation.

His ninth attack began during this liberation, and was more of an irritable manic state than an elated one as before. He was thoroughly suspicious, even accusing the physician, who had befriended him, of mistreatment. He complained of his wife purloining money from his mail, and wrote to the postmaster ; complained of the attendants to the physicians, and of one physician to another. Expansiveness appeared only when he was asked about his business capacity, and then he might so brighten up as to be facetious. The idea had not died within him, for he carried about in his pockets prospective handbills sketched on pieces of toilet paper. This querulous phase lasted for about six weeks.

He was kept in the hospital for four months after this paranoid state had subsided, and was then paroled again. His married daughter had provided money to pay for his transportation to her home, so he was sent to her. This was in September, 1915. A month later, as he had not reported, he was apprehended again, and transferred to another hospital in the State. The notes fail to tell whether his conduct was abnormal at this time or not. He was then lost sight of for nineteen months, after which he returned as a voluntary admission to the Psychiatric Institute.

The following is the story he gave of the development of his tenth attack. At the other hospital he was at once given parole of the grounds, and took

[1] See Chapter XXXIV for explanation of this reaction.

this opportunity to sell fish to the families of the employees. He continued at this for sixteen months, and then was discharged. It is important to note that he then, for the first time, had an opportunity to begin an independent work, safely isolated from family interference, and did not develop a psychosis. On discharge he secured employment in Rochester, but was immediately taken ill with "Inflammatory Rheumatism" and had to stay in a hospital for five weeks. Following this he held a number of odd jobs for periods of a few weeks each, partly in Rochester and partly in New York. Gradually the realization came to him that his business efficiency, "the gleam" he had followed for a generation, was a thing of the past. He was old, his memory was not what it had been, and trade methods had changed. He fought against this, but soon it was a conviction. A broken man, he sought out his wife, and made a last appeal for sympathy. She advised his return to the hospital, and he weekly consented. It was easier than the suicide he planned, but had not the courage to perform.

He was found to be much aged in appearance, with a blood pressure 30 millimeters higher than it had been two years before. Mild sclerotic changes in his retinal vessels, and a haziness in his memory, made a beginning cerebral arteriosclerosis seem probable. This diagnosis was confirmed by a short attack of confusion, which developed three weeks after admission, and was followed by slight right-sided symptoms for several days. He had good basis for his belief in lost efficiency. But he had no philosophy to meet the inevitable burdens of years; how could he have? Had he been able to build up a real sublimation, it would have rewarded him in his old age with financial support and the glow of accomplishment. But his ambitions had been ever more thinly veiled efforts to gain a childish goal. His life had held no guiding star; for over forty years he chased a Will o' the Wisp, and, when it disappeared into the bog, was it surprising that he sought to follow it even there? The world could offer him no more, and so he wished himself out of it. "There is nothing you can do for me. . . . I realize now just what I have done. I am practically dead, but still alive; that's what it meant when I came over here and committed myself." His chief fear was that he would be judged sane and excluded from the hospital. What had been for him a gaol in the years past, the walls that shut him off from the market place, were now his refuge from the Furies howling at the gate. The comedy of the persistent hypomania had closed as a tragedy with an involution melancholia.

CASE 22.[1] *Charles W.* Aged 23, single. Admitted, July 16th, 1908.

The patient was a lad of fair education, but devoid of ambition, rather lazy and given to a feelings of inferiority. He was even-tempered, and, in his normal life, not liable to exaltation or anxiety, but had a strong tendency to depression, which was closely linked with his frequent conviction of inferiority.

When a small boy, as far back as his memory goes, he used to visit at the home of his grandmother in the country on the outskirts of New York, which to his boyish mind represented the height of comfort and wealth. This was apparently the beginning of the ambition, which ran through his boyhood and continued to his adult life, to possess a country house. When asked to give details of this house of his dreams, it was found they were all features of his grandmother's home, which he admitted, when confronted with the

[1] It should be mentioned that, in including this case, I am breaking a rule, otherwise observed in this book, of not publishing cases in which the psychological mechanisms are inferred merely from data supplied by the patient when sane. No verbal utterances were recorded in the scanty notes that are available concerning the psychosis of this patient, which would directly confirm the hypothesis put forward to explain the peculiar reaction to the precipitating cause. This patient, however, was not observed in the Psychiatric Institute.

resemblance, but had never before recognized. When still a boy the house had been sold, the city spread out enveloping the land around it, while the grandmother had become dependent on his father. The importance which this fantastic dream seemed to have for his psychosis will soon be evident.

At the time of puberty he fell a victim to masturbation, and the vicious circle of thoughts and symptoms, which tend to develop in its train. When 21, he fell in love with a girl—or thought he did—and proposed to her. She refused, and he became depressed. This depression was of sufficient severity to justify his commitment to a private sanatorium. The content of this depression centered around his sexual neurasthenia symptoms and his disappointment in love. Apparently he had also some vague idea of the food being poisoned. After his recovery he joined the navy, from which he was discharged after some months on account of inefficiency and inability to get along with his companions. Charges of stealing a number of trifles were preferred against him, but he was never brought to court-martial, because it was thought that the charges might simply be the outcome of his unpopularity. On returning home again, his father shipped him to a farm near Newburg in the hope that agriculture might prove to be his natural vocation. In the meantime he had become enamoured of another girl, and, during the two months in which he was on the farm, he came home every week or two in order to call on this girl. He wanted to marry her, but had obviously no means of support. The family stated that during this period he sometimes seemed a little " strange ".

Then he suddenly developed a manic state with the most interesting precipitating cause. He heard of the death of his grandmother above mentioned, and received the news with apparent calmness. An hour or two later, however, he went to visit his girl and found her out. While still at her home he became suddenly elated, announcing that he was going to get all Rockefeller's money, marry his loved one, have lots of automobiles, and open a legal advice bureau. (His father was a lawyer, but the patient had never studied law). After keeping his family awake all night with his constant talking, he was sent to the Observation Pavilion, where he was noted as being a typical manic, referring continually to his getting money from Rockefeller, and to his most distinguished intellectual talents.

He was admitted to the Mannhattan State Hospital, July 16th, 1908. He was at first very excited, flighty with some distractibility and considerable motor unrest. His talk was almost entirely of the billions he could take from Rockefeller, of the automobiles he was going to buy for his girl, and of his great cleverness. " I could take Rockefeller with all his billions, and take every penny away from him, and put him in the air without a cent." When asked about his girl, he said, " She is the whole thing in this affair. I can prove it because this is the second time. Her name was E.H. This was the first girl that put me on the bum. I had a funny idea too. She put me on the bum, and my father had to send me to S. (the sanatorium)". He was asked if he was going to marry her, to which he replied, " No—yes, but I know it would not do me any good ". He asked twice why he had come there, to which he responded, first, " Because my father is a foolish man," and second, " Because I spoke to Miss A." (the second girl). He talked also of the onset of his elation in the house of this girl, and mentioned that she was not at home at the time.

From the above productions it can be seen that this adult love affair had stimulated the psychotic tendencies, and that he realized the association at the time. Apparently the sequence of events was this. He was desirous of marrying, but had not the means. All his life he had cherished the ambition to own a country house, which was the duplicate of his grandmother's. It is not, therefore, a wild deduction to claim that unconsciously he had a hope of inheriting this property. When his grandmother died, one element of the unconscious fancy reached fulfilment, and when he went to visit his girl the whole unconscious ambition was activated, so he jumped to the conclusion that he had now the necessary means for marriage. This came to conscious expression in the delusion that he was to obtain Rockefeller's fortune (another older person who might be expected to die), and that he was going to buy innumerable automobiles and other luxuries for his intended wife. With this he became universally expansive, and boasted of his intellectual power. But, that more deeply lying ambitions were also represented is suggested by the idea of opening a legal bureau, a plain usurpation of his father's position.

One production shows how the factors operating in his previous depression had not disappeared. In his sexual neurasthenia he had the constant fear of his brain substance being drained away by seminal loss. This association, of psychic force with bodily material, appeared again in his flight when he said, " I cannot get to the toilet now, my brain gives out, it absorbs all the the material—the food stuff. If I am alive I can suffer for God ". The last statement shows excellently how a painful idea can be distorted into a pleasant one in a manic state by putting it in a religious setting. Years later he remembered having in this attack the idea of being a prophet.

During a month he quieted down gradually, but six weeks after admission he had a sudden excitement with resentment at the ward routine. Then came six weeks during which there were occasional periods of excitement, that were found to be associated with masturbation. Three months after admission he had quieted down sufficiently to admit his previous excitements. In discussing his case, he ascribed his depression to the rejection of his first love suit, but expressly denied that the second had anything to do with his excitement. Three weeks later his insight had further improved, and on December 25th he was paroled, and, later on discharged.

The important things to be noted in this case are that a childish ambition was apparently the occasion for a distortion of a painful thought (death of grandmother) into an expansive delusion, and that this only came to consciousness when it was formulated as an adult wish. In other words, the original desire for possession of his grandmother's home was a distinctly infantile ambition ; when it became cloaked as a desire to marry, free outlet was given to it in a setting of elation.

The case now to be discussed shows, like previous ones, a prominence of death ideas that are developed into religious fancies. It is further interesting in showing a religious setting of ideas, which we would classify as distinctly infantile.

CASE 23. *Mary F. B.* Aged 39, married. Admitted November 1st, 1899.
F.H. A paternal aunt was insane for many years and one sister was " hysterical," otherwise her relatives were said to be normal.

P.H. We know little of the patient's personality except for statements, which seem to indicate meticulous devotion to her family with great conscientiousness and religiosity, all of which suggest exaggerated efforts at adaptation. At 23 she had a depression lasting six weeks without known cause. At 24 she was married. At 26, immediately after confinement, she had five weeks of " nervous prostration " followed by six months of a depression with self accusation. This merged over into a psychosis, which seems to have had some stupor features, for she would be cataleptic for periods lasting from ten minutes to one hour. At one time during her psychosis she is said to have had visions of Jesus and her parents.

Two months before admission she was operated upon for repair of injuries received during childbirth, and was in bed until three days before admission. The history states that she then got suddenly out of bed, became " positive," and soon began to talk in a religious strain. She set the table with only bread and water on it. During the first three months she was markedly elated, at times excited and pounding, again standing around but talking incessantly. Sometimes she spoke in a preaching manner, with many religious allusions, but would interrupt this with rhyming nonsense, or comments on the environment. Occasionally she would be silent for considerable periods, but looked around in an alert, elated manner. Her orientation was good, but she mistook persons constantly, calling one physician " Jo C.", and a nurse " Aunt Mary ". It was frequently noted that she was erotic in her behaviour. Following this she was, for a short period only, mildly elated, and then recovered. Retrospectively, she gave an interesting account of the ideas she had had. She stated that she did not actually see the people of whom she talked ; at first she had " impressions ", but later began to hear voices. The bedspread and mattress talked when she moved, and keys would also. Her memory for events at home during the earlier part of her hospital stay was fair, but for the period of her more marked excitement her recollections were quite hazy.

The patient was intelligent enough to be interested in the abnormal ideas she had had and gave the following account of her psychotic experiences. She thought she was going to be laid out and cut up, for which rattling of dishes seemed to be a preparation. This was the only death idea which occurred in a pure form, the others being rather fancies of the other world. Swedenborg came to her and told her that good spirits were all around her. She thought, too, that she was at the Saviour's grave. Infantile ideas also appeared, for her dead father was with her, and possibly as a corollary to this thought, Swedenborg told her to kill her husband. She did attack him once when he came. Then there were expansive religious ideas. Christ came and told her that she was greater than He. When she thought she was at the Saviour's grave, it was as if she were God, or " at His right hand," and she was promised a paradise. When we consider that her conduct was almost always erotic, we can see that, in spite of the brevity of the material, all the common manic formulations are present, including antagonism to the husband, a sexual union with the father, adult erotic tendencies, and a projection into a childlike Heaven, in which the crudity of selfish desires is thinly cloaked by the mask of religion.

Having from her own memory some knowledge of the ideas which raced through her head, we can see how they determine in a very large degree the productions of her flight. The following samples are full of religious references and mention her father, father representatives, and exhibitions of eroticism :

" God—divine love—justice—Christ—triumphant entrance—Cain and Abel —womanhood—saved by grace—unity—harmony—discord—how, why and what ?—water—toil—I try—arrive—strong in death—I arrive—Father, I have sinned—Abraham Lincoln's birthright—strong in death—yes, the ruling passion—the flower fadeth—precious—I begot my birthright—— ".

" Faith, Hope, Charity—I serve my legion—my Lord—I rise to know the truth—I with my servant—I will serve God—King Solomon—king thou art— yes, since Psalm 23 is your motto—behold now the bridegroom cometh— kindness—truth—love of beauty—beatitude for gentleness—I love you— take my hand—thy Saviour, thy pledge, I will lift up my heart to go—I will be the iron law (uncovers herself)—shamefacedness—— ", etc.

Sometimes when she had the tendency to rhyme, she would get into utter nonsense, rhyming such as : " I love Lizzie—I love hope—I love Lizzie and the mope—mope—mope—for the bar bar bar and the dar dar dar—the beta mana—bota, and the da da da—you go to baste and I want waste ".

Later she was more purely distractible, commented on various characteristics of the doctors, but also said, " I am going to run this house—I am the one mighty ". Later, " I am God ". The last quotation but one, " I am going to run this house ", and " I am the one mighty ", presents the core of her ideas, with its crass egotism, foolish ambition, and assumption of divinity.

The following case is that of a woman who was observed in some thirteen attacks which occurred more or less regularly from the age of 24 to her 50th year, since when she has not been observed by us. All of her attacks were more or less pure manic states and the dominant ideas appeared in her flight. It is interesting to note that, although any given sample is disjointed and rather incomprehensible by itself, it is almost impossible to find a single production in the records of any one of the thirteen attacks, which does not contain references to her circumscribed group of ideas. Not only can one see that the productions are consistent in one attack, but the same principle actually holds good for twenty-five years, so that anyone thoroughly familiar with her type of utterances could probably identify a few sentences from one of her histories as belonging to this patient. When all of her ideas are collated, there remains very little which is not explicable in the flight of any given attack. An example of her speech is as follows : " Did you make God's father ? Did you make God's son ? It takes a virgin to make a virgin. A virgin is a purity flag. I can talk to nobody that is alive. My mother was blind when she died. (Closes her eyes and remains still). That is death. I certainly am dead. Can you see the shadow of the ghost ? Well my father was a far better ghost, when he fought in the war with General Grant."

Although her reactions were not always typically manic, the content of her psychosis was produced almost wholly in a setting of elation. Death is the key-note of the varying expressions of this death appearing kaleidescopically. Hers is one of those cases where almost any distressing incident was interpreted as a suggestion of death, and, so soon as this idea came to expression, she would become elated. In her earlier attacks (which are poorly described) there were periods, when she was said to be depressed, confused, dull, stupid, silly, simple or " somewhat demented ". Very occasionally there were crying spells. It seems not improbable that, if observed to-day, these atypical periods would be interpreted as mild stupor reactions with interruptions of anxiety and elation. The impression of dementia, which she several times gave, is probably to be ascribed to apathy, which is such a consistent feature in stupor. Certainly at times there were utterances and conduct, which we have come to realize as highly suggestive of stupor. For instance, she once closed her eyes and said, " This is death " ; again she said, " Death, death " ; or " I am fainting away, fade away ". She repeatedly described the early part of a psychosis as the state of unconsciousness. " I die ; I am completely unconscious." Or she said, " I came to life again ; I came from death " ; " I was dead and came to life," again, " I often felt like going off " ; " I died many times " ; " I have been dead and buried ". She always recovered perfectly.

A detailed description of her attacks would be needlessly tedious, and so a brief summary only will be given.

CASE 24. *Mary E.* was a married woman, 24 years of age in 1888 at the time of her first attack.

F.H. Her family history is bad. Her father, who was a German, died at the age of 35, when the patient was five years old. Little is known of him or his family. Those who were seen were evidently psychopathic. The mother, an Irish woman, was always queer, being so afraid of poison that she would not go out for meals, and constantly tried to separate the patient from her husband. She was alcoholic. The patient's sister had attacks diagnosed as manic-depressive insanity. A brother was also alcoholic, peculiar, and had ideas of poisoning.

P.H. The patient was stated to have been always bright and lively and of a happy disposition. In the intervals of her many attacks she was observed to be quite natural. At 16 and at 18 she gave birth to illegitimate children. She was married at 19 and was said to be a capable housewife. During wedlock she had ten children and no miscarriages.

First Attack : A month after her first confinement she became abnormal, saying she was going to die like a woman next door who had succumbed to consumption. Then she ran to her mother's house, claiming that she heard her dead father calling her to come to Heaven. She began to preach, and at once became elated, with talk about angels and members of her family, claiming that all her friends were dead. This lasted for about ten days or so, after which there were four months during which she was dull and stupid or at times frenzied and noisy or given to religious utterances.

Second Attack : When 28, two months after childbirth, her husband was brought home unconscious, having fallen forty feet from a scaffold. She nursed him for a week, and then, when he was much better, she suddenly began to pray and sing, abused and assaulted her husband, or, again, embraced him. A frank manic state ensued lasting a little over a week, which was full of religious allusions, and then occurred one of these poorly described inactive states in which she was thought to be demented. She recovered, however, and left the hospital after eleven months stay.

Third Attack : When 34, she had a quarrel with her husband and at once became excited, shouting, screaming, crying, singing hymns, and making signs of the cross. For nearly a month she was typically manic with many references to her death and religious ideas. After this there were six months of dulness and " confusion ", after which she again recovered, being in the hospital eight months in all.

Fourth Attack : When 35 years old, ten days after another confinement, she had a quarrel with her sister-in-law and became at once excited and talkative. This state lasted for about a month, with her usual ideas of religious nature, after which she was described as quieter but " silly and simple ", yet she worked industriously. She recovered completely and left the hospital only four months after admission.

Fifth Attack : Eight months following her next pregnancy, when 36 years of age, she tried to wean her child, got " milk fever ", and began to talk and pray. For a month she was excited, shouting, quarrelsome, apparently typically manic, and then quieted down. She seems to have become normal quite quickly, although she was retained in the hospital some six months in all.

Sixth Attack : When 38 years of age she helped to take care of a neighbour's child who died. She also assisted in laying out the corpse for burial. While thus engaged, she began to strike herself on her chest, said the baby's breath was in her lungs, and then began praying and laughing. At once she was in her typical early state of excitement, assaulted her husband and had to be committed. For a month she was frankly elated with her customary productions, then had two weeks during which she is described as being dull, but mischievous, and then got rapidly well, being in the hospital only three months.

Seventh Attack : When 41, a quarrel occurred with a man who lived in the flat about the patient, in the course of which she and her husband punched him and threw him out of the house. The quarrel began either by this man calling her a bad name, or, as she said later, the man accusing his own wife, whereat the patient interfered. She became quite stirred up, but calmed down again. The next day, however, this man's children jeered at her. She became excited at once, commanded the sun to come down, and struck her husband. There followed three months of typical manic excitement. Perhaps it was because of the precipitating cause introducing the idea of immorality that in this attack, in addition to her usual religious content, she included many references to the man who had seduced her and to adultery. She recovered quite quickly, after these three months, and was only three months in the hospital altogether.

Eighth Attack : When 42 years old a neighbour who was the godfather of her daughter died, and the patient with her usual interest in such affairs, helped to lay his body out. For the three days before his burial she talked much and with many tears, about him and his sufferings, and insisted that he was in Heaven. After the funeral she quieted down and remained apparently normal for a week, but then began to talk of the dead man again, speaking of the house being haunted, of death, and of religious wars, and began to preach. As usual she turned against her husband, struck him, and also chased her daughter out of the house. This excitement was typical throughout and lasted for two months.

Ninth Attack : When 43 the patient's daughter had an illegitimate child. She worried over this but did not break down. Two years later her mother told her that her father had had two illegitimate children before his marriage. She became peculiar, repeated the story to her husband, then began to look at the sky, preached out of the window, said she wanted to go to Europe to see her step-brother (one of the above-mentioned children) and had to be committed. Apparently this secret from her father's life stirred up the idea of her own similar history, for, in this excitement, she again referred to her seduction. She was three months in the hospital and was apparently only hypomanic throughout.

Tenth Attack : When 48 she had a quarrel with the landlady, who told her that it was foolish of her to have so many children by such a man as her husband. This hurt her feelings very much and she told the landlady that she would never destroy what the Lord gave her. Subsequently, she said that she took this more to heart than a child's death. She went to bed and thought she was going to die. Then an excitement commenced in which she talked as usual about religion and God. This excitement lasted for three weeks with many religious references and much talk of her own, and of the illegitimate children of her daughter and father. She calmed down for two months and finally was mildly hypomanic, without obvious content, and left the hospital four months after her admission.

Eleventh Attack : When 50 years of age the patient received a letter from her daughter which spoke of the daughter's husband being very ill and probably going to die. In a few days the patient became depressed and inactive, spoke about her unfortunate daughter, the son-in-law's illness and their children. This misfortune of her daughter's evidently stirred up similar unconscious ideas, for, when in the hospital and asked about this precipitating cause, she invariably confused it with the death of her sister, which had occurred a year before. This depression lasted for about a month and was terminated apparently, by her transferring her thoughts from the death of her sister (a potential rival in terms of unconscious attachments) to her father. She suddenly began to talk about her father having made coats for the German army and became excited, elated, and so unruly that she had to be committed. The content of this manic state was essentially the same as in her other attacks. After a month she began to improve but did not recover entirely until after three and one-half months.

Twelfth Attack : When 51 her mother-in-law told her that her husband (that is the patient's father-in-law) had turned her out in the street, and the mother-in-law hoped that the patient would take her in to live with her. The patient, however, would not have her in the house because she drank, and told her not to tell her her troubles because such things upset her. Here again was a situation which stimulated ideas of a misfortune to a rival. Although there is no mention in the notes of her being depressed, it does appear that it was only after three weeks that the elation began. Some time was evidently necessary for an elaboration, below the level of consciousness, of her psychotic ideas into a form, which permitted a free, conscious outlet. This is of some importance because she usually responded to upsetting situations almost immediately whenever these incidents suggested the adult or admissable type of outlet. That the sad plight of her mother-in-law was really the upsetting factor is indicated by the fact that in this attack, in addition to her usual content, she had much to say about her mother-in-law and family antagonisms, which she symbolized as international jealousies. The attack lasted for only a month.

The thirteenth and last attack which was observed occurred three months after her discharge from her twelfth admission. Two weeks before she returned another daughter had a difference with her husband who was drunk, and in the course of the discussion jumped out of a third-storey window and broke her back and legs. When the patient heard of this she talked queerly for a few hours, said this country was going to have a big war, and that her father was a general in the German army. (This was in September, 1914.) The upset was quite temporary. But ten days before admission her husband was mortally injured by a fall. After three days in a hospital, he was brought home dead. She at once began to talk peculiarly about this death and also about her father having been a general. On the day of the funeral she threw her arms about the casket, did not want it to be carried out, said she wanted to go with him, and cried excessively. Evidently the idea of mutual death was stimulated, for four days later she became violent, sang and danced, and had to be taken to the hospital, where she said, " I got upset because my husband died. I kissed him after he was dead. I got the temptation of the embalming into me." The significance of this last statement in connection with the topic of mutual death will be explained shortly. This attack lasted about six weeks, during which she was merely hypomanic and gave expression to practically the same ideas as those of previous episodes.

Having given this brief description of her attacks we may now turn our attention to the ideas which were so consistently present in her excitements. These ideas were, apparently, not merely coincidental with elation, but bore some casual relation to it, inasmuch as elation never appeared until she had commenced talking about one of the topics which dominated her manic episodes. As has been stated, her utterances were frequently disjointed and flighty, and there were a number of expressions the import of which was not clear. It was possible, however, to discover the meaning of these queer phases, because they were constantly being repeated and their significance became plain by correlating the varoius associations in which they appeared. In the following discussion of the patient's ideas the numerals in parentheses represent the attack in which the statement quoted was made.

Death is an idea which is capable of many interpretations. It may be painful or pleasant : the latter when it is associated with thoughts of release from intolerable burdens, or of flight to a haven of rest and glory, or of union with a loved one in another world, where the path of true love presumably runs more smoothly than in this. The death in which this patient was interested was distinctly of this type, as became manifest from her many remarks about it. There is record of her speaking frequently of death in every attack except the fifth, which, however, was not well observed. We have already, in mentioning her stupor-like utterances, referred to numerous statements concerning her own death and need not repeat these again. The elaboration and interpretation of death should interest us more. Sleep and death were repeatedly associated : " The sleeping death " (9) ; " Sleep is the brother of death " (13) ; " Somebody died in this bed ; they have me sleeping in death " (8). Similarly she connected her stay in the hospital, or her insanity, with this delusion : " There is no place nearer death than this " (the hospital) (13) ; " My death is over here " (10) ; " Do you like this side of the world ? [the hospital] ; I think they have destroyed the second world again " (7) ; " I must be crazy or going into the other world " (13).

Death as a medium for the expression of religious ideas is symbolized in the following : " I came in a coffin through Heaven " (3) ; " I think I am here to die ; I am a saint—that is death—I was all right until I took that saintly feeling " (9) ; " I was unconscious, because a saint and God gave me great power " (8) ; " I defy you now, Death, the Father, the Son, the Holy Crown, Death, Death " (6) ; " The Catholics take communion from the dead ; that means you should not murder " (10). When a nurse brought food, " She is cooking death ; she is eating from death, what the child gives in confession, at the altar, at her father's death. Before you go to confession you have to stop eating. You eat after death. You take the sacrament of Jesus Christ " (13) ; Death brought me back this time, the sleeping death, in the tenth commandment, our Lord's supper " (9).

Apparently she gave a sexual significance to the tenth commandment, probably by stressing the injunction against coveting the neighbour's wife. A plainer association between death and sexuality appear in the following : " Ring, marriage, marriage-funeral, marriage in death, marriage in life " (7) ; " Death is sin ; adultery is sin ", (proceding after this statement to speak of an early seduction) (11). Again, in connection with her seduction, she said, " My first sin in Heaven. I came out from death. I am not a murderess ". Again, " I think that is a terrible sin when a man seduces an innocent child ; that is a painful death ; my mother knows that. I have been twice anointed for death " (she was seduced twice) (11) ; " My husband and I have been sleeping for the most part of our lives in death " (7). A vague idea of death as sin is expressed in the following : " Death is not on my mind any more ; I am cleansed from it " (11) ; " I was punished for death " (10).

It is important to note that the sexuality, which is here associated with the death idea, is of the adult type. Close interest in the father appears both directly and in a religious setting, but in neither case is there any reference to, or implication of, what would commonly be termed sexuality.

Her attacks were quite plainly regressive in that evidence was constantly present of her interest being withdrawn from her normal responsibilities and attachments to be placed on that object of infantile, unconscious interest, her father. She spoke directly of her father calling her to Heaven, and repeatedly asseverated her belief that she saw him and heard him call her by name (when " unconscious "). She directly identified herself with him, claiming to look like him, or, " I studied too much with my father's brain " (7) ; " I have my father's brain " (12). She frequently said she was her father's " proof " (11). She magnified him as a great man. He was a general in the German army (13) ; he made coats for the German army (11). Frequently this expansiveness appeared in a patriotic trend which was associated with her father. She spoke much of Washington, Lincoln, Grant, the red, white, and blue. " Father had curly hair like George Washington " (12) ; " I felt death, President Lincoln's death " (13). When asked why she spoke so much of death, she replied, " Why shouldn't I, President Grant's wife ? There is a death in the White House " (this was after her mother's death) ; or again, " Grant's death, his wife is dead " (13). After her attacks, however, she apparently tried to repress thoughts of her father for she was reluctant to speak of him : " I imagine it is not right to think of the father. Let the dead rest " (13).

Her religion was of a primitive order, for in it she quite plainly identified her father with God : " My father was born in Heaven " (5) ; " The father is calling me to Heaven " (immediately beginning to preach) (1) ; " I am fighting for God, for Jesus Christ. I heard a voice from Heaven. I spoke up to Heaven. God has suffered. I talk to the skies where the stars are, to our Saviour. Charles was born on Palm Sunday. (She here associates from God to her son Charles, the significance of which we shall immediately see.) " I have heard God talking to me. He appeared to me in a vision " (15) ; " When you see my father come along with a big cigar, you have the Holy Ghost ;

and you light the light with the light, and that is how it started when I first got sick. The Calvary Chain—and I have been dead and buried " (7). Once she associated her father with the priesthood : " My father was a priest in Rome ; that is where I got my holiness " (7). Just as she identified herself with her father so did she with God : " I don't know who I am except I am God " (5) ; " I have God's face " (5) ; " I am God ; I know more about God than any other person " (3). With such expansive beliefs it is not difficult to understand her elation, and we must remember that there was ample evidence of her religion always being of this self-glorifying type.

Her mother figured very little in her productions. She never thought her mother was dead as many cases do, and only spoke of her death after it actually occurred, but once she said, " My mother is going to be blind (6) ; and, after she had actually died, " She was blind when she died " (13), thus showing some interest in the affliction of her mother. But there were substitutes for her mother, for instance, the nurses. We must remember that her mother was Irish. She said, " They were a lot of wild Irish nurses ; they wanted to control me. They cannot com to America and destroy our flag " (7) ; " They have to draw the flag in, but they cannot get the American flag. New York is in trouble, war with the Queen of State ". (Who is the Queen of State ?) " My daughter, I am the Queen of Europe " (12). In her conduct she showed this antagonism to the mother substitutes. For instance, she turned her mother-in-law out of doors, and in the subsequent attack spoke of starvation in the City of New York. During the onset of her eighth attack she chased her daughter out of the house, claiming that she was the wife of her husband. This is a pretty example of how some patients autistically dispose of two objectionable people by marrying them off.

To her husband she was so antagonistic as to assault him, and when he was dead she spoke quite placidly about him (13). She wanted to be called by her father's name, not Mary E. (1). It is perhaps because of her having focussed on that group of customary manic ideas, which are concerned with death and religion, that she never spoke of having lovers, and was never erotic in her behaviour. On the other hand she had a real situation of this nature to fall back upon, which may have been the reason for her harking back with great frequency to her seductions before marriage. She even ascribed her insanity to this period, and that this interest in her seduction was fundamentally the same as an interest in lovers, is shown by her statement : " Since God made me insane from adultery . . . I broke one of God's commandments ". In one attack (3) she projected her impatience with the marriage bond on to her husband, accusing him of being unfaithful, and swearing she would live with him no more. In only one attack did she speak directly of a former lover : " K. is in Hell roasting ; K., you dirty loafer ! He is off his nut. He ruined me first. To Hell with K." (7). Probably associated with this antagonism towards her seducer was an interest in purity. She spoke of the purity flag, and this was associated with an interest in the Virgin Mary, whom she repeatedly said she had seen (her own name was Mary). " The Virgin is a purity flag " (13). There was probably considerable identification with the Virgin, as she (the patient) said she was the mother of God. Again, " I am the light of Jesus ; I am the light of men " (5).

A husband is, from the standpoint of the development of affection, a surrogate of the father, hence, we can understand the patient's frequent confusion between these two. We can understand, too, how the death of her husband stimulated the idea of mutual death. She freely transposed their names (13). In speaking of her husband's death : " They excited me after my father's death " (13) ; or, in speaking of her father, she said, " I kissed him after embalming " (which she did to her husband) ; or when asked what upset her, replied, " I told you my father's death " (husband's) (13). Once she identified her husband, her father and God together in the following : " Papa put me into the world to love and obey and keep his commandments."

Just as there was an ambivalent attitude towards her husband, friendly in so far as he represented her father, and hostile when he stood for adult responsibilities, so did her ideas represent conflicting emotions about her children. As so many married women do, she had delusions of their loss. For instance, she said, " My mother put me here to steal my money and to take away my children " (5). In several of her attacks the thought of pre-venting conception or producing abortion was quite prominent, inasmuch as she protested many times that she was not a murderess, usually making such statements with reference to her large family. In fact one of her attacks (10) was induced by a suggestion of her landlady during a quarrel that she should not have so many children. That such a suggestion should produce so marked a reaction as insanity must surely indicate that it stimulated potent unconscious tendencies. During the attack she claimed that this remark had hurt her deeply, but it is interesting to note that, when discussing the incident after recovery from her eleventh attack, she denied that the advice about having children affected her deeply, insisting that she was quite upset because the landlady made her move. We may presume that this indicates a repression of the precipitating cause, such as we so frequently see, which is always added evidence of its unconscious significance. She may have associated this imaginary crime with her treatment of her mother-in-law, for, in the attack that followed her turning the old woman from her door, she said, " They have put me down for murder. I never murdered anyone. . . . Starvation in the City of New York " (11). The opposite tendency of the glorification of her children appeared in connection with her religious trend, for she frequently made allusions to her being divine : " I gave birth to eleven children. One will be God before he dies " (10) ; " I had a baby by the name of Christ " (7) ; " I was all right until I heard of the birth of Christ— holy children ". She several times mentioned that her son was born on Palm Sunday. Once, when speaking of her seductions : " That is what I was punished for, insane for. I don't know God was never born yet " (9).

Such were the ideas which this patient expressed, all of which when arranged as we have done, can be seen to fit into a very definite picture. It is important for the reader to know that although we have not quoted all of the paient's ideas in connection with the several topics discussed, we can say with positiveness that nothing was uttered which did not relate itself naturally to one or the other of her dominant themes. In other words, the reconstruction of her ideas has been like the putting together of a mosaic, where meaning has emerged out of chaos, and not one piece remains over when the reconstruction is complete.

The significance of her ideas is not difficult to fathom. Every precipitating cause had in it something painful ; so we can see why the development of an idea of death with its religious implications meant for her a translation from a weary world to one where everything would be as simple and pleasant as in the Golden Age ; hence, the elation. Hence, too, her activity. Con-tact with reality being lost, she had nothing but pleasant ideas to dwell upon, and nothing to inhibit her activity, which was always in keeping with her ideas. So, she sang and laughed, danced and prayed with equal abandon.

The case which is next to be described also showed the dominance of the death idea in a manic state.

CASE 25.—*Celia C.*—Aged 23, single. Admitted to the Psychiatric Institute May 2nd, 1914.
F.H.—Her mother had an attack of insanity from which she recovered a year before this admission. Otherwise nothing is known of the family history.
P.H.—The patient herself was described as bright, sociable, well info.med and very ambitious, but no thorough investigation of her earlier life was made. Her case has already been touched upon briefly above, in reference to the precipitating causes of two attacks, both of these episodes being inaugurated by a quarrel. When 18 years of age, she had a quarrel with her sister in which the accusation was made that she was interfering with the sister's love

affair. From her consequent productions, it could be reasonably inferred that this accusation suggested the stealing of her sister's lover, a rather infantile idea. She became depressed and then gradually passed over into a perplexity state with ideas of being guilty, having destoyed her honour, being a prostitute, and of her mother being dead. This attack lasted for four months. She was quite well for five years, learned stenography and typewriting, and, during the six months preceding her second attack, went to night-school in order to perfect her technical education, having thus very little recreation. She held a secretarial position with a literary man.

Four weeks before the onset of actual symptoms another girl came to work with the patient and they became antagonistic, having several quarrels. A number of these were occasioned by the jealousy of this second girl. The patient visited a dentist professionally, who happened to be the fiancé of the other girl. She was always trying to find out from the patient what the dentist had said to her and, in one of their quarrels, she called the patient a vampire and a " proselyte ". A few days later another discussion arose when the patient wanted her companion to do her work in a certain way and the girl refused. The latter went to their employer and complained that the patient was not nice to her. The patient went home, nervous, talked much about the quarrel, worked in the house in a desultory way, at times down-hearted, or so excited she would have to be restrained. She talked in a rambling way of hypnotism and detectives. Subsequently the patient stated that after the quarrel she had became much upset, called out, " Mama dear ! ' and thought she was going to die.

Her condition soon justified commitment and following admission to the service of the Psychiatric Institute her symptoms for the first two weeks were as follows : She was rather inactive whenever left alone, but talked freely enough when spoken to. She evidently had great difficulty in concentrating, calculated badly, said she felt exhausted, mixed up, sleepy, that she did not feel like herself. She also said she felt sad, but she laughed quite readily. She was somewhat flighty and distractible, and the difficulty in following her trend[1] was increased by the peculiarity of her ideas. Sometimes she suddenly jumped out of bed. Rarely there were depressive utterances, " I want my punishment on earth, not in heaven ", or " I am willing to suffer punishment for what I am accused ". (What is that ?) " A proselyte ". Repeatedly she spoke about dying, and said once, " Death is a beautiful child. If I am going to die, all right, I am satisfied." Once she lay with her eyes closed and would not answer questions, and when asked in the afternoon what she had been doing at the time, she said : " I was suffering with death." " I thought I was melting away ; " or she spoke about a religious fight that was going on. repeatedly spoke of being under ether, of having been operated on by the doctor (at home) ; the doctor cut her hymen, the doctor had intercourse with her, insulted her, and once when asked about the operation, " I don't know what the operation was, people operate on typewriters." This was due to distractibility. The elation broke through at times so that she laughed very readily. Some of the talk is well illustrated by the following : " I get a new wrapper every day. I feel like a washed out rag. I wish I knew what was happening. It is so long since I was in the city. I forget all about myself. I don't know whether I am coming or going." (Why do you get so restless ?)

" I don't know—I jump out of bed—I am restless—I want to go out—I want to exercise—I used to exercise my limbs—I used to exercise—I had a little pamphlet—gee—I am being drawn out a lot. I had a little pamphlet. Well, when I was at home, I used to exercise." She kept on talking about this, then went on, " Then I told you the other day about a scrap with the doctor, and he told me, ' Well, I guess you had better go ', but she does not believe in that. Well, people do once in a while. We went together—we used to eat at the trade union place. I tried to be nice to her. The last time I remember, we worked together, but we scrapped. I went to a nerve hospital. I don't know

[1] See the glossary.

—I must have been operated upon . . . lots of things happened that day. I am darned if I know what they all mean. I was told that I had my choice that day, etc." This well illustrates parts of her trend, the peculiar mixed up talk and her feeling of confusion.

This condition was apparently : a perplexed state; a tendency to stupor reaction and stupor content (inactivity, a difficulty in concentration and ideas of death) ; a tendency also to depression with ideas of sin ; manic episodes with religious and adult sex ideas.

The next few weeks she was frankly manic, singing, rhyming, erotic, though at times irritable and crying. Sometimes she made comments on things around her in an elated way or she rolled on the floor. Unfortunately no notes were made at this time of her dominant ideas. Then she quieted down somewhat and got into a state very much like that of the first two weeks. She sat about in a relaxed manner with a half-puzzled, half-amused air. When interrogated, she was apt to smile, and make a flippant remark, but was usually monosyllabic. Her ideas were evidently diminishing in their intensity, for she evaded answering questions about them, and when pressed would distort them into a little less psychotic form. For instance, although admitting the ideas of being operated upon and of being under ether, when asked if she had been hypnotized she said : " I must have been intoxicated." During the next three months she grew rapidly more normal until her recovery was complete. Her restrospective account showed that she had some memory of her ideas, but disliked talking about them and complained that any discussion of the matter depressed her. Objectively, however, her recovery was perfect.

We may now turn to consider just what the patient's ideas were, remembering that practically all of them were produced when elated, or presenting other manic symptoms. Little content was gathered during the period when she was in a stupor-like state or much perplexed. We may assume, therefore, that what she talked about, when she spoke freely, was intimately associated with the more manic symptoms. We may begin by considering the inner meaning of the precipitating cause and the psychological significance of her reaction to it. In her previous attack a quarrel had also occurred and, as it was with her sister, introduced what was essentially an infantile idea, namely the stealing of the lover of her sister (a natural mother surrogate). In this attack it was evident that similar thoughts were stirred, because she said that in her previous attack she had told the doctor that her sister had called her a prostitute, which was untrue. At the same time, she wished to correct this imaginary mistake, claiming that her sister had called her a " slob " ; but a few days earlier, when more abnormal, she had said the same thing and then associated to " slob ", " fool—bum—bitch ". From this we may presume, therefore, that in the second attack a sexual accusation in a definitely family setting was vaguely stirred so it is not surprising that she said retrospectively that she had fancied during her whole second attack that her mother was dead.

The quarrels which ushered in the second attack were, however, not with a member of the family ; hence the idea of sex transgression was naturally left more on the adult plane, the lover to be stolen, being naturally a legitimate possibility in real life. The psychosis probably occurred on account of its suggesting the more deeply lying strivings, which were directly stimulated in the first attack. The upset apparently began after that quarrel in which the patient was called a vampire. The second " scrap ", which was only about the work, was probably of significance simply because it excited an idea of enmity and hence reopened the other problem. It is quite interesting that during her psychosis the patient mixed up these two quarrels constantly and also included another idea : that she had quarrelled because the girl opened a letter from the patient's lover. After her recovery, she said this had not occurred— not before she was ill at any rate. The significance of the words " vampire " and " proselyte " were amply explained by the patient herself. She said, " Proselyte is a bad woman, a woman who goes out with any man who is not her husband. It also means dying on your own bed . . . I did it." Again she said, " A vampire is a bad woman who wronged somebody, causes them disease or death." At another time : " A bad woman who causes trouble and sorrow, who kills somebody's husband or takes him away." In other words, both vampire and proselyte stand for prostitution, but they also have a peculiar association with killing and with death. For the patient, therefore, we may presume that, when she was called " Vampire " and " Proselyte '" it conveyed to her mind an illicit or adulterous experience, but also suggested dying and killing. We may recall that very soon after her first resentful excitement she thought she was going to die. Throughout she gave almost constantly a sexual significance to death. In a dream, in which she saw a snake with the head of her lover, she was " Writhing with death." When asked about her lover, she said that he was dead and then that she did not want to talk about him and bring him into this . . . : " I don't want to kill the whole nation." Probably there was underlying this association some vague idea of mutual death. She directly associated loss of honour with fear of death . . . : " I was told my honour was gone. Everybody is afraid of death."

Apparently some of her death ideas had to do almost purely with the prostitution fancy (she heard voices calling her a prostitute) and the varying formulations of the sex transgression were constantly merging over into death ideas. She thought she was " traced with a key ", and when asked what " key " made her think of, she said, " Key to your heart—hypnotism ". Now " hypnotism " and " ether " were frequently associated with a persistent delusion that a physician had assaulted her sexually before her admission to the hospital. This trend of ideas led back to death again . . . : " I felt under ether ; I don't know whether I am living or dead." At another time she said, " A key means key to your heart ; Gate of St. Peter ; death."

We may perhaps formulate this case in summary by stating that the patient had death ideas, such as are usually found in the onset to stupors, and that in her psychoses she showed stuporous symptoms at times, but that it was because of an added significance to death, namely, that of adult sexuality, that manic features appear and predominate over all others in her psychoses. At the same time, the fundamental disturbance, that which accounted for her having a psychosis at all, is probably to be assigned to the stirring up of her deeper lying infantile yearnings.

The following case shows how ideas of death may be the occasion for manic excitement, which occurred in this instance, even although the pleasanter formulations of death, such as religious and erotic fancies, were merely indicated rather than openly expressed.

CASE 26. The patient, *Sara K.*, was a married Jewess, aged 51 at the time she came under observation, which was some twenty years ago. From our present standpoint the case was insufficiently observed, and, consequently, we have indulged in more inference as to the meaning of some of her productions and behaviour, than would probably be necessary had more extensive notes been made. She is said to have been normal in health and temperament. When 23 she had a child, was troubled with insomnia for some months following, and then developed a typical manic state which lasted four months. She remained well for five years, when following the birth of another child, there was precisely the same sequence of events. The attack to be considered developed as follows :

About three months before admission she was supposed to have received an electric shock while turning on a light, and to have fallen unconscious to the floor. At all events she was found unconscious and the lighting company found some disorder about the switch. She remained unconscious for half an hour. Whether this loss of consciousness was in part a psychogenic reaction cannot be stated definitely. At any rate she at once began to be nervous, and the idea of an electric shock certainly made some impression on her mind, for it reappeared in her psychosis. It is not improbable that there was a suggestion of death in this incident, to which the insomnia that developed immediately was a response[1]. This insomnia, with its accompanying diurnal nervousness, increased in severity, and she soon began to complain of various sensations, such as numbness and a prickling in her arms and legs. The meaning of these sensations may be an expression of the idea of the electricity, or have been an hysterical manifestation of a still unconscious idea of death. More probably they represented the latter. In her psychosis sensations were certainly described as evidence of mortification. With increasing restlessness she began to be depressed, until the week before admission, when there was an accentuation of her symptoms. She spoke of fear of having to go to an institution again. The following day she was talkative and happy. The contents of her speech betrayed the typical manic combination of regression and imaginary plans. She related stories of twenty years ago, talked about her mother's, father's and brother's deaths. She cried over this, but also spent much time in planning a trip to the mountains. Three days before admission she became irritable, lost her temper, scolded and abused her children. With this last there was evidence of the tendency we commonly see, to resent the responsibilities of her married life. The following morning she was completely mixed up in both her behaviour and speech. She did not seem to appreciate her surroundings, and talked constantly in uncomprehensible flight. There were occasional terrifying hallucinations. For instance, she tore about the house trying to escape from a black dog, and required several men to restrain her.

It was in this condition of excitement, with disorientation and confused productions, that she was admitted to the hospital. For two months she was erratic in her behaviour, usually with considerable motor excitement ; was often destructive, spat at the nurses, and talked or sang for long periods of time on end. Occasionally, for a short while, she would become quiet and tractable. During the third month of her residence these periods of diminished excitement became more frequent, and by the fourth she was usually docile, having only occasional outbreaks in which she sang, danced and was noisy and careless in her appearance. By the end of the fifth month she had recovered. Her orientation during the acme of her excitements was apparently nil, although she occasionally made statements quite irrelevantly, which showed appreciation of the fact that she was in the hospital and attended by doctors and nurses. On recovery she claimed to have always known where she was, although she had very slight memory of her ideas.

During all of her excitements her productions were quite disjointed, so that it was impossible to follow the thread of them at any one interview. It is of interest, however, that almost everything which is recorded referred directly to ideas of death, or to what may be interpreted as elaborations of such ideas. Only once did she mention antagonism to her children, when she said in the middle of her flight, " I have children, and they are frozen ". Regression to her childhood appeared frequently in misidentification of those in her environment as relatives or old-time acquaintances. When her excitement first became marked she said, " Put me on ice," and it was at this time that she had the hallucination of the black dog, whom it is possible to consider an agent of death.

On admission she seemed very sleepy, yawned constantly and complained of the heat and bad odour in the room, and insisted on having the windows open. These complaints are so frequently heard in claustrophobia, that it is not unreasonable to presume that they were associated with ideas of death and burial, to which she gave such frequent expression. When asked, "Where are you ? " she replied, " Buried in the ground," and then to " How long

[1] See Chapter XVIII.

have you been there ? " " Years, and years and years ". This idea of being buried was repeated over and over again. She several times complained of pinching sensations, which she interpreted as the evidence of worms in her body. But she was not alone in this grave. She spoke very frequently of the dead members of her family, usually her father or brother, once of a sister. Quite often she hallucinated a vision of her father and spoke to him. Once she said, on looking fixedly at the ceiling, " Look ! That is my father ; I see him with mine eyes now ! " Several times she imitated her father, as when she said, " Farder lays like that " (with her hands outstretched). Again beating with her hands on the bed she remarked, " That was farder's way, like that ". Association between her father and herself is well shown in the following productions : " I was in the ground buried and I have to put a stone in my farder's name." Again, " Doctor he die in my house. Oh ! Ah ! Yah ! Mother know, and when the doctor came they had to run away from him. You cannot save me, and I am so hoarse. Let me die here to the ground "—this followed by unintelligible singing. But there is a suggestion of birth being combined with death in some of her productions, for she referred quite frequently to the 22nd of February (Washington's birthday). For example, she said, " My old papa is buried ". (When did he die ?). " Oh ! ah ! George name 22nd of February." At the same interview she was asked what month it was, and she replied, " 22nd of February, 22nd of February. My son was still dead ten years ago, not even twenty years ago. I could not see him ". She repeatedly answered, " February 22nd," when asked the month, which was quite incorrect. After recovery she spoke of remembering queer sensations when lying down as if flying or falling, which are, perhaps, to be correlated with the delusions of another existence.

The elaborations of these ideas were not extensive—or at least few are noted. Once there was an expansive interpretation with an association of treasure. She said, " I am a Jewess. I want my farder," and pointing to a corner of the room, said, " See the gold and diamonds ". A moment later, while rubbing her hands, rolling her eyes, and at the same time spitting, said, " There is glass and diamonds in my spit ". This idea of wealth was quite isolated. A religious setting which one expects to meet with an association of death ideas was present only in a form which her utterances sometimes took, when she would intone them in a sing-song way, resembling the fashion of service used in the Jewish synagogue. Erotic tendencies were manifested in her behaviour, with frequent efforts to expose herself, in talk of wedding rings and an interest in the details of the examining physician's dress and toilet, which was more acute than any she had for the other details of her environment.

The interesting point in this case is that associated with a manic excitement there is a constant repetition of the idea of death, and that this death is apparently a mutual one, inasmuch as almost invariably the thoughts of her father's death or being with him is mentioned. The development of the psychosis is also instructive. She begins her abnormality with an accident, which would naturally suggest death, and has at first a neurotic reaction, such as frequently is associated with fear of a personal death. This continues, increasing in severity, until there is a sudden change from a neurotic to a psychotic state, as her thoughts regressed to childhood. From then on the idea of death comes into consciousness, dramatized as companionship with her father. On recovery, the precipitating cause suddenly reappeared again in an hysterical symptom. She began to complain of pains in her right side, her chest and right arm, and of a weakness in her right arm, all of which she attributed to the electric shock, although she admitted there had been no pain up to the time of recovery from her psychosis. Needless to say, careful physical examination revealed absolutely no abnormalities. The symptoms were, apparently, a mild substitution for the death idea which had been a dominating factor in the productions of her psychosis.

The following case is also one that was observed some twenty years ago, and was, of course, not described with the modern interest in the ideational content. It is now included, however, to show how the general principles, of which we have been speaking, appear even in a meagre record. The case is one in which elation is definitely associated with delusions as to supreme capacity, with veiled indications of infantile factors being at work.

CASE 27. *Lawrence P.* Aged 24, single.

F.H. Information as to the family is limited to a statement that the father was a dilapidated drunkard, although in good circumstances.

P.H. The previous history of the patient himself is also meagre, but it is stated that he was always a spoiled child, and that he had had two brief attacks of depression prior to the excitement which caused his commitment. The dates of these depressions are not stated.

The attack in question commenced six weeks before admission, when the patient became much incensed over a certain article in a newspaper, the contents of which is unfortunately not mentioned. The excitement began with a threat to horsewhip the editor, and his consequent acts all seem to indicate a tendency to dominate those in authority. He demanded that the newspaper should no longer appear at a well-known club of which he was a member, and, when this order was not obeyed, he wrote an insulting letter to the president of the club. Apparently he had some king-making fancies, for he announced that he was going into politics and would make his father mayor. He went to Washington to see the President. Soon his behaviour was so abnormal that he had to be commited to a hospital.

Under observation, his mood and behaviour were highly typical of a hypomanic state. He was loquacious, taking the lead in all conversation, and not hesitating to be quite rude. To the physicians he was patronizing or critical, talking about their mediocrity and lack of culture, or he treated them " de haut en bas," speaking of himself as a man of the world with experience, such as the physicians had not had, claiming that a temperament like his could not be understood by pedants. At times he was unduly familiar, and flattered those about him in a coarse manner. To the nurses he was rude, and talked about " family matters in a highly indelicate fashion ". He showed considerable restlessness, both physically and in his speech. Although there was strikingly little flight of ideas, he tended constantly to shift from one topic to another. Judgment as to the validity of his claims was absent, yet he could always see a logical weakness on the part of his opponent in conservation, so that a physician had to be constantly on his guard, lest he should be tripped up.

The productions were concerned almost entirely with boasts of his ability. He often compared himself to " Poor Byron," who also was put into a mad-house. He wrote poetry and essays, which he considered excellent, and he spoke of certain of his theories, which he wished to investigate scientifically. In telling these he would walk up and down the room, look very serious, and deliver something like the following, the absurdity of which did not strike him : " Syphilis is in reality the manure of humanity. It improves the race in many individuals, in others it has a destructive action." In order to prove this he wished to go to the chemical laboratory to study the effects of strong acids upon animal, vegetable, and mineral matter, etc.

The indication of infantile tendencies appeared in an abuse of his father, whom he did not hesitate publicly to call a drunkard, and also in a typically manic production, an essay on love, which he wrote for the alleged edification of some young lady. Although this essay was mainly composed of banalities, it contained some startling statements about mother love, which showed a sublimation of what were probably his own inner cravings. One feels justified in making such a claim, because his thoughts on this subject were so highly unconventional. It is usual enough to read panegyrics of maternal affection and filial piety, but the patient went quite beyond this in his productions, so that it seemed as if he had projected, in a literary effort, ideas normally unconscious, which only appear in consciousness during the most disintegrating mental disturbances.   By projecting these ideas in a literary form they are not consciously associated with himself, and, hence, are sublimations. The following is a literal transcription of his outpourings on this subject :

" After giving full play to my imaginative faculty, I turn [term ?] mother love unique, extraordinary and grotesque.   Sometimes it is platonic friendship ;   often it is animal passion, but most of all it is human, and sensible to the most important of human feelings, pain, pride and love.   Its conception is animal love, the realization of which is painful truth, from which time of pride engulfs everything until death comes to the mother."

CHAPTER XXII

EMOTIONS IN MANIC STATES OTHER THAN ELATION

WE have considered a sufficient number of typical manic cases to show how limited is the range of ideas in this group. We find in the foreground: First, constant talk of sublimations (using that term in its narrower sense of natural activities). These are psychotic, because the element of personal ambition is so stressed as to exclude other considerations and therefore causes a lack of judgment as to the propriety or expedience of these schemes. Second, there may be engrossing religious ideas, which, as a rule, show a primitive and child-like egocentricity, and are often a vehicle for crude expansiveness. Third, the patients may merely luxuriate in fancies of unconventional but adult love affairs. Finally, we hear them speak of a return to childhood with fantastic re-establishment of the nursery attachments in which the element of sex (in its commoner meaning) is eliminated. Then in the background there are scattered references to ideas, necessarily related to the above, of getting rid of those responsibilities, which bind the patient to his adult routine duty. Sometimes these thoughts are not directly expressed, but may be easily inferred from the conduct of the patient, as when a wife becomes highly irritable, perhaps assaultive, towards her husband or children, or when a man abandons his business having antagonism towards his employers and associates in it. These less prominent ideas are not part of the manic content *per se*, but are " vestigial embryonic rests ", as it were, which betray the infantile source of the dominant ideas. In other words, these less pleasant or pleasure-producing ideas do not belong to the manic picture as such, but are related casually with the psychotic origin of the manic content and prove that the manic fancies do not come into being full-fledged, but are intimately related with the unconscious roots of the personality of the patient. It is the maladjustment of this personality, which produces the insanity, and, consequently, sporadic utterances or anomalies of conduct betray the fact that maladjustment is present, while the typical manic ideas and behaviour represent one type of psychotic solution of the difficulties in which the unstable personality finds itself.

Our next task is to consider the relation of the typical manic content to the other more obvious symptoms : in other words, to those features of the disease which usually are taken as the basis for diagnosis and description—what we may term the formal aspects of the disease. First we must consider that which is the most prominent symptom, as a rule—the mental and physical over-activity. This is easily explained. In our normal life our activity is inhibited, as has been explained in Chapter XIX, both by instinctive and conventional repressions. We are usually little aware of the former, but any introspectionist knows how much he is blocked by consideration of what Mrs. Grundy would say. As we have seen, the attention of the manic patient is exclusively directed to ideas which evade the instinctive repressions and, because he is engrossed in thoughts divorced from reality, he gives little heed to his environment and is not affected by considerations of the feelings or criticisms of his associates or of his society. Hence his energy is flowing fairly directly from its unconscious sources and gaining an unhampered outlet. He feels happy and has no more consideration of the social impropriety of his acts when he gesticulates, stamps, pounds, or runs around, than has a child or puppy. We may quite properly compare his condition to the excited phase of alcoholic intoxication, where precisely similar activity is in evidence, so soon as the subject's inhibition is removed by the drug and he ceases to consider what other people think of him ; hence the half truth of *in vino veritas*, the personality which is not an artificial product of convention being crudely displayed. It would be a whole truth were it not that conventionality is an integral part of the personality of each of us.

Other anomalies of conduct are similarly explicable. Free from the restraint of social criticism, the manic patient entertains quite impolite ideas, hence he may be rude, mischievous, untidy or destructive, according to the whim of the moment. Irritability may be simply explained. It seems pretty generally to be a protective tendency. When conscience would bid us recognize our own shortcomings, we try to evade the issue by searching for similar or worse derelictions in others, so, with sharpened eyes, we see and criticize the mistakes of those about us. Usually the process is hampered by our more or less complete recognition of this being none of our business, but the manic individual knows no such inhibition, consequently he tends constantly to correct the defects of his own system of ideas by discovering faults in others. This postulates a certain contact with environment, of course, and, as a matter of fact, we do not see irritability in those cases who are so wholly engrossed in their psychotic thoughts as completely to neglect the environment. It is in just those cases, where the patient endeavours to force attention on his egocentric ideas, that we find a manic irritability ; in fact one may say that this symptom is always suggestive of a certain rudimentary insight. The patient repels interference because it implies criticism, which in a dim way he feels he ought to apply to himself.

Another type of irritability is seen in cases where introversion is marked. Patients who become entirely absorbed in their own interests, their own thoughts, often resent any reminder that another world exists. Then, like children in a bad temper, they ward off the approach of others with physical or verbal abuse. This is negativism (see Chapter 18).

Although elation is the commonest of moods in the manic state, it is far from being the only one, and to understand the emotionality of these patients we must remember that even the simplest emotion is rather a complex affair. It contains at least two components, subjective and objective. The subjective is the more difficult to describe. I can feel happy, sad, lonesome, fearful, or guilty, without betraying my feeling to any observer in the environment. This deception is possible only in so far as I inhibit the tendency to display the other component, the external manifestation of my feelings. The former, the feeling tone of any thought, the *affect*, is an intensely personal thing. It can only be expressed to another individual in symbols which is probably one of the tasks of art. We constantly gauge the emotions of a companion from his facial expression, bodily movements and speech. We infer from these signs a subjective feeling tone, which may even be engendered in ourselves. For instance we are stirred by the intonations and gestures of an actor. If coldly critical, we realize all the time that he himself is not suffering, merely acting. If, however, he be very skilful, we may forget that we are viewing a stage, and an artificial production, and feel real sympathy with the actor's mood. In such a way we make a false inference. Now when we are observing a patient, who is, of necessity, very largely out of contact with his fellows, we judge of the feeling tone of his ideas from his words and speech. The normal man inhibits these expressions in proportion to his conventionality and the customs of his society. Probably all civilized people inhibit emotional expression to some degree. The manic, patient, however, is largely free from these inhibitions, hence with every slight change in the formulations of his ideas there appears a marked variation in his expression, speech and movements. He appears to us, " emotional ", hence we find patients crying, scolding, whining, in spite of their being generally quite elated.

In some cases the tendency to a variegated emotional reaction is more characteristic than their elation, and in such patients the type of mood presented seems to follow quite definitely the prominence of one or another topic. As an example, we may cite our next case. She was a woman whose behaviour was typically manic and who, although generally elated would become fractious, scolding and crying whenever she mentioned her husband. Ordinarily, when manic patients express ideas suggesting the undesirability of their marriage partners, they do so in rather fleeting references. Complaints of this woman's husband, however, always absorbed her in long accounts of his abuse, and, consequently, irritability was a marked feature of her case.

CASE 28.—*Catherine D.*—Aged 40. Admitted to the Psychiatric Institute, June 17th, 1912.

She had been married for many years and had had nine children, four of whom died when small. The oldest was thirteen years of age, and the youngest was ten months. A limited anamnesis stated that she was quiet and sociable, not given to worrying, and a hard worker. She plainly had had a very hard life with an Irish husband who drank and probably abused her. No matter how stable or unstable her make-up may have been, she certainly had ample occasion to worry over the many burdens of her married life.

She was born in Ireland and came to this country at the age of 15. Apparently, like many of her country folk, she was litigious and thought a good deal about gaining benefits by legal means. For some seven years there had been trouble over a will by which she hoped to gain some property. Two months before admission, one of her boys dislocated his arm and she thought the doctor who attended him did not display the requisite skill and could therefore be sued for damages. Two weeks before admission, another boy was very ill. She took care of him and had no sleep for three days, being naturally much worried. At the same time there had been a quarrel going on with the janitor's family and there was talk of the daughter of the janitor having thrown a lighted match into her baby's perambulator. She claimed subsequently that she was not able to sleep at this time for fear that the janitor's daughter would set fire and burn up her children. This probably was her first symptom, for absurd anxiety over the safety of children is a frequent early manifestation of a developing psychosis. On the night of June 2nd the boy was so ill that he was not expected to live and a priest was called. The next day another child received a post-card with a picture of a ship on it. This same day she became quite excited, began to sing, was very talkative and elated, speaking constantly of her early life.

The significance, for her psychosis, of the illness of her son, and the receipt of the postcard soon became evident in her productions.

The patient talked much of the events immediately preceding her commitment, always distorting and giving them a psychotic meaning. Apparently the son's illness suggested the idea of mutual death, for she spoke a great deal of having been killed and brought to life again. The killing was at times the work of her husband, again, the doctor gave her powders [undoubtedly for insomnia], or she was chloroformed, put into a pack and thrown into the river. The idea of being put into the water [a frequent symbol of death, or return to the Nirvana from which we came] probably originated in her trip across the water to the hospital. She gave many versions to this, but common to them all, was the idea of being drowned and then rescued by a lover. This is where the postcard with the picture of a ship got its significance. Mere death alone without any suggestion of new life does not seem to be a manic content. The ship, however, suggested two things to her. It was the boat, in which she had been rescued by a lover (an idea initiating fancies of adult lovers), and, secondly, it brought to her mind the expression " When my ship comes in ". So she interpreted the postcard as a sign that she would be successful in her lawsuits and that a fortune was coming to her. This explains how the melancholy thought of her son's death was distorted through successive steps into pleasing fancies ; first, she died herself ; secondly she was brought to life again by a lover ; and third, she inherited a fortune.

For the first month of her hospital stay, she was in a state of marked emotional disturbance, often with plain elation, when she would sing happy songs, occupying herself with the physicians, calling them her lovers, and wanting to be kissed ; but more often she was angry and crying, especially when talking of her husband. As this tended to be her dominant topic, she was fractious and unruly. But if she were distracted from this theme, her mood would at once become that of elation ; she would be good-natured and amorous. Her productions were more disjointed and rambling than truly flighty, for there was little evidence of sound associations or distractibility. It seemed more as if there were certain groups of ideas, which she had to think and talk about, and her speech was essentially a broken stream of exposition of these thoughts. After a month or six weeks she became more elated and continued in this state for about two years and four months. occasionally quieting down or, again, becoming more excited. Rarely, she assaulted the nurses. The greater her excitement, the more exclusively would she confine herself to her trend of ideas. When quieter she could be brought to talk quite rationally on other affairs, although it was never possible to bring her to speak of her husband without many complaints of his treatment.

The ideas she presented were quite typical of a manic state. In the first place, there was constant evidence of regression to her girlhood. She sang Irish ballads and was continually identifying those around her as companions of her childhood. Secondly, she spoke, usually in retrospect, of her death— a more marked regression. She was fond of telling how she had been chloroformed and thrown into the water, rehearsing the tale of her rescue and of being taken to the " Tombs ". Naturally this regression implied a dissolution of her marriage bonds ; she constantly talked of how her husband ill-treated her—insisted that he had broken their vows, or, quite frequently, she alleged she was not married to him at all, but to one MacB. Sometimes other lovers were substituted for MacB. We can probably account for the great prominence of scolding by the quite conscious and obsessing antagonism she had for her husband. In most cases we see fleeting references to delusions of the death, or removal, of the husband and such cases are not irritable, except when in the presence of the husband. This woman, however, was solving her problem by assigning all responsibility for the unhappiness of her married state to her husband, hence the necessity of her reiterating the story of his abuse and infidelity. It is probable, of course, that there was some basis of fact for her criticism, but the energy that went into her tirades seemed to come from the projection of her own unfaithfulness on to him.

There were also ideas which we might term progressive. The first of these was her fancy of lovers. These were most of them men whom she had known in childhood, who had died and who, she insisted, had come to life again. This shows how divorced from reality and how truly unconscious in origin were these delusions. Secondly, she had expansive ideas of her new life. These were concerned essentially with the wealth she was to inherit or receive from lawsuits, but she was also fond of saying she was " Queen of the world and the fifth generation." Finally there were delusions of simple wish fulfilments, put in a religious form, which appeared in scattered reference to the Virgin or a saint crowning her ; or the heavenly being would tell her that she owned a grocery store or something of that kind.

Through all of her psychoses there were suggestions of a plain infantile motive. This appeared in the identification of those around her as relatives, or her consistently calling the doctor " Father ". Occasionally she addressed the physicians as " Father " and spoke as if she were talking to a priest. That her lovers were but father substitutes, appeared from her habit of calling the doctors " Father " and saying that they were her lovers. It also appeared in such associations as the following : " There were twelve lovers that are buried in Killebeg's graveyard. . . when my father had all [?] buried and you are one of them."

The dominance of these ideas in her productions and the form in which they appeared can possibly be shown best by the quotation of the actual notes taken at one interview. (Well, Mrs D., how are you feeling ?)—" I am not Mrs D., I am Mrs McB. I have a lover, he was to be my husband and he can't get to Heaven until I am happy. I married your brother [to stenographer] Miles McB. I certainly did, he was the only lover I ever liked." (And who is this man D. ?)—" O Lord, sure he broke the bonds, I married him in St. Catherine's Church, he broke the bonds . . . I always had to work for my living." Who are these people here ?)—" You are Edward C. [addressing one of the physicians], you are my second cousin and she [nurse]is Father O'D., Johnny O'D.'s son from South Africa." (Do you hear talk about you ?)—" Yes, I hear my husband indeed." (Do you hear any talk ?)—" I do not, they are gone away." (Do you see things ?)—"Indeed I was afraid at first, they murdered me and I came to life again, they tied me up in packs and everything, they carried me out at the hour of midnight." (Where ?)—"On 348th Street, D. wanted to get rid of me, to murder me." (Who am I ?)—"You are Edward C., my second cousin." (What place is this ?)—"North Brother Island, the House of Records." (What's the matter with these people ?)— "They wanted to get my money, God damn them, they cannot get it, I am Queen of the world and the 5th generation." (What place is this ?)—"North Brother Island." (Month ?)—"July 24th, 1913." (August 8th, 1912). (Day of week ?)—"Thursday the 24th of July—what do you take me for, you God damn bastard." (My name ?)—"Edward the 2nd." (My business ?) "You went to be a priest, didn't you ?" (When did you come here ?)— "I left home the 4th of June." (Where did you go then ?)—"They took me and brought parties and everything to murder me, I went to Westchester with my lovers and then they took me to Bellevue." (How long there ?)—"Then I went to City Hall." (From where did you come here ?)—"From the City Hall, 7th June." (How get here ?)—"They took me up here on a boat a prisoner." (How get here ? ") "From the boat, my uncle brought me." (How did you come ?)—"I come in a wagon." (Did you come right up here ?)—"No, I was taken in below." [Correct.] (What ward ?)— "Downstairs, I don't know what ward it was, part of this ward, I don't know when, I don't care. It is the House of Records." (This is Manhattan State Hospital.) "I never was in no hospital." (How long downstairs ?)—"Until I came here, only a couple of hours, I met St. Anne down there, she said, 'Come here dear, they will not kill you' ; she took off the cap off herself and put it on me and said, 'Now I will crown you '." (How many children ?)— "I got nine, I don't know how many ' misses ', I have nine living, I have four in Heaven and a miscarriage. I have five living, four dead." (What age is the oldest ?)—"Going on 15 ; the youngest will be a year the 2nd day of August." (The oldest was born ?)—"13th of June." (Do you feel sad or happy ?)—"I certainly feel happy, I am Miles McB.'s wife." (When married to him ?)—"The 26th of June." (Does the Virgin Mary talk to you now ?)— "I see her dressed up as Susan K. She comes over and shakes hands with me and sits on the table with me ; she looks like your sister Susan." (How long here ?)—"They took me away from home the 3rd of June, now this is the 24th of July." (How long would that be ?)—"How long would that be ? I can't tell you." (Have you been mixed up in your head ?)—"I certainly was, he brought me poison and everything." (Are you mixed up now ?)—"I am not, I am a prisoner here, he took me to the House of Records." (What place did I tell you this was ?)—"I don't care what you told me, it is North Brother Island, it belongs to the State, I know it's North Brother Island, this is the House of Records, this is where they put everyone with all kinds of diseases, consumption, diphtheria and everything else."

This case illustrates the principle of which we have just stated, of a particular type of idea producing a dominant irritability, because that idea itself is dominant. Examples could, of course, be given showing that other emotional expressions such as crying or whining are similarly determined, but the principle is probably sufficiently plain for it to be recognized in descriptions of cases cited for other purposes. The point to be borne in mind is that, in manic states, the emotionality in general is an expression of poor contact with the environment and its accompaniment of disregard of convention, while the particular mood shown is determined directly by the coincident ideational content.

CHAPTER XXIII

THE PRINCIPLE OF DISTRACTION OF THOUGHT

OUR next problem is to consider the factors which produce flight, distractibility, disorientation and such disturbances of normal processes of thinking. All these anomalies can finally be reduced to the influence of introversion of attention. In a word, one may say that orderly thinking is affected whenever there tends to be preoccupation with thoughts of highly personal interest.

It must be admitted, of course, that psychiatrists have usually considered that there is some inherent tendency to disintegration of logical thinking in the manic state. It would usually be considered a primary symptom of the disease. Most text-books speak of these disturbances of thinking, as if ideas, normally present in logical relation to one another, were all jumbled in the mind of the manic, much as playing cards are disarranged when shuffled. If this view were accepted we could never find any law which would govern the appearance of ideas in their speech. Nothing but chance could account for their words. As a matter of fact, however, manic patients of all types are not multifariously productive ; their speech tends to be confined to prevalent topics. This is a phenomenon which is, of course, recognized in hypomanic states, where the patient insists on always publishing his views on some given subject, continually makes the same boast or expresses some chronic antagonism.

With patients who are definitely flighty, however, an impression is certainly given of their productions being disjointed and haphazard in the extreme. It seems as if nothing but accident led them to rouse from their memory totally unrelated ideas, or to be distracted by observations on their environment, which have the appearance of complete irrelevancy. Nevertheless, if one takes the pains to secure complete stenographic records of the productions of these patients at different interviews, it is discovered that the range of topics in their talk is really limited, the same ideas occurring time and time again, even the comments on the environment often being identical. Reference to this internal consistency has already been made in the case of Mary E. described above. As will be recalled her productions, apparently haphazard, were really confined to a small group of ideas and reappeared consistently in thirteen attacks during twenty-seven years. As an example of this dominance of the circumscribed number of ideas in speech which was quite rambling, we may quote the following utterances of a Jewish girl during the attacks which were separated by two years of normal mental health.

(What happened this time to get you in here?) " I myself does not know what the trouble is ; if you don't know, I certainly don't. I am under your care. My temperature wasn't taken. I can read and write English language and no other language. I didn't take no bath, wasn't weighed, nor nothing. I don't know unless you people are so great that through your stenographer you discover everything. The first time I came here I went to Miss K.'s [the stenographer] office. I touched the machine, and that dumb patient Kittie pushed me away ; but there was a patient here, the second time I came, and her name was M.M., she was deaf and dumb, and there was another little Jewish girl. I went and spoke to them in their own language, and they naturally like me. But I can read and write English too. I wonder why I can't have wisdom teeth? But Dr. Bliss said he wanted to protect the physicians. I said to him he should take all the cops. I paid £5 for a gold tooth. I said he treated my sister. I lost my love for H.S. [a Jew] because any young man who doesn't take my interest in a sister, we were sisters and brother in the same society—I've grown a little older and I have met other men. I am trying to study my sickness. Dr. A. has my history. He is the only physician that could cure my brain. I have relations in this hospital. I want to know if it is inherited. I have studied it ever since I went out, to find why people go insane. If a woman becomes insane and she is pregnant, the child naturally becomes insane. I want to clear myself from insanity before I get married, and I want to clear my sister Molly. She is worse than I am, when I told her that she was wild."

In this production there are some ten different topics that appear without any obvious internal relationship. The next quotation from the attack two years later is about the same length. In it seven of these same topics reappear, while the other three which are not seen in this particular example did occur in this second attack time and time again. In this second example there are some six ideas not present in the first productions, but these again echo many ideas expressed in the former attack, and all of them were dominant throughout the second.

The second example is as follows : " This is Miss K. She used to be stenographer for Dr. A., Dr. B., Dr. C., and Dr. D. I was very much interested in insanity since I left this island, and they told me that A.M. died. I'd like to know why I didn't die. I'd like to know why any Jew wouldn't marry an insane girl. I never went for any physician. I was arrested by my own brother, taken from an orphan asylum. I am going to be 28 years the 19th of May. My father will have to tell me what men and women diseases are. I am only a member, but no man can study law, and no man can tell me where I was found. I am a member of the maternal tree, that means deaf and dumb asylum. If I could make people understand me! This time I come to the hospital for an English company without U.S. money. My brother was born . . . Dr. A. told me I talked too much. There are many histories, too many generations. I know too much anarchism and socialism. Everything must go to the insolvent bank. That's the trouble. If I was only deaf and dumb and blind I would be better off. Why didn't I have my picture taken, I would like to know? I am only a patient." (Are you happy?) " Never, never confess my heart's concern, never confess my troubles since the day I left here, doctor. I have been a sin to my nation. I never wanted to love a Jewish man, not that I loved Dr. A. I told him that at the staff."

Anyone, who is interested in the observation and study of what patients actually say, is soon quite familiar with this phenomenon of the dominance of certain topics, which are continually not only reappearing, but often seem to be the only ideas present. These have some special personal significance, which we believe to be related to the obvious anomalies in the thinking processes of our manic patients. We would term this disturbance DISTRACTION OF THOUGHT, because we believe the trouble is caused by attention being withdrawn from the environment to be placed exclusively on the dominant trend of personal ideas. The patient is distracted from consideration of his environment to an absorption in his own fantasies. Etymologically the term is appropriate, because we find that it is an old term for insanity, which survives to-day in the word " distraught ".

To understand how distraction of thought disturbs the clarity of speech, we have only to turn to our own daily experience. Spoken or written speech depends for its comprehensibility on a wish to be understood, and a consequent intellectual control of the productions. It is a commonplace of life that anyone, who is excited, and has his attention concentrated on some particular event or idea, is apt to be incoherent or, at best, can be understood only with great difficulty. Quite similarly, when we concentrate our attention on some problem, and answer a remark addressed to us irrelevantly or incorrectly, we are said to be absent-minded. What happens then is that our attention is simply directed to our own thoughts, and we are not putting sufficient interest into the intelligibility or what we say. Possibly the finest examples of normal distraction of thought are seen in drowsiness, where fatigue prevents us from focussing our attention sharply on our environment. We may then be guilty of uttering most ridiculous statements, some of which may be determined by actual dreams from which we are disturbed by a question.

Very often, too, in normal life the logical train of our thoughts is interrupted by some external stimulus, which we usually blame for the interruption. As a matter of fact it is a difficult matter for us to

R

give unwavering attention to any given subject. It is much easier to let our thoughts drift on topics of internal, personal interest or to let our minds be distracted and give attention to something which does not demand the same effort of concentration. Very frequently, however, there is an unconscious meaning attached to the stimulus which breaks up the logical train of our thoughts. For instance, the author was one day studying the case of a patient C. He had been working for some hours and was growing weary, a condition naturally favoring relaxation of concentration. Suddenly his attention was attracted to a calendar on the wall opposite him, bearing the face of a woman whose features suddenly fascinated his attention. His thoughts were : " That face is familiar ; she resembles someone ; it is Mrs. X. Before marriage her name was C." With the last thought the explanation of this distractibility was clear. For six weeks the calendar had been in the same place on the wall opposite his desk. He had observed it casually thousands of times, and had quite probably noted the resemblance to Mrs. X. unconsciously. When he became weary, and his mental tension was defective, he unconsciously began to associate freely from the name of the patient, whose case he was reading. The patient C. made him think, we presume, of his friend Mrs. X. At this point the picture before him became suddenly familiar and riveted his attention. Without an interest in such phenomena this example of distractibility would have been regarded as purely accidental.

How much the desire to be understood makes our everyday speech logical and intelligible is clearly seen in studying the phenomena of free association. When once an individual succeeds in relinquishing his normal critique, his thoughts flow in a highly illogical way, and, as a matter of fact, actually duplicate the features of manic flight. In free association we see two forces at work : first, the influence of superficial associations, such as those of time and place of events in our memory, or of contiguity of objects spread before us, and less often a superficial association which comes from similar sounds in words. A cursory study of free associations might lead us to suppose that these are the only factors, but more careful scrutiny reveals that in many, if not in all, cases there is an unconscious bond also linking the thoughts which come into consciousness. In fact, during the process of psychoanalysis, a patient becomes so trained in letting his thoughts flow freely and " illogically," that his associations tend to reach a goal in some deep-lying unconscious idea, which, when reached, is seen to be a motif running through all his productions. When this is discovered it gives a logic to his utterances, which they previously lacked, and is particularly useful in explaining those jumps from one topic to another which seemed on the surface to be quite unrelated. In truth, the more that logical criticism of one's thoughts is abandoned, the more transparent does the unconscious bond become. Patients during the course of an analysis not infrequently become aware of ideas, so far removed from consciousness, that they slip away even with the effort of finding words in which they may be expressed.

A few examples may make this clearer. A patient who was being treated for homosexuality had a dream in which, accompanied by his chief homosexual friend, he was watching his own funeral. He particularly noted the casket. When asked to associate to "casket," his thoughts proceeded as follows : "Casket—my grandmother's funeral—cypress trees—poplars—Riverside Drive—homosexuals whom I have met on Riverside Drive." .It may be noted that all of these are perfectly "natural" associations, but, that there was a deeper trend to them, became evident from the relationship, that was immediately shown between his grandmother's death and his homosexuality. He recalled that his grandmother of whom he had been inordinately fond, died at Christmas time. After her death he was very lonely, and escaped from that loneliness only by beginning friendships with men in the spring of the ensuing year, which soon developed into homosexuality. He had never before related these two events in his life, but was unconsciously aware of them, and it was this unconscious connection which determined the association from death to his grandmother and from that by easy transition to the thought of homosexuality. If this sequence had been purely a matter of superficial connections between the ideas expressed, any one of them might have led to a thousand different ideas, but his thoughts were really not free. The unconscious connection, between sorrow for his grandmother's loss and comfort from a new type of emotional contact, drove his thoughts relentlessly along one path only.

As an example of sound associations which seemed to be superficial in the extreme, but were determined by an underlying idea, I may quote the following : A patient wrote down a dream she had the night before in which "Epsom salts" occurred. In writing this she misspelled Epsom, putting an n for the m. When asked to associate to "Epson," she gave the following : "E P S O N, E P S I L O N, E L S O N, N E L S O N." The moment she uttered the word Nelson, there flashed into her mind the memory of another dream, she had had during the night, which concerned an individual named Nelson. It is a simple matter to see how this name first caused the replacement of m by n in her writing, and then made her, in her rhyming, inevitably change epson into Nelson.

The following gives an example of how associations may be utterly illogical on the surface, although clearly related when the unconscious common denominator of them all is evident. A patient had a dream in which dish-washing occurred. Her associations from this word began with quite intelligible superficial connections, but then suddenly became utterly illogical. They were as follows : "Dish-washing—routine—sameness of type—independence of women—Mona Lisa—the Sphinx—children do not understand their mother." Any one who has read Freud's "Eine

Kindheitserrinnerung des Leonardo de Vinci " will see at once how these last three associations may be united, because in this paper he deals with the probability of childish curiosity concerning the mother, being expressed in the riddle of the Sphinx and in the inscrutable smile of La Giaconda. These associations are all the more startling coming from a patient who, so far as I was able to discover, had never even heard of Freud's paper, was totally unfamiliar with German, and with whom the topic of sex curiosity had never been discussed. For our present purposes, however, we could admit the possibility of her having gained knowledge unwittingly of Freud's theory, without invalidating the principle of unconscious guidance of free associations.

In one patient, with a tendency to hysterical clouding and dissociation of consciousness, whom I have studied, free associations, at times, became totally independent of external relations, and appeared as pure unconscious memories. When this process reached its acme, she would be amnesic for all that she had said. In fact mere concentration of her attention, on a topic of intense unconscious significance, frequently led to her developing a somnambulic state, in which she was oblivious of the environment. This shows very nicely how contact with environment, and logical sequence of thought (that is, in terms of conscious logic) are intimately bound together.

Our theory, then, could be stated thus. Leaving aside for the moment the question of the mood reaction, the essence of the manic state would be an absorption of the patient's attention on autistic thoughts. In milder hypomanic cases these thoughts would appear in a fairly adaptive form, implying contact with the environment, so that the train of thought could easily be followed and not appear markedly illogical. In more florid manic states the autistic ideas would tend to present themselves in less adaptive form and, the patient's attention being riveted on something quite out-of-keeping with the environment, he would suffer from an apparent disturbance of his intellectual function. Finally, if a complete or almost complete divorce from reality in the patient's thoughts were encountered, contact with environment would be totally lost, the patient would become non-productive, and be in practically the same condition as one who dreams, his mind filled with the images of his dream, living in imagination, through scenes of much activity, but objectively saying not a word and showing no change of expression. This last stage would, of course, imply a profound disintegration of the intellectual processes so far as they could be studied. We shall shortly endeavour to show from case material that these principles are sound, and that the rationality of a patient's utterances, intelligibility of his conduct, and disturbance of orientation are all directly proportionate to the degree of absorption in thoughts of unconscious origin.

Formal psychiatrists have already noted a number of these

features, which are mentioned by Kraepelin in his text-book. For instance, he speaks of there being in mania a diminished sensitiveness to external stimuli, even painful ones. It is not difficult to interpret this as a distraction of attention from external to internal events. He speaks of a subjective appreciation of flight, such as when a patient remarks, " I am not master of my thoughts ". This is a clear statement of the pressure of internal thoughts being too great for them to be controlled consciously. He says, too, that difficulties of apprehension are largely due to distractibility of attention, the grasp of the environment being faulty, not because of a primary defect of apprehension, but rather because of a defect of attention. This is, of course, the kernel of our theory. Isserlin[1], in his studies of continuous associations, noted that in the normal individual there is a change in the direction, while in mania this change occurs in 1.6 to 1.7 seconds. This is merely an arithmetical measurement of the degree to which the normal compulsion to give logical sequence to our thoughts is relaxed in the manic state. Kraepelin notes further that, with an increase of excitement, the train of thought becomes very fragmentary. We may infer from this, that enhancement of the manic process is correlated with exaggeration of the intellectual loss.

Whether an idea appears to us as an imagination which we recognize as unreal, as a dream thought which we know to have been unreal when we awake, or as a delusion which seems real to us even while awake—all this depends on the degree to which we devote our attention to the idea. So long as we are completely absorbed in such an idea, we cannot devote our critical faculties to an examination of its reality. To do so, we must deflect our interest from the idea itself to a consideration of the facts of experience, with which we compare it, in order to determine whether it be fantastic or reasonable.

It is not surprising, therefore, that Kraepelin observes that cases with definite delusions are apt to have consciousness mildly clouded, so that they are uncertain of time relations, apt to misidentify persons, and do not understand the environment fully. The acme of this process is observed in the delirious states, which Kraepelin describes, where he notes fantastic, confused hallucinations and delusions, associated with deep dream-like clouding. He also records the fact that patients in giving retrospective accounts are, at times, uncertain as to whether their experiences were real or dreams.

[1] Isserlin, *Monatsschr. f. Psych. u. Neurol.*, XXII, 302, p. 1197.

CHAPTER XXIV

W E shall now consider the various stages in the development of distraction of thought. The first phase is naturally to be seen in hypomania, where, as we have said, attention is directed to thoughts of activity fairly well in keeping with the environment, so that the patient does not lose contact with reality in any marked way. One notes with these cases that their distraction proceeds only to that point, where there are dominant topics of conversation. They speak continually of their capacity, their wealth, or the importance of their schemes. They are fully oriented and in no way show any gross defect of intelligence, but the underlying principle, of preponderate attention being given to autistic rather than to critical thinking, does affect their intelligence at one point. Judgment as to the practicability, the expedience, of their plans, is weak or absent.

When we leave the mild hypomanic cases to approach those with some flight, we find that the most marked characteristic of their speech is a jumping from one topic to another, on the basis, apparently, of the most flimsy, superficial association. As a matter of fact, it is frequently possible to show that an underlying trend of ideas is responsible for these transitions, and that a greater unity can really be demonstrated, than appears on the surface. In other words, the sequence of thoughts is quite similar to that seen in free association during psychoanalysis. Some examples may make this clear.

As has been stated, clarity or obscurity of a patient's flight seems to depend on the degree in which his dominant ideas are objectivated. When we pass from the mild hypomanias whose attention is given to a single or very few ideas to those engrossed in a greater complication of fantasy, we begin to meet with genuine flight in the patient's productions. In cases where the ideas are sufficiently objectivated to be easily understood the flight is orderly, and one can follow with ease what the patient says.

For instance, we may quote the case of *James L.*, a married man of 52 (CASE 29), who, in a second manic attack, was absorbed in the idea that he had a religious mission to perform, that he was appointed to investigate Harvard University secretly, and that he understood and could control many natural phenomena, particularly those connected with electricity. All these are well objectivated fantasies and consequently the patient was consistently oriented. He even had some insight into his flightiness, fcr he said that he had difficulty in arranging his many thoughts. A representative sample of his talk follows :

As he stumbled over the carpet, and at the same time heard a railroad whistle, he said, " There, I must be on guard to break the current, or else that switch won't be set. Switch ! Switch ! See, that whistle threw me off from what I was talking about. My thoughts switch around and around like the trainman swings his lantern. Now it's the devil that does it. It was the devil that made the engineer go past the signal in the New York tunnel and kill so many people. The devil has the power over life and death. Life and death ! What can I do with life and death ? [Seeing a palm] How can I make that palm grow ? " Then he compared the palm to his daughter, spoke next of his wife, his father, son, their education, his own education, his fraternity life at Harvard University, and went on to talk of being watched on one side and threatened on the other, etc., etc. This is an example of moderate flight where practically nothing occurs, which has not an understandable reference. Moreover, the ideas are all so well objectivated that most of the transitions from one to another are transparent.

The next extract, from the record of another patient, shows the extension of distraction of thought to a point where attention is further removed from reality, so that the productions are less easy to follow. (The orientation in this case was not consistently good.) In the following continuous production one discerns religious ideas, appearing in an identification with Christ or the devil, as well as a marked father antagonism. Further, there are suggestions of erotism. The statements, which seem to be determined by the trend of his dominating ideas, appear in italics.

(When did you come here ?)   " I don't know ; I've been sick— perhaps crazy. *If God knows me he is my father. It is a wise man that knows his father.* I don't know what sent me or through what agency. *Maybe it was my Father. I thought I knew my father. He never had such a Judas. Christ knew him better than I. If I am the devil I want to go to hell because it is full.* Are you an American ? You are not the wisest man in the world. Who was the wisest man three weeks ago and he's now dead ? [A local congressman died the day before.] Did you ever hear of the old lady and how she died ? It is criminal libel, isn't it ? Who was that queen that came to see him ? *I thought I saw the Queen of Sheba but I've seen better.* She came from New Brunswick—don't laugh [the physician smiled] ; I've never been in a theatre in my life only three times, and then I was dragged in. You've seen Shylock ? *I've beaten every Jew I've met. Do you know my father—my father in heaven or hell ?* I don't believe they are there. I'm not an Irishman but I can tell an Irish joke."

The degree, to which his absorption in inner thoughts prevented his grasp on externals, is well shown by a reading test, to which it was impossible for him to give sufficient attention for accurate reading, largely on account of his tendency to go off on a side track whenever a word reminded him of some egocentric interest. He, was given the following clipping to read : " In considering the steel strike it must be borne in mind that the strike is not over wages or hours. The union scale has been accepted. It is not over the right of labour to unite. It turns on the unionizing of certain mills in which local lodges have been formed since this trouble began. The corporation has recognized every man's free right to join a union, coupled with a refusal to unionize men against their wishes." He read slowly and carefully, but stopped to comment on many phrases in this manner : " It was a strike. I was struck, and grappled and mauled." At the word " corporation ", he said, " Corporation, corporal, big-belly, corporal punishment " ; and at the phrase " every man's free right to join a union " he said, " especially a marriage coupled ".

The dominance of special topics is more marked in our next example.

CASE 30.—*Robert S.* was a married man, 24 years of age, who was observed more than twenty years ago. Naturally little effort was made at that time to understand or study his productions. Nevertheless it was possible to demonstrate certain dominant topics, which affected his productions materially. His mind was apparently engrossed with autistic religious experiences, which centred around delusions of ascent to Heaven and identification of his father with God. Secondly, there were numerous ideas of the " constructive delusions " type, which showed many fantastic speculations concerning metals, electricity, magnetism and fortifications, all of which were somehow further associated with his religious ideas, although the exact connection cannot be made out from the meagre notes. Finally, there were sporadic references to a homosexual trend. When his attention could be secured, he gave the gross data of orientation correctly except for repeated mis-identification of persons.

The following is a literal transcription of a continuous production which seems superficially to be rambling and quite inconsequent. In the right hand column an explanation is given, which shows the close latent association between the various topics touched upon. For one statement only is there no explanation obtainable from the history, but, if fuller notes had been taken, the great probability is that the significance of this too would be manifest.

My prayers are answered . . . and I see everything like the lady and the man at the Brocton Fair. It was sent up very far, you know; the lady fell first, but the man went out of sight, then they fired at me just like the other night, I saw my father in the cemetery across the street. . . .

Religious.

The patient had the idea that he had been sent up by a golden cartridge to Heaven where he had talked with his dead father and God. Hence his interest in the balloon ascension and his confusion in the account by intrusion of his own autistic experience.

I prayed for Dr. P. . . .

Possibly a father surrogate. He later said that he had been married to Dr. P.

I had a letter from the F. people.

No explanation.

Why, it's just as clear as the kite, the kite the electrician sent up, just as the electricity I feel now. Can't you feel it? Well, that's because you haven't any brass about you, you don't wear a badge (showing one of his suspenders).

Constellation of ideas about metals, electricity and ascension.

The people on the cars feel it. I am putting electricity in my home just like the cable to England. The plumber at Harvard Square put hot water into my house. . . .

These thoughts are centred disconnectedly around an incident, in which Harvard Square and street cars figured.

He painted it gold. I noticed the new terminal station in Boston was in silver.

Interest in metals.

These accidents have happened just because I have been on the car; just as I saw my father's grave in the cemetery. . . .

Association of electricity (car) and heaven.

I started my fortifications the next morning. I had a magnet in one corner and a ring in another, and I had electricity in the four corners of the room.

One formulation of his " constructive " fantasies concerned fortifications, with corners and electricity.

Just as Longfellow writes, I shot an arrow into the air; just like the rainbow up in the air where they say the gold fields are.

Association from electricity to ideas of ascension, heaven and gold.

The following productions are from a patient whose case need not be otherwise described than to state that her productions were concerned very largely with ideas of death, her own and her father's. The first quotation shows how sound associations which superficially are the occasion for the linking of different words, serve only to facilitate the presentation of different death formulations. " My mind is weak, thirsting for blood, to-kill, to-arms, too brave they are, two angels, two saints, they go, one black angel, one black Joe, two angels, too wise you are for me, what is grave, two you gave." This was produced in answer to the question, How is your mind ? Her inner thoughts ran, apparently, as follows : " My mind is weak, weakness is due to poor blood, I need more blood, blood thirstiness, killing, soldiers, virtue, heavenly virtue, heaven and death." The second quotation shows how distractibility may be a cover for internal associations to a dominant theme, in this case, that of death, both her own and her father's. On seeing a butterfly she said, " There is a butterfly. Let it die now. That letter [seen] is mine, Toledo, Ohio [on the letter] is all right if it is spelled right. Paradise [sees word " paradox "] Alley is where my father was killed. That is the knife [shown] you killed me with." Here every transition is explicable on other grounds than those of pure distractibility, except the reference to the letter and Toledo. The probability is that, if she had been asked about this, her associations would have betrayed the relationship of the letter and Toledo to her dominant ideas.

The disturbance of intellectual function occasioned by distraction of thought is most easily seen in cases where there are variations in intensity of the process. Some patients, although usually in fair contact with their environment, may tend to become absorbed in their own thoughts and at such times show evidence of definite falsification of external impressions. For instance, the case, Ellen D., whose history will be abstracted briefly a little later, when reading over a test, consisting of a short story about a baby elephant and its mother, became absorbed in an absent-minded sort of way. When asked what she was thinking of, she replied, " Thinking of a story, a woman going into the woods with a young girl. Before night there was a new baby in the house. She was out working in the field, harvest time. Before night God had sent her a gift. I read it." When the remark was made to her, " There is not much point to it, is there ? " she replied, " No, but hard work to it. The woman was laborious."

When a patient becomes entirely absorbed in his inner thoughts, he has, of course, no attention whatever to pay to his environment, and is completely unproductive. Before that stage is reached, however, there is often a phase where questions are answered in the most superficial, haphazard way. The situation is directly analogous to that, which we see in everyday life among normal people who are " absent-minded ". Such persons answer a question irrelevantly because they say the " first thing that comes into their minds ". The " first thing ", naturally, may come from within, as a fragment of their engrossing thoughts, or may be picked at random from the environment. Precisely the same factors seem to operate in manic states. We have been quoting examples which show obtrusion of inner thoughts. The following examples will illustrate how indifference to the task of intelligibility, or inability to concentrate on it, leads to the utterance of mere words that have no pertinence and no deeper meaning.

For instance, a manic case was given the following story to read :

" In the jungles of India there lived a mother elephant with her baby, a little elephant only one year old. One day the baby elephant ran away from home, and the mother, almost wild with grief, went out to find the lost baby. After a while she came to the top of a hill, and looking down, saw her darling asleep in the grass just at the foot of the hill, while a hungry lion was creeping along almost ready to spring upon the sleeping baby elephant. The lion stopped a moment just below the place where the mother stood. Then more quickly than it can be told the mother elephant rolled herself into a ball and rolled quickly down the hill. The lion never knew what struck him, he was completely crushed. The baby elephant was taken home and given a scolding."

She placed the cardboard about ten inches from the eyes and read in a slow, painstaking manner : " In the jealousy of Indiana lived an elephant, who showed wonderful satisfaction, and the mother-in-law for her offspring one day, underless it has absent, reaching for the top of the hill, and took Willie's foot along, at not a great distance was a mountain lion, the mother was at her world's ends. She, realizing that the baby would not have the ghost of a chance, and banging of this lion, she every memory was drawing nearer to his destined end. The lion had tended directly a moment and stood. More quickly than can be told, the elephant rolled into a hog ball and leaned down the hill. The lion never know what struck him, his feelings were completely outstretched--and Willie the baby elephant was led home where he no doubt got a severe scolding for going without his mother's permissionary." (What have you just read ?) " It was about an elephant in the North Pole—you know as well as I do the rest."

One can see on comparing the original with the inimitable non-sense of the reproduction that the patient's thoughts were far from the task at hand, except in so far as it gave her a chance to be facetious. Here and there she picks out a word which she reads correctly. Here and there, although reading incorrectly, she absorbs an idea which she presents in a distorted form. At no time is there the slightest evidence of her grasping the significance of the story as a whole. Her thoughts were so far from the problem at hand that she could not mechanically reproduce the words in front of her.

The following is a case which shows well that degree of distraction of thought, where the patient becomes almost completely inaccessible, is disoriented, hallucinates, and produces either irrelevant nonsense or fragments from her inner thoughts. In other words it is a condition where the patient, although awake, acts very much as if she were living in a dream.

CASE 31,—*Charlotte R.* was a single woman, a teacher of 29, whose case was observed twenty years ago. In make-up she had always been slightly abnormal, being easily worried and inclined to be hypochondriacal. Now and then she had what were called hysterical attacks of laughing and crying. For two years she had been in love, but encountered much opposition on the part of her mother. Two and a half weeks before the onset of her mental symptoms, she had an intense, " nervous " headache, and soon after developed an ulceration of the jaw, which necessitated the administration of hyonotics and the attendance of a nurse. Then, only three days before admission, she began to talk much about her lover, at first in a rather normal way, but soon with an increasing excitement and demands to see him, insisting that he was in the house. She became so unmanageable that she had to be taken to a psychiatric hospital.

When first examined, she was found to be well nourished and to have no physical disability, except some sordes of the teeth and a coated tongue. She knew the name of the hospital, the date, how long she had been there, and called a physician " doctor ", but knew no names.

By the next day her orientation was apparently gone. She denied having seen the physician before, and, to questions about the place, said one time that she was in another town, and again that she was at her cousin's home ; but most orientation questions were not answered. For a few days she indulged in a good deal of acting. She would say, " Now I will show you something else ", and, assuming a beseeching attitude, would raise her arms in the air with the words " Come to me, oh come to me ", etc. Again she might crouch down like a Mohammedan in prayer. Sometimes she whispered. In her beseeching attitude she would repeat phrases, such as the following, four or five, even six times : " Oh, I see it, we all see it, don't we ? Why, I will stop. We all see with our eyes, don't we ? So simple. Why was it given to me in Bangor, in Maine, we know that, Mr. E." She also indulged in religious utterances with which were associated thoughts of her lover and of maternity. For instance : "'O God, you God, you, [throwing kisses into the air] love me, love me, God, I love God. He made this beautiful world. I love God [dancing about] ; I thank God for giving me a child, a child, a child." Once she was heard saying the following : " Harry ! Harry ! [the name of her lover] He says that I can make all these gestures I want to, Harry, Harry, say, say I can come from Heaven to you ! I went to Heaven last night. I see it all now. I must suffer some terrible dream ; but it is all for the best. Christ suffered. I can bear more than he did. God, God, come, come." All her acting was performed only when she was observed. Then again she might get into tantrums, screaming and kicking. But, as to this, she said herself, " See what I can do to prove my sanity ", and then would begin to rage, so that it was probably in part, at least, assumed. One evidence of her absorption and indifference to external stimuli was in the fact that she could be pricked with a pin without wincing, although she might make remarks about it. This phase of acting lasted a couple of weeks.

She then became still less accessible, with a good deal of bounding and stamping, pulling her bed to pieces, singing, dancing, and talking volubly, often in a sing-song manner and rhyming freely. It became quite difficult to attract her attention, and, when it was gained, her replies seemed to indicate that she thought she was in the house of her cousin. It seemed certain that she did not know the name of a single person in her environment. Her productions may be illustrated by the following : She was rocking a pillow in her arms, singing, " I had a baby last night, a dear little baby, help, help . . .

I'll help you, Harry, the purest, the sweetest, the dearest, the best, *take it and I'll attend to the rest."* Or, again : " I hate them, I hate them, I hate them, I do, if I had a knife I'd run it through . . . For we loved it, for we loved it, why don't you. *Doughnut, doughnut,* 1, 2, 3, *a big pail full don't you see.* It was God who saved the girls in the country to-day ", etc. The italicized words are probably pure nonsense ; the others are rather plainly expressions of her dominating ideas.

In the third week of her admission, she stripped herself and refused feeding. When asked why she did these things, she replied, " God told me to ", but this was submerged in other talk. The next six weeks her condition was, in general, the same, except that she became untidy[1] and seemed to express her tendency to introversion in a very positive way, for she often scratched anyone who attempted to do anything for her. She continued to be disoriented, and from her frequent references she seemed to have the idea that she was surrounded by Unitarian ministers. Her talk became still more ridiculous, owing to the purely verbal elaboration of her trend of thoughts. For example, she said, ' Father, father [often repeated with various intonations] I am not the daughter of the mother of the son of the mother of the armies of the generals of Christianity of Christianity and the power of one of my father of the rainbow of a lover of the time of a mother." One sees in this specimen evidence of her thoughts turning to her father, of a denial of her mother, of interest in her lover and in religion, but the sentence, if it can be called a sentence, is merely a hash, as it were, of these ideas.

Some two months after admission, she quieted down for a week or so and, although far from normal, she became accessible to the extent that she was able to say that she had thought all along that she was in another town, and that she was surrounded by the Unitarian Association. She called the physician " Sam E. ", and could only with difficulty be convinced that he was not he. She wanted to give him a message and wrote the following down : " Do you know me, Sam E., and are you strong enough to take care of me now and will you find Mr. B. Find Mr. B. of Worcester or President Unitarian Association. Sam, will you marry me now ? Your father and you weren't strong enough to marry me and I have been here all alone for a long time. Did you know you were the only lover I have left. I have been here all alone all day, Sam is that Nurse Katie H. Take my hand you father has a message [see above.] Will you get me out of this bondage if you are sane and send at once to C. R. N. W. Rice and Company, Boston, N. Brattle Street. Will you take care of me now. If you have read the papers you will know who I am, and Rev. Spofford Brooks will you and it seems that I have been brought . . ." These sentences are lucid in comparison with the productions quoted above and are mainly delusional in origin. At this time she also said : " I have been in heaven and on earth ; I have been dreaming."

After this quieter interlude, she again became excited and entered into a condition, which lasted for a number of months, in which she was much quieter, often sitting in a chair rocking to and fro, and talking continuously in a sing-song manner, her productions being usually nonsensical. The only evidence of contact with her environment came from the fact that she would sometimes weave words, which she heard spoken, into her productions. Her mood throughout was one of distinct exhilaration with a mischievous perversity but no real silliness. Occasionally the monotony of her behaviour was interrupted by sudden actions like jumping up and slamming the door, or throwing a chair over. All evidence seemed to point to her being completely disoriented. How far she was from contact with reality is shown by the fact that, when her lover and her mother came to see her, she paid no attention to them whatever.

Some nine months after admission, her condition had somewhat improved, so that it was possible to gain her attention quite frequently. She remained disoriented but was apt to read a short test story fairly well, but the way she

---

[1] See the glossary.

did it illustrated her general condition quite well.   She frequently interrupted the progress of a sentence to read the numeral at the head of a page, or a word on a different part of the page would catch her eye and she would comment on it ; for instance,.she said, " I have taken cold," on seeing the word " cold." When asked to give the gist of the story, she recalled several of the ideas in it, but without any logical connection between them whatever.   During the next four months her improvement continued steadily until complete recovery resulted, but for quite a while, after she seemed superficially to be well, she retained a resentment toward certain nurses, had difficulty in believing that one of the nurses was not her cousin, and, for a long time, insisted that she received messages from one B. . . . all of this showed the persistence of her ideas.

Her retrospe .tive account is of interest, because it confirmed the impression, which had been previously gathered, that she had been quite disoriented. She stated that from the second to the fifth month of her admission her mind was a complete blank.   She said she had had beautiful dreams during her sickness, thinking that all the Unitarian ministers, she had ever heard of, were near her ; and that she had communion with many dead.   A less pleasant idea was that urine had been thrown at her through the register.   Thoughts that used to come to her, and which she regarded as wireless telegraphy, she realised to have been hallucinations.   It is interesting that the notes state nothing of her remembering her talk about her father, mother, lover and baby.   It would seem probable that ideas closely related to deep unconscious trends were repressed and that she recalled only such objectivated fantasies as the religious ones.   How completely out of touch she had been with her environment was evident from the fact that she thought one physician was a reporter, another a Pullman car conductor.   At times she fancied she was in a prison.   Again, the reception room was a court room, and a friend who was there at the time was a railroad lawyer.   Up to a month of her complete recovery she realized that one of the physicians was a doctor, only because he had once treated her throat.

To recapitulate then, we may say that this case shows a marked manic state, wherein the patient quickly becomes absorbed in her own delusional ideas and in this introversion loses contact with her environment to such an extent that she becomes totally disoriented, nonsensical in her speech, saving such references as obviously refer to her delusions, and is subsequently amnesic for the period of her greatest excitement, except for some memory of her false ideas.   In retrospect, her experiences appeared to her like a dream, and we have every reason to believe that her situation was psychologically closely analogous to that of dreaming.

Reading tests, including their reproduction from memory, often furnish us with an excellent record of the distraction of a patient's thoughts.   The following example, for instance, shows how a patient may reproduce very little indeed, that is actually in the extract given him to read, but only loosely associated thoughts, which items in the extract suggest to him.   The test was the following newspaper paragraph : " In the absence of Gov. Roosevelt from Albany on his personal electioneering business, Lieut. Gov. Woodruff seems to be acting governor only in business of a minor and routine character.   Important matters are waiting to be acted upon by the actual governor when he can get released by the National Committee to give his attention to them."   He read this correctly.   When asked to give the gist, said : " Oh, I've read about the history of all the great generals in the country and all

over the world, and I'm glad to listen." Urged, he continued :
" Well, there should be not a monarchy nor a republic but a kind
of equality and some one should rule." When further urged he
said it was about " Teddy ". " A good sort of a chap." " Well,
I read that he was rather a hearty chap, a rough rider, a good fellow
in his generation." (What else ?) " That he was going to be
elected for Governor." On a second reading he said, when questioned what he read, " Well, we are carrying a corpse between us.
There will be three men," etc. When urged, " Oh, Teddy Roosevelt
was a rough rider before he got to be a saint." Finally he said,
" I cannot connect it all. There was Lopez and an undertaker of
Chelsea, and the doctors. I read it all but I cannot connect it."

The next case is a good one to illustrate the principle of distraction
of thought. Almost from the outset the patient was disoriented.
At the beginning he showed a slight degree of contact with his
environment by commenting freely on it, weaving his observations
inappropriately into his productions. This seemed to be true
distractibility in the ordinary sense of the term, for there was little
evidence that what he saw in the environment had any deep personal
meaning. But he quickly settled into a state of confusion, quite
marked both objectively and subjectively, and continued in this
for more than two months. He then began gradually to recover.
Unfortunately no effort was made (his case was observed more than
twenty years ago) to collect and compare his productions so as to
study his trend, but it seems that his mind was engrossed with
plans for business, and ruminations about such things as education
and the effects of tobacco and alcohol.

CASE 32—*Frank C.* was a clerk, single, age 19 at the time of his attack.
Little is known of his make-up, it being merely stated that he was always well
and naturally active. In May, 1900, he took an eight weeks' trip through
Europe. On his return on the first of July he appeared very thin, but presented no other abnormality. On the fourth of July, however, he became
unusually active, talkative, making many calls, being out late at night,
and began to talk a great deal about a certain patent, which he was promoting.
After two weeks of this overactivity, he became convinced that some people
were trying to steal the patent from him and went to a police station for
protection. At once he became quite expansive about his schemes, and also
thought that some customers at his shop were detectives watching him on
account of this patent. He was then brought to the hospital.

For the first few days he was decidedly exhilarated, with considerable
physical expression of his excitement, was continuously talking in a definite
flight, rambling from subject to subject, and distracted by remarks or
occurrences about him. He was at this stage perfectly oriented. After a few
days his excitement became more intense and he was occasionally untidy.

It was often difficult to get him to answer questions. His productions at
this time may be illustrated by the following : " Did you ever see McKinley
and Hanna ? I had a girl called Hannah, but I called her Anna for short, but I
added a ban and called her Bananna, then I shortened it down to Nan and
shook her." Again : " I want a drink. I want phosphates. I don't want
any root beer. I don't like the name of beer. They might think the root
is the root of all evil." Again : " The rose is red, the pink is pink, I love you,
I don't think. Give me a gavel and I will travel. I have brain fever on my
upper lip. Am I a mason or a stone layer ? " etc.

Shortly after this he became more subdued, deliberate in his movements, spoke less, appeared to be confused. He looked puzzled, calculated very poorly and seemed to have no control over the ideas which he expressed For instance, he said : " If Mr. . . . would come and ask me a question about Odd Fellows, what kind of a chart would you make for me ? " The reference to the chart seemed to come from the fact that the physician at that moment had picked up a temperature chart. The intrusion of irrelevant ideas is well shown during his calculaion test (7 from 100 ?) He said slowly " 93 ", then " 24." (93-7 ?) " Oh, yes, you want me to spell my name backward." He had been spelling a short time before. (93-7 ?) After thinking, " 16." (16-7 ?) " Well, that's a cigarette cure and there is a God in Heaven ", etc.

During the next week this confusion increased. He wandered about a great deal, rolled up his bed clothes and carried them about with him and defecated into his pitcher. This condition persisted for nearly two months with some variations. At times he would calculate quite well, and, although normally unobtrusive and quiet, he would occasionally be mischievous. He was consistently disoriented. On his better days he could play a little golf, and at times played the piano continuously and well.

The following illustrates his mental processes nicely : He was given this paragraph to read :—" One influence that is making itself strongly felt in favour of the retention of our troops in China is the missionary interests. From the missionary boards in all parts of the country letters are now pouring in, begging the Administration not to lessen the protection afforded to the Christian workers in China and to their native converts. While these appeals are now mostly from official boards, it is expected that they are but the precursor of a general demand from the clergy and laity of the evangelical churches of the country." He read it thus : " Well, about—a missionary fund—that is to say—about how it is raised—how money is raised to carry on the work." (What else ?) " Well, the method of a—method of—" (Well, of raising what ?) " Well, the—how the work is done." (What work ?) " Of helping people—that is—educational work." (Tell me what you really read ?) " Well I forgot what to start—I formed an idea in reading the paper just now about a certain kind of work—" (and ?) " That prices were just the same—about that line of thought." On second reading gave after a long pause : " The present situation—well, practically—of the world—and, well, whether one country has a right to interfere with another country unless there's a good cause for it and who shall decide what the cause shall be."

Abruptly he then said : " There is one point in history I always want to know, that is, the last treaty the U.S. made." (Now let me understand that you know what I want ; I want you to read, then reproduce from memory what you have read.) " In other words, then, I did not read that article right ? " (Now read it again and give me what you read.) " Word for word ? " (No, the gist.) Third reading : " Well . . ." (Can't you give it to me ?) " Yes, sir. Well, it's a question whether the U.S. can hold the fortifications in China and if so on what ground . . ." (Is that all ?) " And who shall decide what share—who the high officials are—in the world."

Some of his statements are quite significant as to the nature of his mental state. For instance : " *Lots of things seem to run through my head and I don't know just where I stand.*" Later he said : " I took up this book and that made me think of my uncle and that of Boston and the old man. I had—well, that makes me think of the village down here and so lots of things go through my head."

In spite of this marked confusion, he was capable at times of quite accurate accounts of past events. For instance, he could give a detailed and accurate description of his travels in Europe. It was interesting that once, when talking quite connectedly, the topic led to the mention of his mother and he at once became confused. This was but an example of his general tendency towards confusion, when anything reminded him of an affective interest. He would then immediately become absorbed and mixed up in his talk.

During the last month of his psychosis, he cleared up gradually, his recovery apparently proceeding without any marked alteration in his mood or conduct, normality returning as his contact with the environment grew, and his intellectual processes became less clouded. During this period he was able to give a meagre account of his condition during the previous months.

He remembered that, when he first came to the hospital, he was afraid of the idea of insanity. He thought that a patient might get so bad that he would be killed, and interpreted the movements of attendants and physicians as evidence of some such hostile purpose. He had a fancy, too, that anything he said or wrote would be used against him. It is important to note in connection with this retrospect of fearful ideas that his expression on admission was occasionally that of anxiety. We shall have occasion to comment on this later, as it is of theoretic importance. It was clear that his intellectual processes had been markedly disturbed. He could remember fairly well the incidents that occurred at the time of his entry to the hospital, and it will be recalled that at the outset he was well oriented. His memory for the rest of his attack was vague, however. He could recall occasional interviews and remembered a number of his misidentifications. For instance, he thought that one of the physicians looked like a special police officer he had known in New York, and that this man had come to see him in reference to the case of a former employee, who had got into trouble. That his mental condition was analogous to that of one who sleeps and dreams is shown by one remark : " I have written and said so much, I talked a lot in my sleep." He was bothered with a vague idea that smoking and drinking had put him into this condition, possibly also sexual promiscuity, but his mind was so confused as to all that had been going on, both internally and externally, that he never was able to form any clear idea of what the nature of his illness had been.

The next case to be briefly described is that of a girl whose psychosis was characterized by rather violent excitements alternating with inaccessible periods, during which she made no replies to questions or answered them irrelevantly, had apparently a good many hallucinations, and whose orientation varied markedly, even at the same interview.

CASE 33. *Isabel U.* was a single Hebrew girl, age 24 at the time of the attack in question. She is said to have been good natured, but more quiet than the other children in the family. She did well at school, and showed some ambition, after a year and a half in high school, by learning stenography in the evenings. She then worked quite efficiently for three years, but from 18 years of age on she was nervous, hypochondriacal, had periods when there would be frequent crying spells, and began to shift a good deal from one business position to another.

Her father died a year and a half before her admission. The family expected her to break down, because she had been so much attached to him, but she did not seem more depressed than the other children. After her attack, however, she ascribed her illness to this event, and said that she had worried inwardly about it until it became too much for her. Seventeen days before admission she attended the wedding of a girl friend, and there met a young man who had the reputation of being a Don Juan. Two days later she begged her sister to accompany her to a musical show, during which she cried softly, and said she did not feel well. From then on she went out every day alone to the theatre, particularly to vaudeville entertainments, or some place, which, she said, would enliven her. She began to consult fortune-tellers, who told her she was going to be married soon, have good luck and so on. She seems then to have begun mentioning the names of young men, with whom she had been friendly at various times, especially the reputed Don Juan.

A week before admission she woke her sister at 4 a.m., and said, " I have

S

something I want to ask you ; " but, when the sister turned on the light, the patient said she had changed her mind, and would not tell what she was thinking of. An hour later, however, she began to scream, said her father was in the next room, and that she knew he was alive. She kept saying " Papa is in the closet, he is not dead," and also alleged that her father was going to pour cold water on her, and that she could not stand it. She could not be persuaded that her father was not in the house. After a few hours of excited and anxious screaming, she began to get out of bed, and slide round on the floor as if she were on skates, laughing and singing. When a physician was called, she said he was her father's brother, whom she had never seen. When a policeman called at the house, she thought he was her brother, who had been away three years, and she misidentified a neighbour woman as her step-mother's sister or her own mother's sister, she did not know which.

After a few days she had to be removed to the hospital, where at first she showed a typical elation, mischievous playfulness, and a noisy, restless excitement. She was over-talkative with a distinct flight of ideas. This excitement persisted for twelve days, and was at times seve e enough to demand treatment with packs. Then she became quieter in one of the abstracted periods, which were a peculiarity of her psychosis. In these she would at times seem quite natural, again look rather blank. Occasionally she would comment on things going on around her, or seem a little annoyed by sounds. She gave the impression of having great trouble in gathering her thoughts, looking abstracted, and sometimes made such a remark as " I can't say anything more. This is overtaxing my mind ". She spoke with a good deal of hesitancy, and sometimes closed her eyes. Frequently she would be speaking clearly enough, and then, apparently, become sidetracked and confused. For instance, after showing quite a clear orientation, she suddenly confused the hospital with places where she had worked, or, again, said, " I have been here all my life ". She tried to answer promptly, but seemed to have a tendency to block. All of this is highly suggestive of her mind be ng in that state, where free associational thinking is substituted for a normal control of the stream of thought. It is interesting that she could give a fair account of her past life until recent events were touched upon, when she became quite mixed up.

This condition lasted for about five months, although for the last month of this time there was some improvement. She might become quite violently excited with no apparent cause, and remain in this condition for a few hours or a few days, but, as a rule, she was in this more abstracted state. At times she could not be induced to speak at all, although this gave the impression of being a caprice. Again, she might be stimulated to a sentence or two of typical manic flight. The following is an example of such productions : (What's the matter ?) " Nothing," opening her eyes wide, " nothing. I have the measles. I got the measles." (Where ?) " I can't recollect, you ought to know more about it than I do." (Sick ?) " I have a toothache." (Anything else ?) " Hip disease, brain fever, meningitis, erysipelas." (What else ?) " Oh, I can't think—money in the bank—slippers (she kicks off slipper), if you want them you can have them." (What's the matter ?) Seeing a blue blotter, she says, " I am colour blind." (What else ?) " I am swallowing something, coke or something, I am a ' coke ' fiend, I am swallowing some now, this place is filled with ' coke '." She laughs. (Anything else been given to you ?) " I refuse to talk." (What else give you ?) " ' Coke ' and candy and everything nice." (Any one talking about you ?) " I don't know, and I don't care whether they are or not." Again, when asked the question, she says, " Can I pose instead of talking ? " Often there was a good deal of posing, grimacing, and turning her eyes about. She would apparently watch the stenographer, for instance, but not with a gaze of interest, because, when she looked in another direction, at the wall or door, she would have the same expression, as when looking in the direction of the stenographer. At times she would make believe to telephone to people, and might often answer other patients, who were talkative or noisy. Occasionally there seemed no doubt whatever that she answered hallucinated voices. As her psychosis progressed she became quite untidy and occasionally masturbated. It is striking, too, that in the periods of her greatest abstraction there was little evidence of any emotion whatever. Her mood of elation or whimsical mischievousness would come out when something attracted her attention. Recovery was gradual, in that she got more and more in contact with her environment, and her periods of excitement became less marked.

Naturally, in a case as inaccessible as this one was, it is impossible to study in any detail or any completeness the ideas in which the patient is absorbed. Nevertheless, from her scattered remarks, one discovers that the usual manic content was present. In the first place, of course, we note in the onset the delusion of her father's return to life, and probably closely related to her interest in her father was the idea of death. She spoke of this from time to time with apparent irrelevance. Once she remarked. " You need not try to bring me back to life ". Again, apropos of nothing, she said, " You are taking my strength away from me," which quite possibly is connected with her death fancy. On the other hand, evidence of adult sex interest was not lacking. She said once, " I think I am so beautiful no one is allowed to stare at me ". Quite frequently she spoke of " Eddie ". When one adds to this that her conduct in the presence of physicians was occasionally erotic, we see that the usual fundamental manic ideas were present. To what extent and in what direction they may have been elaborated internally, we can, of course, form no conjecture. It is important to note, however, that, when we eliminate from her productions purely superficial references to the environment, there is nothing left which does not fit in with the ideas just related.

The anomalies of orientation produced by distraction of thought are worthy of discussion. Naturally no one who gives all his attention to internal mental events is capable of noting and registering his environment. Consequently, in the gravest types of thought distraction, we meet with complete disorientation and complete amnesia for the period of the psychosis ; but many of these patients are capable of being roused from their dreams to take some cognizance of what goes on about them. These cases may give the impression of always being oriented, because they are capable of answering questions for such data, whenever they are put, but they are amnesic for a large part of their hospital residence, owing to the fact that, when not stimulated, they sink back into the world of fancy and hence do not register and retain the environmental data. Sometimes there is disorientation with amnesia for the environment but a memory of the autistic experiences. The patient Elizabeth K., whose history was described at some length above, as the first of the typical cases to be quoted, belongs to this group. It will be remembered that for most of her hospital stay she was quite confused, but had quite detailed memories of her imaginary experiences and of the distortions she made of the environment. The case of Ellen D., to be described immediately, is particularly interesting in this connection. Her psychoses were always characterized by a strong tendency to absorption with many hallucinations. It was almost always possible to attract her attention, and, when this was accomplished, she would usually give the date and place with accuracy and always knew the examiner was a physician. But, as such periods of clarity represented but a very short space of time, relative to the hours she spent communing with herself, it was not surprising to find that, on recovery, her memories of where she had been and of what had been happening were very vague.

She was a woman who had some eight attacks from the ages of 20 to 46 which were apparently all quite similar, being characterized by absorption with evidence of distractibility, bursts of elation, and often irritability in connection with specific topics. Only one attack—her seventh—will be described. They seem all to have been quite alike, and this happens to be the one in which her condition was most carefully noted. One of the most interesting features brought out in this attack was that she had a strong tendency to become absorbed when certain topics were mentioned.

CASE 34. *Ellen D.* was a single woman, age 45 at the time of this seventh attack. She is said to have had a happy disposition, and to have been enthusiastic in everything she did. On the other hand, she was inclined to worry over other people's difficulties and to take them on herself. She was bright in her school work, and later quite efficient as a stenographer. There were definite seclusive tendencies, however. She never cared to go out to parties, although she did like to entertain at home. She chose for her friends older people, and never cared much for the company of men. Her most constant companion and friend was her father, and it is important to note that she became violently antagonistic to him, with the onset of each of her mental attacks. Her previous psychoses, which were not well described, occurred, one in her teens, and then at the ages of 20, 28, 31, 35 and 40. All of these were, apparently, manic states, and she was sometimes quite violent ; but often there was an obtrusion of other emotional reactions, such as fear or depression. In all of them she seems to have become easily absorbed, and, on recovery from her seventh attack, she said that when ill she always hallucinated.

Her seventh attack began at 45 with apparent abruptness. In bed one night she had a severe attack of vomiting, was irritable, cross. Two days later she became destructive, tore up clothing, books, papers, threw things at people, spat in her father's face, and would have nothing to do with him. She complained that one of her sisters got everything and that she got nothing. She had an hallucination of her mother, and called out to her to come back.

On admission she was found to be rather thin and generally somewhat below par physically, but with no specific somatic ailments. There then followed a psychosis, which lasted for four months, in which her condition was usually as follows. When left to herself she was absorbed, would talk in a low tone to herself, occasionally saying something that was audible. Very frequently she would hallucinate in an obvious manner, and address imaginary companions. After her recovery she stated that she had been surrounded by many persons of ordinary appearance, but floating around her in the air, distracting and irritating her through their conversation. When examined her reactions varied. Occasionally something seemed to interest her, and she would show a mood of elation. When occupied with a definite task, such as fancy work, or making a calculation, she might appear rather normal. As a rule, however, she seemed to resent any interference and chafed under questioning. She frequently would put the examiner off with totally irrelevant remarks, often drawn from observation of her environment, in fact she was extremely distractible. Very frequently, too, she would dismiss the questions with some such statement as " I think of too much together to write it down," or other references to preoccupation with her thoughts. That the pressure of these thoughts was rather intense, like that of the ordinary manic case, was shown by the fact that she frequently would lie nearly all night long talking to herself in bed, apparently totally oblivious to her real environment, but surrounded by imaginary persons. Her orientation was usually surprisingly good, but this was evidently due to the capacity she had of being roused from her reveries. This was also shown by her ability to calculate accurately and fairly rapidly. During the calculation she might be distracted by a question which she would acknowledge briefly. She would finish her calculation, and then answer the question quite rationally, which showed that this stimulus—a professional activity—had roused her to a higher intellectual level. The same question put to her in her ordinary state would have to be repeated several times before she would make some such response as " What did you ask ? "

It was, of course, impossible to gain any complete idea of what her absorbing ideas were ; but, from her chance remarks, one can collect enough to see that her dominant topics were limited in number and were analogous to ideas such as we usually meet in manic states. In the first place, there were a good many remarks about her mother's marriage and her father's re-marriage, and about her mother's death. She insisted that she was the only one in the family who kept the latter's grave in repair. There were frequent references to death and to funerals. Retrospectively, she accounted for some of these by saying that she had attended the funeral of an old friend of her father, shortly before she was taken ill. Interest in adult outlets was shown in protestations of her stenographic ability, and in her interest in marriage. Once, when absorbed, she was questioned as to what she was thinking of and admitted that she was wishing she might become the bride of a man who had recently lost his wife. She had many remarks to make about marriage, mostly about people who were unhappily married. For instance, she professed much annoyance with the case of a Dr. C., whose marriage was unhappy because he had no children. There were not infrequently such remarks as " She killed her husband."

Complaints took up a large part of her attention. There were vague complaints of ill-treatment both at home and in the hospital. She railed against her poverty (without justification). One source of irritation recurred time and time again and this had to do with some families from Buffalo who visited annually at her home in New York. She explained once that these people had turned up immediately after her mother's death, camped on her family, and ate them out of house and home. When this subject came into her mind she almost always became abusive, apparently hallucinating the presence of some of these odious people, and would usually become absorbed.

It is important to note that this patient, who was never frankly and continuously elated, had other ideas than those which we have come to associate definitely with manic states. The topics which we have just outlined include typical manic ideas, it is true, but she was evidently obsessed with many thoughts that were painful and caused her a great deal of annoyance. Like the scolding manics, her ideas were not preponderately pleasant. The prominence of these other fancies are of theoretic importance, as we shall see when the relationship of these conditions with much distraction of thought to other types of manic-depressive reaction is considered.

In order to give a clear picture of the variations in her condition and their relationship to the thoughts that she expressed, we cannot do better than quote from the notes of one interview which took place some six weeks after her admission : " Her condition during the interview varied from a state in which she made pert remarks, very often inspired by the environment and somewhat flighty, to peculiar, absorbed states in which she sat, usually looking to the side, totally ignoring questions, shaking or nodding her head, muttering something at times. There seems very little question that these spells are apt to occur more when certain topics are approached. Once when another physician came in she was quite elated and made a number of flighty remarks. It was also noted that when she began to do some fancy work during the interview, she was more natural. As she came into the office, she said, shaking hands, ' I don't get any mail. My hand is cold. What do they say ? —a cold hand and a warm heart '. Then she spoke of the telephone which was ringing ; then of two people she saw outside, thus going from topic to topic and being distractable.   When a previous production is read to her, ' My godmother was not a witness to my mother's marriage ', etc., she gets quite irritated, says ' It is lies ', and becomes, for the first time, quite absorbed in the manner described above ; then breaks out, ' I don't like September first '. (Why not ?)   ' Because I don't like people to have their anniversaries on that day.   A young lady and a very young gentleman have birthdays on that day, and one person has a death on that date '.   Then she again gets absorbed, looks to the side, says ' Go to hell '.   (To whom did you say that ?)   ' The one who is to go to hell.   His grandfather was Peter.   He has a farm, an adjacent farm in Angola [this in very stilted tones], they had to have bonfires.   They didn't have the Maine smudge.   Do you know what the Maine smudge is ?   I have never been in Maine.   I have never been in Maine.   I've been in Saratoga, I've been in Canada, I've been in California, I have been to see the Brock's monument '.   Here she again got absorbed and when asked to tell what she was thinking about, said ' I hate people because they live on us '.   (Who ?) ' An ex-sheriff of Buffalo, Smith ;   he was born in Troy ;   he lived there with his trollops '.   (Who are they ?)   ' His wife and two daughters and the wife's sister.' "

The stimulus which led to this last absorption is interesting, there being quite evidently free associations leading to the dominant topic of the hated visitors.   These associations, as can be seen, were Maine, travelling in Maine, travelling to Saratoga, to Canada, to California, seeing Brock's monument. At this point she became absorbed.   Now Brock's monument is on the Niagara River, within the distance of an easy excursion from Buffalo.   Apparently, when she thought of Brock's monument, that brought up a memory of Buffalo and naturally of the odious Buffalo people.   At this point her attention was distracted from her environment to her dominating internal thoughts.

During the last month of her residence she gradually improved, finally recovering completely, as she had always done before.   Retrospectively she stated that her memories were hazy for about the first three months of her psychosis.   She remembered distinctly having had many hallucinations and knew that they distracted her attention.   She gave the impression of reticence when discussing her various productions that were retailed to her. Some of these she recalled, others she had forgotten.   It was difficult to make out whether her memory really failed for these ideas or whether it was too unpleasant a topic for her to discuss.

CHAPTER XXV

DISTRACTION OF THOUGHT AND ANOMALIES OF MANIC STATES.

IT is a commonplace of everyday life that our intellectual operations concerned with problems which interest us are more accurate and keen than is the operation of our minds when forced to attend to that which bores us. This is probably due to the greater concentration of attention that goes with greater interest. In spite of the simplicity of this principle, little use has been made of it practically in psychiatry, yet in some conditions it is apparently a psychological factor of primary importance. For example, it is not difficult to show that the deterioration of intelligence in epileptic dementia is rigidly correlated with a loss of interest[1]. The same principle is capable of explaining some of the anomalous features in many attacks.

As has been mentioned before, all manic cases show a certain intellectual defect, if it be only in that mild disorder of judgment which appears in those hypomanics who give undue credence to their fanciful schemes or theories. As we pass from one stage to another, we find in the more excitable cases evidence of disorientation, the genuineness of which is sometimes in doubt ; but, when we approach the cases that are deeply absorbed, there can be no question as to their total inability to judge of the nature of the environment, and even quite simple intellectual problems are plainly beyond them. These are the cases which show a marked thinking disorder, in fact, they seem to grade very insensibly into states, which, for the time being, seem almost identical clinically with deliria, and many of these cases, if seen only once, might be so diagnosed. They are completely out of contact with the environment, give nonsensical answers to questions, are incapable of performing such simple tasks as adding five and six together, and often seem to have their apprehension so disintegrated, that they cannot be roused at all, and are seemingly totally oblivious to their surroundings. Such cases are apt, like the delirious, to hallucinate freely and, as a rule, after recovery, are almost completely amnesic for the time when their abstraction was most profound. At most they recall fragments of their delusional experiences.

Two cases may be cited to illustrate this condition of profound thinking disorder.

[1] MacCurdy, " A Clinical Study of Epileptic Deterioration ", *Psychiatric Bulletin*, April, 1916.

CASE 35.—*Clara B.* was a single woman, age 21, a post office clerk, whose case was observed twenty-five years ago. A meagre anamnesis showed nothing of interest in her family history and stated that she had always been perfectly natural and capable. Six weeks before admission she was taken ill with what was called influenza. She had some fever and complained of much weakness. At the end of a week she had become a little excitable, laughed easily, and slept poorly, so that hypnotics were given her. At the end of another week she became talkative, with the items of her productions poorly connected. Then this talkativeness diminished, although she began to show more motor excitement, and, too, would repeat such irrelevant words as " Buster ", or " silver up." With this there was definite exhilaration and some evidence of mischievousness. She continued in this condition for three weeks, when her admission to the hospital was necessary.

Under Observation : For two days she showed considerable physical activity, jumping up and down in bed, moving furniture around, playing with her handkerchief. At the same time she talked a great deal in many independent sentences, which were separated by much laughter, by singing or by physical activity For example, she would say such things as " Are you going to shoot or fly, don't bother me. My goodness, is it right or not, shoo, shoo, shoo", etc. The next day she was quieter, remaining in bed, gesturing a good deal, frequently bursting out in laughter and again, as suddenly, crying. Contact with her environment seemed to be confined to speaking, when questions were asked, without much evidence of there being comprehension of the question. There was often some rhythm in her answers. For example, when asked what the place was, she said, " I will, I will once more, but if you wish I will." (Well, what place is it ?)—" Yes, I will once more say no." (Tell me where you are.)—" I will, I will, why I will once more, and if you are, I wish you once more where I am. I don't know, and if you know I wish you would." Again she might simply say, " Silver up and silver on, I will once more, I will once more, it is mine."

The following day she was more inactive physically, but talked almost continuously, as is illustrated by the following sample : " It's all right, it's no matter—Oh ! please don't ! Oh ! Dear ! I don't know, I said, that's all ! It's nothing more. Yes, I know it . . ." " It is not, that's all. Perhaps it is. That's enough—It is my last ! It's nothing, just the same, pass it on.— I should have said it might have been. It's all I wish, it's not too much. It's ever so much !—I will tell you nothing—Oh, yes ! certainly !! All right ! Let it pass ! Do you think as much as I do ? Too many for once ! Let her rip it up if she likes ! I have got enough for once. It's neither mine, it's neither hers ! If it's yours, pass it over. Very well. Rather countrified. Do you mistake this country evenings ? Foolish, isn't it ?—I will if you ask it ! I will any way, I don't care ! Don't say any more, that's enough ! It is not my way ! You know it too well !—There ! that's enough ! I don't care, do you ? Never mind. Now I go, don't I ?—I suppose so—that's nothing ! I am sure it isn't, we will fix it all right—Oh ! carry on ! I can't carry on, I'm sick (crying). I don't know, you know too well ! What do you think is the better man, I don't . . . Got your seat yet ? Never mind.—Supper up, down the hollow (singing). I don't know, do you think of Joe ?—Will you please pass me over or push me under ?—First one ! Present ? Yes, no ma'am—once I was, once I wasn't, if you wish it ! Don't care anything about it now."

There is a striking resemblance in the above productions to the snatches of conversation which one hears at some social gathering, where all the guests are talking at once in groups. This resemblance is probably not without significance. It suggests that many thoughts were racing through her mind and that some of them came to expression in words, which, apparently, had no relation to what she had said just before. Unfortunately no large collection of these utterances was made, or it might have been possible to discover certain dominant topics.

At the time when these productions were noted, she was lying in bed, moving her head from side to side, her eyes closed most of the time, and opened only when anyone entered, or when some noise attracted her attention momentarily. She could not be made to follow any commands, and most replies were completely irrelevant and stereotyped. Yet occasionally it seemed as if something of the sense of the question had perhaps, attracted her attention, as for example, when she was coaxed to tell the name of the place, she said, " Yes, I would if I were you, it is nothing more," etc.

This physical inactivity lasted for only five days, and then the appearance of dullness disappeared. She left her bed, and for two months was in the following condition : She would walk much about the ward with a good deal of gesturing, take other patients by the hand, make sweeping bows to them, sing and laugh a good deal, but all the time remained quite inaccessible to questioning and incomprehensible in her speech. There were variations in the latter. Sometimes she spoke little of her own accord, although she would always begin to talk when addressed. At other times it was difficult to get her to open her mouth at all. Her answers were nonsensical, and often seemed to indicate a disinclination to think, a desire to take the path of least resistance, although she was not externally distractible. Questions involving mental effort, such as demands for simple calculations, would often lead her to say " I don't know ". Again, she might, apparently, make an effort to think, but gave it up as impossible. This condition is best shown by transcription of an actual note.

When asked the day she said, " First time, one year ". (When did you come ?) " Thursday." (What month ?) " April " (correct). (What day in April ?) " First day." When asked who the nurse was she gave a wrong name, and then said, " It reminds me of my school days ". One physician she called " my cousin from New York," and again " a post-office inspector ". The other physician, " my cousin Charles ". When asked 7 from 100, she said " Nothing ". (9 x 8 ?) " That means to me study. For me it is a French word, I think ; or just nothing. French word, one." (5 x 7 ?) " 2, I should say 14." When asked to give the alphabet, she said " x, y, z," and when told to begin with a, b, c, she said " a, b, i, I be, is to you one French word" etc., and, when immediately after this, she was asked what she thought was the matter with her, she said " I should say French words ". Very striking was the fact that when asked how old she was, she said " 4—1—15— I cannot get my mind to you," and again, " I cannot th'nk ". It may be added that especially with calculation questions she really seemed to think, contracted her brow, but often ended up by saying, " I cannot think ".

Once during this period it was reported by a nurse that for one evening she brightened up, asked where she was, confessed to mental confusion, and said she must have been chloroformed. A month later she again cleared for a couple of hours, and was examined during the interval. She was very flighty, becoming more so during the interval. It was found that she was quite disoriented, could not say what she had done the day before, did not know how long she had been there, but knew in a vague way that she had seen the physician before.

Ten weeks after admission these clearer periods began to occur more frequently. In the first one, during which she was examined, she knew the name of the place, but could not tell how long she had been there. She said, when asked to describe the kind of a place it was, that it was " as near a gaol as anything else," and the people were " about as crazy as they could be," both of which statements indicated some grasp of the surroundings. She recognized the examiner as one whom she had seen before, and even recollected having seen him in the garden, but did not know his name. The name of another physician A she thought was either A or B. Her efforts with calculation were highly interesting. It was evident that she was capable of performing the simpler operations, but was unable to concentrate her attention sufficiently to make continuous effort, and to avoid this effort she would swing in a flighty way to a simpler problem : When asked to substract 7 from 100 she laughed boisterously, and said " 93 ". (8 x 5 ?) " 5 x 8 is 40, so I suppose 8 x 5 is 40, did you ever take ether ? " (laughing). When asked to substract 7 from 100 serially, she said " 93, 86, 75, no, it's hard to go by 7's and 9's ; 7 and 9 make 16 ".   Again, " 7 and 9 get me mixed up, 7 times 9 make 63, and 7 makes 70, that is 70% ".   It is not difficult to see that an extension of these mental processes, the nature of which is so transparent, would lead to the complete irrelevance which characterized her usual state of abstraction.

Most of these clearer periods lasted only for an hour or two.   In one of them she complained of her confusion, and in another stated that there was a constant succession of thoughts in her mind.   These two statements probably furnish an explanation for her whole condition.

After a month, during which these intervals of relative lucidity appeared, she began to improve steadily, and showed a decided tendency to occupy herself.   While still exhilarated and decidedly flighty in her conversation, she became fully oriented.   There then followed a few weeks, during which she was still exhilarated without definite flightiness, and then she returned to complete normality.   The entire psychosis lasted for six months.   Retrospectively she claimed to have no memory at all for her psychosis, except that there were very vague memories of the time when she was still at home. She could recall a little also of the periods when she was clearer.   For the first four months of her psychosis she thought that she was in a gaol, otherwise she had no memory at all for internal or external events.

Physically there was nothing to suggest that she was in a toxic state.   She had from the time of her admission, a normal pulse, respiration and temperature.   She had lost some weight and slept little, so it was not surprising that her weight, until she began to improve, was ten or fifteen pounds below normal.   Slight paleness and a coated tongue, with this loss of weight, were the only evidence of any physical disturbance whatever, so we are probably safe in assuming that this was a psychogenic and not a toxic psychosis.

The next case is that of a man who went through four phases in his attack.   In the first he seemed typically manic, talking much nonsense which was probably an echo of his engrossing ideas.   In the second stage he was silent with manic behaviour, a good deal of grimacing and, not infrequently, smearing[1].   In the third stage he was languid with manic behaviour in bursts.   Finally he expressed an interest in his environment, recovered quickly and fully with an almost complete amnesia for his psychosis.   During the second and third phases there was a marked thinking disorder.

CASE 36.   *Frank S.*, whose case was observed twenty-five years ago, was a married physician, age 30.   He is said to have been normal, his disposition naturally bright and full of fun.   Up to five years before his mental attack he had been physically well, but at this time he developed signs of incipient pulmonary tuberculosis, and was ordered away from his practice for a year. On his return he had gained forty pounds, and was pronounced entirely recovered by a competent internist.   Following that he did well in active practice.

Six weeks before admission he went to a military camp to act as physician, and, on his return, it was noted that he had become unusually loquacious. Moreover, he attracted attention at home by making the servants greet him with military salutes.   In spite of his volubility, however, his talk was rational, he did not lose the thread of it, and admitted himself that he was thinking aloud.   He appreciated his condition to the extent that he asked a colleague to treat him for nervousness.   After four or five days he became extremely active, sent many telephone messages, and was unnecessarily busy.   This over-activity increased until two weeks before admission, when his actions

[1] See glossary.

became quite abnormal. He bought some property, and made plans for a house with a hospital attachment, even going so far as to buy tools for the building and wall paper for the house. He conferred busily with lawyers and architects. At the same time he became over-active in regard to a corporation of which he was a member, wrote many letters, had circulars printed, and once even went so far as to wake his wife in the middle of the night to dictate to her. Not unnaturally he neglected his patients. Finally he became so disturbed that commitment was necessary. In all this we see a typical manic case, with an absorption in normal activities which became abnormal, when he lost his sense of the relative importance of his interests, and expansiveness and undue optimism appeared.

On admission his physical condition was found to be excellent. Mentally he exhibited the symptoms of a typical manic state with much talking, gesticulation, whistling and laughing. At times he shouted loudly. His talk was distinctly flighty, but it was possible to break into it at times and force a relevant answer ; but even then he would switch off immediately into flighty productions. He was oriented for place, but could give neither the month nor the day. His talk may be illustrated by the following . . . " Are you in private or official business ? I will use the Grand Seal of Massachusetts. Those may be exaltations. It is none of your business, and I am too ready to go, and you two boys better hurry up. There is some man pacing the corridor now. If you can remember how I found that out, go ahead and do it. I am a visitor in this hospital, locked up, and they will hold a consultation, but I will not hold you responsible for any package left in your care, and they won't find it because I don't know where it is myself. What is your hand in that pocket for ? [to the nurse]. They have it at the other end now. Connections are good when you once put out your feet, and I'll give you all of the tests, the mirror test is the best . . . You make every one of your changes too prominent, I'll sit up here and tire them out, because I am not talking rationally. Now they have got me on my cranky subject, and I'll stop." Unfortunately sufficient of the productions were not recorded to enable me to discriminate between that which is purely superficial and what came as an expression of his inner thoughts. It may be noted, however, that a flavour of expansiveness runs through these utterances, and there are references suggesting a delusion of some government connections or of official importance.

After two days his physical activity began to diminish slightly, and at the same time it was possible to interrupt his talk. This, however, had become even more irrelevant. For instance, when asked when he had seen the physician before, he said, " Yes, Sir, in disguise," and to a repetition of the question, replied " Northeast, southwest, no I have not, Sir ". Both of these statements suggest an irrelevance produced by the intrusion of dominating ideas. References to points of the compass were very frequent in his productions. When asked, " Did you see any doctors yesterday ? " he answered, " I was left uncovered in Boston," and then went on, " I raise it by twos and square it by twos. They are going to be packed into that hole. I am working on the full tension to please you ". When told that he knew more than his answers would indicate he said, " I have an anthropomorphitic brain. I am run between two and three ".

Four days later it was noted that he was still quieter, talking less, but chanting and whistling more. His tendency to gesticulate was more marked. At times he would have quiet intervals, then began to whistle, sing, or make comical grimaces and cock his eyes. Simple questions which involved no thinking were answered promptly and correctly ; others in an absurd manner, occasionally as a result of distractibility.

A note made two weeks later shows that he was much quieter but with the same tendency to mischievousness and other manic behaviour. His talk was interrupted by many pauses and was so slow that the greater part of it could be taken down in longhand. His intellectual state is evident from the following productions : He was asked what month it was and replied, " It looks like an autumn month ", seeing the dry leaves outside. (What month ?) " August, September, October 13 would be the date [October 7]. August 3 to the 9 was when I was in camp and when the breakdown came. *The various sounds that distract me and those which I have said and done* ; and this centre in the signs of the red Indian . . . [pause], east, west, north, south, uniting finally and the various ages coming together, and it must be of such an order that the entomologists and others would rather go to the south antipodal regions, and once I was sent to the south because . . [pause]—*I don't know what I am talking about I am blurred* [pause]. Yes, I spoke about oval and ovoid shape, which a certain bicycle track takes in those things, which centre about honour ", etc.

Two things are of interest in these productions. First, there is evidence of dominant ideas in his reference to points of the compass, scientific matters and wheels ; secondly, he interprets his own mental state in the statements which are italicized. The first of these is particularly interesting, as he evidently refers to distraction of his thoughts, both by internal and external events.

During the next three weeks his tendency to inactivity increased, so that he became rather chronically silent, so far as speech was concerned, although his exhilarated mood was obvious and an inner restlessness was manifested by much grimacing, laughter, whistling, and such acts as picking up paper and buttons and stuffing his pockets full of them or chewing them. In eating he was slow and mixed his food up. When left alone in his room he was apt to smear his faeces about. Mischievousness was frequent. For example, he was once found carefully scrutinizing another patient's head and acted like a monkey picking fleas. During an examination when he did not answer any questions, there was nevertheless behaviour which suggested a primitive type of contact with his environment. It seemed as if he were substituting actions for speech, in other words using what might be called a sign language. For instance, immediately on seeing the physicians enter the ward he came to them, pointed his fingers at them, made faces and took hold of their hands. When put in a chair, he sat there and continued to whistle as he had been doing, but made all sorts of grimaces and moved his hands almost continually. These motions were quite multiform in character : he would point from one to the other of the physicians, take hold of them, pick up his chair and turn it around, pull his shirt over his head and move his head about in it very quickly. He was attracted by the buttons on the physician's coat, then fumbled with the buttons on his own, pulling off one and placing it in his mouth and biting it to pieces. When the physician snapped his fingers, he did the same. When a large circle was made in the air before him, he quickly made a small circle on the physician's knee, and then immediately continued with his own motions. When, among other things, he was told that he was a doctor, he responded by immediately feeling the physician's pulse.

This condition endured for about a month. Then it was noted that the multiformity of his movements was less, although he still had a twinkle in his eye and twisted and turned his body in a comical manner. Although usually silent, he would at times answer questions, which answers seemed to be mischievously irrelevant, but closer study showed to be the result of a grave thinking disorder.

For the next three months his condition remained practically the same, although his inactivity began to assume an appearance of languidness, and he would sit for an hour in a chair absolutely unoccupied, or would walk about without associating with others. When he did speak, he affected a comical drawl and always had a twinkle in his eye. His capacity for thinking in this stage is represented by the following note : He was asked how long it had been since he was engaged in practice and answered as follows : " How long since I was in practice ? Well, I went into practice some other time ago, I—I forget." (How long have you been in practice ?)—" I have been in practice for—er—for—er—for er—for er." (Where do you live ?)—" Why I live—in er—in—er —Jerusalem." He was unable to give the symptoms of typhoid fever. When asked the dose of strychnia, he said, " Strychnia—strychnia is a hundred—

strychnia strychnia is a hundred sixtieth of a grain." (What is the dose of morphia ?—" One dose of morphia is—well I don't know—it makes a difference whether morphia—or—murphia—or—what is my name ? " (What is morphia the alkaloid of ?—" Of opium." (9x3 ?—" 9 times 3 are 27." (7x 8 ?)—" 7 x 8 are 92." (9 x 8 ?)..." 9 x 8 are 92." (5 x 6 ?)—" 5 x 6 is 30." (100—7 ?)—" 92, 93, 93."

With this increasing inactivity he steadily put on more weight.

The languid stage lasted for about three months. It seemed as if, during it all, he had so little interest in the outside world that there was no desire even for physical activity. He always had to be compelled to get out of bed, but would then dress himself, which he did very slowly. He ate well but for quite awhile had to be led into the dining room. When he undressed he was apt to put his collar button into his mouth and then swallow it which shows the degree of his absent-mindedness. At times he would whistle or might knock a table over, occasionally, he would walk slowly up the ward. As a rule, he would be found stretched out in a chair looking lazily out of the window, answering questions with great carelessness, and frequently yawning. While in this state at one examination, although still much mixed up and apparently indifferent, his answers to some questions exhibited some trace of new life. For instance, when asked if he did not want to go home, he said, " Well, it gets monotonous walking around here all the time." When asked the usual orientation questions, he answered most of them with stereotyped " Can't tell you ", but mentioned the name of the hospital and the year, interspersed with wrong answers, so that it seemed as if the necessary information was in his mind, but that he could not, or would not, concentrate sufficiently to make himself actually conscious of his environment. His awakening interest was shown by his spontaneously remarking, " You ask me the same quesions every time." When he made this statement the physician asked him, " Why do I ask you these questions ? " and he replied, " I have my ideas, I'll keep them to myself, I don't tell all I know." When pressed further to say why he did not answer better, he remarked " Often times I don't care to answer ", and when catechized as to the month, he answered with a little irritation, " I don't know, I never hear the mouth spoken of about here. When I say I don't know, why don't you believe me ? My word has always been taken before." All of this is strongly suggestive of a reawakening, and it is also interesting in that it gives some indication of what his mental state was. It shows that his mind was not such a blank as it appeared to be, and that lack of interest was responsible for his poor orientation. It is not surprising that at this interview he did simple multiplications promptly, and was able to subtract 7 from 100 serially with one mistake in 65 seconds, and immediately afterward, without a mistake in 130 seconds. This was by far the best performance that he had made so far.

Two days later he suddenly asked for a newspaper, and a little later for a book to read. He then began to ask many questions about the hospital, spoke of some of the incidents which he remembered and also of his first night and asked whether he had not been brought to the State House before he was taken to the hospital. It was later found that this idea was a misinterpretation of the Administration Building of the hospital. Two days after this he was given a careful examination and found to be perfectly well. He said that the whole time up to two weeks before was almost a blank to him, because, although he could remember many incidents, there was no connection between any of them. It is noteworthy that he recalled some of the examinations when he had made such a poor performance, and assured the physician that he really could not have given better answers and that the calculation tests were really difficult.

To recapitulate : we may say that the interesting features of this case were that he began as a typical manic, and then became gradually more and more abstracted ; that this abstraction was correlated with a profound thinking disorder and a concomitant retardation of activity both in speech and in movement. Further, he made a number of remarks which showed that his mind was inactive only in so far as its operations could become externally manifest. His attitude was one of indifference because his interest was being put on internal mental events.

That excitement, both physical and mental, marked emotionality and the apparently opposite tendencies to inactivity and absorption, are all part of the manic picture, is best shown by studying those cases where transitions from one state to another are observed. Superficially, one would certainly think that a hilarious manic state was an entirely different psychosis from that of the patient who remains rather consistently unoccupied, says very little, and seems very stupid ; but, when one of these conditions merges over into the other by easy gradations, and, when one can see that the same fundamental factors may produce the two conditions, their basic unity becomes apparent. The possibility of transitions from one of these states to another has not remained unnoted, for Kraepelin says that " unproductive manics " tend to become more excited and productive if placed in an exciting environment. We would say of such cases that interest, which had been placed on internal events, is in part turned to the environment, which is more stimulating, and that so soon as attention is given to the environment, contact is established with it by speech and movement.

A change of attention from external to internal pre-occupation is not merely accompanied by alteration in intellectual capacity. Mood changes are always present. The most prominent of these is subsidence of elation and of the behaviouristic symptoms, which we associate with exhilaration. As patients become more absorbed, the exuberance of their joy diminishes. They become less active, less mischievous, make fewer jokes, and so on. All these tendencies seem, then, to be exhibited much more in little spurts than continuously, but this is not the only mood change which may be observed. As has been stated many times, the franker, more productive manics have ideas which, by their nature, imply a contact with the environment and grant a free and pleasurable outlet to fancy. With increased introversion the ideas are less objectivated and, consequently, approach more nearly the type of primitive unconscious fancies divorced from reality and therefore productive of neither activity nor elation. These thoughts seem to flow in continuous free associations. Now in free associations we find, as a rule, a dominant latent content which is being expressed in different conscious formulations. The nearer the free associations are to the original unconscious theme, the greater is the likelihood of their being presented in unpleasant forms. Hence we observe sporadic outbursts of anxiety, evidences of depression, or, if the patient tries to examine his own mental processes, perplexity.

The following examples will demonstrate these transitions in the objective conditions of manic patients, associated with changes in the degree of preoccupation and in the type of content.

The patient, Alfred J., whose case will be given in greater detail a little later in reviewing this part of our subject, was a cyclic case, whose clinical condition varied directly with the degree to which his attention was given to his ideas. In his exhilarated phases he was only hypomanic, but even then his obvious symptoms appeared and disappeared according to this principle. This was objectively noted and later confirmed by the patient, a man of excellent education and an accurate introspectionist, who gave a long and highly interesting account of his psychotic career.

His ambitions ran along academic lines, and, when events suggested a recognition of his ability with consequent academic advancement, he would become hypomanic with exaggerated ideas of his capacity, achievements and prospects. For instance, he would regard himself as the coming president of Harvard University, the adviser of kings, and so on. While in the hospital, he one day got himself quite worked up in conversation with a nurse, whom he promised to send to college, and otherwise patronize. An hour later the patient said, " I wish that man hadn't come in. Then I would not have talked all that nonsense for half-an-hour. I thought it was all right when I spoke, but I know now that it was all nonsense." In these phases of greater excitement he would become so voluble as to be distinctly flighty, become physically overactive, and at the same time have a firm belief that his boasts were fully justified in fact. When questioned about this, he claimed that he was always able to gauge the intensity of his psychotic condition by the way in which he adhered to or relinquished the exaggerated ideas of his own importance. But his ideas were not limited to egotistic trends, for he stated that, when exalted, he always felt a great hate for his father, although, when normal, he had a reasonable view of his relations with him. This shows how preoccupation with psychotic ideas leads to the release of the more deep-lying unconscious tendencies.

This case was particularly interesting inasmuch as it was possible experimentally to verify the principle under discussion. When he was apparently quite normal, one could produce all the symptoms of a hypomanic state merely by getting him to discuss his prospects. The change was not merely in the production of symptoms of excitement, for such profound alteration in his judgment was induced, that he would quickly give himself over to ideas sufficiently divorced from the truth to be called genuine delusions. And all this would disappear again when he was left to himself.

The case of Robert S., which has been described above gives a number of pretty examples of this tendency. When quite flighty, and incapable of reacting normally to his environment, he could still give a perfectly clear connected account of incidents in his past life, which had impressed themselves on him. For instance, he was asked to describe a " cane rush " which he had witnessed in Boston, and produced a clear account of about three hundred words. This was a topic which turned his attention from autistic ideas to something of objective reality. On another occasion, while quite flighty, he gave a delusional story of a conversation with his dead father and of seeing him sitting on a white throne. When questioned about this, however, he was roused from this dreamy state and the delusion faded somewhat, for he said that he could communicate with his father only by prayer and that he could see him when he closed his eyes. During that same interview, while his talk was disconnected and flighty, his stream of thought led to his business troubles. He began to cry and gave a long coherent account of his difficulties. This again was a topic of objective reality and is, further, an interesting example of the change in mood brought about by the emergence of an unpleasant thought in the course of his free associations. Later this patient became quite absorbed, so that his intellectual processes deteriorated and his utterances seemed haphazard. In this state, when general distraction of thought was obvious, he gave voice to an isolated, definite homosexual delusion of being married to one of the physicians at the hospital. This again shows the tendency of cruder unconscious fancies to come to expression, when there is marked preoccupation with psychotic ideas, rather than with environmental reality.

In the case of Elizabeth K., whose history was cited as the first of our typical manic cases, an exquisite example of a sudden change in the clinical picture has already been described. It will be recalled that this patient immediately on entrance to the hospital became quite absorbed and apparently lost all contact with her surroundings. Prominent among the ideas which dominated her attention were thoughts of death that were not formulated in any unpleasant way. The third night after her admission, however, there was a sudden episode, when these death ideas took the form of a descent to the infernal regions. This episode is best described in terms of the note made at the time : " In the midst of her excitement she seemed frightened, screamed loudly, saying, ' Look at the picture on the wall. See it move. Now look, it's going around the room. Oh, *I am so frightened. I am going down, down through the earth. See, I'm sinking.* Look at that imp coming out of my closet. Look at him. Why am I alone here ? No light, all dark.' Then she threw herself on her knees and said, ' *O, my God, what have I done that I should suffer so ?* Where is my Red Cross nurse ? Oh, they have left me alone in this cell. Won't someone come to me ? ' When the nurse went in, the patient calmed down and asked her if she thought she had had delusions or was it real ? Later she slept, and on awaking began singing and pounding as usual." There are two striking features to be noted here. In the first place her manic excitement changed to typical distressed anxiety, when her idea of death appeared in this painful form ; and, secondly, she became partially oriented for the time being. Not only did she realize her environment to the extent of knowing that she had a nurse, but she also gained slight insight, as shown by her question as to whether

her experience was a delusion or real. One is struck here by the close analogy to a dream, where the appearance of a terrifying experience may cause an awakening and a return to contact with reality.

The reader will recall that this patient showed throughout her attack the symptoms which we have described of distraction of thought. Her recovery gives an exquisite example of the transition which we are now discussing. In her psychotic experiences she went through various phases in which the world was destroyed and finally was to begin over again with her. This last formulation tended to direct her attention to the outside world. A confused idea that she was in a hospital appeared and she tore up the sheets to make bandages. Finally something in the environment established contact between the inner and the outer world. The guard on the window looked to her eye like a cross. This directed her thoughts to religion and, rather abruptly, she became well with excellent insight.

The case of Frank C., which also has been described, shows again the influence of a dominant topic on the picture of the psychosis. Usually quite confused, he was able to answer questions quite clearly, when they referred to anything which happened before his illness, or to something with which he was quite familiar. For instance, he was able to give an excellent account of a trip abroad with much detail and no flightiness or rambling. Once, however, after giving such an account, he was immediately asked how long ago his mother had been to see him. This evidently distracted his attention to his more psychotic thoughts—the ideas of unconscious origin—for he at once became confused, said he could not tell, and added, "There are a lot of things you notice and again things you don't—I really don't know. I start to say something and I don't know what to say. I am muddled. One thing leads to another. I don't know what to say."

Isabel U., whose tendency to become blocked and to change from normal to free associational thinking, has been described, could give a fair account of her past life until recent events were touched upon, when she would become confused. These events had stimulated psychotic reactions, so, naturally enough, both reality and fantasy were recalled together and the latter led to further ruminations of an antistic order. Absorption in these produced an interference with her intellectual operations.

The case of Ellen D. furnishes some beautiful examples of this principle. After recovery she stated that she had been distracted by hallucinations of people floating around her in the air and talking. Definite tasks, such as fancy work or making a calculation, might produce an appearance of normality. It was particularly interesting that when roused by a stimulus of her professional activity—calculation—she would be able to answer questions quite rationally, that, in her usual state, would have to be repeated many times before her attention could be gained—and even then could not be answered.

T

A description has been given of how certain topics would tend to produce absorbed spells and in one example the mechanism was transparently that of a free associational process.

To demonstrate these transitions we have so far given examples of temporary changes in the condition of our manic patients, which have been correlated with an increase, or diminution, of the introspective tendency. The next case shows this same principle marking off long-continued stages in a manic attack. The patient went through various phases which lasted weeks or months : first, of a mild hypomanic state, where there were no delusional ideas but a preoccupation in various activities, that could be correlated with the later developing delusions ; next, there was a period of restrained elation and other hypomanic symptoms occurring with fairly well-adapted ideas ; thirdly, the excitement increased as the ideas became less adaptive ; and, finally, there was a very marked excitement coincident with wild religious and erotic ideas.

CASE 37. *Ruth C.*—The patient was a married woman 33 years old when her case was observed twenty-five years ago. Her mother had an attack of melancholia at the menopause. Her father was a spiritualist. Otherwise there was no evidence of abnormality in the family history. She was said to have been a normal child of an open make-up and received a collegiate education. She was married at 25, but had no children, which caused her considerable sorrow. The same year she was married, she had a fall from a horse which resulted in uterine displacement. For this there was an operation and at the same time an ovarian tumour was discovered, which was removed, the other ovary being left in place. Later, another operation was necessary to correct a hernia. At 27 she had another fall, which is said to have been followed by a renewed uterine displacement. Again there was an operation. There is no account of any mental trouble in connection with these operations, but that there should have been recourse to surgical treatment a third time suggests the possibility of hypochondria.

Fourteen months before admission the patient became depressed with considerable loss of energy, sadness and crying. She remained in this state for four months ; no special false ideas were reported. From then on she seems to have been in a cyclic state. This depression was followed by an elation of six months duration which was at first moderate. While visiting at her father-in-law's house she lost her rings and got quite excited and headstrong in prosecuting a search for them. She was sent to her mother's and there became stirred up about her brother being out late at night. Five months before admission, depression set in again and this state continued for three months after coming under observation, constituting an attack of eight months in all.

This second depression was characterized by a feeling of inadequacy, lack of energy and some distress over her loss of affection, of feeling, and of interest in anything. During the latter months she was obsessed with thoughts of suicide. She later said that she could think of nothing else than that she was " too wicked to live and afraid to die." Several times she was quite excited by the idea that she had poisoned herself, although on each occasion it was found that her belief was really delusional. All of this suggests that, throughout this depression, ideas of death were in the foreground. When we recall what we have learned from studying stupors, namely, that death represents, psychologically, a regression of which loss of feeling and interest may be but partial stages, we can see that the death ideas probably contributed in large measure to the psychosis. Unfortunately this highly interesting case was observed at a time when no effort was made to establish psychological connections between different psychotic stages in a patient's career. It is possible that if efforts along this line had been made, definite evidence would have been secured of the depression changing into an elation with the metamorphosis of this death idea. We know at least that she later developed religious ideas, which in many patients appear as a sequel to delusions of death. For lack of proof this must remain merely a conjecture in this case.

At any rate her depression slowly lifted and for three weeks the onset of a manic phase was shown by a gradual increase of activity and of cheerfulness. Then she began to complain of the food and insisted upon cheering the other patients up. She grew so insistent that she was daily threatening to report alleged irregularities in the hospital to the superintendent. Considered by themselves these complaints and her ambition to cheer the other patients would mean little, but in the light of subsequent ideas it becomes plain that they represented an increased idea of her own importance (food was not good enough for *her*) and the beginning of the belief in her having a special mission to perform. When examined at this time she was euphoric and voluble, insisting on giving the physician a detailed account of her case ; in other words, she presented the picture of a very mild hypomanic condition.

The next five weeks saw the development of another phase. During two weeks her excitement gradually increased until she began to protest that she would reform the hospital, and assumed command of all the nurses in her ward. She was by this time so disturbed that she had to be removed to a ward designed for the care of more unruly cases, which transfer she interpreted as an evidence of her influence over the hospital superintendent. Coincidentally she became quite flighty in her talk, with an open elation and a tendency to such excitement that it was difficult to manage her. Her plans were becoming more definite, her conceit more inflated. She wrote poetry, began to compare herself with Goethe and Dante, who had done their best work at her age. She talked much of the nature of the reforms which she would inaugurate. She was going to see the trustees of the hospital, raise $2,000,000 for the physical improvement of the institution and take charge of it herself. It is interesting to note, before we proceed further, that her ideas, so far, represent merely exaggerations of what might be quite normal interests or ambitions. A desire to cheer her fellow patients is certainly a commendable idea, so is the wish to reform the hospital, provided the need for a reform existed. She begins, of course, to be definitely psychotic at the point where she is convinced of this need and it is just here that her euphoria and volubility appear. As the more reckless ideas of raising $2,000,000 and of taking charge of the hospital herself, came to expression, her excitement increased, but still it was well within the limits of what we would term hypomania.

Almost at once she passed over into a more definitely manic state which lasted for a week, in which she was typically flighty, although she was able in spite of her constant wanderings from the subject to return to her main topics. Physically, she was constantly active, moving things about, walking about the room, and all the time talking incessantly. This increase of excitement was correlated definitely with a change in her ideas. The notion of reforming the hospital developed into a ridiculously expansive idea. A greater conception came to her. Not only should the institution be a great hospital for people tired nervously, but she would found a great city, on the hill where the hospital was, and there all people interested in the welfare of humanity could come. It was to be a very great and wonderful city and be called the " New Philadelphia " or " The City of Brotherly Love." Just in proportion as her ideas lost contact with reality, in the same degree did her unconscious fancies come nearer to conscious expression. After announcing this new city she began to read her Bible and soon stated that she was the Christ. It was the second coming and the end of the world was close at hand.

A certain contact with her environment was, however, evidenced in an attempt to adapt these ideas to her surroundings. The Bible said that the temple was to be upon a hill, so she discovered that this was the hill where the great temple was to be erected. Similarly she went back over the story of Christ and His earthly doings, and tried to pick out people about her who corresponded to His contemporaries. Thus she identified the different doctors as Herod, Paul, St. John, Barabbas, and so on. Certain nurses against whom she felt bitter she dubbed the five foolish virgins. To identify herself further with Christ, she said that on a Friday she would be crucified, not as Christ had been, but in some new way. Her soul would leave her body and journey three days with the souls of all the great religious teachers, and on Sunday there would be a great transformation on the hill. Her soul would come back and wise men would come, attracted by spiritual forces. Chief among these she named three noted philosophers of Harvard. A less adaptive idea was that Christ's life and death had been an expression of paternal love and that she would represent the maternal. This came to her as a vision to her soul and heart, but not to her eyes. Some months before she had been unconsciously affected by one of the physicians, while more recently her husband, by means of a " spiritual communication " or an " unconscious cerebration ", said to her the time had come for an expression of maternal love. Later in this week she announced that she was about to give birth to Christ. She meant this literally and wrote a letter to one of the physicians inviting him to witness the event. On the other hand, she attempted to make these religious fancies fit in with her environment by writing to a certain clergyman, whose name appeared a great deal in her productions, demanding that he come to the hospital to preach. She said, too, that her poems would be published and the proceeds devoted to the buying of pictures and books for the hospital.

Sexual ideas were suggested not merely in her claim of personifying maternal love. Similarly tendencies were concealed in various schemes for determining affiinities, at which she worked at times quite busily. She would make charts, connecting different dots by lines, and saying that the whole scheme could be worked out mathematically. Again, she would put down the names of men and women whom she knew in two columns, and connecting them by lines and numbers would demonstrate these to have natural affinity. The inspiration for these schemes she claimed to have derived from spirits, yet in her description of the communications it appeared that she did not actually hallucinate (this came later). She felt a pressure in her head as if the spirits were forcing an impression upon her brain, and, when the conception suddenly became clear, the pressure would depart, and with it, she presumed, the spirits left. Further, she said that she had heard noises in the bathroom, and, when she had gone to look, had found no one there. This she interpreted again as the work of the spirits. The definite relationship between absorption in these more riotous fancies and her flight were betrayed by her own statement. When referring to a letter she had written, she said that the thoughts came so fast that she could not put them down, and added, " I go like a sewing-machine ". It is important to note, as an example of the wavering of attention between reality and her autistic thoughts, that she frequently referred to her ideas as symbolical. Thus she said that she suffered, as Christ did, because of her thoughts, and went through the " hell " of her depression. Then came the " resurrection," by which she meant that the doctors and nurses whom she loved put sunlight into her soul. The rising of the sun was a promise that the soul should rise, and so on. At other times however, her ideas seemed to have a literal meaning to her.

The next phase of her psychosis lasted, with some variations, for about nine months. During this period there were displayed all the symptoms, which we have come to regard as evidence of internal distraction of thought. Hallucinations were frequent, if not more or less constant, while she seemed to be living continuously in a world of delusion. Because her attention was removed from the environment, so that she lost interest in making herself understood, her delusions seemed more confused than heretofore. It was possible as a rule to see that all her conduct was determined by her false ideas, and it varied constantly with the changes in her imaginations.

At first a violent excitement was present. She would screech at the top of her lungs, while keeping up a constant flow of talk, dance, sing, pound the walls, beat her arms to her side, or attack the nurses savagely, saying she must kill their bodies to save their souls. Often she would stand in the middle of the room, stretching her arms out towards the electric light, and staring fixedly at it for long periods, claiming that it was the middle of the universe. With this marked excitement there was very little laughter and no distinct exhilaration. It was much more a condition of strong, pure excitement. A little later she would become so absorbed in her ideas that her activity was reduced, and also the volume of her speech. She might even talk quite deliberately. At such times she appeared dull, yet to have a decided exhilaration, and, in these periods, she seemed to have little grasp of her environment. Not infrequently, when her ideas assumed anxious or depressive colouring, she would react with anxiety or tears. Some times she might whistle all night, which she explained as the method of protecting herself from mutilation at the hands of the Turks. When quieter she occasionally seemed silly, and undoubtedly there were many times that she was thought to be demented. As time went on, her conduct became still more unreasonable, as she would not keep on any clothes, and very frequently would smear food and faeces about. Toward the end of this nine months she often posed and decorated herself with leaves and flowers, or covered herself up with blankets. In spite of this tendency to decorate herself however, she could not be persuaded to wear ordinary clothes, although she would usually keep on a linen gown. Even this she would often tear, and was constantly exposing herself, showing no modesty whatever. In general, then, we may say that her conduct varied a great deal, as did her productivity ; that all her actions, practically, were abnormal, because she reacted to constantly shifting thoughts, all of which were psychotic. In spite of her variations, however, the most constant mood was that of exhilaration, or, perhaps we should more accurately say, the most constant thing was a marked emotionality.

There were, of course, corresponding changes in her intellectual functions. With the onset of this more " distracted " phase, her talk became very much more flighty, more difficult to follow, and strung together more by internal than external associations. Comments on the environment were made but rarely. The following sample will show typical productions of this period :

" They are trying to make me believe by suggestion that what I say to you is not right. I must keep the maternity instinct in me—I heard birds singing last night in a pure atmosphere—They cannot control my mind like father. F—F is father ; all is nothing ; life is all ; everything is wrong ; there are no children in the world ; there are no flowers like Plato tells of ; there are no colleges ; no men, no women ; so investigate, go on to new science. Find other men and women and make them hear. They tell me a war is going on outside, war between Ham and Shem. I never heard anything like it. I have never read a paper. The beginning is the end. The outside is the inside. No one can teach me love, because I am a biological affinity. I may be the one but I may not be. The natural end is to produce many children. They tell us they go by twos and produce eights. [She dances up and down now, slapping her sides violently]. I am going to be an old woman. I am going to see my grandmother. Oh Lord I have found maternity and I disappeared from the world. That letter writing was in a later world, and when I came here I found a baby [at this point she turns her head around and shrieks angrily as to a voice]. Stop your influence ! You are my son ! You are beneath my feet ! Herod, you cannot conceive yourself. Herod, you are the end, the A B and you've crossed the F and P and the L and the M ! Investigate science, investigate the law ! Read Plato ! We all have soul tragedies. We come at three months when the men defile us, and we leave at seven months. They defile the body which was meant to be something holy. I say it was a man. The women are men, men produced by the five heads of the church," etc.

When quieter and apparently more absorbed in her ideas, there appeared idle repetitions, purely superficial in character, which seemed to satisfy the desire to talk without the expenditure of any intellectual effort. At the same time the internal connections preponderated to such an extent that the conceptual connections could only be determined by studious analysis of all her ideas. The following is an example : (Who is this ?) (A nurse) " She is the daughter of would-be mother of Peter the Great, who never was Peter the Great, never is Peter the Great, never shall be Peter the Great, until he becomes Peter the Small, Peter the Little, typefying the truth of first the soul, then the birth of love—the telegraph is giving and carrying a message just around here as fast as it can go, but I like it, I love it—my head will be too big, it will hold the earth " (laughs). (Peter the Great may have been suggested by the somewhat Slavish look of the nurse). " Does the gentleman whom you work for, whom I work for, ever allow his patients, who are patients, who become patients, the father and the children of that doctor of law—no, no, of the heaven of law and then of love, who going backward knew absolutely nothing of the things of soul, which typefy the things of the truth going around my brain which circle in the universe, surrounds as soul every other small soul [laughs] like it, it is lovely to be telegraphed. That man will have to take me or he will have to get off the earth."

As she began to improve, and get more in contact with her environment, her talk was sometimes quite clear, but during an interview when vexed or excited by talking about her ideas, she would again become very flighty.

On account of the constant variations in her condition, her orientation was changing all the time. As a rule she seemed to recognize the nature of her environment in a partial way, for she would usually address the physician as doctor, and often spoke of the institution as a hospital. She would even know the names of the physicians and nurses, but at the same interview would insist that they were other people or that the building was a prison. The idea that she was at Oberammergau playing a rôle in the Passion Play was very insistent. During most of this period she refused to answer orientation questions with any interest whatever, but, as her condition improved, she would do so, and it was then found that she knew the day, the month and the year, could remember the date of her admission and the different wards that she had been in.

As would be expected, there were frequent evidences of confusion, part of which was delusional in its origin, and part of it due to her distraction of thought. For instance, she complained not infrequently with some distress of being changed around all the time, which was a delusional idea, but paralleling this were statements expressing obvious perplexity; for instance, she said that she could not tell whether it was real life or the play, and went on : " Everything is mixed. Is that the door I came in ? Then everything is turned round. Oh yes this is the stage. My brain goes just like a tram car. How would you like to be in a room that goes round and round ? This room is not in the same place all the time. It mixes you up. I don't know where I am. They make it go round so I am in Hades." As has been stated, towards the latter part of this phase, increasing excitement would lead from clarity of utterance to considerable confusion in her talk. As we have seen with other patients a definitely objective and real interest might lead her to give consistently intelligent accounts at a time when she appeared otherwise much mixed up. For instance, she once, while in such a state, gave a perfectly clear account about a boil from which she had suffered.

If we turn to examine the ideas which this woman presented, when the manic processes were most in evidence, we find a number of interesting points. First, delusions, reference to which she was constantly making, were apparently always present, and there were a good many of them. If we can judge by her speech, her attention was shifting constantly to one or another of her imaginations and to variations of them. Second, ideas which one might suspect to have initiated (by operating unconsciously) the reactions and thoughts of the earlier part of her psychosis, now came to plain expression. Third, although this case was examined twenty-five years ago, and observed by three or four different physicians, none of whom had any interest in, or knowledge of, psychoanalytic principles, still the notes show in a remarkable way the type of content which we have described as being typical of the manic state. Finally, in spite of the fact that her stream of thought was so scattered as to be incomprehensible in short quotations, the collation of the ideas expressed nevertheless makes plain practically every word which she uttered. To understand her delusions properly, it is best to consider them under different headings.

It may be recalled that in the depression which immediately preceded her manic attack the patient was obsessed with thoughts of death, a matter that has already received comment. Some significance of this may now be demonstrated. She made many references to death, or to her being dead ; for instance, " I have been taken out of the world, and I died because of death ; of course you will kill me, but it does not make any difference to me. I care nothing for the body ; I have been nothing since coming into the world ". She spoke of seeing the fire of hell, and said she was burning up. Such state-ments as these were repeated many times, but with them there were other remarks which suggested strongly the conception of rebirth ; for instance, " I am going to do something to return to life, I woke up in the autumn " (her depression lifted, and gave way to elation in the autumn). Again, " I came into this world this morning ". She spoke of dying and of being re-surrected or reincarnated every seven years. We shall see immediately that a dominant note of her productions was the thought of a new world, a new scheme of things in which she would play a leading rôle, and she connected this life quite definitely with a resurrection fantasy.

The reader may remember that this patient had been married for many years, but had been childless, which was a grief both to herself and to her husband. In her psychosis she had an opportunity to enjoy autistically that which reality had denied her, consequently there were innumerable references to maternity in general, and to her motherhood in particular. Some of her ideas were very literal ; for instance, at one time she wanted the scissors in order to open her pillow in which her baby was. She claimed that she had had two babies, but had never known it. Such statements as " I know of maternity, of women, and I must keep the maternity instinct within me," are typical of her reiterated remarks on this subject.

As is usual in our cases, there was antagonism to her husband, in her case directed particularly against the idea of carnal union with him. Thought of spiritual union she did not deny. Consequently in many of her remarks there is a denial of physiological conception combined with an insistence on her maternity. Naturally such ideas are closely allied to her religious delu-sions of being the mother of Christ. She repeated many times that a child had been taken from her womb and then conceived. Sometimes she stated bluntly that she had a child by spiritual union. The following productions contain the kernel of her psychosis in that they speak of her death, her assumption of maternity on coming back to life, and the related scientific or philosophical schemes which bulked so largely in her new world. And it all begins with the statement which reflects her own childlessness : " There are are no children in the world ; there are no flowers like Plato tells of ; there are no colleges, no men, no women ; so investigate, go on to new science. O Lord, I have found maternity ! I disappeared from the world ; I am the great mother of all ! "

She talked a great deal about science, philosophical schemes, and her ambitious rôle in the new scheme of things. A number of remarks seemed to indicate that this reconstructed world represented a solution of two great difficulties, namely, her childlessness and her antagonism to marital obligations. For instance, " by biological affinity, the source of all life, I have discovered the end ". Again, " Some one said, the first one was to be made by chemistry, but it is not so. I say all science is tending toward this in-vestigation to make new science. O Lord, I feel love. I hear it go by twos, and this is my testament ". (At other times she gave to " twos " a definitely mating significance). Of course the elaboration of these philosophical ideas

claimed that one of the doctors had assured her she would never see her husband again.

The first indications of recovery appeared in a greater variability of her condition. First at longer intervals, and later about every third day, she would have a few hours in which she was quiet, amiable, and would talk reasonably but still with definite flight. When interviewed at such times, she would always become irritable and work herself up into a fresh excitement. Every two or three weeks she would have a depressed spell during which she would cry a good deal but say nothing. Before other evidence of definite improvement was at all striking, her orientation became quite good except for an insistence on her having been in that ward for five years. Then, quite suddenly, she became less irritable and quarrelsome when interfered with. At the same time her talk became more connected, and her behaviour in general improved, in fact she became quite decorous and tidy in her dress and habits. Depressive episodes became a little more frequent, but in general a manic flavour persisted, as she decorated herself, laughed readily and whenever interviewed would tend to work herself up and become definitely flighty.

During the next month this improvement continued so that she no longer misidentified people and made in general a perfectly normal impression. Again in this period, when interviewed one day, she said she felt blue and lonesome, people said things to her which gave her ideas, but she knew she was not hypnotized, and went on to correct many of her delusions quite satisfactorily. But suddenly she said, " I want to get away from here so much. I was talking with my brother this morning, and he says he is coming to take me away ". A little cross-questioning then led her to speak quite freely of ideas which still persisted. She believed herself to be in spiritualistic communication with many people, partly with her father, and gave quite an account of how she had lately learned that he had been poisoned by an aunt, taken to Chicago and buried. But he had talked to her from his coffin, she proceeded, assured her that he was not dead, then she had gone to Chicago, had taken him out of his coffin, and they had gone off together. All this she said she had learned quite recently from these spiritual communications. Further, these voices told her that her alleged father was really her uncle, that her mother was adopted, her real mother being a woman professor in a western university. Then she spoke of her aversion to the doctor about whom she had had so many sexual ideas. She hated him, not because she had thought he had mesmerized her, but because he had tried to seduce her, and she claimed to have told his ten-year old daughter about it telepathically. Further, she expatiated on her dislike for her husband, alleging that he had abused her in their marriage relations.

This is, theoretically, an important episode. Talking of her ideas in retrospect attracted her interest to them, whereupon their reality returned and in a few minutes she gave a digest of her psychotic ideas including statements of antagonism to her husband, reiteration of adult sex delusions, a denial of blood relationship with her mother, a shifting of the relationship with her father so as to make her attachment to him a little less scandalous, and finally a delusion of union with her father after death. This recrudescence of psychotic ideas was not accomplished without a reappearance of other symptoms, for with the recital, she became quite flighty and began to complain of the abuse she had suffered at the hands of the nurses, although a few minutes before she had seemed at peace with her environment. As the physician was about to leave she made a remark showing the pressure exerted by these ideas more or less against her will. She said, " I suppose my confession makes you think I am crazy and that it will cause me another year's stay in this place, but I cannot help it, it is all true."

Two days later she seemed to realise in some degree that her ideas had been unnaturally peculiar, but was not quite in a position to recognise their complete falsity. She was worried by them, for she said spontaneously to the physician, " You think it was crazy, but, if you had been shut up as long as I, all by yourself, you might understand how one could have such peculiar thoughts."

During the next two weeks she seemed to recover completely from her manic phase with perfect insight into the fact that she had been insane and that her ideas were all delusions. Most important of all, perhaps, her antagonism to her husband disappeared. She was willing to see him, when he came, and treated him well for the first time in more than a year. She remained in the hospital two weeks longer, during which time she became mildly depressed, and it was interesting that remorse was now centred on the weakness of her wifely love. This is highly suggestive of the mechanism of cyclothymia being a change in the conscious formulation of the same unconscious ideas.

We may summarize this study of transitions from one phase to another of manic states by saying that apparently the fundamental variant is the direction of attention. The hypothetically normal individual directs all his attention to the outside world and has a complete grasp on reality. In manic states attention tends to be turned from the environment to the patient's inner thoughts and, theoretically, should ultimately lead to absolute absorption in the inner mental life and entire ignorance of the existence of anything but the patient's imaginations. As has been shown, the intellectual capacity of the individual varies proportionately with the degree to which attention is intro- or extro-verted. We judge of this intellectual capacity by the ability which the patient shows to speak logically and connectedly, by the accuracy of his orientation and by his capacity to perform set intellectual tests such as arithmetical calculations, spelling, and so on. This relationship between attention and intelligence is easy to understand.

A more difficult problem arises when one studies the changes in the conative reactions of our patients, that is, the changes in physical activity, in productivity of speech and in the degree of emotional expression. One would perhaps assume quite naturally that these conative reactions would vary directly with the degree of contact with the environment, inasmuch as they all express contact with the environment. As a matter of fact, however, we find an apparently paradoxical relationship to exist, as we have seen, a hypomanic case becomes more disturbed, productive and emotional, with an increase of absorption in his thoughts. On the other hand, if his introversion continues still further, all these exhibitions diminish so that he becomes steadily quieter, as his interest is more exclusively centred in his own creations. This changing picture is, apparently, the result of the combined action of the two factors—direction of attention and intellectual capacity.

We are all aware that normally our recognition of propriety in behaviour, and of the necessity for logical expression, inhibit our tendency to act and speak as our inner impulse would dictate. We keep up the appearance of normality, in fact we *are* normal, just in so far as our intelligence enables us to make our speech and actions adaptable to the immediate situation. A hypomanic case begins to lose this inhibition when he obtrudes his dominating thoughts on his fellows. As these thoughts compel his attention still more, he makes less effort to render them intelligible in speech and becomes flighty. Finally, a point is reached where all insight vanishes and his productions become incomprehensible. Proceeding *pari passu* in this change, there is a progressive loss in inhibition of bodily and emotional expression, so that the patient, as he becomes more manic, suffers from a greater activity, increasing queerness in his conduct and a more unbridled emotionality. Beginning at the point where insight vanishes, as contact with the environment diminishes, the tendency to externalize thoughts in speech or translate them into action steadily decreases ; consequently all the conative reactions decrease with the introversion of attention, and the patient becomes quieter and more apathetic, in the same proportion as his intellectual capacity is deteriorating.

The accompanying diagram (Fig. 1) represents these processes in a rough schematic way. The brown portion of the rectangle shows introversion of attention, while the yellow exhibits the corresponding extroversion. As one increases, the other decreases. The blue lines represent the degrees of intellectual contact with reality, which reach a theoretic maximum at the lefthand side of the diagram, which stands for normality, and fade away to a theoretical zero at the right hand extremity, which is the point where extroversion of attention disappears. At each stage along the line F E the intellectual capacity is directly proportionate to the degree of extroversion of attention. The red lines represent the conative reactions which increase from the normal at A to the hypomanic stage at B and reach their maximum in the florid manic state of C. From there on, the excitement and verbal productivity diminish proportionately with the loss of intellectual capacity and the increasing introversion of attention. The triangle F A C shows the insight, the vertical blue lines of intelligence meeting the red lines of expression, so as to show the diminishing inhibition which proceeds along the line A B C.

If one now compares with this diagram the observations made on any one of the cases, which we have just been describing, where transitions were evident, the reactions may appear more comprehensible. For instance, when the normal man at A becomes dominated with some idea, in so far as this engrosses his attention, he loses contact with his environment and, to the same degree, his intellectual judgment. Consequently his intellectual critique is weakened and he expresses himself more forcibly than conventionally. In brief, he becomes hypomanic, and all these mechanisms are represented by imagining him to move from A toward B. Then if we consider a case of hypomania who is stimulated to talk about his ideas, we can see that, in so far as he gives more attention to these thoughts, he will move up toward C, becoming less critical, more productive, more excited. On the other hand, C, who is a florid manic, has lost all insight, and consequently greater absorption in his ideas (which we can now safely call delusions) leads at the same time to a loss of expression and a proportionate loss of his intellectual faculties. The quieter he becomes, the more sodden he is, the more incomprehensible in his speech. Finally, if this process proceeds to the point E, it will reach a condition of complete non-productivity and complete apathy, and a total disregard of the existence of the environment. In other words, the objective symptoms are, for the time being, identical with those of stupor. We shall later discuss the theoretic importance of this tendency, when we consider the inter-relations of the various psychoses in the manic-depressive group.

Similar changes in the other direction may also be followed. We have given many examples to show how the patient at D—an "absorbed" manic—becomes, not only more rational, but also more productive in speech and action, when his attention is directed away from his thoughts and is forced on to something environmental. Conversely, the effect on the excited patient at C, when he is brought down to earth, so to speak, is to decrease his excitement, decrease his productivity, while his intellectual judgment improves. The hypomanic case at B, if distracted from his dominant thoughts, so far loses his exaggerated activity in speech and conduct, and regains his normal judgment to such an extent that he takes up his place at A and is quite normal for the time being.

CHAPTER XXVI

S O far, in our discussion of the manic states, there has been no mention made of the occurrence of elation without expressed content. Yet all psychiatrists are familiar not only with hypomanic conditions, where the patient expresses no delusional ideas, but also with phases of manic-depressive attacks during which elation is present without obvious content, and, finally, we all know that in normal life we have our ups and downs, so that one day we are happy, everything seems pleasant, even the sun shines more brightly, although we are unaware of anything peculiarly pleasant having happened to cheer us up. Either these states of elation must be explicable by an extension of our theory or else the theory is unsound. As a matter of fact, it is not difficult to understand how the manic reactions may occur without any relation to any conscious or expressed content.

In many of the absorbed cases which have been described above, manic behaviour was noted when the patients would interrupt their usual quietness with sudden singing, laughter, mischievousness, and so on. When one has studied the development of ideas in such cases, it is not difficult to imagine how this behaviour may be determined by thoughts in which the patient was engrossed although he did not utter them. Somewhat similarly in the last case described, the patient emerged from depression to a gradually increasing elation, that was manifest before any definitely delusional ideas came to the surface. But in her case we know that there had been, during the depression, an absorbing interest in the topic of death ; in her later more florid manic state that she spoke freely of both resurrection and a mission to establish a new world. During this hypomanic phase she had an exaggerated sense of her own importance, as evidenced by her constant criticism of the hospital, and her ambition to cheer other patients up. This criticism, and an apparent desire to aid others in the institution, passed gradually over into her craze to reform the hospital, which in turn grew into the full-blown delusions of a new world.

In such a case we are surely justified in assuming that her highly expansive ideas, which later came to expression, were lurking on the fringes of consciousness during a hypomanic state. It was these which determined her energy, and the mood, we presume, broke through into consciousness, although not accompanied there by the fully developed ideas that later appeared. Careful study of all cases of hypomania without apparent content, that we have been able to examine, has shown similar mechanisms. For instance, the reader may refer again to the description of the case of William A. W., the second one whose history is given as exemplifying typical manic states.

Probably the commonest condition, which we see in our hospitals for the insane, where elation is present without content, is that observed in cases of stupor, or of stupor-like reactions, which, emerging from their period of sodden unproductivity, return to normality through a phase of hypomania. Since our theories of the psychology of these reactions have been formulated, we have not had an opportunity to study any of these cases closely as we have the hypomanics just mentioned. Consequently, our views are mere assumptions to explain this condition. We know however that many stupor cases make an autistic journey to heaven and return to earth with delusions of an expansive religious order. These cases are then manic. We are probably not doing violence to the facts in assuming that those cases, who have no content, owe their hypomanic reactions to similar ideas, which do not come definitely into consciousness, but which operate at the threshold of awareness. If one talked to such patients about their hopes, aspirations or ambitions, it is probable that some evidence of this could be obtained.

The problem of elation in everyday life that is independent of any obvious cause for extreme happiness will be discussed later in chapter 48. It will be shown that a dream in which an unconscious idea is formulated, as are the manic delusions, may be forgotten by the dreamer but still determine his mood through the following day.

CHAPTER XXVII

EXPLANATION OF MOOD VARIATIONS IN MANIC STATES

PSYCHIATRISTS, ever since the manic-depressive classification was adopted, have been puzzled by the so-called mixed conditions. The psychological mechanisms which seem to determine these reactions, will be discussed more fully later, when the interrelation of the various manic-depressive psychoses is considered. At this point, however, it may be well, in order to round out our description of manic states, to mention some of the more atypical cases where anomalous reactions apparently occur.

Essential features of mania are held to be elation and over activity. Loss of activity with sadness, anxiety, apathy or perplexity seem to belong essentially to other manic-depressive reactions. How can we explain their occurrence in manic states? We must bear in mind, as has been shown above, that elation alone is not the only fundamental characteristic of the manic state. An equally important characteristic is what we have termed " distraction of thought ", that is, the domination of the patient's attention by internal mental events, rather than by the environment. As has been stated, the greater the degree of distraction of thought, the less marked is the mood reaction, which of itself is a form of contact with the environment. Hence, full development of distraction implies a reduction of the elation. At the same time, with greater abstraction, the tendency of unconscious fancies to assume more primitive form is magnified. Naturally, when these ideas are reduced to their original crudity, they tend constantly to be reformulated. Hence they are apt to appear as ideas of danger, with a mood of anxiety ; in an anti-social form, which gives rise to depression ; as a death idea that leads to a stupor-like behaviour, and so on. In other words the tendency to distraction of thought, when well developed, leads back to that kind of matrix, as it were, from which all manic-depressive ideas and reactions arise. A patient in this condition may, therefore, laugh one minute and cry the next. The whole picture of the psychosis may consequently seem to be a mixture of different moods. As a matter of fact, no true mixture seems ever to be present. What we do observe is an alternation of moods, or a reduction of the intensity of elation which corresponds to the patient's further divorce from reality.

Even in cases where distraction of thought is not a prominent symptom, there may be a kaleidoscopic changing of formulation which will give rise to the same picture of alternation of moods. For instance, we may refer to the case of Annie D., previously described, who showed after the death of her employer mainly a manic reaction. But it was characterized by many references to death, as well as erotic remarks. Frequently the death ideas were formulated as thoughts of suicide ; or of being killed on account of her sins, when she was depressed ; of being killed, when she had a whining reaction, with prayers not to be killed ; or she showed stuporous symptoms, when she was apparently dominated with ideas of being dead.

Another case will be described in greater detail, not only for a demonstration of this principle of change of mood corresponding to change of formulation, but also because her whole history demonstrates well the fundamental principles of our manic-depressive theory. Her case was studied rather intensively in 1914 when she was in her ninth attack.

CASE 38. *Mary S.* was a single Jewish girl, age 26 years at the time of her last observed attack. The family history was negative for three generations, so far as information could be gathered. She was born in Roumania and brought to America when three years of age. Her mother had died five days after she was born. Of four other children, one brother was drowned in 1902, and another married in 1907. Of two sisters the eldest married in 1902, and the second lived with the patient. As family situations bulked largely in her psychoses, it is important to bear these circumstances in mind.

The patient herself was an efficient saleswoman, quiet and very proper in her behaviour, inclined to worry over her material situation, but otherwise, superficially considered, was normal. She admitted a great attachment to her father and to the brother who was drowned, but in her normal life she evidently showed no pathological attachment to the other members of the family, except for the fact that she preferred to live and stay at home rather than to indulge in social relaxation with strangers. Briefly then, she was rather of the seclusive type, although intellectually probably a little above the average. Other features of her make-up will be discussed later.

Her surviving brother, who was a good observer, gave the following general description of her attacks. She always had a certain amount of worry about holding her positions. An increase in this worry invariably marked the incubation of an attack and she would begin to speak about the likelihood of her being discharged. With this she was rather depressed and, at times, irritable, quarrelling with the sister with whom she lived. Then gradually a restlessness would set in. She would depart from her normal stay-at-home habit by visiting various girl friends, whom she otherwise never saw, remaining with each one only ten or fifteen minutes, and boasting about her love affairs. These affairs never had any foundation in fact, and the slightest incident was sufficient to justify her in establishing any chance acquaintance as an imaginary lover. For example, one of her " lovers " was a clerk who had sold her a pair of shoes and with whom she had no other contact. With this restless visiting she developed an excitement and sleeplessness. She would also frequent theatres and read exciting novels, which normally held no interest for her. Occasionally her attacks went no further than this, but often the excitement and irrationality of her speech and conduct reached the point where commitment to a hospital was necessary. During the recoveries she always went through the reverse process of losing her insane ideas and became at the same time quieter, until finally she would be depressed for a few weeks, staying at home, doing no work, and talking only with great effort.

We may next give a more detailed description of her attacks.

When ten years of age she was awakened suddenly by an alarm clock,

U

became much frightened and thought the house was on fire. For the following two weeks she was sleepless and easily startled and worried lest something should happen to her brother whenever he was late coming home. This was probably her first psychotic episode.

In April, 1900 (when the patient was 12), her father died. When she was told of this, she became very excited and screamed. When she saw the body in the coffin she ran to it and shook the coffin so that the body moved. Then she shouted that he was still alive. Following the funeral she was sleepless and depressed for two weeks, complaining constantly that the body should have been kept longer before it was buried. The family thought that following this incident she had an attack in the autumn of every second year which would last about two weeks and be terminated by depression, but this could not be definitely confirmed.

The next marked attack was in July, 1902, when the patient was 14. Her brother, to whom she was especially attached, was drowned while bathing. It happened that she had stolen a bathing suit from the house and given it to him before he went swimming. On first hearing the news, she was agitated and, so soon as she saw the body, insisted for half an hour that he looked to be still alive. Then for a week she was depressed, but after this period was for two months sleepless, laughed and cried a good deal and spent much time walking the streets. From then until the age of 16 she kept house for her family, but at that time took up her present occupation as saleswoman.

In the autumn of 1905, when 17 years of age, she had a longer attack than usual, but nothing is known of it.

When 19 years of age, in June, 1907, her surviving brother married suddenly. She at once became depressed, quarrelled with her sister and worried over what she and her sister would do lacking the brother's support. Her distress gradually passed over to a nervous sleepless condition with decreased efficiency. With this, she began to talk about her lovers, and was much put out when her brother criticized her for receiving a letter from a man. Finally, in October, the firm for which she was working dismissed her on her brother's request. Immediately she became more restless. Three days later she heard someone say General S.'s monument is on 150th Street. She began at once walking the street looking for the monument of her dead brother, and finally collapsed in a drug store, whence she was removed to the hospital. A note made in her case in this attack states that she was very restless, talking continuously under considerable tension, rambling, occasionally with true flight. When speaking of her troubles she cried, but when talking of her many lovers she was elated, and at times, erotic in her behaviour. By the end of January of the following year she had quieted down sufficiently to be paroled, and then remained for six weeks at home, during which time she was probably depressed.

In September, 1909, when 21, she had another attack of which we know little. It was apparently characterized by depression and loss of ambition, lasting for some weeks.

The following year she began to worry about getting a rise in salary which had been promised, and blamed herself for inefficiency. On March 5 she was told that A. (a man whom she had known casually in a Hebrew social society) was engaged. Immediately she became excited, quarrelled with her sister, grew more talkative and sleepless and began her rounds of visitation. On March 11 she became more excited and went to see A. The day following she was discharged from her position and some four days later was removed to the hospital. Her condition on this admission was essentially the same as on the last, but she gave voice to many more ideas, or perhaps more care was taken in recording them. She spoke of being married to A., or of having been married to A. with an elaborate ceremony. The doctor had hypnotized her. There was much erotic talk. She insisted on calling herself "Mrs." and was angry when addressed as "Miss." In addition she was much exercised over the family affairs of the manager at her store. After five months she had quieted down sufficiently to be allowed parole. It was noted that she had very little memory of her symptoms, although she could recall external events perfectly.

Her next attack was in June, 1912, when she was 24 years of age. She was promised an advance in wages which she did not get. She worried more and more over this, soon feared she would lose her job, and this as usual passed over into her restless excitement, visiting and amorous boasting. She was nearly two months in working up her excitement to the point where commitment was necessary and her attack, which was essentially the same as the others, quieted down again after five months.

Four months later, she was downhearted and sleepless for a short time, the cause of which was not determined.

In the fall of that same year there was a failure and change of management at the store in which she worked. Although there was no occasion for it, she began to think she would be discharged. Around Christmas time, failure of the new management was discussed in the press, which much increased her worry. Excitement also began and this increased gradually up to the time of her commitment on March 20, 1914.

As this is the attack which was studied in special detail, it may be well to mention some other incidents which occurred during this last period. On February 10 her brother's first child was born. She had worried over her sister-in-law's ability to carry the baby and was anxious at the time of delivery, according to her retrospective account. Objectively, however, there was no change in her condition, which was already quite abnormal, for she was making her visits, restless, extravagant, and occasionally screaming during the day and restless at night. This incident may have had something to do with her next psychotic development. The day following the birth she telephoned to the one who had been her autistic husband in a former attack and told him to congratulate her. He thought at once that she was engaged but was much relieved, she said later, when he learned what the congratulation was for. He told her that she ought to " become civilized " now that she was an aunt, which she interpreted as meaning that she ought to be married. Two weeks later she met A. by appointment, according to her statement at the hospital, because he wanted to assure himself that she was still single. On March 14 the store was closed. There had been some suspicion of dishonesty on the part of the new owner, and before leaving the shop she signed a petition with other employees asking that their employer should not be put in gaol. Immediately her symptoms became accentuated. She quarrelled with her sister, talked much of her father and brother and had an idea that she might be put into prison " for something " and also because she was related to her late employer. This excitement demanded her commitment.

At first she was excited and tense, rather than being distinctly elated. She talked incessantly in a rambling way but always confined herself to the same topics. After three weeks her behaviour was quieter, but she was still over talkative, decorated herself a good deal and was slightly erotic in her behaviour with physicians. About June 1 she had quieted down almost to normality. She was never at any time in a comfortable, happy, open mood of a typical manic elation ; she seemed to be more in a state of continued tenseness, with variations in her mood corresponding to her utterances. For instance, when she mentioned certain topics she cried or gave some other sign of being ill at ease ; she was nearest to true elation when she was speaking of her imagined lovers.

Although her talk was so rambling as to seem, superficially, to be merely a jumble of reminiscences, there was nevertheless a certain consistency of reference at different periods. For the first three weeks her talk was frankly sexual with many references to marriage, of a gynecological examination, which had been made, which she insisted had shown that she had lost her virginity. She spoke much of venereal disease and made many erotic references to the physicians. At this same period she had much to say about the different members of her family, at times stating that her father was alive and visited her at nights. She was much interested in the situation of her married sister and her sister-in-law, claiming that they were incapable of having children, and so on. These, with occasional tedious accounts of the failure of her firm, made up her entire trend of ideas at this time.   As she became quieter her frankly sexual references became less frequent, while the same ideas were repeated in politer language.   She continued, too, in her talk about the members in her family, but it was much more superficial.   Finally, when she was definitely recovering, she had little to say beyond wearying repetitions of the failure of the firm.   This same development was shown well in her statements about A.   At the period of her greatest excitement, she declared unreservedly that she was married to him.   When she began to quiet down this had been reduced to a simple engagement.   Later, when she had practically her normal mood, she said she would marry him if she would marry anybody.   Finally she claimed that he meant nothing to her at all.

Her lack of insight on recovery was striking.   She admitted that she had been ill, but was amnesic for her false ideas and would never make a full admission of her mental abnormality.   Even when her history was read to her she not only failed to recognize many of her absurd ideas, but even claimed that there must have been a mistake.   In these instances she would substitute some perfectly innocent statement, which she claimed was what she had said.   These statements were interesting in that they apparently represented her normal, sane formulations of unconscious ideas which came to much franker expression in her psychosis.   For instance, in her attack she said that her sister-in-law called her a prostitute.   Her explanation for this was that she once said to her that if she lost her job she would be on the street.   Again, she explained a remark, to the effect that her brother " ran her name down " and made her a street walker, by saying that her brother's sudden marriage had left her without a home.   There were many examples of this.

This patient's ideas were of particular interest, because it was possible to demonstrate that both her normal life and her psychoses were under the influence of the same dominating, unconscious trend.   She was a girl, who was very prim and proper, meticulously careful about her surroundings and associates, dressed very quietly, and avoided all amusements which she did not consider dignified.   With men she was distinctly shy, and avoided meeting them except under circumstances of complete propriety.   For example, she would not go out with them in the evening, nor let them call on her at any place but her brother's home.   On the other hand, she had the constant worry of not being able to dress as well as Christian or American girls.   Further, she thought she was not so attractive to Gentiles, because she was a foreigner.   Finally, she was troubled with a constant anxiety lest she lose her position, and be left without any means of support.   For this last there was no reasonable excuse, as her family were always willing and able to look after her, and she was an exceptionally efficient saleswoman who could always secure employment.   The inner meaning of all these worries became apparent when her psychoses were studied analytically.   Her marked aversion to anything suggesting social freedom or license would indicate a reaction against a strong unconscious tendency to licentious indulgence.   In other words, she had a strong unconscious inclination toward prostitution, while her whole conscious life was an expression of antagonism to this.

This assumption makes the development of her typical attacks quite clear. The first one came on a number of months after her brother married suddenly, but her mental abnormality plainly began with that marriage.   She was sad at losing her brother, but immediately gave a personal twist to the event by worrying about her financial situation, fearful of poverty without his support. Then gradually she began her restless visiting, boasting of her lovers, and became, in a literal sense only, a " street-walker ".   By the time she was committed she was frankly elated, with constant talk of her lovers.   In the last attack she said that her brother had forced her to become a prostitute, and later explained that it was his sudden withdrawal of support, which meant that she would be put on the street.   We may presume, therefore, that this same prostitution fancy existed from the beginning.   The loss of the brother's support led to the worry over her financial situation, and, as long as the content was purely financial, her mood remained that of distress.

As soon as the conscious prostitution idea developed, however, excitement set in, and when the definite delusion of having lovers was formulated she became elated.

In her next admission, worry over failure to receive an increase of wages and self-reproach for inefficiency began the psychotic story. The worry changed to excitement when she heard that her autistic lover A. was engaged. This precipitating cause was constantly echoed throughout her manic attack in frequent erotic references to A.

In the next admission, disappointment over failure to advance in business led to the same worry, and the same change of mood to excitement, so soon as her ideas underwent a displacement from the financial to the erotic field.

In her last attack the transparency of this development was complete. With the first mention of the failure of the store where she was employed, she became worried. As soon as the business actually went into the receivers' hands, her restless visiting began. When her sister-in-law's baby was born some weeks later, her maternal instincts were stimulated (for she identified herself in her attack with her sister-in-law). This led her to re-establish communication with A., which excited her still further. When the store was finally closed, her excitement reached a pitch that demanded commitment. For several days she had actually spent most of her time on the streets, and had been away from home every night almost until morning.

A number of her delusional ideas were definitely associated with this prostitution trend. For instance, in several of her admissions she boasted of her knowledge of a number of foreign languages and her attractiveness. She talked, too, of her marriage to a Gentile, which was another evidence of her superior attractiveness. She thus compensated for her normal feeling of sex inferiority by autistically endowing herself with those attractions which fate had denied her. As recorded in nearly all the admission notes, she commented freely on the stenographer. The significance of this became clear during her last attack, when she said that her sister-in-law had asked her why she did not become a stenographer. To this she had replied that, if she did so, she would only become some old gentleman's darling (and then passed on to speaking of a man who reminded her of her father). In other words, a stenographer's position implied sexual accessibility in her, which probably accounted for her interest in that occupation. The evidence for the existence of this prostitution trend became unequivocal during her last attack. She spoke frequently of being called a prostitute—" I am more vicious, I did not use to be, but they made me different." She talked much of the maternal tree and of having babies—" My aim is for maternity." There were constant references to her virginity being lost, and once she said the men were going crazy because they could not have her hymen. She claimed that all the girls working at her store were thought to be impure. Some man had intimated to her that she was getting money from outside sources. In connection with one of her remarks, " If I do not sleep I know I am old enough to get married," it is interesting to recall that she was sleepless during her periods of worry even before other evidences of excitement were present. All these data have to do with prostitution in general. In addition there were innumerable references to definite lovers.

Although these erotic fancies were the core of her psychoses, there were recorded, as in all our well-observed cases, many references which seem to show that family attachments provided a real dynamic element underlying her prostitution trend. Her family stated that she loved her father and the brother who was drowned more than any other people in the world. That some of this attachment was transferred to her surviving brother seems probable from the fact that, although she invariably quarrelled with and hated her sisters during the incubation periods of her attacks, she never showed any hate toward this brother. At these periods she always began to talk of her father and brother. When her father died, and again when her brother was drowned, it was difficult to convince her that life was really gone.

During her psychoses she would refer to them as being still alive, very often confusing them.

The corollary of this attachment for her father and brother was naturally to be found in jealousy of the female members of her family. Her antagonism to her sisters, that came to open expression when she was insane, has already been mentioned. The jealousy she felt for her brother's wife demands some comment. During her normal periods this was cloaked by great solicitude. She was very apprehensive during the sister-in-law's pregnancy, and said that at times she almost wished that the child were dead, rather than the mother's health should be endangered (a rather transparent expression of the unconscious wish for the sister-in-law's death). When the child was finally born, it (a girl) looked so like her brother, who had been drowned that the patient could not look at it. In her attacks this jealousy came to more open expression. She declared that her brother should divorce this woman, because she had not been a virgin when married. She also had a good deal to say about the unfitness for marriage both of her sister-in-law and of her older sister, because they had been wedded for so many years and had only had miscarriages, and so on. This topic was particularly important during the last attack because the birth of her brother's child seems to have been a definite precipitating factor and throughout her psychosis she had much to say about maternity.

Any one interested in the development of her ideas could find ample proof of there being a close unconscious connection between her prostitution fancies and her attachment to father and brother. This connection was evidenced mainly in the sequence of ideas in her rambling flight. For instance, she frequently associated venereal disease with her father. He had died of blood poisoning and kidney disease, and she rarely spoke of venereal infections (a constant topic) without passing over directly to talk of her father. Once the association was still closer when she said " My father used to tell me about men's diseases ". A variant of the same thought appeared in statements about an old man who acted like a father to her and who told her about men's and women's diseases. Another intimate association occurred in the remark " I am afraid of men, I am even afraid of my brother, who has such filthy ideas ". She constantly implied licentious habits to her father, speaking frequently of his having lived with a woman to whom he was never married. Her lovers seemed images of her father or brother. A., she claimed, was a great friend of her brother who was drowned, went to school with him, and followed the profession that he was going to follow. She called the physicians " father," behaved in an erotic way with them, and repeatedly claimed that she had been married to some of them. In her 1910 admission she wrote a letter to A. in which she addressed him as husband, and said, " Dr. G. is your brother, as Dr. K. is my brother ". Dr. K. was one of the most frequent imaginary husbands. Finally, she stated in one of her attacks that she had always slept with her father until menstruation began, at which time he put her from his bed.

The position of employer has, of course, some analogy to that of paternity. It was not unnatural, therefore, that this father attachment should be transferred to her employer. During her last admission she had a great deal to say about her having been mistaken for the daughter of her employer. Sometimes she called herself his wife. Elaborations of this same thought were that she might be put in prison because she was a relative of her employer ; that her complaints received no attention from the receivers, because they thought she was his relative. The same constellation of ideas, probably accounted for her interminable talk about the manager of the store. In one of her earlier admissions she worried a great deal about the death of his wife or daughter, and in her last attack she thought that she was taken to the hospital by his son disguised as a chauffeur.

The most important feature of her attacks has still to be discussed, that is, the relation between the particular form, which these ideas assumed, and the accompanying mood reaction. In fact she was observed during her last attack with particular care because all her psychoses had been characterized with much crying, in spite of their being manic attacks, and an effort was made to see whether there ever was such a thing as a true mixture of her moods, or whether it was always a matter of alternation. The latter was found to be the case. It was possible to show that without exception each mood reaction was correlated definitely with a specific autistic formulation.

In the first place, as has been remarked, her excitement, and what genuine elation she showed, came on only when she began to imagine that she had lovers. When under observation her elation invariably ceased abruptly at any time when her reference changed from a love affair to any definite trouble. For instance, she cried when speaking of the fact that she was called a prostitute, but laughed when talking of A. This contrast was always present. Prostitution to her mind was invariably associated with the idea of wickedness or of social censure, and, whenever prostitution as such was mentioned, her emotional reaction expressed pain. The position of a lover, on the other hand, was closely related to her idea of marriage, and was therefore a pleasant idea to which she gave free rein in a setting of elation. References to her financial situation were always accompanied by signs of distress. She was apt to be sad when talking of her family relations, and at one time she remarked that her father always appeared to her when she was " worrying ". When she made the remark, quoted above, that she was afraid of her brother, she cried.

In reviewing the history of her attacks we find that when they were precipitated by some family trouble, her reaction was of a depressive nature, so long as her thoughts remained centred on the family. Finally, in this connection, we should mention that during recovery she had a depressive tendency, and she repeatedly claimed that any effort to discuss her previous ideas made her sad. When we consider to what a degree her memory of her attacks was affected, we realize how much repression there must have been at the close of each attack. Apparently the depression which rang down the curtain on each of her manic episodes was definitely associated with repression.

We may summarize all these conclusions as follows : We have seen that there is some fundamental father or brother attachment appearing under different disguises and that there is as much difference between these disguises as there is between the corresponding moods. The mood is, therefore, in a definite relation to the form in which the unconscious wish comes to expression. When attention is focussed on one of the original infantile objects of affection or hate (family troubles) the mood is one of depression. Similarly, when she attempts to rid her mind of her insane ideas, there is again a depression. When, however, her affection has been transferred in imagination to one who is a permissible object (although at the same time a father surrogate) she is elated. On the other hand, if this outlet takes the specific form of prostitution, which is socially frowned upon, she is distressed, and, when this prostitution fancy is cloaked in the form of solicitude about her pecuniary situation, the emotion is, appropriately, that of anxiety. In a word, her mood is in a definite relation to the manifest rather than the latent content of the delusional idea, and we can see that her elation is connected only with the idea of obtaining a sexual outlet in a socially permissible manner. A case, therefore, which superficially observed seems anomalous, offers on closer observation a detailed proof of our thesis.

CHAPTER XXVIII

NORMAL HAPPINESS AND HYPOMANIA

BEFORE leaving the problem of psychology of elation, it might be well to speak of the bearing of our theories on normal happiness. It may be recalled that the discussion of manic states was initiated with some remarks on normal exhilaration, so it is not out of place to conclude by reciprocal application of the principles gained in the study of frankly psychotic condition to those of everyday life. This subject will be discussed more fully in a later chapter, when the relation of dreams to the mood of the following day is considered. Now, however, we may take up those slight elations which would not be regarded as partaking of the psychotic were it not for their occurrence in individuals who are prone to develop definite manic attacks.

For this purpose we are fortunate in having the record of a patient of rare intelligence, a keen introspectionist, who, after suffering from two circular attacks, wrote a description of his symptoms, in which he dealt, not only with those exaltations and depressions which were objectively evident, but paid equal attention to such minor exhibitions of these tendencies as remained purely subjective. From his own statements it is easy to see how these " normal " variations were really manic-depressive episodes. His record is also interesting in another respect. It was written twenty years ago by one totally unacquainted with any psychopathological theories, and yet it is possible to show how all the phenomena, which we have been describing in our cases of marked mania, were present in his milder attacks. In fact, by making slight assumptions, and what we consider to be justifiable interpretations, it is possible to see the working of such deep-lying unconscious forces as come to frank expression in the more florid psychoses which form the bulk of our material.

CASE 39. *Alfred J.* was born of well-to-do parents who were able to give him an excellent education. In disposition he was said to be active and self-confident, with the desire to rule. His intelligence was decidedly above the average, and, although somewhat " artistic " in his temperament, yet he had considerable business ability. When seventeen years of age he had a severe attack of diphtheria. His father claimed that following this illness the patient was different, but he himself said that he simply became more self-assertive and followed the dictates of his own judgment rather than relying on his parents for guidance. It would seem probable that this was a normal adolescent development.

After passing through preparatory school, the patient entered a university, where he was consistently successful in his studies up to his third year, when hhe was 23 years old. At the beginning of te following semester, he spent much time in reading with a young woman and consequently neglected his college work. He began to feel that he was getting behind in his studies. This worry apparently precipitated a depression that marked the beginning of his psychotic career. In the light of what we have learned about the importance of various adaptations in healthy instinctive development, this precipitating factor is of importance. As we shall later see, his depressions and elations were all concerned with his feeling of success or failure in various undertakings, chiefly academic.

A normal individual, who puts a reasonable amount of energy into his various sublimations, remains normal, because these sublimations give him a productive outlet and exist for themselves alone. It is the fate of the psychotic individual, on the other hand, to concentrate on various ambitions, which are a means to an end rather than an end to themselves. We may recall the case of William A.W., whose desire to go into business for himself was merely a cover for a life-long ambition to be the sole support of his mother. This patient (we may presume) was unable to get a normal outlet in his friendship with a young woman and to carry on another sublimation, his studies, at the same time. The probability is that he felt himself inadequate to the problem of marriage (he was still unmarried at the age of 34) and transferred this inadequacy to his studies. His academic work became symbolic of his incapacity and maladaptation in the sex field and hence appeared as the content of his depression. Having unconsciously transferred his sex interest to another activity, the latter gained a heightened significance. Success or failure in academic work meant achievement or incompetence in his more important instinctive life and, in consequence, from this time on, progress in his studies had a profound meaning to him and determined his mental health or abnormality. At any rate, with this precipitating cause he passed into a mild retarded depression for some five months.

He emerged from this depression with an elation that was severe enough to cause his removal from the university. It lasted altogether six months, part of which time he spent at a sanatorium. This was apparently a hypomanic state in which he was overactive, full of schemes and extravagant. This depression and elation were the most severe attacks that he had. On leaving the sanatorium he was already beginning to be a little depressed, but, as he had made up his mind to go abroad before re-entering Harvard, he began the trip accompanied by a nurse, although he had great difficulty in travelling on account of his retardation. This depression lasted in its turn six months and reached its acme three months after it had begun. As he improved he returned from Europe to America and again in the spring became exhilarated. This elation continued for another six months, after which time he remained well for five years. Immediately on his return to normality he went to Germany for a year and a half, where he studied, and then returned and finished his university course successfully. In the autumn of 1898, the year of his graduation, he made up his mind to go to Paris, which he did on his own resources, with the result that he found himself with only 60 francs in his pockets on his arrival at that city. His capacity was then demonstrated by his tutoring various persons, among others the Prince of an Eastern Kingdom. He made enough money to work his way through the University. While there he evidently lived a Bohemian life, but did good work, so that eventually he got his Ph.D. at the Sorbonne *summa cum laude.*

With the prospect of this degree ahead, after six years of normality, he again became exhilarated in April, 1901. He was slow in recognizing the abnormality of his condition because it did not begin with a depression as had his previous hypomanic episodes. In time, however, he did realise that he was abnormal and, aware of the curve which his attacks followed, expected the height of his excitement to come in the beginning of July. For this reason he postponed his examination till the end of that month and then, while still exhilarated, passed it.   At the end of August he returned to America, when he again became depressed.   This was never a severe retardation, but lasted some eighteen months in all.   It was when he passed from this depression to the inevitable elation that he came under observation as a voluntary patient.

In the spring he went into the lobster business and made $750 inside of three months, but he became exhilarated, wanted to control the firm alone, and was forced to leave.   His father hearing of his conduct sent a doctor for him.   At first he wished to fight, but later agreed to follow.   For two weeks he lived near this doctor in the city and was well controlled until a few days before admission, when he was guilty of a typical indiscretion.   He employed a locksmith to visit his father's home and made a key for the door.   While thus engaged the locksmith was unfortunately discovered and this led to a grave rupture of relations between father and son.   Following this he was persuaded to come to the hospital.

Under observation he showed a typical hypomanic state with occasional physical over-activity and always a tendency to over-productiveness in speech. He was boastful.   He was constantly euphoric, although never intractable, and at times irritable.   As to his stream of thought it seemed to be more a matter of loquaciousness than of definite flight, although there was a slight tendency to get sidetracked.   Invariably, however, he would return to the subject in hand.   This exhilaration lasted for seven months and was terminated by two months of very mild depression, after which he passed from observation.

As has been stated, this patient wrote for the physicians a long account of his attacks, and it is in this account we are now interested, because it demonstrates the existence of the various ideas and mechanisms, which we have been describing from objective material.   In this case they were objectively not apparent, but subjectively recognised.   In other words, we find evidence in his story of the same principles being applicable to those milder disturbances of mood which grade over into normal variations.

First as to the content of his elation he wrote : " The exhilarated condition is essentially creative and synthetical and has as its characteristic a desire for composition."   This is, presumably, his formulation of what we would call sublimated activity.   His normal ambitions were inflated, his capacity exaggerated, and his prospective achievements were so magnified as to give him a feeling of success not justified either by the realities of the situation or by his potential ability.   To quote from him : " The exhilarated condition is characterized by an abnormal desire on my part for starting enterprises, a strong feeling of power for accomplishing and an abnormal adequacy, together with a craving for command.   All of this usually culminates, in spite of various side schemes and ambitions, in an intense desire for intellectual activity and organisation.   And the fact is characteristic that it is invariably I, who has to be the leader and, eventually, the President, of the University."   In connection with this ambition, he spent a great deal of time in prospecting for professors to serve under him, and he told how he would catechise almost every one he met in order to discover his general capability and special training for a position.   When at the height of an attack he would so far lose his judgment as to make an immediate promise of a teaching position *under him*.   The gross egotism of his ambition betrays its weakness as a true sublimation, but that both the selfish and altruistic motives were combined in his fancies is nicely demonstrated by these words : " During the entire conversation I am, sub-consciously, speculating as to the exact number of cents and dollars I shall economise by this new acquisition of trained and educated, but comparatively cheap, labour, to my service in the enterprise I am about to undertake.   Though, at the same time, I have a most earnest and unselfish desire to elevate the individual and through him mankind."

When under observation his boasting overstepped the boundaries of mere academic renown.   He talked of having degrees from Harvard, Dublin, an English University, and the Sorbonne ; but he also claimed that he had crossed the Atlantic twenty-five times ; once he had commanded an ocean liner and took four thousand people across the ocean ; that he had been employed by the King of England and at that time made $19,000. All this was told to a nurse. To the physician the same characteristic was shown, although in a less crude way, his bragging being closer to the limits of possibility, that is, he would boast about his relations to noted men, the importance of his work in early English and French literature, and so on. Again, he magnified his influence over the Prince (whom he had tutored in Paris) until he made it appear that he controlled both the external and internal politics of the latter's kingdom.

With this was a feeling of increased power of perception, so that he felt that he had an insight into men, nature and even God, which was many times his normal capacity. He read poetry with a feeling that it had a new significance and could find inner meanings, which had been hidden from him before. One sentence is interesting : " I think I perceive an almost mathematical unity and interdependence in all things." This seems to be an echo of the delusions which we have noted so often of scientific and philosophical solution of the riddle of the universe, ideas which we have termed constructive delusions and which seem quite frequent, particularly among men patients. At another place he wrote : " I may perhaps be said metaphorically to have got glimpses of the infinite."

We have been constantly describing the religious delusions of the manic, pointing out how selfish they are, and how crudely they sometimes identify themselves with the Divinity. This patient came very close to such identification in the following rhapsody. It is interesting, too, that in this paragraph he includes the other important manic content, namely, adult love.

" Were the restless activity of this powerful mental delirium not so ineffably wearying, and its individual points of light not so ephemeral, its ecstatic pleasure would be comparable to that of the old Greek Gods. Indeed, as it is, my mental insight, my perceptions, sensibilities, observation, intuition, my power of ' Anschauung '—all seem intensified and to take heroic proportions. And just as my sufferings, during a depression are abnormally great, so, I sometimes questioned if any ordinary mortal ever experiences such intensity and depth of pleasurable sensation, as those which fired my abnormally stimulated imagination during my first exhilaration. Of any highly excited states of mind or transports, of enthusiasm, frenzy, or madness, that might be brought about through alcoholic intoxication or by the drug habit, I know absolutely nothing either from experience or observation, and the only sane state of mind which I know at all comparable to this exhilarated condition is that of a person deeply in love. Under the stimulation of the two conditions, dormant sensibilities seemed awakened, and the exalted being commences to wonder if he has really ever heard, or felt, or seen before. He realizes capacities for pleasure of which he has never previously suspected the existence. He sees beauty everywhere, and takes a supreme enjoyment in everything he sees or does ; and he is incessantly fired by an ambitious desire to extend this happiness, not only in the one case of her, but in both to all he meets. In fact, confining myself, for the moment, to my experience with the disease alone, I am, when exhilarated, even incommoded myself and embarrassed others by the very intensity and generosity of my feelings, whose essence is kindliness and good-will towards men. But this benevolence is no longer administered according to the dictates of reasoning sympathy ; it has rather become an exaggerated, insane beneficence or an all embracing wildly extravagant munificence. The original sympathetic desire for the sharing of joy, happiness and well-being has run mad."

This factor in his elation is more pointedly stated in these words : " I crave strongly companionship, sympathy, and love, and being filled with a longing to possess some object upon which to bestow my affection, I am then more prone to fall in love than at any other time. It is then, too, that my solitary, lonely life seems to me most irksome and unsatisfactory. As a matter of fact each of my various exhilarations has had a woman in one way

or another connected with it ; and good women they have been, too ! And
when, as may thus perchance have happened, the poor innocent mortal finds
himself, at one and the same time, under the combined influence of the Goddess
of Love, and the Spirit of exhilaration, the resulting gratification of subdued
longings, and the intoxicating effect upon his brain, beggar description.''

Almost always a manic-depressive patient sooner or later makes some
remarks which give a hint as to the unconscious motivation of their ideas.
Naturally such remarks are most frequent where mental balance is most
upset, and, consequently, we would not expect to find any direct references
to such matters in this patient's story.   Traces are, however, to be discovered.
He speaks of his admiration for his mother, and the belief that he had inherited a gift in repartee from her.   On the other hand, he devoted a whole
chapter to the relation between himself and his father.   These attitudes
were strained, largely on account of the patient's tendency towards extravagance.   He took some pains to demonstrate that his father's attitude
in money matters was wrong, and evidently derived some satisfaction from
being able to quote an uncle on this subject.   When normal he was able to
adapt himself to his father's alleged peculiarity, but when exhilarated this
enraged him and led to recurring ruptures.   In his attacks he not only lost
sight of his father's characteristics, but would make unusual demands upon
him and expect him to meet them.   To quote his own words : " Under the
influence of the exhilaration I apparently forgot that the portion of my own
personal income, over which I have control, is not sufficient to allow me to
indulge very extensively these impulses ; and further, that my father, upon
whom I must usually fall back to pay the bills, does not view money matters
by no means as I do.''   In this statement it appears pretty plainly that in his
attacks the patient assumed a right to his father's property, which we are
perhaps justified in suggesting may be an echo of the deeper-lying, unconscious wish to supersede his father.

What this gifted observer had to say about the onset of his elations is again
interesting as giving evidence of the operation of a rebirth fancy.   This does
not occur as a crude delusion such as we have so frequently noted, but is
represented by the opinion that his feeling was like that which *would* go with
rebirth and return to childhood.   His own words express this with great
clearness.   After speaking of his obsession during the depressed period with
thoughts of his own folly and turpitude, he mentions that a time comes when
he realizes these feelings to be pathological.   He then goes on to say : " Directly I have made the ' break ' or ' plunge,' and given up and realized that
the whole disease is a force, now, at least, largely beyond my control, and
not to be regarded as my fault, and that there is some excuse for my apparently morally, cowardly actions, I at once begin to feel less remorse, and to
suffer less.   As already intimated a relaxation of tension ensues.

" Very soon a soothing, domestic, home-loving feeling sets in, and I am
in somewhat such a frame of mind as I knew as a child, when my mother put
me to bed with the measles, and cared for me tenderly, reading to me all day
until I was rather glad I was sick, and that I could have my own way and
domineer and be waited upon by inches, and that nothing was expected of
me, not even good humour.   In fact, at this stage of the disease, the loving
and interested care of some sympathetic person, now that the important
decisions have been made and the great steps taken, preferably a woman,
is almost craved for, and may be of inestimable advantage.   Above all one
wants then to be petted, nursed along, and relieved of all personal responsibility in the whole matter.

" I soon feel almost as if I had been born again.   The things about me,
and what is going on around me, assume new relations to myself.   And with,
of course, the obvious differences, caused by former associations, accumulated
experience, memory, etc., etc., my surroundings appear to me, to make
somewhat the same impressions upon my recuperating brain, as they seem
to produce upon the awakening and developing intellect of the child.

" I most assuredly have a certain restless, inquisitive, and at the same time, timid and withal decidedly childish interest in the objects about me, which is much more healthy and normal than my gloomy views and attitudes of the more acute period, which was much like a wreck of my normal self.

" This interest assumes, as my initiatory powers increase, with gaining strength of will, a more active form. I begin to desire to occupy myself with those objects, subjects or pursuits, for which I have manifested a healthy interest in my normal condition, and being a great believer in the force of habit, and in a regular, gradual development along natural lines, I humour these feelings and reaching-out aspirations all I can, with a desire to help myself along." This rather forced interest soon became spontaneous and then enthusiastic as the definite exhilaration commenced to show itself.

Another point which we have made in the introduction of our discussion of manic states, namely, that we are normally elated over prospective rather than completed achievements, is well borne out in these sentences : " The first attack came during the relaxation following some time after the realization of success, in the form of a depression. The second attack came as the pinnacle of success was being approached, during the very heat of the struggle, in the form of an exhilaration." These statements betray the abnormality of his sublimation. A normal sublimation provides a progressive outlet, wherein achievement is always satisfying, but when the sublimation is a symbolic outlet for tendencies not properly controlled by the individual, success in it naturally fails to solve the other problems, which leads, of course, to the feeling of failure. On the other hand, the prospect of success being of itself imaginary, carries with it the feeling of success not only in the specific activities in question, but also in those others which are the real problem of the individual.

This patient also furnished many descriptions of that psychological principle which we have termed distraction of thought. A few quotations will bear this out :

" On the whole, I feel that when I am exhilarated, my mind occupies itself, for the most part, with its own affairs. And its inspiration and motives for action are self-creative and come from within. It is, as a rule, too busy, and in too much of a hurry, to stop and make minute, rational, and detailed account in passing of external objects. Its tendency is towards flightiness." No better statement of the determinants of flight could be given. The way in which this process may be interrupted is also described with accuracy, for he goes on to say : " Though, of course, if observation be for the moment, its special occupation, as when acting as a coast pilot [he did this once successfully], it might be capable of observing and regarding with abnormal minuteness and accuracy." The next quotations give an exquisite statement of the psychology of inspiration, a problem akin to that of mania. As most introspectionists would agree, original thought occurs when we relax our critique of reality. This thought must then be criticied in order to determine its practical availability. In other words, there must be an alternate relaxation and application of the test of reality. The unconscious must be free from inhibition in order to initiate the new thought. Secondly, that which comes into consciousness must be examined to see if it shall be retained in consciousness or not. As this patient said, " The point seems to be, so far as I grasp it, that during an exhilaration the mind penetrates infinitely more deeply into all things, and receives flashes of almost divine light and wisdom, which open to it, momentarily, regions of thought hitherto difficult or impos ible of penetration. But, except in the milder form of the exhilaration, the mind's own restlessness, and impatient activity, interfere, for the time being at least, with the just application and the rational and appropriate, not to say the sane, use of what it has thus acquired." Normal inspiration passes over into psychopathic fantasy-building just at that point where the tendency of the unconscious to express itself overmasters the capacity of the individual's critique—" Naturally the more exhilarated I become the more difficult it is for me to reason to myself and to admit the insanity of my projects and hence to be willing to renounce or break away from them." When he was asked how he gauged his degree of abnormality in the absence of such external evidence, as loquaciousness, for example, would furnish, he answered that he based his opinion chiefly upon the way in which he had adhered to or relinquished the exaggerated ideas which he had formed, when more psychotic.

As his was a state in which he never completely lost contact with his environment, the latter could always affect his clinical condition. For instance, when, at the height of his exhilaration a few days before admission, he was in a car accident where a man was hurt, he was able to pull himself together for the time being and take charge of the affair in a perfectly sensible manner. Another example of environmental influence has already been mentioned in connection with his boasting. When in the company of those of good education his boasting was moderate and confined within the limits of possibility, if not probability, whereas, when talking to the hospital attendants, he would indulge in a much wilder expansiveness. Further examples of environmental influence may be of interest. He said, for instance, that tendency to talk seemed to increase rapidly in proportion as the circle of those with whom he came in contact was enlarged. Conversely, when his daily life brought him in in relation with but a few people, he would become in a week or ten days much quieter. He therefore concluded that isolation was the best form of treatment for his exhilaration. When excited by an audience, he found himself inspired to give didactic talks whose content was rational enough. But, that in his excitement evidence of loss of contact with the true demands of the situation was present, is shown by the following : " These talks are usually perfectly logical, correct, and instructive, and are often much appreciated by my hearers. They are not, however, always appropriate to the occasion, and their most striking abnormality lies in the superabundance of meat or information which they contain ; for my heated imagination conjures up far more material than the average person could possibly take in, and assimilate at one time, much less retain. A rational, experienced instructor would give shorter, less varied lessons."

The close relationship between psychotic expansiveness and normal business imagination is demonstrated in this example of accurate introspection : " During the heat of the telling I may be said, in a limited degree, and momentarily, to believe my own stories. I am not, however, sufficiently carried away to prevent my taking account of stock soon afterwards, and to separate the truth from the falsehood and to experience a definite regret for the latter. I have sometimes asked myself by what stretch of the imagination and silencing of my own conscience I could possibly, for example, aver ownership to real estate which I had in reality merely viewed and talked of buying ; or assert a complete mastery of branches of learning whose merest rudiments I was perfectly well aware only to have examined superficially. And I have, at such times, detected myself explaining it all to my conscience in some such way as the following : ' That I could easily, should occasion require, or were it in any way to become necessary for me to back up my statements, buy the land in question, or study the subject under consideration until I had mastered it.' Thus I try to soothe my conscience with the thought that I never assert things which are not, at least, within my power, and which I might not perfectly well have done, or indeed can do if necessary, or may even at the time perhaps fully intend to do. And in this way I excuse myself to myself, by imagining that I am in somewhat the same category as the merchant or broker, who undertakes to deliver, at some future time, articles which he has not yet bought, or makes prices on things which do not belong to him. For, we both undoubtedly think that we can produce the goods when called upon to do so."

As a further example of this he says : " Still it is interesting to note, however, that in spite of certain flightiness and volatility which have, at times, characterized me in this particular respect, I have later, by dint of months or years of persistence and application, succeeded in carrying out very much as I have planned ideas originally conceived in these heated ecstasies of the brain." The counter-tendency away from reality he proceeds to describe :

[Continuing this last quotation] " but during such exhilarated times themselves I rush on and on, stopping for very little real reflection or analysis, having lost, as it seems to me, the power of myself to check or restrain my impulses and ambitions ; though I am well aware even at the time, that the irresistible, insistent motive force often impels me to do things of which my reason does not then approve, and which I may regret bitterly later." As we have several times stated, just in so far as contact with environment is lost, and with it the desire to appear conventionally natural goes,—just to the same extent does emotionality appear in the behaviour of the manic patient. " During my worst and most severe exhilaration I had a tendency to become very emotional, hysterical, and even at times to break down and cry."

All these quotations show that his abnormality and normality appeared just in proportion to his loss or gain of contact with his environment. One objective observation was made which was highly important in this connection. When in the hospital it was noted that on the first day in which his behaviour was perfectly normal, he showed an unselfish interest in those about him for the first time. This demonstrates the existence of a dynamic emotional factor of much greater importance th n that of intellectual contact. So long as the patient's interest was self-centred, contact with his environment was forced, unnatural, and hence difficult to maintain. When, however, his emotional balance redirected his instinctive interest to a normal altruism, contact with those about him became no longer a matter of artificial effort but a natural thing. This was the true sign of recovery.

CHAPTER XXIX

THE PROGNOSIS OF MANIC STATES

HAVING now discussed the psychology of manic states at some length, it may be well in closing to view the question from a somewhat different angle. In so far as our work has been a matter of observation and correlation of observations, and not merely speculation, in just that degree have we been engaged in studying the symptomatology of manic-depressive insanity. One would expect that the more that was known about the symptoms and therefore of the disease process, the more secure would be the position of psychiatrists in predicting the outcome. In this respect we feel that some advance may be claimed, or, at least, indicated.

This study has, of course, been merely a preliminary one. For each problem solved, a dozen have sprung into existence. One of these is, What information may be gained from one attack which would enable the observer to predict recurrence or the frequence of recurrence ? Unfortunately we are not in a position to give any definite answer to this question, which will probably only be solved after many years of work. It is our opinion, however, that in all probability the patient, who presents during the psychosis many delusional ideas and on recovery is amnesic for them, is likely to have another attack whenever his imperfect make-up is subjected to a strain at all similar to the one which produced the original breakdown.

Occasionally we see patients who have been apparently normal for many years and who finally break down with a psychosis in which many abnormal tendencies come to expression. Some of these cases seem positively to luxuriate in this free outlet to the unconscious and appear to blow off steam, as it were, so that upon recovery they remain well for many years. Others, after an attack in which their unconscious tendencies are betrayed, have an intelligent interest in learning of their abnormal interests and seem to gain, from a discussion of the psychosis, a self-knowledge which prevents a recurrence of their trouble. Although we have not sufficient cases to prove our point, it seems probable that those individuals who have many attacks and forget their abnormal thoughts are just those who cannot derive any benefit from the psychosis. They are like sedentary dwellers on the banks of a river that periodically floods the valley. The inundation is regarded as an act of fate ; the river is never traced to its source and channels dug to supply alternate outlets when storm clouds burst.

If we consider, for instance, the case of Mary S., described above, who protested, when her productions were read to her, that there must have been some mistake, and who was merely depressed by any mention of her insane ideas, we can see how inevitable it was that she should have many attacks. Each attack seemed quite definitely the product of her pathological make-up and consequent inability to adapt herself to situations which were bound to recur. It was impossible to put her on her guard because all the information, which her psychosis laid bare to us, was meaningless to her.

More has been learned of definite practical value in connection with the problem of differentiating dementia praecox from the manic-depressive reactions. In dementia praecox, although the typical case shows a poverty or dissociation of affect, there are many cases that for many months appear to have a genuine elation, and it is these cases in which mistakes in diagnosis are probably most frequently made.

We have already mentioned that the prevailing content in the true manic state is of a sublimation, infantile ideas being transformed into an adult setting, or, if the infantile object of affection be brought directly into the spoken productions of the patient, no definite reference is made to this attachment being sexual, in the everyday use of the term. In other words, friendship, sympathy, communion of spirit in this or the other world, or desire for a Platonic relationship, is expressed. It is true that we find almost universally, when careful records are made, that a more definitely sexual interest is suggested, through free association, or in virtue of an identification of the infantile with the adult object, but the short circuit, as it were, is never made. Moreover, the dominant note in the true manic state seems to be interest in the sexual *relationship* with the adult object rather than in the specific *act*.

If we now compare this content with that observed in the manic-like dementia praecox patients, we find that the latter sooner or later make definite references to the infantile object as a sex object, and that the physical side of sexuality bulks much larger than in the manic depressive case. Further than that, the type of sex outlet is apt to be of the infantile order, representing what are perversions. The patients' autistic thoughts centre, therefore, around what are termed, in psychoanalytic literature, the secondary erogenous zones, rather than focussing on the genital regions.

Now we find that when a psychosis, seeming to be typical mania, contains ideas of this infantile type, the prognosis is bad. Either the attack in question goes on to a definite deterioration, or, after an apparent recovery, the patient deteriorates in a subsequent attack. Some examples of this may be cited. For instance, there is the case, which I reported some years ago[1], as a clear example of

[1] *Journal of Abnormal Psychology*, February, 1914.

psychoanalytic principles appearing in the delusional content of a psychosis. This patient presented a typical manic state, so far as the onset, genuine elation, manic behaviour and flight were concerned, but at no time was he considered to be a true manic case on account of the extreme infantilism of his productions. He lived under observation for 19 months, during which time there was no essential change in his clinical condition. There is no reason to suppose that had he lived ten years longer there would have been any change, consequently we are justified in regarding his psychosis as a chronic rather than a benign one. Another case may be mentioned which has appeared in the literature. In 1909 Dr. Ernest Jones[1] had reported the content of a similar psychosis for the purpose of demonstrating Freudian principles. According to his descriptions there was nothing to indicate that this woman suffered from dementia praecox, but we felt so sure that no manic-depressive case could utter the thoughts which she expressed, that inquiries were made in 1914 as to the outcome. Dr. C. K. Clarke, of Toronto, very kindly looked up the case and reported that she was at that time in a state of apparently chronic deterioration.

Both these cases presented quite florid infantile ideas. The following case is of more interest, inasmuch as the infantile references were not prominent and might not have been recorded and not great pains been taken in her examination. Her psychoses were not always typically manic, yet she apparently made such good recoveries that she was always diagnosed as a manic-depressive case or " allied to manic-depressive ".

CASE 40. *Margaret W.* was a woman born in 1875 who had her first attack in 1904 at the age of 29. She had been married at that time for a number of years and had had four children and one miscarriage. The family history, it is stated, had been negative for any evidence of nervous or mental disease. As to her make-up, she was always sensitive, much inclined to brood over, and to worry about things, especially after her marriage. She was suspicious, having a tendency to think that people were talking about her, although she would never divulge what she thought the neighbours said. In her married life, her husband claimed, she was affectionate except during her attacks. He further stated that at the time he first met her, although she was outwardly jolly and lively, she really took life seriously.

First Attack : About six weeks before the birth of her fourth child—in 1904 —she became nervous, biting her finger nails, clenching and unclenching her hands, as if she were brooding, and distressed about something. A few days after the childbirth, she suddenly became excited, calling " police, police," and ordered her husband out of the house. He was in his shirt sleeves at the time. When he put on his hat and coat, she did not know him. According to another account, this excitement appeared when one of her babies had a convulsion. Excited by the spectacle, she threw her wedding ring into the stove and turned against her husband. If we accept this account, we have at the very outset an indication of a reaction which is atypical for manic-depressive insanity. Injury to a child is, as we have so frequently observed, an infantile wish-fulfilment which is not accepted freely by a patient whose psychosis is benign. Such an event should lead to a depression or a depressed

---

[1] Ernest Jones, " Notes on a Case of Hypomania," *American Journal of Insanity*, October, 1909.

anxiety state. Excitement with manic features such as immediately appeared imply a certain acceptance of the idea on the part of the personality, which is more of the dementia praecox reaction. This psychosis seems to have been characterized by a rambling, incoherent speech, with much distractibility and at times, definite flight. She was noisy and excited. In nine months, she had apparently recovered completely.

Following this attack she was always more suspicious of her neighbours than she had been before. She also became more moody, being one day jolly, the next day morose and irritable. With the latter spells she frequently complained of headaches. She continued to take good care of her home and children, however, and was sexually normal except during her attacks, when she would not only have nothing to do with her husband, but would not even let him come near her.

Second Attack : At 33 years of age, when eight months pregnant, a second cousin, a priest, committed suicide. When she heard the news she became slow, languid, and depressed. She was apparently in this condition when the childbirth occurred, but showed no other reaction for some two months. Then, one week before admission, without known cause, she suddenly turned against her husband, accusing him of unfaithfulness and insisting the children were not hers.

In the hospital she remained for two months in an anomalous state, where she seemed puzzled, but was too inaccessible to determine the actual degree of her confusion. She was quiet, but had occasional outbursts of irritability. Two months after admission she became brighter, apparently in better contact with her environment, but at this time made the following extra-ordinary remark, " When my baby was buried that queer feeling came over me. I thought I saw my child in a bad place, some animal is in my inside eating it up." This is the second anomalous feature from a psychological standpoint. The idea of having an animal inside one is so fantastic as to make one think at once of dementia praecox. But there is a more important point than that. We have here another example of an infantile wish-fulfilment this time manufactured by the patient herself and not an actual event. Such an idea, according to our observations, should only appear in a state of marked anxiety or depression. To have it come into consciousness at a time when the speaker had a normal or nearly normal mood implies an independence of the patient's autistic life from the personality as a whole, that is strongly suggestive of the " splitting " of the schizophrenic reaction. Before becoming completely normal, she assigned her trouble to a fright, telling of a telephone message which she interpreted as news of her father's death. Retrospectively she stated that throughout the attack she had had ideas of her husband's infidelity, of her father and husband quarrelling, and that she had heard her father and brother talking together, During the psychosis there were isolated examples of flight and distractibility. On the whole, the reaction looked like that of either an absorbed manic state or a partial stupor reaction.

Third Attack : This attack occurred when she was 37 years of age and was poorly observed. After a sudden onset she was apparently rather typically manic for six months. The only note made on the content stated that she was " expensive." When she cleared up, the examining physician suspected that she still had some ideas of infidelity, although she was officially recorded as " recovered."

Fourth Attack : Ten months after discharge from the hospital, when she was 39 years of age, another attack occurred. According to her husband's account, there was a sudden onset without known cause a week before she came to the hospital. She was nervous for several days, biting her nails. Then she became excited, wanting him to pay $600 for the house where they lived. She accused him of infidelity. A doctor, who was summoned, she thought was a lawyer and wanted him to call a second lawyer, so that they might together settle an estate of $75,000 which she thought belonged to her husband. She also talked of being an actress. According to her own statement given when she was quite clear, there had been for a long time trouble with a neighbour woman (the delusion was that this woman wanted to get the patient's house). Six months before, she had found herself pregnant and wanted to have an abortion performed. A month before the attack she said that the children had diphtheria, that the husband was ill with bronchitis and was failing. She nursed him, became quite worn out and then had a quarrel with her husband that caused her excitement. Here again we have mentioned a situation suggesting an infantile wish-fulfilment (illness of children and husband) to which she reacted with an excitement instead of a depression as one would expect in a true manic-depressive case.

While still at home she began singing nonsense, was very restless and slept poorly. At the Observation Pavilion she was noted as being restless, irritable, excited and flighty. Interesting, in view of her subsequent emotional reaction, was some preoccupation, at this time, with ideas of death, for she identified one of the physicians as an undertaker's helper and asked whether there were blue bells or red bells on the corpse. When admitted, she was quiet and agreeable for several days, being apparently rather natural. The third night, however, she was restless and, when ordered to return to bed, became assaultive. As soon as she got into her bed she was quite quiet and as natural as if nothing had happened. There then followed two months, during which her condition suggested a partial stupor reaction, which we may perhaps correlate with the ideas of death mentioned before. She seemed languid, tired and had poor attention. She was agreeable but sometimes irritable and rarely jocular. She complained of drowsiness and said she was trying to put her troubles out of her mind. This last statement would be incompatible with the stupor reaction, where one expects to find with the apathy a vacancy in the patient's mind, and the appearance of ideas, if they do emerge, only in episodes. She made isolated statements of a highly psychotic nature. She said, for instance, that one of the nurses was going with her husband, that she had no children, or again that the doctor was going with another woman. These seemed to be ideas, that suddenly came so strongly into consciousness, that they had to be expressed. On the other hand, she was invariably evasive when asked if she were married or not.

She then gave birth to a healthy child, after which her condition remained for some three weeks as it had been in the previous two months, although during this latter period she cried occasionally and seemed depressed. For the following month there was a mild exhilaration in which she was flighty, flippant and gradually more and more intractable. She acted as if she thought she owned and managed the hospital. At times her utterances were so disjointed as to seem almost scattered and, what was stranger, was the fact that these incomprehensible utterances were made at periods when there was no marked emotional disturbance, but at a time when she seemed pretty well in contact with her environment. As an example of this she suddenly said, when speaking of someone bothering her during the period when she was pregnant, " Now if you were size, you could X and I's and get a lawyer and take some other person's children away. Mrs. F. she calls herself, I guess her name is C. I take sympathy with her, she buried a daughter. When you are good to people it never does you any good." The first sentence of this is a significant one, but the latter part she at once explains, so that it appears to be quite a normal flight. Mrs. F. was a neighbour who bothered her and she had the delusion that she had married a Dr. C., but the reference to size and X and I remains totally inexplicable and, therefore, seems like scattered speech. At this time she also made vague references to divorce, disinheriting children and to her shooting a man (no particular emotional reaction) and, quite rarely, she made frankly erotic remarks to the physicians.

Then her behaviour improved somewhat, and while still given to a very mild flight she talked about her psychosis. She explained the statement at the Observation Pavilion about the undertaker by saying that she identified a man there as an undertaker whom she had known in Albany and thought he had come to bury her. She stated that she had " thoughts " not exactly voices in each attack. She spoke of her enemies both in and out of the hospital.

Further she had a good deal to say about property she owned, a house for instance, and thought people had given her shops and various presents. She claimed that the hospital belonged to her and was an actress' home. When mentioning this she made another statement highly suggestive of a dementia praecox utterance, " Income of 56 billion times 18 years ; it is a study in analysis however ; it is sort of a civil service course ; 18 times 18, condense it and it means that father wants me to marry some smart man."

At this same interview she proceeded quite calmly to detail ideas of that degree of infantility which we consider to be incompatible with a good prognosis. She said that her father had been wanting to marry her for thirty years (she said this quite unconcernedly). With more evasiveness, she admitted having the same ideas about her brother. When asked about her mother, she said " I guess she is dead." Then went on to say that she had died in 1880, but sometimes she thought she was alive, and that she did not know whether her brother was older than she or not. Further she stated that there were a lot of men who wanted to marry her, but also many girls wished to do the same. Her father and brother wished to marry her in the same sense that her husband married her. It was different, she explained, with the girls. She would go around with them and have a good time, live with them, sleep with them. Her mother, she thought, also wished to go around with her ; she said she would live with her but would not sleep with her.

Following this she was for a month rather more elated and frequently assaultive. Then for three months her condition showed a gradual improvement. Finally she was thought to have completely recovered. When she left the hospital she denied her false ideas, but still blamed her husband for her commitment, and was apparently inclined to entertain suspicions of him.

The patient remained superficially well for some twenty months after leaving the hospital, but when she was again returned her husband stated that right from the time of her first attack she was chronically suspicious of the neighbours talking of her, and that this tendency seemed to be stronger after each attack. She had also been gradually growing more moody, one day jolly, the next day morose, irritable. In spite of this, however, she worked well and took good care of her home and children.

Fifth attack : Seven days before her readmission in her fifth attack (then aged 40) her husband asked her if she had found $2 which he had mislaïd. She replied that she had not. We have seen that an actual quarrel with her husband was sufficient to precipitate a psychotic reaction. How much more unstable her condition had become was shown by the fact that, although there was no accusation and no quarrel, when her husband asked this simple question, the possibility of an accusation being made was enough to stir her up. She was restless for three days, although she said nothing, but on the evening of the first day her son remarked to his father that his mother was going to have another " spell ". Four days before admission her husband told her that he was going out for a walk, to which she rejoined, " Don't you come back unless you bring $25 ". On his return he discovered the house locked. He entered through a window, and found her sitting at a table in an abstracted way. She asked, " Did you get that money ? " On his replying in the negative, she at once became angrily excited, and forbade him to stay in the house unless he produced the $25. She accused him of non-support, and wanted to have him arrested. She was taken at once to the Observation Pavilion.

There, as before, she was noted as being rather typically manic, although by the time she had reached the hospital she was quiet, in fact, throughout this entire admission, which lasted for some seven months, she at no time showed any definite mood reaction of a manic type. As a rule she preferred to sit apart from the other patients, and, even when with them, would not converse. Although she often objected to going to meals or going out for walks, she never offered any physical resist ,nce to such orders. When observed from a distance she had a subdued, meditative expression, although there were occasionally quick movements of the eyes, as if she were covertly following the movements of those around her. When questioned she usually brightened up and smiled naturally, responding promptly to the questions. She might even be stimulated to become quite bright, with natural laughter and evident mirth, but this was also transitory. A more striking phenomenon was her frequent, obstinate refusal to answer questions, or, when apparently accessible to examination, a sudden protest against some quite ordinary question which she criticized as being personal. Quite rarely some topic of conversation with the physician would move her to tears, as, for instance, on one occasion when she spoke of her husband wanting to get rid of her and perhaps kill her. In the latter part of her stay she cried more frequently. This seemed to be at that period when her ideas were diminished, so far as their insistence was concerned, and when she was more concerned with the possibility of her returning home.

She gave the impression of always being very clearly oriented. Five weeks after admission, however, she insisted that it was Indian summer instead of midsummer, and that she had been there for three months. A moment before, however, she had given the month correctly, and it seems not impossible that this was a definitely delusional distortion. She seemed to know the names of only a few people around her. In other ways her orientation showed no defect. Four months later, when her ideas had receded a little, she gave all the data of orientation without hesitation or mistake. It is certain that her contact with the environment was quite keen, even at times when she was living in a riot of delusions. For example, at such times she spoke of reading people's thoughts. It was then asked if she could tell what the physician and stenographer were thinking of, to which she replied that they were thinking that she was crazy and making very silly claims. This accurate observation of hers is important diagnostically because, as we have seen in our typical manic cases, delusional ideas in any great profusion do not flourish except when the patient becomes absorbed and rather thoroughly divorced from reality.

Her productions were rarely flighty, more often they were clear enough in sequence, although obscure on account of their delusional reference. This process at times went to the point of positive scattering; for instance, when asked about her daughter, she became rather excited, and said, " Now you are going to have her here under the same bubbles that you have got me ".

In response to inquiries she gave utterance to a great many ideas, some of them systematized, others rather incomprehensible. As before, fancies of her having money and houses appeared. At times she connected this property with her father's alleged wealth, and once she stated he owned Ward's Island, where the hospital was situated. Other rather expansive actions were that she could nominate any one for governor or for mayor. A possible expansive notion was contained in this isolated statement : " They say I am the Statue of Liberty, and the Statue of Liberty is taxes."

As usual there was much preoccupation with sex. She had a great deal to say about the immorality of various women outside, while not infrequently she was violently assaultive toward nurses or fellow patients whom she accused of going with her husband. Once she stated that she knew of it by electrical sensations and by feelings which she had in her genital region whenever such an act took place. Similarly she claimed to have such sensations whenever her husband thought of her. In explanation of this she said that she thought " something " must have been left inside of her at the time of her last confinement (a frequent idea in dementia praecox). Quite often she spoke of clairvoyant powers. At times it was her husband who was gifted so. He belonged to a secret society, and had a watch of magic powers. Again, she could read the thoughts of those around her. For instance, she claimed to know all about the family affairs of the physician. Perhaps connected with this theme was a complicated idea about a nurse in another hospital being a detective who was working to have the New York Central Railroad take a certain man into its employ.

Throughout there was a great antagonism against her husband. She thought he wished to kill her, and continually denied that he was her husband, with many accusations against his faithfulness. As to who her autistic husband was there was much confusion. At times it was her father, again different men by the same name, or men whom she had known in her girlhood, friends of her father. This confusion extended itself to all the family relationships. She was doubtful as to who her father was or her mother, and even could not tell the relative ages of her brothers and sisters. She spoke sometimes of her father being governor or of his being a priest. At other times she expatiated on his luxurious life on Fifth Avenue, where she alleged he was living with a well-known society woman. Occasionally she talked of hearing her father's and brother's voices. Her mother, she claimed, was still alive, and was a most attractive woman. Sometimes she fancied that she was a Catholic sister, having become so after returning to life. A rather isolated delusion was that some vague employer ordered her to behave the way she did, and that she obeyed him because he was paying her to do so.

Four months after her admission her delusional ideas began to be less insistent. This was shown first in her capacity to discuss them a little more objectively, later to her capacity to deny them. Finally a point was reached where she said that she had been insane, and quite evidently was amnesic for some of her earlier statements. She passed through a phase in which she explained the origin of a good many of her ideas, although she still adhered to them. For instance, when asked about a statement to the effect that she could live in the governor's mansion if she wished, she replied, " They said my brother was ringleader in Albany, and could get anything he wanted. He belongs to some Masonic Lodge. They say they can do anything they want ". At the same time she recognized quite definitely that her ideas were looked upon as insane, for she remarked, " How can I keep well so that I will not get such ideas ? I cannot afford to be sick ". But on the same day that she made this statement she continued to abuse her husband, and express the notion that she belonged to the same Masonic Lodge as did he. So, although her psychotic ideas were under some control, they had not really disappeared. She made such a normal impression, however, that she was allowed parole and returned to her husband.

Sixth attack : She was able to maintain an outward appearance of sanity for only four weeks. The circumstances were as follows : Soon after returning home she was told that her father had recently died. As we have seen, many of her ideas centred around the acquisition of property, which she believed her father to own. As a matter of fact, he did leave a small estate, but disinherited both the patient and a brother in his will. She brooded over this, and soon began to have spells of abstraction, accompanied by heavy sighing, and was irritable when aroused from these spells. Three weeks after she had left the hospital, she got the idea that they must move to another flat, and, while her husband was away at work, picked out one and paid a deposit on it. The landlord, however, suspected her sanity, and refused to go further with the negotiations. In the course of her talk with him, she said she would have to go to Albany to see her mother. Considering that her mother had been dead since the patient was five years old, this was regarded by her family as being pretty definite evidence of her being again insane. The day following this she left home, but came back on the morrow, when she explained that she had abandoned her family, because she was afraid she would be returned to the hospital. This shows pretty well her type of insight. She evidently recognized that her ideas were getting the better of her, in the sense that she was becoming unable to keep them to herself, and knew that they were considered by others to be insane. A few days later her conduct became more irrational, with her usual antagonism to her husband, and it was necessary to return her to the hospital. This could not be accomplished without force.

For two days she lay quietly in her bed, seldom speaking, and rarely doing more than shaking her head in response to a question. She had a number of crying spells, and tears were apt to come when she was spoken to. When an effort was made to examine her, she refused to answer practically all questions, and when pressed became vituperative, profane, obscene.

The next two months her condition was so much like that of her previous attacks that no further description is needed. During this time she made a most tell-tale statement. While her case was being discussed between the physicians, the remark was dropped that her condition was about the same as it had been in former attacks. She interrupted to say " *Well, I tell you facts when I come, but I have to smooth it over in order to get out* ". The significance of this statement lies not merely in that it was confirmatory of the suspicion already held that she made a conscious effort to appear normal at the time of her improvement, but much more in the use of the word " fact ". Apparently she was never really free from delusions. Her ideas were always facts to her, and her improvement consisted merely in the capacity to disregard the existence of these " facts " until they were again impressed on her mind by a renewed association with her family and the outside world.

This improvement began a couple of months after her return to the hospital, and six weeks later she was again paroled to the care of her husband, and left the service of the Psychiatric Institute. Her career since then has been as follows : After being home for ten days she deserted her husband, and her whereabouts were not known. A month after her parole, a letter was received from her, in which she refused to give her address, stating that her husband had driven her out of the house without any money, and she had gone to seek employment, which she had secured, and was working regularly. Three and a half months later she was again returned to the hospital, where she remained for six months, and was again paroled, but was able to get along outside only for five weeks. After another ten months in the hospital she was paroled again, but this time stayed out only for a week. At the time of writing she is still a patient in the hospital. So for nearly four years her name has not been off the list of the hospital patients, and it is safe to assume that her condition is really chronic.

We may look, therefore, on her psychosis as being of a malignant type, and resembled manic-depressive insanity chiefly in that it was characterized throughout by exacerbations and remissions, and that in some of the earlier attacks there were mood reactions resembling those of the benign psychoses. On the other hand, correlated with the malignancy of the disease process, there were, as has been pointed out, two features that we would regard as having important dynamic significance. First, there was the appearance of infantile ideas, and, secondly, the existence of delusions in a setting of almost perfect contact with the environment.

The following case is of particular interest, since clinically, her appearance on admission was much more typical than that of the woman, whom we have just been describing. Further than that, her infantile sexuality appeared in gross form only once, and in only one other instance was there a definite stressing of the physical rather than of the mental aspect of this attachment. This case was regarded as an exception to our general rule, which correlates infantile sexuality with dementia praecox, until the subsequent history of the patient was learned.

CASE 41. *Margaret L.* was a single woman aged 36 at the time she came under observation in April, 1915. The history stated that she had had a former attack at the age of 23 with a perfect recovery and had since been efficient. The second attack was said to have developed when her father lost his position. This psychosis was, symptomatically, a typical manic state, with marked elation and flight, some overactivity, an important point being that her affect at first was quite natural and in harmony with her actions and productions. Her ideas may be briefly detailed as follows :

The usual interest in adult love and marriage was represented by much talk of a former lover ; she called the examiner and also another doctor by his name. Once she spoke of identification with him : " He is in me now, I close my eyes and realise he is." At another time she said : " Did we dream those nights together, or did the devil get them ? " Two other men she also spoke of as her lovers. She talked of the marriage room and said people ought to get married in spite of the " darn churches."

There were, too, a good many religious references in which a transformation of her father into God was indicated : " I have been in heaven, I saw what was a realization of the Deity." Her father's Holy Spirit guided her to say that he was highly regarded by the priests. Again she remarked : " Call no man on earth father, the Bible says." She spoke of the crucifixion. Finally the customary expansiveness appeared in statements that she was the Madonna.

In most of her talk abut her family (which was considerable) her statements were rather a type which we expect to meet in a manic state. She spoke a good deal of her father directly and said the doctor was he. At other times, of course, she said the doctor was her lover, but this type of alternate identification is what we usually find in manic-depressive cases. Once, however, there was a suspicious literalness about this identification when she remarked to the physician, " You are his body, you know." Her antagonism to her mother came out, when she spoke of a dream in which she had killed her mother and in much talk of her being a foster child, the daughter of another woman. She also identified herself with her sister (a mother substitute), a similar mechanism to that of identification with the Madonna. Dissatisfaction with the marriage of her father and mother was reflected in repeated statements about Napoleon and Josephine, he having been unfaithful to the latter. Napoleon, whom she alternately named as Jesus, was calling to her frequently.

As we have seen time and again, a common expression for union with the father is the fantasy of mutual death. In our patient this idea was indicated, but became the medium for a definitely infantile sexual delusion. She said : " I thought papa's torso or body was beside me ; it was just as if he lay beside me in bed. . . . I kissed him so he would live." But then she added, " I said this is the way I kissed J. (her former lover), I put my tongue into his mouth." It was this notion of fellatoristic contact with her father which we regarded as highly suspicious.

Her subsequent career was as follows : Three months after admission she became resistive, turbulent, but talked very little. Such productions as were noted were quite incoherent. She was assaultive, interfered with the nurses, frequently disrobed, exposing herself thoroughly, and constantly masturbated. In her speech she was obscene and erotic. This condition, which was much more indicative of dementia praecox than of manic-depressive insanity, continued for some six months, while she remained in perfect physical condition. Then she began to belch gas and lose weight. Three months later her hair began to come out and sores appeared on her lips. She became untidy and seclusive, talking very little. Then a urinary examination indicated parenchymatous nephritis. Two years and three months after admission she was sent to a disturbed ward. Five months later a diarrhoea developed. At this time she did not reply to questions, made peculiar guttural sounds in her throat, and did not seem to appreciate messages sent from her father and mother. As there was no evidence of profound toxemia, the probability is that this was an indication of deterioration rather than of organic dementia. Three years and three months after admission she received a laceration of the scalp. This became infected. She continued to deteriorate and finally died six weeks later from aspiration pneumonia.

As the symptoms of deterioration preceded the appearance of physical disease by some six months, and as this deterioration consistently developed much in advance of the symptoms of somatic illness, we feel justified in claiming that the mental picture was essentially that of dementia praecox. An important point to bear in mind in this connection is that typical manic-depressive cases who die of intercurrent physical diseases show no such tendency to deterioration in the dementia praecox sense.

The following case is of interest because the principle of non-appearance of definitely infantile sexual ideas in a true manic state was utilized in making a diagnosis, which the subsequent course of the psychosis justified. After a rather acute onset, the patient presented a typical manic appearance, and there was considerable division of opinion as to the prognosis. It is in just such a case that a new principle, such as we put forward, is of value.

CASE 42. *Eva M.* was an unmarried girl 22 years of age when she came under observation. Her family history was negative, so far as nervous and mental disease was concerned. As a child she had been active, but after the age of 12 became rather seclusive, preferring to spend much time in reading rather than in social activity. She was not talkative but reticent. At school she was a hard and successful student, and was a regular church-goer. As a child she was friendly with men, but later became shy with them. In school she was sensitive and afraid of being laughed at. She was over-conscientious. As she grew older her antagonism to men became plain to her family, as she had no love affairs and was always finding fault with any man of her acquaintance. At one year of age she had " marasmus ", but subsequently was physically healthy, except for menstrual irregularities. Menstruation began at 13½ years of age, was always irregular, painful, accompanied by twitching of her face, and a complaint of things being " black." Occasionally she appeared to lose consciousness for a few minutes, but would come back to life with administration of smelling-salts. This disturbance continued until she was 21, when she was advised to put her feet in hot water, and this treatment seemed to do away with these manifestations, which were, possibly, mainly neurotic.

Mental abnormality began when she was 16. Her father one day asked why she had forgotten the meat for dinner (she was not to blame). She at once had an attack of hysterical crying and screaming, her body stiffened, her hands clenched, she seemed in terror of her father. A year later, after having a term at the high school, she had an attack of what was called " nervous prostration ", which her physician ascribed to overstudy. For a whole summer she had spells of depression with some crying. She stayed at home, doing little or no work, and was very quiet. In the autumn her condition improved and she returned to school, but only for three or four weeks. Her last day in school she handed in a composition which won a silver medal. Three days later she suddenly screamed, and when her mother went to her, said she could not help it. From that time on, she was kept at home, although she once attended a course in millinery at the Y.W.C.A. At home she did a good deal of embroidery, went out walking and occasionally to the theatres. The family felt that she was in a somewhat nervous condition and watched her rather closely. During this period of four or five years she would have crying spells about the beginning of each year, the occasion for which she could never explain. This crying became more frequent during the year and a half before admission. During the last twelve months she read less than she had before, and had occasional laughing spells at inappropriate times, such as at church. She seemed more moody and had more of a desire to avoid company. Occasionally she would talk to herself. For the last few months it seemed as if she were less grown up ; she would kick her feet around, was not so ladylike as before. Sometimes also she would talk in a babyish voice.

More definite symptoms set in about a month before admission. She began to have spells of talking at night as if carrying on a conversation and occasionally made quite peculiar remarks. For instance, she walked about ten miles one day, and when asked why she did not ride, said she did not have the " power ", although she saw taxis and trolley-cars (she had money with her).

Three days before admission she wished to go out, but was advised not to, so she sat down by the front window, and later said that she wished she had gone out. The following day she went again to the same window, and her father, fearing that she might jump out, asked her to close the window. She at once became excited, angry, told him that it was not his home. When her mother tried to quiet her, she flew at him, scratching and kicking, and then attacked her mother also. They could do nothing with her, but when she was left alone she gradually quieted down, and began to talk to herself, saying such words as " baby monkey, want to eat grass, papa monkey." The following day she behaved fairly normally and went to bed at four in the afternoon. In the middle of the night she was heard talking as if carrying on conversation with someone, but her talk was very disconnected. When her father went into her room and wished to give her some aromatic spirits of ammonia, she became very angry. Half an hour later she began to talk out of the window, using very vulgar and profane language. She then got up, dressed, and left the house. Her father followed her. She refused to have him stay with her and screamed so that the police came, and she was taken to the Observation Pavilion.

On admission she was somewhat over-active, apt to be playful, and talked and acted in an elated way. Occasionally she cried when speaking of a desire to go home. Her mood was always appropriate to the content of her talk. Her orientation seemed perfect, except that she might say it was Friday instead of Saturday ; although she frequently misidentified those about her in the course of her flight, she seemed to know them perfectly when questioned directly. Her productions were given in what seemed to be a quite typical flight, but were so rapid that it was impossible to get any long connected samples stenographically. She was always distractible, as could be demonstrated at any time by presenting any new object before her, on which she would comment. Much of her productions were put in the past tense and she usually spoke of herself as " she ". A sample of her flight may be quoted : " God damn it who wants to beg, borrow or steal—they tell me I had a baby, and it looks like you. I says I have good sense . . . She knows hieroglyphics—parallelogram—the baby can walk why don't you . . . they do love to entertain the gentlemen—she's a bitch if there ever was one— she says who's Grace Wilson, I said she's a society woman— on the advice of my grandmother I reported it, that's inherited information—the National Suit Co. will corroborate . . . That's what she is, a law student, she's got glasses (looking at stenographer)—down with the Trust Company . . . I said your belongings, she says don't bother, you're not a reader—she says I keep a disorderly house, I got to support a man and a woman—not necessarily—I says did you ever hear of the vaccination—so you don't care for the position—I said I will steal my face picture—in the name of God who invented lies . . . That girl over there don't know how to write—take a text book in your hands, and read now if you like, show her what you can do—the only thing I can do is to sit with a gimpy leg," etc.

On account of the difficulty in recording all that she said, the trend of her ideas had to be pieced together from the short statements, which it was possible to record. These were mainly statements which were constantly being reiterated. For instance, there was much talk of antagonism against both her parents, with a denial of their existence, and a claim that she had no home. She had a great deal to say about menstruation, about its being produced in various queer ways, about its being " unlawful ". She spoke often of going naked. She was to have children. Masturbation was often mentioned. Rarely she made allusion to death and coffins. Once she said something about being in love with Jesus Christ, and then immediately added, " I wonder who's my father ". Again, she remarked : " The devil says I am the resurrection and the light ". A most striking feature in her productions was its obscenity. Much of this on examination proved to be definitely infantile sexuality. For instance, she talked continually of some one putting a bean in her rectum, or of some man putting a revolver up her rectum and shooting. This seemed to have some connection with her menstruation.

This condition continued for about three months with slight variations, when she would become more intractable, and during the latter part of this period she wet the bed and masturbated, both without shame. During this time she made other remarks of infantile type. She said, for instance, that her mother was a prostitute, and spoke of having been castrated by her. She said she had a child inside, she could hear its voice. Once in reply to the question as to what made her nervous she answered that she could feel people having sexual contact with her, although she could not see them, and went on to talk as if this had caused her menstruation.

After these three months, spontaneous speech very largely disappeared, although she would sometimes talk after much urging, and when she did, her productions seemed to show more scattering than pure flight. Contact with the environment was very largely lost ; she indulged in a great deal of silly laughter without real elation, and presented, on the whole, an appearance quite typical of dementia praecox. There was no essential change in her condition in more than five years, during which we had the opportunity of seeing her. It may be worth mentioning that a positive diagnosis of dementia praecox was made a day or two after her admission, when it was noted that she spoke of having a bean put in her rectum.

The most fundamental principle in our theory of manic-depressive insanity is the correlation of the mood reaction with the content. Ordinarily we consider as content, those ideas which we conclude are in the patient's mind, after studying his productions and actions. If he reacts to these in a certain way, we consider the case to be one of manic-depressive insanity. As a matter of fact, and in a wide sense, the content should not be confined to these alone but should include situations, as well as ideas, which determine the patient's behaviour. This, then, includes the precipitating causes. There are certain situations which, to the normal individual, are depressing or produce anxiety or elation. Such events should call forth similar reactions in a psychosis if the disease process is benign. We have already, in one of the cases cited above, noted that the patient became elated when the life of her child was threatened, and we stated that this reaction was anomalous for manic-depressive insanity and therefore suggestive of dementia praecox. Sometimes we can gather a hint as to the gravity of the psychotic process from the reaction to the precipitating cause alone. If a situation arises which represents an infantile wish-fulfilment and the patient reacts to this with elation rather than with depression or anxiety, it implies an acceptance of the suggestion which should, according to our theory, only occur in the profounder psychotic condition of dementia praecox. The following case illustrates this.

A young man whose mother was a patient in a hospital for the insane had a quarrel with the others in his family, which arose from his criticism of their neglect of the mother. He announced to them that, even though they might all abandon her he would not, and promptly developed a typical manic state. In this instance the situation implied an intimacy between himself and his mother in which the rest of the family were not included ; in other words, the way was left open for him to assume a proprietorship of his mother. This would naturally be an infantile wish-fulfilment. When the case came to our attention he had already made, apparently, a complete recovery, but we were so convinced that this was a malignant rather than a benign type of reaction to this situation, that he was given a careful examination to see how complete this recovery really was. No amount of questioning could adduce any evidence of his being insane until the conversation, more or less by chance, turned to the question of his sex development, and it was then found that he had a mass of definite delusions about his sex organs and their functions. We felt justified, therefore, in concluding that he was really suffering from dementia praecox in a mild form and that the manic state simply represented an exacerbation of the psychosis. Of course, had he been examined during the period of elation, with a view to discovering all the ideas which were present in his mind, it is quite possible that a definite praecox type of content might have been elicited.

As can be seen in a critical reading of the cases which we have just been quoting, infantility of content in a manic state is rarely present without there being something slightly unusual about the other symptoms, although these other irregularities would normally not be sufficiently obvious to justify a diagnosis. The irregularity which we have most frequently noted is a lack of proportion between the luxuriance of psychotic ideas and the degree of distraction of thought. In our typical manic cases, when the patient betrays the existence of many delusions, he also shows evidence of being in poor contact with his environment. We therefore now regard the presence of many delusions with perfect orientation as a bad prognostic sign. If the patient gives utterance to many false ideas but is quite clear in his speech and plainly in good contact with his immediate environment, that is evidence of a mental splitting, the essential feature of the schizophrenic reaction. The dementia praecox patient is living at the same time in two worlds of which one is fantastic and the other is the world of actuality ; the nature of the latter he grasps and with it he is in contact. The typical manic case, on the other hand, gives more or less completely undivided attention to his psychotic ideas, and if these are of the type which are divorced from reality, he loses all contact with his environment.

The following case is of interest in this connection. For the first week or two of observation no diagnosis was made. Dementia praecox was, of course, suspected, but the cardinal symptoms were not present in sufficiently marked degree to be impressive, and there was no infantility in the content. On reviewing the case, however, we saw that there had been a marked discrepancy between the degree in which his speech was dominated by psychotic thoughts and the clearness of his orientation. This should have enabled us to make a diagnosis at the outset.

CASE 43. *Salvatore L.* was an Italian, married, and aged 30 when he came under observation some eight years ago. The onset was sudden, one week before admission, according to his wife, who stated that he was worrying over the love affair of a sister-in-law. Then he became restless and talkative, going to many theatres, but not showing any marked elation or excitement. On admission he seemed rather dull and absorbed, and spoke hesitatingly, as if he were groping for his ideas. All his utterances were poorly connected and irrelevant to the external situation. Recurrent topics were his innocence, his relations with his wife, the father's death, going out with girls, his not having wronged any girl, and other boys fooling. A stenographic sample of his productions at this time was as follows : " Well, I cannot understand what is going on. Somebody made me believe my father died. Then I said . . . three weeks later a letter said my old man was dead . . . I was wearing mourning." (When was that ?) " I can't hear that." (When did your father die ?) " On . . . about a couple of years " (What are they saying ?) " They were saying ' Your father is dead. Why don't you wear mourning ? ' I could not stay home three days. I cried very much . . . I was married two weeks . . . my mother came over and said, ' Youı father died.' " (What else happened ?) " We were two friends playing pool. Nothing happened between two . . . nothing wrong between one another . . . a ball jumped out and hit me in the mouth." (What else ?) " Some boys, you know, fool around. I said ' Don't fool with my . . . but I think there is nothing wrong in that . . . I was sleeping home, I was sleeping with my wife, he saw me, he said, ' Get up, I want to talk to you. I was sorry,' he says to me, ' I was thinking on one way ' . . . I says ' You are a single fellow, I am married. You stay for you, I stay for me, that was all . . . there is nothing between two orothers against one mother, there is nothing to trouble " (What have they said about you ?) " I was pencil writing (seeing physician's pencil), and my boss said ' When you see a pencil like this buy me one. They look like silver,' " etc.

As will be observed, these productions are not unlike the utterances of an absorbed manic indulging in reminiscences, and probably full of delusional thoughts. Distractibility also would be quite natural in an absorbed manic. An interesting thing was, however, that, when his attention could be secured, he was found to be well oriented, and that he could perform simple arithmetical tests with very few mistakes. This, of course, might also occur with an absorbed manic, but if it did, it would be accompanied by signs of closer contact with the environment, as evidenced by a heightened mood, a greater productivity of speech, and a greater lucidity. With this patient, however, evidence of intellectual contact with the environment appeared without there being any change whatever in his mood or type of productions.

For some weeks he remained in this condition, never at any time showing any frank elation, but at times given to irrational behaviour with some excitement and infrequent assaultiveness. Then progressive deterioration set in, and he soon became a typically dilapidated dementia praecox, in which condition he has remained.

PART VI

ANXIETY STATES

Wenn Phantasie sich sonst mit kühnem Flug
Und hoffnungsvoll zum Ewigen erweitert,
So ist ein kleiner Raum ihr nun genug,
Wenn Glück auf Glück im Zeitenstrudel scheitert.
Die Sorge nistet gleich im tiefen Herzen,
Dort wirket sie geheime Schmerzen,
Unruhig wiegt sie sich und störet Lust und Ruh ;
Sie deckt sich stets mit neuen Masken zu,
Sie mag als Haus und Hof, als Weib und Kind esrcheinen,
Als Feuer, Wasser, Dolch, und Gift ;
Du bebst vor allom, was nicht trifft,
Und was Du nie verlierst, das musst Du stets beweinen.
Faust, Scene I. Goethe.

CHAPTER XXX

THEORIES OF ANXIETY

IN the Psychological Introduction mention has been made of the prominence given to anxiety in psychopathological studies of emotions. We may recall that many hypotheses have been advanced to account for pathological fear on somatic grounds. The argument is as follows : That which distinguishes normal fear from its morbid analogue anxiety is the independence of the latter of any, or of an adequate exciting cause. If the James-Lange theory holds true, the visceral sensations constituting anxiety may be the result of bodily abnormality, not of a psychic stimulus. To supply the physical etiology there are as many anomalies assumed as there are writers. One reads, for instance, of cerebral ischaemia, of special excitability of subcortical, spinal and sympathetic centres, of excitability of vasomotor-secretory-visceral centres, of over-excitability of the vasomotor nerves of the heart, and so on.

No real evidence is ever produced to substantiate these pure assumptions. All may be characterized as " neurologizing tautology ", to use Meyer's effective phrase. Against all these views it may be urged that *all* the physical symptoms of anxiety are symptoms of excessive functioning of the sympathetic-adrenal system, which Cannon and his associates have shown conclusively to be the *results* of psychically induced fear. The variations in clinical pictures may with safety be looked on as products of chronic repetition of the stimulus and idiosyncrasies of the patients. Since these physical phenomena, summoned as *causes* of anxiety, are shown to be *results* of normal fear, these speculations can surely have little value. Further, as Janet[1] has pointed out, organic disease may produce the appropriate physical symptoms in marked form without anxiety being present, or in hysterical states, a patient may be subjectively and emotionally undisturbed although exhibiting the bodily manifestations of fear.

We may therefore turn our attention to the purely psychological theories. Most authors agree in ascribing to mental factors at least a provoking agency. Dubois holds the curious view that it is a defective judgment and moral weakness on the part of the patient which allow him to be afraid of certain things. Since so many sufferers begin their story with the plaint that they know the ridiculousness of the fear, it seems unprofitable to discuss such a view. Further, many anxiety cases show rare courage in the face of real danger. More serious students have attempted to explain the phenomena as occasioned by instinctive or unconscious factors. Janet, for instance, holds that owing to a lack of " mental tension " the patient is unable to meet a new situation adequately on a logical basis and falls back on instinct. The question as to why the reaction should then be of anxiety rather than any other emotion, he answers rather tautologically with the statement that this is the peculiar and habitual reaction of the patient. Quite similar views have been held by other French writers.

Such a theory merely raises fresh problems. What is the basis of the " fear habit " ? What is there in the novelty of a situation that calls forth the emotion ? One might call these the remote and immediate causes. Two different schools have attempted more or less complete answers to these questions. Psychoanalysis offers a hypothesis for the first, while the hypnotic school, represented best by Morton Prince, furnishes an explanation for the second.

The earliest Freudian work was based on a definitely somatic conception of what was termed " Anxiety Neurosis ". Insufficient physical outlet for sex impulses was held to lead to an accumulation of sexual excitement, which was transformed from the primary physical and sexual manifestations to psychic and anxiety phenomena. In support of the physical etiology, Freud claimed (as have many non-psychoanalytic authorities) that abstinence, coitus interruptus, coitus reservatus and ejaculatio praecox were always present when his syndrome of symptoms appeared and that amelior-

---

[1] Janet, *Les Obsessions et la Psychasthenie*, 1908, tome I, p. 472, *seq.*

ation of the morbid state occurred when normal coitus was established.

This was in 1895. Evidence rapidly accumulated to show that this formula was far too simple to meet clinical conditions. Abstinence and incomplete copulatory acts were often found to exist with mental comfort or, at least, without anxiety. Secondly, anxiety was frequently present when the sex life of the patient was physically normal. These facts led in 1908 to Freud's splitting off a group called " Anxiety Hysteria ", in which the etiology was mental rather than physical, the mechanism being hysterical, *i.e.*, in the Freudian sense, the work of a perverted psychosexual development. According to this view a warp begun in childhood prevents the sex instincts from adequate outlet in adult life. There results, then, a mental rather than a physical accumulation of energy, which constitutes a danger. The ego recognizes this and reacts with fear. A third change in these theories was brought about through the independent observations of a number of psychoanalysts who found that the mechanisms of " Anxiety Hysteria " were present in many cases of apparently pure " Anxiety Neurosis ". Thus it has resulted that morbid fear is now generally held to be the result of psychosexual distortions, in other words, of unconscious, infantile impulses. Jones sums up as follows : " [Sex] Desire that can find no direct expression [*i.e.*, as a result of circumstances or of conflicts which prevent the coming in to consciousness of the desire] is 'introverted' and the dread that arises is really the patient's dread of an outburst of his own buried desire. In other words, morbid anxiety subserves the same biological function as normal fear, in that it protects the organism against mental processes of which it is afraid[1]."

If one accepts the evidences which the psychoanalysts furnish of unhealthy sex instincts in the lives of these patients—and the writer finds it difficult not to—this final theory offers a good explanation for the push, the *dunamis*, of a morbid emotion. But it does not account adequately for the type of emotion and is, in fact, inconsistent with other Freudian teachings. The tendency of psychoanalysis is to find in the unconscious definite wishes or impulses and definite mental images of childish simplicity and, so divorced from reality and consciousness, as to be free from ethical control. It is characteristic of morbid anxiety that its origin is hidden from consciousness, hence it must arise in the unconscious. It is therefore inconsistent to have an unethical unconscious, normally concerned with ideas of the concrete, rebel against a highly abstract and conscious type of idea, such as a conception of a mental process. In fact, the incompleteness of his theory is evidenced by psychoanalytic claims themselves. This etiology is found in anxiety neurosis, in anxiety hysteria, in hysteria and in manic-depressive depression.[2]

---

[1] Further elaborations of Freud's hypotheses about fear, I have discussed in *Problems in Dynamic Psychology*, pp. 75-89.

[2] The last is from a personal communication of Dr. Ernest Jones.

THE PSYCHOLOGY OF EMOTION

Plainly, then, the struggle for expression of repressed sex impulses provides an *Anlage* for many different types of neurotic and psychotic reactions. Some other ractor must be invoked, the introduction of which crystallizes the morbid mental processes into a specific clinical type.

Stekel, who has written more fully of morbid anxiety[1] than any other psychoanalyst, seems to feel this difficulty and has some generalizations to meet it. His views are, in brief, these : Fear is an expectation of discomfort and it can always be reduced to dread of the unknown, which is symbolized and epitomized in the concept of death. [This provides a definite something to be afraid of.] All psychic forces are ambivalent (bipolar is his term). Running hand in hand with the death idea, therefore, is a desire for death, unconscious as a rule, of course. On the other hand, the strongest impulse of life is for creation, *i.e.*, the sexual impulse, which may be viewed teleologically as actuated by a fear of death of the species. This, he says, accounts for the relationship of death and sex ideas. Shame is the inhibitive emotion that goes with conscious sex excitement, while fear acts against unrecognized sex cravings. The unconscious formulates a fantasy of outlet which involves the idea of sin, which produces an ethical or religious conflict and ideas of punishment, the last coming into consciousness as fear. Most of the typical phobias, he claims, can be reduced to religious and superstitious notions of punishment (death). He therefore accepts and confirms Freud's claim that repressed sexuality returns as anxiety but has a specific mechanism to account for the latter.

There are several criticisms justifying a rejection of this theory. In the first place, knowledge of a connection between copulation and pregnancy is quite a recent discovery in human history. Many savages are to-day ignorant of this[2]. To prove the relationship of death to sex, therefore, Stekel should first show that such savages never suffer from morbid anxiety. Secondly, his evidence is not sufficiently objective to be compelling. Death ideas are probably universally present in the human unconscious ; it is one thing to bring them to light in the course of a psychoanalysis and quite another to demonstrate their specific connection with fear. The therapeutic aim of modern psychoanalysis is to reduce the pressure of deep unconscious tendencies, it is not directed towards the discovery of the immediate determination of symptoms. It was only in the early days when quasi-hypnotic methods were used that sufficient stress was laid on the immediate occasions for symptoms for much objective evidence to be obtained on this point. As a therapeutic method the aim of psychoanalysis is to cut off abnormal tendencies at their source rather than to dally with academic problems of specific determination. Hence, if during a course of treatment anxiety disappears, one cannot assign the recovery to the

[1] *Nervöse Angstzustände*, Urban & Schwarzenberg, Berlin & Vienna, 1912.
[2] Hartland, E. S., *Primitive Paternity*, David Nutt, London, 1909.

ventilation of death ideas unless these alone are discovered, which is never the case. Finally, as we shall see, his mechanism is much more that of depression than of anxiety. Psychoanalysis, therefore, cannot be held to have shown more than the remote and fundamental causes of anxiety, having merely demonstrated that unconscious sex conflicts exist which somehow mediate the energy appearing in the conscious anxiety.

A specific factor has, however, been demonstrated sporadically by a number of hypnotists, pre-eminently by Morton Prince. In his work on " The Unconscious " he gives examples of attacks of anxiety which were shown under hypnosis to be due to " co-conscious images ". Co-conscious images are thoughts of which the patient is not consciously aware, which dominate his automatic behaviour and determine his affective reactions, when these are not fully accounted for by his conscious purpose. The mechanism can best be understood by an example. One of his patients had a phobia of church bells. Under hypnosis it was demonstrated that any reminder of church bells roused a co-conscious image of a painful experience twenty-five years before, when this emotion was prominent and, under the circumstances, natural. In her attacks, therefore, she was co-consciously living this experience over again and only the emotion of it reached into consciousness, being felt as a fear of the perfectly harmless bells. Such a discovery accounts fully for the type of emotion observed ; it makes the fear an understandable, even logical, reaction, and Prince gives many examples of similar findings.

So far, so good. But why should this memory have such dynamic power ? It is in answering this question of the ultimate pathology that Prince fails, wandering from the objective and demonstrable, to speculate about pure assumptions. The co-conscious image in this case was of praying in church for the recovery of her mother, who was mortally ill. The ringing of the bells interrupted her prayers and she felt that if she were not persistent in her petitions her mother would die, and she, the patient, would be responsible. Prince found that from the age of 5 or 6 on the patient had been given to self-blame, hence the importance of this incident, which merely symbolized a life-long tendency. One naturally asks at this point, why the life-long habit of self-blame ? If one can account for that, he has discovered the dynamic cause of the phobia. Prince's answer is simply to adopt McDougall's tautological psychology and say the self-blame is the result of an " instinct of self-abasement " and a " self-regarding " instinct. In other words, instincts are manufactured *ad hoc* to account for what is otherwise inexplicable[1].

From this review, then, we might be justified in assuming that a correct theory would contain elements of both Freud's and Prince's

---

[1] As a matter of fact, the " Phobia " Prince describes was a complicated emotional state of which fear was only one, and, probably, a minor component. This, however, does not invalidate the theoretic considerations just discussed.

psychology : Ultimately, the abnormal emotion is due to insufficient emotional (specifically sexual) outlet, which creates a powerful unconscious pressure. This is projected in a co-conscious image, having a form which is *of its own nature* fearful and produces the anxiety. The latter alone penetrates consciousness but has back of it all the force of the deep-lying unconscious cravings. We shall now look to the psychoses to see what information they give in support of this composite hypothesis.

CHAPTER XXXI

ANXIETY CASES

THE most typical, protracted, anxiety states seem to be those associated with a fear of death, all of which belong essentially to the involution group. In looking over a large material it was striking to find how regularly other kinds of anxiety states were transitory. In fact, up to late middle age, anxiety seems to be a mood merely of onsets or interruptions in manic, depressive, stuporous or perplexity psychoses. Since the involution cases have already been considered, the clinical material still to be discussed may be exemplified by brief resumés of some anxiety phases initial to more protracted psychoses.

In the involution group the pathological mood is part of a reaction to a delusion of approaching death. Sometimes this is merely a fear of dissolution in a vague way, but often one sees a vivid and hallucinatory dramatization of physical aggression—the victims are to be killed in various ways. In the briefer anxiety states an analogous notion of bodily injury is usually the dominant one, as the following cases show. We shall also see in them that these aggressions frequently furnish another variant of adult sex interest ; they are veiled—sometimes open—sex attacks.

CASE 44. *Anna H.* was an unmarried woman of 27 when she came under observation 13 years ago. She was described as very religious, a devout Roman Catholic, quiet, reserved and dignified. Her sense of propriety was probably morbidly exaggerated, for she was wont to remark on the foolish behaviour of others. That this was connected with a rather " old-maidish " sex antagonism is suggested by her having had a young man call on her for six years without this acquaintance ripening into any more intimate attachment. He was apparently, her only male friend.

We often find that such prudish characteristics are reactions against a strong unconscious impulse to unlicensed sex activity. When such a person is put under the kind of strain which is liable to stimulate deep-lying infantile ideas, prostitution fancies are apt to emerge (cf. the case of Mary S. in chapter 27). Six months before admission the patient's mother was found to be suffering from carcinoma. During this illness the patient nursed her, which was both a physical and mental strain. Ten days before admission she was downhearted, blamed herself for neglect of her mother and begged the latter's forgiveness, all of which was uncalled for. Her actual psychosis was introduced abruptly by a projected sex idea. On her way to church, she heard two men on the street say : " There goes the whore of Amsterdam Avenue." Then came an anxiety state with fear of social punishment and, more specifically, of physical and sex aggression. She stayed at home, not even going to church, lest she be ejected as a bad girl. She thought the police were watching her and the tenants in the same building talking about her. Her young man also played a rôle in these delusions, for she imagined he had set spies to watch her. Finally she was in terror of a physical examination attempted by the family physician. After a few days she began to be depressed and was taken to the Observation Pavilion. With the depression all these fancies disappeared, in fact only one false idea was expressed and it of an infantile order. When asked about her parents, she said : " I have a father [dead] but no mother [still living]." The depression lasted for some ten months, at the end of which time she was well enough to return home. Then she developed a mild hypomanic state, the ideational content of which was not reported.

The next case is more complicated, inasmuch as the observed attack merged over into a stupor, which reaction seems to have coloured the anxiety state preceding it so that the patient's utterances were not always clear. As troubles with the step-children appeared as precipitating causes of her attacks, it may be well to note that persons in such a relationship are facile substitutes for original infantile objects of attachment or antagonism, so that any disturbing incident in connection with the step-child (or step-parent) is apt to stir up the deep unconscious tendencies.

CASE 45. *Leona W.* was a married negress, aged 28, when she came under observation, about 20 years ago, in her second attack. Her family history indicates a considerable mental instability. Her father was an evangelist, who deserted his wife and disappeared with another woman. After this incident the mother became melancholy for several years and then died at the age of 40 from unknown cause. A sister of this woman, who herself had fainting spells, gave birth to three children, each of whom had an attack of excitement with recovery. The patient had one brother who was said to be well.

Nothing was learned about the early life of the patient, except that she married a widower with grown up children when she was 20 years of age. With these children she did not get on well. Moreover, she was jealous of her husband and generally highly strung. Particularly at menstruation she was apt to have frequent headaches or " depressed " feelings in her forehead. She had four children.

First Attack : When 26, a year after the birth of a third child whom she was still nursing, she became much run down as a result of malarial infection (the family were living in Florida at that time). Quarrels developed with a neighbour woman and then with the stepchildren, the husband siding with the latter. Shortly after this she saw a snake crawl out from under the house and was convinced that the neighbour woman had put it there. Within a few days the attack began suddenly. She woke one morning with anxiety, being afraid of her husband, thinking that the neighbour woman wanted to kill her and hearing the latter's voice saying, " I have got you now." That this antagonism was a vehicle for expression of unconscious notions of jealousy is suggested by her accusing her stepdaughter of trying to get money from her (the patient's) husband. These fragments were all that could be obtained in the history concerning this attack, except that it lasted for three weeks, terminating with perfect insight.

For two years she remained well, during which time the family moved from Florida to New York, leaving the stepdaughters in the former place. Four months before admission a fourth child was born, and soon after this she suffered from a feeling of vague depression with hot flashes and headaches. Two weeks after the birth her husband had to leave for a long trip, and, during his absence, one of the stepsons made indecent proposals to her. Symptoms of an anxiety neurosis appeared at once. She felt sick, nervous, and sensitive to noise. This state continued until three weeks before admission, when psychotic symptoms were added. She began to sleep badly and heard remarks to the effect that she was going to be dispossessed (the idea was unwarranted. Next came an interesting phase in which she was vaguely aware of malign agencies, for she had vague fears that " something " was after her and felt " like a person a long way off." Everything looked dark and gloomy, even the furniture seeming to be different.

She was removed to the Observation Pavilion, by which time a definite anxiety had developed. She appeared confused, anxious and exposed herself, saying : " Oh, don't do it ! What is it you want to put in my stomach ? " After transference to the Psychiatric Institute a picture of agitated anxiety. Her expression was one of distress and anxiety, and she was in constant motion, now clutching at her throat or various parts of her body, now pulling the sheets about, grasping at the bystanders or anything she could get hold of, and aimlessly resisting any attention. Often she breathed irregularly, with trembling, and momentarily assumed attitudes of prayer or supplication. For one day her excitement was more intense, when she grunted, rolled over, flinched, strained, jerked her limbs, while her facial expression changed from whining to disgust, sneering or smiles. Throughout the entire period there was often marked muscular tension. Sometimes she held her body stiff, with her hands in a claw-like position over her chest, while sometimes she writhed and squirmed almost in opisthotonic attitudes. With all this variation in her movements, however, her mood was, with the exception of the one day noted, a rather consistent distress and anxiety.

Considerable explanation for this behaviour and emotion was gathered from her remarks. Once while a physical examination was being made she spoke more or less connectedly about the attempted assault on the part of her stepson. She said : " He sat on the bed just like that (indicating doctor)— the other children were gone to school—he said get in bed—O Lord, I don't deserve it —O Lord, have mercy—nurse I am telling the truth—O doctor and nurse, if I had to tell—he did approach me and he said he would tell his father that I felt him first—I said I would tell my husband—O Lord, it is true I done nothing." Apparently she was, as a rule, living in a delirious-like repetition of this experience or of imaginary incidents of a similar nature to which her thoughts turned. For instance, she confused her husband and the stepson : " That is my husband talking—no, I know it is not my husband, it is Thomas " (stepson).

But as a rule her remarks were not as clear as this, the following examples giving fragmentary insight into the painful thoughts which dominated her disturbed consciousness. These, apparently, were elaborations of the thought of the assault, with an introduction of the jealous fancy, for the antagonism and death of some women is spoken of. " O Lord, have mercy—oh me—O Lord "—or " My God, don't let them fight—wait a minute "—or " O wait, wait, no, he will have to come back and take the whole family " (probably her husband and the stepchildren). " O Lord, he wanted to make me say ' Lord '—and got me, pumping another way—no, I am not going down "— " They are going to kill me." " I know you are going to shoot." " Please have mercy—no, that's not it—no, no, I don't know when she died." " My bed is turning under me," or again : " I know, but then I paid her back for what I done for her—O, please Missus—I forgive you—yes, please—now they would not let me go back," or " You grabbed me around the leg—I feel you ".

Then rather suddenly this state merged over into a stupor of some months duration. This terminated with a period of about two months, during which she was somewhat languid and complained of " a kind of dumb feeling ". At this time she still heard voices, as she had for a period of five days at the beginning of the stupor. The content of these hallucinations was mainly the vulgar talk of men and the voice of S., a man who came to see her and who fought with her husband. Shortly before recovery, she said spontaneously that she thought it would do her good to sleep with her husband again, from which one might gather that she realized that sexual thoughts were disturbing her. She remembered coming to the hospital, and so on, but forgot all about her anxiety and the accompanying false ideas. She had good insight, however, and claimed to feel better than she had for years, remarking that the pain in her head was gone. This last statement makes one fancy that in the psychosis she had quite possibly relieved an abnormal unconscious pressure that had earlier expressed itself in a neurotic symptom— the headache.

In the following case the anxiety state was not so dramatic in its outward exhibitions, and lasted for only about a week or ten days as an onset to a slightly perplexed depression of two months.

CASE 46. *Elizabeth W.* was an unmarried girl of only 14 years of age when she came under observation 13 years ago. The family was low both in the economic and moral scale. Her father was a drunkard, who had deserted his family eight months before the patient's psychosis broke out, but he returned at times intoxicated, praying his wife to take him back. The latter seems to have been no better than her husband, for she was not only loose in morals, but sufficiently careless of this to allow the patient to witness her intercourse with a stranger.

As one would expect, this family was able to give little information about the make-up of the patient beyond saying that she was natural in her de- meanour, good at school, rather quiet in temperament. About the time her father deserted, she went to work in a laundry.

The onset of her psychosis she herself described on recovery as follows : She had been worrying about her father and mother, and for six months had lost flesh and complained of dizziness. Later she worried, in addition, about a syphilitic infection which her sister had contracted in marriage. Two weeks before admission she began to complain of headache and occasional nose- bleeding. The first definitely psychotic incidents were in the form of pro- jected ideas of failure and appropriate worry about them. She thought the girls in the laundry were laughing at her because she was so thin, and that they indicated her as one who would be discharged (reduction of help was actually under consideration). Then she thought that an inspector was there to find out her real age, which she had alleged was 16 instead of 14.

A week before admission ideas with less basis in fact appeared, and with these there developed a definite, rather mild, anxiety state. She came home from work one day with the report that her head felt light, and that she was going crazy. During the following week she appeared preoccupied and frightened ; when at the Observation Pavilion she was already rather dull, while by the time she reached the Psychiatric Institute all evidence of anxiety had disappeared, so far as her demeanour was concerned, and her fearful ideas were reduced to hypochondriacal complaints.

The ideas that she expressed during this brief anxiety phase were of adult sex aggression, of infection, or else infantile in type. At home she thought that a man who lived on the same floor was trying to break in the door. At the Observation Pavilion she thought she was in a Chinese building. After recovery she explained this by saying that she had read of girls being kid- napped by Chinese. Apparently she had some notion of moral or physical defilement, for she was suspicious of the doctor's medicine, and thought that the food given her was poisoned by a bad woman upstairs. She also did not want her sister's baby to eat of the food for the same reason. Intimately associated with these fears of pollution or poisoning were those of infection. Inasmuch as she had learned from her sister of the latter's syphilitic infection, it is probable that the latter gave her some information about mercurial treatment, or at least of its complications. At any rate this would readily explain a number of her ideas. She spoke of her teeth falling out, or of a bad taste in her mouth, she feared that medicine would destroy her teeth. Before going to the Observation Pavilion she was sent to a general hospital, where she was much frightened, and could not understand why they asked her about contagious diseases, thinking that they wanted to make out that she had a contagious disease. Here, too, she was frightened at a coloured woman in the next bed, and had a sensation of water running around in her stomach.

There was no explanation for these ideas in any of her other utterances. It is possible that the second represented a symbolized pregnancy.

Infantile ideas concerned her father only. Even before the anxiety appeared she heard her father's voice call her. When she was taken to the Observation Pavilion, she said, " I am where my father went ". After recovery she explained that she thought for a time that she was in a prison to which her father had been sent for wife-beating. Further, she made an all but overt association between her father and the fear of sex aggression. When she spoke of the Chinese building, she said, " This is a Chinese building. My father brought me here ".

This brief anxiety state, then, had all the elements we have come to expect ; an evidence of psychotic attachment to the father, and an association between this and the fantasies of adult sex aggression, the last occurring in the idea of a physical attack and in fear of poisoning and of infection, the nature of the last two being strongly suggestive of the sexual.

We may recall at this point the onset of the rather prolonged stupor of Charlotte W., which is described in full in Chapter 14. A year before admission she had an abortion performed and another four months later. A month after the latter one she confessed these delinquencies to the priest, who reproved her. Three weeks later an anxiety state developed rather suddenly after some burglars had broken into a nearby church. She would not stay at home, saying that she feared the burglars would return and kill someone in the house. Later, when reviewing this period, she said that she was afraid someone would take her honour away and that the burglars had taken her wedding dress. These references are plain enough as expressions of dissolution of her marriage, whereas the notion of sex aggression is merely hinted at, but when giving this account she added, " I then thought I would run away and lead a bad life, but I didn't want to bring disgrace to the family ". It is important to note that this last idea was accepted and, appropriately, there was no anxiety with it. The clinical condition changed, however, for she then became depressed.

This case differs somewhat from the others cited above in that the threatened danger affects something which the patient is vitally interested in rather than herself directly and exclusively. We frequently find mild anxiety episodes associated with such ideas : a woman, for instance, being anxious about the safety of her children, the life of her husband, and so on, but it is characteristic of these worries, however, that they are transitory or are apt to be mere worries rather than true anxiety states.

Finally we may describe briefly a psychosis which stands rather as a transition between the involution melancholic and the anxiety states described above.

CASE 47. *Mary K.* was a single woman 27 years of age at the time of her psychosis, which was observed 15 years ago. Her father was an alcoholic, who died when the patient was 20. One brother out of eight siblings was alcoholic, and a paternal uncle had a depression, otherwise the family history was negative. The patient herself was described as a bright, sociable and jolly domestic servant, who had been living in the United States for seven years.

For two years she had been acquainted with a young man to whom she was to be married some four months before admission. After recovery she claimed that she had become engaged at his insistance, although she never really cared much for him, preferring someone else. Shortly before the wedding was to take place, this young man left and a week later sent a letter stating that he could not marry her as his mother objected to his bride being a Roman Catholic. In spite of this rupture they continued to correspond for a while. The patient, however, began to worry at once, slept poorly and appeared nervous. Retrospectively she said that her worry was about what her friends would think and say.

Two months before admission she went to a fortune teller, who told her the young man would come back, if she took his picture and talked to it. She followed these instructions. Then a friend informed her that a fortune teller had once tried to bring back a lover, but succeeded in summoning the devil. This information produced further worry, and then she began to wonder if the fortune teller had not perhaps put a charm on her. At the same time she was unhappy because her friends spoke to her pityingly about her broken engagement. She thought she would rather die than have her friends talking in this way, and then began to fear that she was going to die.

In this unhappy state she dragged on for some months, and then suddenly became markedly anxious, paced the floor, was cold and tremulous, with numbness from her knees down, and a feeling as if her whole body was going up through her head. She thought she was dying, and wanted the priest called. Her condition was such that commitment was necessary.

On admission she looked anxious, constantly rubbing her feet, groaning and sighing. She had little to say, but when she did speak, repeated such statements as " Oh, do something for me, I am going to die, my feet are wet, that means I am going to die ". Then she would ask for the priest. This anxiety seemed to be directed definitely against the death idea, but she also spoke of somatic sensations so analogous to pregnancy and parturition that their origin could hardly be mistaken. She said she had a pain in her abdomen and a swelling sensation, that something had burst inside there and passed away with her menstrual flow. Finally she spoke of being sinful. Like an involution case, she was given to irritability when questioned.

This condition lasted for a week, and then, for a seven or eight day period, she was somewhat better, admitted that the feelings in her stomach must have been imagination, and spoke less of dying. However she became rather worse again, with renewed restlessness and occasional references to death, while a remarkable carelessness in her appearance was also evident. Following this there were renewed pains and fears of dissolution, and when this subsided she appeared dull, although restless, said that her head felt heavy, the time went slowly, " she was dead in herself " and had no life in her. With this rather dilapidated depression, she also masturbated. Three months after admission she improved rapidly, and soon was quite normal again with good insight.

CHAPTER XXXII

WE have described (Part IV) marked and prolonged anxiety states such as occur in involution melancholia and some examples have also been given of briefer fear states in which the emotional reaction is sometimes not very dramatic. Our material, therefore, includes all variations of anxiety psychoses. It is time to see what generalizations can be made, which might further understanding of this emotional reaction.

In the first place, in all cases there is evidence of regression to primary objects of interest—an infantile content—which, because it occurs in all manic-depressive psychoses and does not appear in normal or merely neurotic states, we assume to be associated fundamentally with the origin of the psychosis. This is a general factor and, according to our hypothesis, is the vehicle of energy expression in the abnormal reaction of any functional insanity. In other words, this finding relates anxiety to other forms of mental disease but fails to account for its specific symptoms.

A peculiarity is found in the ideational content, however. In all cases there are found expectations of some danger—violent death, bodily injury, burglary, sexual assault, loss of property, health or honour—and in each case the mood reaction is, roughly, appropriate to the situation imagined. In other words, the insane woman who hears a man trying to break in the door of her room has just about the same emotion as her normal sister would feel, were she in such a real predicament. So generally is this true that it seems foolish to seek for any further explanation of the affective reaction. The fear is *not* abnormal but normal. What is pathological is the vivid delusion or hallucination against which the anxiety reacts.

This leads, in turn, to an examination of the disturbing thoughts. The first observation we make is that they are all of them prospective dangers. When the imaginary evils are formulated as already having happened, the mood is no longer one of anxiety but of depression or stupor. For instance, expectation of moral ruin or death produces fear, while a delusion of death or accomplished ruin occurs respectively in a setting of stupor or depression.

A more important question is, of course, what determines these ideas. One forms an idea of a real burglar from seeing and hearing the man with his mask, gun or club. But why conjure up such an image ? An explanation can be gained from analysis and correlation of the attendant fancies. Let us consider the episodic manic-depressive cases first. Dissatisfaction with life as it is initiates regression to the infantile outlets which are hinted at. Acceptance of these implies a more profound mental disintegration than characterizes the manic-depressive psychoses, wherein such strivings are transformed into adult form. In anxiety states it seems that the mechanism of *projection* is in operation : the sexual opportunity is represented as being forced by outsiders on the patient. Hence in most of the histories given in this chapter sexual aggression, plain or implied, appears as a delusion. This seems to be unacceptable even to the changed personality, and a further distortion takes place whereby the attack is symbolized as a de-sexualized assault. It seems to be mainly these last imaginations which stimulate the fear, while the vividness of their presentation is due to their being manifestations of potent, unconscious lusts.

A critic might urge at this point that cases of women only have been cited. What of the anxiety states in men ? It should be stated that factors of pure expedience have restricted us largely to the study of functional psychoses in women. Nevertheless a considerable number of male cases have also been investigated, and it seems that (outside of the involution group) the anxiety states seem to be rare. We have a suspicion that the masculine analogue to a prostitution fancy is the thought of homosexuality. The greater repugnance people have for " degeneracy " than " license " may account for the rarity of anxiety states in men. Some other formulation of an adult outlet to infantile cravings is chosen and a different clinical picture results.

As fine an example as we know of anxiety occurs, however, in acute alcoholic hallucinoses. It is true that this psychosis is usually classified with the toxic group, but Kirby[1] has shown how close is its clinical relationship to the functional insanities with sufficient cogency to justify us in regarding it as a psychogenic reaction usually liberated by alcoholic excess but not necessarily so. It has a simple clinical picture : the patient is terrified by the sound of guns, the clank of arms and words of men whom he hears plotting to attack him. At the same time voices accuse him of homosexual practices. If we assume that the attack of the assassins is a symbolic sexual assault, the whole clinical picture becomes consistent. In analogous hallucinoses in dementia praecox the necessary transitions are often patently present so that one can trace the regression to the infantile content, its growth into homosexual ideas and then their transformation into fears of physical attack. For our theory it is important to note that women with acute alcoholic hallucinoses hear heterosexual, in place of homosexual, accusations.

[1] Kirby, George H. " Alcoholic Hallucinosis, with Special Reference to Prognosis and Relation to Other Psychoses ", *Psychiatric Bulletin*, July, 1916.

At this point the curious behaviour of anxiety symptoms in a non-psychotic patient may be mentioned. This man was for years timid, afraid of strange men, of horses and, particularly, of burglars, the last amounting to a phobia. His cowardice resulted in his evading service in the war in spite of some disgrace. He had what Janet or Prince would call a dominating fear instinct. Analysis showed that many, if not all, the objects of his fear were symbols of homosexual aggression. Now it happened that he was seeking treatment, not for his anxiety, but for attacks of compulsive homosexuality. He had the normal disgust for such practices, but was, from time to time, when approached by male prostitutes, impelled to fall in with their suggestions. When indulging in any perverse act, he felt nothing but disgust, but was powerless to control his actions. The interesting phenomenon was that in some of his escapades he took into his home obviously armed and desperate gangsters and, of them, for the time being, he felt no fear. The compulsive nature of these escapades proves that they were unconsciously demanded. The craving, receiving direct satisfaction, had no necessity for symbolic subterfuge, hence there was no attention given to the potential danger of the situations. Such a case proves (so far as one case can prove anything) that anxiety is directed against a conscious (or co-conscious) image of danger, while the concentration of attention to it is derived from the unconscious backing of the offensive symbol.

As to the reasons for choice of a projection mechanism, we can offer only speculations. A number of factors are probably involved which have varying importance in different cases or combine in operation. One of these is an egotism which leads the patient to think that others are more interested in him and his fate than they really are. This is probably more prominent in cases of what we call paranoia, than in the latent paranoid mechanism of anxiety states. A second factor may be masochism, a perverse delight in suffering. Both Jones and Stekel emphasize the frequency of such an unconscious tendency in their anxiety cases (on a homosexual basis in men). This, in turn, is probably not a primary instinctive entity but a product of simpler forces, such as a laziness, which prefers a passive to an active rôle—a desire for intense feeling without energy to seek it. Biologically, too, it is probably an integral part of female psychology, present also in the male in so far as he is bisexual in psycho-sexual constitution. Finally, projection is favoured by certain moral influences. All of us prefer to have others responsible for our misdeeds ; it is more comfortable to be sinned against than to sin. The transformation of the idea of sex aggression to symbolic physical attack is favoured by such ethical considerations. Many people prefer physical or material injury to loss of honour. Hence there is less pain in the thought of being stabbed than in the anticipation of sexual assault. An implacable unconscious demands gratification of antisocial cravings. By means of projection this is obtained, indirectly, it is true, but with economy of effort and moral comfort. Fear is preferable to shame.

In this discussion we have considered only the briefer anxiety states which are incidents in other manic-depressive psychoses as a rule. The terror observed in involution psychoses is more dramatic and these conditions are clinically more important. But their psychology is simple. The sufferer is dominated by thoughts of imminent dissolution and shows a fear of this which is appropriate to the intensity of the mental image. Projection frequently causes delusions and hallucinations of murder and torture to appear which make the fearful thoughts more vivid than the abstract picture of death. The origin of these death ideas as regressive fancies has been fully discussed in Chapter 18, and need not be repeated here. A word as to the difference in content in the two groups there discussed may not be out of place.

In contrasting stupor and involution melancholia we have suggested that probably the thought of death is less welcome as age advances, since it becomes a more real danger. At the same time failing strength forces a desire (unconsciously) for relaxation of the effort at living. Similar factors tend to make the anxiety states of youth and early middle age essentially sexual (in the popular sense of the terms). From puberty to the climacteric, sex is physiologically a dominant force and, in common experience, a more potent instinct than that of self-preservation. As involution of the gonads proceeds, maintenance of life becomes more important than its procreation. Biologically the individual becomes selfish. There is no germ of altruism in the wish for death, while it is always present in sexual fantasies and reproductive acts.

To recapitulate : We found from a survey of the literature that one should expect a competent theory of anxiety both to explain appropriately the occasion for the fear and to account adequately for the energy of the reaction. In the psychotic material described above (and in Part IV) we have data, the analysis of which enables one to formulate such a theory. The anxiety is directed against mental images of a dangerous nature which in the psychoses come into full consciousness. The fear, as such, is rational, if the reality of the stimulus were only granted. The vividness of the delusion or hallucination is explicable from its history as traced by study of the attendant ideas. There is in the psychosis (regardless of its particular type) a regression to primitive interests, normally unconscious. These are sufficiently energized to demand expression, which is secured in a roundabout symbolic form, in the imagination of something which is dangerous. The intensity of the emotion is proportionate to the intensity of the mental image which, in turn, is an expression of primitive, instinctive and unconscious force, acting more directly than in normal life.

There remains for discussions the psychological factors of the secondary symptoms of anxiety states. Only one of these is sufficiently conspicuous and constant to demand consideration. This is restlessness, largely muscular, but sometimes betrayed in speech as well. The outstanding characteristics of this unrest is the purposelessness of the movements. It seems that such motions tend to appear with unwelcome thoughts, for we find them, not only in involution melancholia and ordinary anxiety states, but also with perplexity. In depression, as we shall see, there is little or no content ; in mania, the thoughts are welcome and lead to a different type of motor restlessness with purposeful motions. One tends naturally to force a solution of any unpleasant situation, and when this is impossible a state of tenseness results. Then, as a substitute for directed action, a meaningless motor discharge relieves the tension. " The Devil's Tattoo " of normal life is a good example of this. In insomnia and epilepsy[1] these movements are, perhaps, attempts at the maintenance of consciousness, but their immediate purpose, as in fear states, is to distract the subject's attention from his painful thoughts. It is a futile effort at escape. There is some biological foundation for this view. Darwin[2] suggests that writhing in pain is a relic of more or less reflex efforts to escape from a noxious stimulus, an instinctive muscular action originally associated with useful behaviour. In the condition we are discussing the pain is mental rather than physical, but the principle is probably quite the same.

[1] See Chapter XVIII.
[2] Darwin, *Expressions of the Emotions in Man and Animals.*

PART VII

DEPRESSION

The eldest of the three is named *Mater Lachrymarum,* Our Lady of Tears. She it is that night and day raves and moans, calling for vanished faces. . . . Her eyes are sweet and subtle, wild and sleepy, by turns ; oftentimes rising to the clouds, oftentimes challenging the heavens. She wears a diadem round her head. . . .

The second sister is called *Mater Suspiriorum,* Our Lady of Sighs. She never scales the clouds, nor walks abroad upon the winds. She wears no diadem. And her eyes, if they were ever seen, would be neither sweet nor subtle ; no man could read their story ; they would be filled with perishing dreams, and with wrecks of forgotten delirium. But she raises not her eyes ; her head, on which sits a dilapidated turban, droops for ever, for ever fastens on the dust. She weeps not. She groans not. But she sighs inaudibly at intervals. Her sister, Madonna, is often stormy and frantic, raging in the highest against heaven, and demanding back her darlings. But Our Lady of Sighs never clamours, never defies, dreams not of rebellious aspirations. She is humble to abjectness. Hers is the meekness that belongs to the hopeless. Murmur she may, but it is in her sleep. Whisper she may, but it is to herself in the twilight. Mutter she does at times, but it is in solitary places that are desolate as she is desolate, in ruined cities, and when the sun has gone down to rest.

Levana and Our Ladies of Sorrow—De Quincey.

CHAPTER XXXIII

ANALYSIS OF THE SYMPTOMS OF DEPRESSION

DEPRESSION is perhaps the most important of abnormal emotions because it is the commonest. There is probably no one capable of introspection who has not experienced it. We have all been happy too, but we do not regard that state of mind as morbid, while any real sinking of spirits we think of as unhealthy. Moreover, there is no mood of which introspection teaches us less ; the victim feels he is under a curse and at the best can invent only inadequate reasons for it.

The psychological mechanisms, as opposed to the symptoms, of depressions, have received extraordinarily little attention from psychopathologists. Most psychiatrists, like Kraepelin, are content with statements and statistical proofs of there being a constitutional tendency in these patients to look on the dark side of the picture. A few psychoanalysts have published articles on the psychology of the condition, but none of them have worked with enough cases to justify generalizations.

Maeder[1] is the first of these. In 1910 he published the case of a man who had been troubled for months with feelings of unworthiness, incapacity and indecision in his business. In childhood and youth he was rather feminine in his reactions and seclusive, shy with girls. At 24 years of age he married because it was the thing to do but had difficulty in performing his sexual duties. At 42 he came for treatment and had then been impotent for years. A brief analysis revealed strong unconscious homosexual tendencies which appeared symbolically in many dreams and frequently in bald form in pollution dreams. As this was all dragged out and the situation explained, he recovered. As to the mechanism, Maeder suggests that the homosexual tendency caused the depression under the influence of repression and wisely refrains from drawing any further conclusions as to depression in general.

In 1911 Brill[2] published one case out of three which he said were similar. This was of a married Jewess, aged 38, who had had five previous attacks, each occurring in the autumn of the five previous years. The first, fifth and sixth attacks were characterized by anxiety, depression and sleeplessness. The second, third and fourth were milder and lacked the symptoms of anxiety. A brief analysis showed that her first attack came on when, in the absence of her husband, she found herself sexually excited by a man whom she thereafter feared. It was possible to trace the significance of this relationship back to sexual experiences of early childhood. The recurrence of these upsets coincided with the Jewish Day of Atonement. It was on this day that she first realized the sexual nature of her behaviour. Brill's conclusion is that she was unconsciously celebrating the anniversary of this painful discovery. Because of its painful nature, she repressed and forgot the original event, but " The affect belonging to it came to light and produced the depressive condition ". From this one might conclude that Brill believes depression to be a feeling of guilt originating in a repressed memory of sin. In the description of his analysis he says, " —her periodic attacks of depression represented only the earlier libido changed by

[1] Maeder, " Psychoanalyse bei einer melancholischen Depression ", *Zentralbl. f. Nervenheilkunde u. Psychiatrie*, 1910.
[2] Brill, " Ein Fall von periodischer Depression mit psychogenen Ursprungs ", *Zentralbl. f. Psychoanalyse*, Jahrg. I.

repression into depression ". But, since he later says that the anxiety (in a nightmare) came from the repression of the libido, he apparently does not attempt to ascribe any specific influence of repression in producing depression. In the article there is no effort made to discriminate between factors producing anxiety and those leading to depression. In fact, he says his diagnosis was " Anxiety Hysteria ".

Abraham's[1] work on manic mechanisms has already been cited. In the same paper he discusses the psychology of depressions. These he lays at the door of unconscious sadism. What he means by this term is clear enough from his theoretic discussion—a desire to injure the object of love or a change from love to hate—but in the only case, of which he gives a description, not one shred of evidence is adduced showing that the objects of hate were anything but rivals. This is surely a perversion of the term. Would one say that a bull moose fighting another was giving a sadistic outlet to homosexual attraction ? An impulse to injure is there and it is associated with sex, but to be sadistic it should be a substitute for, or an immediate accompaniment of, the sex act. This extension of the meaning of the term enables him to fabricate a theory having no contact with clinical material.

Briefly his scheme is as follows : The tendency to hate inhibits normal application of the libido, so that the individual lives an unhappy, incomplete life. Some situation arises in which the hate finally paralyzes the capacity to love and regression takes place. This is like the psychology of compulsion neuroses up to this point. Instead of choosing a substitutive sexual goal, the sadism is projected. The stages are these : The unconscious says " I can't love, so I must hate ", which gives a feeling of insufficiency that may be attached to physical or mental defects. Then a transference of the enmity is made as the first step in projection. " I am not loved ; people hate me." This, in turn, is connected with defects—" I am regarded as defective." This mechanism explains the various symptoms. The feeling of guilt is a recognition of an unconscious tendency to violent acts which should disprove the inferiority. The inhibition is a product of unconscious regression to a state of auto-erotic exclusion of the world, which inhibits the application of libido. The feeling of insufficiency belongs to the stage before the regression when the patient feels himself unable to love. Finally, he believes that the depressed individual takes a morbid pleasure in his woe, which he ascribes to masochism.

There is more to criticize than applaud in this theory. He reports one factor of importance, namely, that these people give a history of enmities and supply evidence of unconscious tendencies to indulge these in acts of violence. When he calls this sadism and elaborates a hypothesis on this basis, he begins at once to do violence

[1] Abraham, *Zentrabll. f. Psychoanalyse*, Jahr. II., s. 302.

to clinical facts. His first case showed no sadism, in the proper sense of the term, and his breakdown was not occasioned by a situation of hate but by a reminder of his inferiority. This was based on his masturbatory history and warnings in childhood that the practice would ruin him. As a matter of fact, the type of depression described is not a retarded depression (the purest type of the depressive reaction) but rather the neurasthenic kind, which frequently, if not always, is based on conscious, or nearly conscious, sexual and social insufficiency. In such cases there often is a revelling in sorrow, but this is absent in typical deep depressions. Finally, except in the irritability of a manic phase, he offers no clinical evidence of anything that could be called a sadistic symptom. In a word, he gives us no proof from case material to substantiate an intricate and not too plausible theory.

Stekel in his book on nervous anxiety-states has a chapter on four cases of melancholia, two of which he describes at some length. He adduces no special mechanism for depression but emphasizes that thoughts of crime were present in all his cases. Further, he claims that suicide is always the product of a wish to kill someone else. It is the Talion. It should be remarked that Stekel's cases were peculiar in that each had real crime or indiscretion to disturb her conscience.

More recently Freud has elaborated a complicated hypothesis to account for certain symptoms which he finds in "melancholia"[1]. It has to do with transference to the ego of impulses normally directed towards objects of affection, and is, in a measure, an amplification of Abraham's suggestions. Discussion of this theory of Freud would carry us into the maze of his ego psychology, so, as I have already criticized it elsewhere[2], it may be dismissed with this mention. It seems inadequate and irrelevant to clinical facts.

The most, therefore, that we can gather from a sparse literature is a suggestion here or there. No satisfactory hypothesis for depression has yet been offered. Moreover, these writers have dealt with quite various clinical pictures, being none of them (with the exception of Maeder) primarily psychiatrists. Those with much experience know that one frequently meets with patients who, on a background mood of depression, show intermittently and sometimes prominently, symptoms of other reactions. For instance, there may be episodes of anxiety, hypochondria or painful excitement. The uncritical analyst is apt to investigate these phenomena and assume that the psychological mechanisms, he finds, account for the dominant depression. It is safer to study pure depressions as they are seen in retarded states, and then test any hypothesis, that may be formed, by applying it to the more complicated cases as well.

In this attempt we may begin by analyzing the typical symptoms

---

[1] *Trauer und Melancholie, Sammlung Kleiner Schriften zur Neurosenlehre, Vierte Folge*, 1918, Hugo Heller, Leipzig and Vienna.
[2] *Problems in Dynamic Psychology.*

of retarded depression. It is not a simple state but compounded of a variety of feelings, some of which are so exquisitely subjective that description is difficult. A gifted introspectionist like De Quincey may give some picture in metaphor of this complicated mood with which so many of us are familiar. But figures of speech are too cumbrous for scientific purposes. Fortunately in psychotic depression the patients often illumine the facets of this emotional structure with delusional or semi-delusional utterances, which gives us more tangible conceptions, enabling us to separate off the inter-related symptoms.

The first of these is a feeling of *sadness*. Like most terms of everyday speech, this is hard to analyse. By many it would be taken to be synonymous with depression itself and, indeed, it describes pretty well a normal sinking of spirits. We can gain a hint as to its essence from its derivation. It has the same root as appears in the Latin *satis*, or the English *satiated*, with a meaning of full to repletion, heavy. This significance comes out in the term " sad iron ", which is merely a heavy iron, or in the adjective *sodden*. The particular shade of meaning given to this root as an emotional term seems to be that of lack of desire or of ambition. The same etymological tendency to compare general with nutritional appetite appears in the contemporary slang " fed up ". In " sadness " the idea of lethargy is accentuated rather than repletion. It is Alexander weeping because there are no more worlds to conquer. As the sight of food to one who has over-eaten is distasteful or repulsive so, when one is sad, normal stimuli do not quicken to activity but merely remind the sufferer of his sluggishness.

It may be objected that to be depressed as Alexander was, according to the fable, is so unusual as to be fantastic ; that the common cause of sadness is grief over some loss of friend or property or pity for a loved one who suffers from a similar deprivation. This is quite true. But grief and pity are not the same as sadness. Both the former lead to action, to measures of relief actual or fancied. It is impossible to pity one's self or another without at least fancying some alleviation of the distress. Grief is not a state of mute, inactive suffering. Relief is attempted in restless movements (*cf.* the restlessness of anxiety states) which represents, apparently, a primitive tendency to do something about it. Similarly the cries of grief are instinctive protests or demands for assistance. Sadness appears when these perturbations cease with a sodden acceptance of the situation. The characteristic inaccessibility to stimuli is then comparable to the loss of physical appetite and accounts for the etymology of the word " sad ". The advent of *hopelessness* ends grief and produces sadness ; so hopelessness is an essential factor in the production of the state, for a painful lack of energy and of susceptibility to stimulus is felt, which constitutes sadness.

The mechanism of hopelessness might not be apparent to intro-spection, but a prominent symptom of psychotic depression makes it easily understood. This is a *feeling of unreality*. The patients complain that the sun does not shine as it used to, the woods are not so green, even bodily sensations have lost their acuity, their legs and arms are wooden, and so on. There can be no hope in such a world.

" Turn whereso'er I may
By night or day,
The things which I have seen I now can see no more.

" The Rainbow comes and goes,
And lovely is the Rose.
The Moon doth with delight
Look round her when the heavens are bare ;
Waters on a starry night
Are beautiful and fair ;
The sunshine is a glorious birth ;
But yet I know, where'er I go,
That there hath past away a glory from the earth."

As a rule, the patient (like the poet) knows intellectually that the environment is not altered but only his affective relationship to it. Now the vividness of any idea in our consciousness is proportionate to the amount of interest it excites. For instance, most of us are probably more disturbed by seeing a horse cruelly beaten than by reading of a massacre in Russia. One is a " real " atrocity, the other happens too far off to excite our horror, we form no vivid picture of it in our minds. We are not inhuman, we simply have too little anterior interest in the Russian victims for them to be anything but intellectual abstractions. But let a dear friend or relative fall in the way of that foreign mob and the whole scene can become a moving mental picture. Such examples, which could be repeated endlessly, prove the truth of the rule given above that the feeling of the reality attaching to any idea is proportionate to our emotional interest in it. Loss of the feeling of reality is, then, only a manifestation of loss of interest, which is, in turn, related to the loss of energy and stimulus susceptibility.

It is now easy to analyse hopelessness. When we hope for anything, we have a mental image of it which gives us comfort just to that degree in which we are able to imagine the vision to be an actuality. If vitalizing interest is lost, it will affect the future first, since this is normally illumined by the excess of energy remaining over from that used in adaptation to the present environment. Our beliefs in the intangible, present or future, are actuated by unfulfilled desire. When our interest, mental energy, libido—call it what you will—is unexhausted, it expresses itself in a wish for something further and beyond. that is satisfying only in so far as the vision of the desideratum gives a feeling of reality. All these elements are compressed into that peerless definition of faith " —the substance of things hoped for, the evidence of things not seen as yet." It is significant that no truly depressed person can pray. Without the capacity of personifying the idea of creator and benefactor, without the energy to wish fervently, God becomes a graven image and petitions mere words. One could define depression as a loss of faith so extreme that it affects one's belief in the visible as well as in the invisible.

While we are on the topic of unreality a remark as to its clinical significance may be in order. In the ordinary benign depression the feeling of unreality is accompanied by insight. That is, the patient makes complaints similar to those of Wordsworth quoted above. When actual delusions develop and beliefs appear that the sun has actually ceased to shine or that a limb has really turned to wood, the prognosis is affected. If the ideas are not fantastically absurd, recovery may merely be prolonged, while, if as in many cases of involution melancholia, palpable absurdities are reiterated, the probability is that the patient will not regain his sanity. It is not hard to explain this contrast. In the benign cases the *feeling*, but not the *sense*, of reality is lost. The latter disappears only when such a profound introversion of interest and attention takes place that intelligence itself is affected. This introversion is the foundation of functional insanity ; loss of the feeling of reality and loss of the sense of reality are reflections of it. We have suggested a comparison between the sturdiness of religious belief and general emotional contact with the world ; similar factors underlie both. These two aspects of the feeling of reality appear in analogous delusions which frequently initiate depressions and dementia praecox respectively. The depressed patient suddenly thinks that his soul is lost, while the schizophrenic imagines that the world is destroyed. Both these ideas are dramatizations, as it were, of a sudden loss of interest, of emotional contact with the environment or, in psychoanalytic terms, of an introversion of the libido.

The next symptom, and the one most pathognomic of deep psychotic depression, is *retardation*. Of this no better description is to be found than that of St. John of Damascus[1] " . . . a sorrowfulness so weighing down the mind that there is no good it likes to do. It has attached to it as its inseparable comrade a distress and weariness of soul, and a sluggishness in all good works, which plunges the whole man into lazy languor, and works in him a constant bitterness. And out of this vehement woe springs silence and a flagging of the voice, because the soul is so absorbed and taken up with its own indolent dejection, that it has no energy for utterance, but is cramped and hampered and imprisoned in its own confused bewilderment, and has not a word to say."

The other phenomena we have analysed were seen to be related to deficient psychic energy. The retardation seems quite plainly

[1] " *De Orth. Fid.*", II., 14, quoted by Paget in *The Spirit of Discipline*. Longmans, 1911.

to be a direct expression of this. It, too, is frequently present in everyday life. We all know the effort it requires to think or move actively on first awakening, particularly if we are called to duties that seem onerous. Even in mild depressions this slowness persists for hours. Normally, however, when once really awakened and out of bed, our minds work actively enough except under special circumstances. These are of great theoretic importance. Every acute instrospectionist knows that his intelligence is keen when it is engaged in solving a welcome problem but that distasteful mental exercises are laboured. From this we can gain a hint as to the etiology of retardation—that painful thoughts are slow. Routine examinations of depressions show the same phenomena : when the patient is questioned about neutral matters, such as facts of orientation, the answers may be prompt enough, but, when personal troubles are touched on, the retardation appears promptly. Often in our daily lives the thought of something unpleasant suddenly " blocks " our mental processes and we are temporarily incompetent. Fear of such a reaction leads one to say of a suggested topic of conversation, " Oh, I can't think of that ! " We shall shortly cite some examples of painful ideas producing a sudden blocking when they tend to enter consciousness. Such a sudden inhibition is a miniature depression, which can occur either in normal life or during the course of a psychosis. When *any* personal topic produces such an interference with thought, the reaction has developed to a definitely psychotic degree. In the deepest depressions retardation is so extensive as to affect all thinking and even bodily movements. But at no point is there a change in its nature ; it simply becomes more frequent, more inclusive. At first only specific mental presentations result in inhibition, then any affective idea produces it, finally all thinking is consistently slowed. One might say that the extension of the process is merely a lowering of the threshold for mental pain, so to speak, until any psychic event is painful. We shall see later that by viewing retardation from this angle it becomes a simple matter to explain the nature of psychological processes in depression.

Sometimes a dominant symptom is a feeling of *inadequacy*. It is always present, and occasionally is expressed, in delusions of mental and physical incapacity. Apparently inadequacy is not a primary symptom. It seems to be simply a pathological insight, as it were, a recognition of the lack of energy and interest discussed above, which is morbidly exaggerated into a feeling of utter impotence. No new element in the depression complex is introduced with inadequacy.

If we consider together the symptoms so far discussed—sadness, hopelessness, unreality feeling and diminished emotional response, retardation and inadequacy—we find that all of them have, as a common characteristic, a lack of " psychic energy "—a kind of mental anæmia—in fact, each symptom presents a different aspect of this deficiency. If one subtracted this factor, very little if anything of the symptoms would be left. Such a condition also prevails in stupor where absence of interest and energy account for most of the psychosis. The depressive and stupor processes are so alike that some authors, such as Kraepelin, regard the latter as a mere exaggeration of the former. There is, however, a vital difference between them. The tendency of the stupor reaction is for the energy to disappear entirely ; in depression some is always left, although it may not be applied to the environment and so fail of detection by an observer. It remains, however, in an introverted form, for the patient is always intensely interested in himself and acutely conscious of his disability. In fact, all the symptoms, with the exception of retardation (which, with the facial expression of sorrow, is the only objective symptom), are painful recognitions of the inadequacy. The stupor patient is indifferent, the depressed patient suffers acutely. This phenomenon of preoccupation with conative incompetence suggests that mental activity is not cut off at its source, that it is not non-existent, but rather that it is constantly striving for expression against some inhibitive force which persistently represses it. The patient feels the conflict or, rather, feels the paralysis resulting from the deadlock reached between expression and repression. But why repression ?

The argument, up to this point, may be summed up as follows : the kernel of depression is a lack of motive of which the patient is poignantly aware. This deficiency is best manifested in retardation, which seems to be a blocking in response to milder and milder occasions for mental pain as the depression increases in gravity. Anything which would explain why thoughts are intolerable would explain retardation. The preoccupation of the patient's attention with his disability suggests that repression is in operation. Since we normally repress the painful, it may be that the explanations of repression and retardation are the same. Some X is wanted, some factor which tends to make all thoughts painful and, to banish which, repression is invoked. To discover this we turn to a consideration of the only feature of depression not already discussed, namely, the ideational content.

When one has made a conscientious effort to note all that depressed patients say, a striking fact appears. In contradistinction to all other forms of emotional insanity, with the exception of deep stupor, the material recovered is meagre. Apart from productions indicating the subjective distress of the patient, there are references only to convictions of wickedness rarely projected as accusations of crime. Sometimes these are accompanied by shame or remorse, which should therefore have been discussed with the other emotional symptoms above, but it is far from constant and in deeply retarded (the most typical) depression is entirely absent. We have seen that the autistic ideas in involution melancholia, stupor, mania and anxiety are quite definite affairs. Here, however, the complaints or confessions are either vague or irrelevant and inadequate to explain the profound disturbance of affect. The patient says, "I am very wicked ; I have committed a mortal sin ", and is unable to state what that sin is, or else alleges some trivial peccadillo or a bit of mischief in childhood. These allegations are of misdemeanours whose gravity is so incommensurate with the affective crisis they are said to have produced, that one is forced to regard them as rationalizations. They are laboured excuses dragged out to excuse the abnormal state of mind. One gets the impression that the patient himself has no knowledge of what saddens him. If we accept the hypothesis of psychic determinism, we must assume that, somewhere outside of the sphere of the patient's awareness, there is a painful thought which causes his suffering and that this thought is cf something morally repugnant to his personality. Grant a co-conscious idea of crime and the whole reaction is explicable. We shall see at once that there is evidence for this.

It should be remarked parenthetically that there are depressions that appear after great mental shocks and trials, which are constantly on the patient's mind. These troubles are more or less adequate causes for emotional disturbance. Such " Reactive Depressions " seem on the surface to upset the argument just made, but it should be borne in mind that they are clinically different from the retarded depressions now under discussion. They will be considered later.

According to our hypothesis if, in the course of a benign psychosis, the content should change from some adultified form to a purely infantile presentation, we would have a symptom of dementia praecox. [See Chapter 29.] In other words, it is significant of the manic-depressive mechanism that anti-social, infantile ideas are taboo. If, then, they tend to appear, they must be repressed and, so long as repression operates, there would be depression and absence of significant content. In brief depressions this mechanism can easily be inferred, while in momentary blocking it may be transparent. Such momentary depressions often occur in perplexity states, where there is a dominance of free associational thinking, with its tendency to reach an infantile goal in ideas which are normally deeply unconscious. [See Part VIII.]

As an example of this we may cite an episode in a case of perplexity[1]. The patient had dreams of her mother and sister being dead or dying, which disturbed her greatly. The meaning of such ideas is clear to one who has read the foregoing chapters. This is part of an infantile wish-fulfilment, for the completion of which the idea of union with the father should appear. Once, however, she also spoke of her father being dead, but added, " I dreamed he was dead and came to life for someone else ". Evidently this paternal death was some kind of arrangement for a family readjustment. If her father were to be united with someone else (plainly herself as

---

[1] Described in the *Annual Report of the Director of the Psychiatric Institute of the New York State Hospitals*, 1913, p. 23.

gathered from many utterances), her mother would have to be got rid of. The latter's disappearance, therefore, would be a natural free association from the thought of her father's remarriage. But this idea is the quintessence of anti-social infantility, which explains her reaction. When she made the statement about her father's return for someone else, she was asked, " What do you mean ? " She at once became blocked, the question had to be repeated several times, when she finally said, " I dreamed my mother died ". During this short time when she " could not think " the idea of her mother's death was being slightly elaborated, until it was merely a dream, a little less harsh a presentation. This elaboration then proceeded further in the next statement which came spontaneously : " They had a quarrel." (Who ?) " My mother and father." This is a highly instructive observation. Had she not been repeatedly questioned it is probable that this thought of her mother's death, which was hovering on the fringe of consciousness, would not have been recovered ; an effort conquered the repression which was temporarily paralysing her conscious faculties. She spoke fairly freely both before and after the blocking, at which times the utterances were, only by inference, of the infantile order. On the other hand, her speech was inhibited during the short period when expression of the thought of her mother's death was in conflict with repression.

Arguing by analogy, we might assume that the same mechanisms account for the absence of any trend during depressive phases of psychoses in which definite content is obtained before and after the depression. Some examples of this have already been given. For instance, in Chapter 31, such a sequence in the psychosis of Annie H. was described. In an anxiety phase she gave utterance to fears of sex assault and heard herself accused of prostitution. Then came a depression in which all content disappeared except for one remark of a definitely infantile order that slipped out apparently as the result of an unchecked free association. When asked about her parents, she said, " I have a father [dead] but no mother " [still living]. At the end of ten months of depression she developed a hypomanic state ; its content was not noted because it occurred after returning home.

Similar observations were made in the case of Elizabeth W., whose case was also cited in Chapter 31. During the onset of her psychosis, in a setting of anxiety, she spoke of adult sex aggressions and of contagious diseases (venereal ?). Depressive symptoms had begun by the time she reached the Observation Pavilion and the content had become restricted to hypochondriacal complaints and one isolated remark about a Chinese building and abduction which constituted an all but conscious association of sexuality with her father. It was probably this infantile tendency which was being repressed and producing the depression. When under observation at the Institute, in addition to her whining hypochondriacal remarks, she had the typical depressive ideas of trivial misdemeanours, such as having gossiped, eaten too much ice cream, and spied on her mother in the sexual act. So the adult sex content had disappeared. The subsequent course of her psychosis is of interest. This depression lasted for only three days after arrival at the Institute followed by a remission of three days, when she was practically normal. Then for a little more than a month she was in what seems to have been mainly a mild perplexity state. During it, occasional ideas of death appeared with anxiety. Whenever she was questioned about external affairs, she answered freely enough ; but when topics of a personal nature were introduced, she always became retarded. This definitely depressive symptom reflected a general tendency in the same direction, for she was usually inactive and somewhat dull and gloomy in her facial expression. At the end of this time she cleared up rapidly with good insight. During the admission she gained 14 pounds.

If depression represents repression, the occurrence of the former at the end of a manic or anxiety phase can easily be understood, particularly when ideas of infantile flavour have been present during the florid psychosis. Sometimes the relationship between memory of distasteful ideas and depression can be seen to be specific. For instance, Celia C. (Chapter 21) became depressed if one attempted, after her recovery, to discuss the ideational content of her psychosis. During it, in addition to many crudely sexual fancies, she believed her mother to be dead. The case of Mary S. (Chapter 27) is even more instructive. All her manic episodes were terminated by depression and she was invariably amnesic for her false ideas. Moreover she complained that examinations, aimed at getting retrospective accounts, made her feel sad.

This principle—of the trend disappearing during a depressive phase, presumably as a result of repression—could be illustrated by innumerable examples. Two more may be cited.

CASE 48. *Hilda T.* was a married woman, aged 24 when she came under observation. Her father was still alive, living in Sweden. Her mother died when the patient was 7 years old. The family history revealed nothing of any importance. The patient was said to have been bright, efficient, sociable but somewhat hot tempered. At the age of 21 she married a widower with two children and in the three years before her psychosis had had two children of her own.

The second of these children was born eight months before admission and she was still nursing that baby when she was taken ill. She never felt well after this childbirth. Two months before admission she became religious, hanging up religious pictures, gazing at them, praying and reading devotional literature. Subsequently she stated that she felt she was not good, thought she was going to die and had a longing for the Old Country. Two days before her mental disturbance became acute she heard two children sing the hymn " Come let us go." Although she knew these children she thought angels had put this into their minds and so took her baby and ran out of the house, thinking she was going to the Old Country to see her father. This led to her commitment, as it was thought that she wished to commit suicide.

The trend of her ideas can easily be interpreted. Relief from the dissatisfaction of her life was first formulated in a religious setting and then in a somewhat more direct form in a desire for the home of her childhood. Naturally, according to our hypothesis, as this was approaching an infantile formulation, ideas of wickedness appeared. As we have seen frequently, there is a close relation between ideas of Heaven, childhood and union with the favourite parent. The children's hymn seemed to stimulate all these ideas, particularly that of turning to her father. At this point a depression developed abruptly. Under observation she showed decided reduction of activity and mental retardation with some whimpering. Once she gave utterance to the typical isolated idea of crime when she said : " I thought I killed so many in my thoughts, where I was lying—I thought it was true when I took up some dead persons." Retrospectively she was able to explain this only by saying that she felt as if she had killed someone, and that on two nights she thought she saw some of her dead girl friends from the Old Country (mother substitutes ?) lying on a boat outside. Apparently the depression was connected with that aspect of avoiding adult responsibilities which demands destruction of adult ties or of natural unconscious rivals. When asked if she was married, she said " I was married ", and retrospectively she remembered having had a vision of her baby with wings.

This depression was not entirely consistent, however. Occasionally she would smile a little and sometimes smiled or even laughed when questioned. As has been noted frequently in Part V, religious formulations belong quite definitely to the manic reaction. Since the patient began with such notions, one can imagine that two tendencies were present : one for a dwelling on the crude infantile desires, and the other to warp these into a religious form. The former she had to repress and would then be depressed, while the latter may easily have accounted for her sporadic smiling. The dénouement supports this view, for after two months she suddenly became active, worked, talked a good deal, said she felt very well, and she had no longer any " funny ideas." The cause of this elation was apparently preoccupation with religion in a de-personalized form. She wrote many gushing letters, full of religious references, effervescing with gratitude and love, and calling down blessings on the recipients. Sometimes she wrote down whole hymns. This hypomanic phase lasted for a few weeks, then, after a short period when she was rather lazy, she recovered entirely.

To sum up then, this patient began with religious ideas and fancies of returning to her childhood and father. When the last became a dominant thought, all the ideas disappeared in a depressive phase, except for rare utterances which had to do entirely with abolition of her marriage, death of her baby, and killing " somebody." When religious ideas only dominated her consciousness, she became hypomanic.

The case of Charlotte W. has already been described in connection with stupor and anxiety. It will be recalled that her psychosis began with an anxiety state in which she feared burglars, who might kill " someone " in the house, take her honour away, and that they had stolen her wedding dress. A month before admission her husband moved the household. She then became depressed and all these ideas disappeared. In their place she complained of her incapacity to work and blamed herself for having had abortions performed. An infantile content was limited to an idea, she had at the Observation Pavilion, that her children were cut up (a retrospective statement). Three days after admission a stupor developed with many interruptions of an anxious, depressive or hypomanic character. In these a copious trend was gathered, including ideas of the death of her husband and children, of her death and translation to Heaven, of being Queen of the World, together with erotic fancies. During the periods when she talked at all, there was only a period of a month when a definite trend was not present and she was then depressed. The only truly delusional thought she had at this time was of a frankly infantile order—an isolated instance when repression failed.

These cases show that the signal for repression may be the descent of the patient's ideas to a more infantile level. Naturally the psychosis may begin with such a content so that there is no introductory phase. Such attacks often seem to come out of a clear sky, but this is probably not so. In the first place, we believe that careful anamneses will always reveal a preliminary mental disturbance, although relatives tend to minimize the early symptoms which by contrast seem insignificant. Secondly, in many cases, it is likely that the infantile ideas may occur in dreams or the semi-conscious state following sleep, so that these thoughts are neither uttered nor remembered. Morton Prince has shown clearly that emotional reactions may be connected with co-conscious ideas alone, and in a later chapter we shall show how frequently dream fancies may persist during the day just beyond the fringe of awareness, producing abnormal moods, particularly depression. The effort to repress them to a deeper unconscious level becomes general, so that all energy is repressed and depression results.

Forel[1] and Janet[2] give examples of this mechanism in depressions, although neither of them draw any conclusions of a general nature. The former quotes two dreams which were associated with subsequent depression : one of these was of bigamous marriage ; the other, the dream of a woman that her brother was dead. (In the experience of the author the memories of dreams which seem to be associated with depression are incomplete. There is always a part repressed and, when this is dragged into consciousness, the depression disappears.) A third dream-depression which he quotes from O. Vogt illustrates our contention nicely. " Miss St. dreamed that her father was dead, and had been buried. She was sad during the whole morning, but only in the afternoon did she remember her dream. She became uneasy. She felt homesick, although she had never before felt like it. Added to this, her head began to ache. The patient, after receiving a suggestion that she should be amnesic and in good spirits, declared that she was happy, and that she had been sad and anxious during the afternoon on account of a dream, which she had, however, completely forgotten. The second suggestion produced complete amnesia." Evidently in this case there was a co-conscious image which was tending to come into consciousness and constantly calling for repression. When by strong suggestion this image was forced into a deeper level of the unconscious, the necessity for repression at an upper level was unnecessary.

[1] Forel, *Hypnotism or Suggestion and Psychotherapy*. Rebman Company, New York, 1907, 323 p.
[2] Janet, *L' état mental des hystériques*. 2nd Ed., Paris, 1911, pp. 248-9.

Janet's case is of greater interest, since the same mechanisms were demonstrated, as we claim to be productive of depressions, and the content is just what we find in our cases. In his chapter on unconscious fixed ideas he cites the case of " Isabelle ". She came to be treated for hysterical anorexia. It was found that this was the result of an unconscious vision of her mother, who chided her for some sin, told her she was unworthy to live, should not join her in Heaven and bade her not to eat. Janet remarks that this vision was associated with quite a sequence of earlier events, from which one might suspect the patient's mother played an important part in the girl's unconscious life. It would not be surprising to find such a psychopath disturbed by death wishes in connection with her mother or some surrogate of the latter. Such an attack did come, which Janet graphically described :

" Behold her for a week sombre and sad, she hides and does not want to speak to anyone. I have trouble in getting her to say a few words, which she utters in a low voice and with downcast eyes : ' I am unworthy to speak with others—I am quite ashamed, there is a weight which suffocates me, like a frightful, gnawing remorse—.' ' Remorse about what ? ' ' Ah ! that is just what I'm looking for day and night. What could I have done last week ? For I wasn't like this before. Tell me truly, did I do something very wrong last week ? ' This time, as one sees, it is not a question of behaviour but of feeling, of a general emotional state which she expresses with the term remorse. She is equally incapable of understanding or expressing the fixed idea which determines this feeling. By distracting her attention it is possible to elicit automatic writing and her hand writes ceaselessly a name which is always the same, it is that of Isabelle's sister, who died a short time ago. During her attacks and during her somnambulisms, we come upon a complicated dream in which this poor young girl regards herself as the murderess of her sister. It may be said that this is a common enough delirium [content, we would say], yes, but it appears in a manner quite curious for a hysteric ; she suffers only from the *contre coup*, she feels its emotional atmosphere but knows nothing of the delirium [content] itself, which remains subconscious. . . . From this last example it may be seen that, in certain cases, a small part of the fixed idea can be conscious. Isabelle felt remorse without knowing about what." This last explains the trifling sins with which depressed patients seek to justify their feeling of wickedness.

I can quote a somewhat similar instance from my own practice. A woman who had long been a patient of mine appeared one day in deep depression. The details of her preliminary symptoms and of the untoward circumstances precipitating her illness are complicated and irrelevant. It is sufficient to say that her father and then her mother had died within a day or two of each other when the patient was only three years old. Subsequently her lot was cast with unsympathetic people, she had grown cumulatively more unhappy and, for some time, had had several attacks a year of incapacitating depression.

At this visit she was so retarded that it sometimes took her a full minute to answer a simple question. Nevertheless an effort was made to find the cause of her suffering by the free association method. Asked what had been on her mind, she said a patient named D. was much in her thoughts (she was a professional nurse). She associated from D. to a Miss D. to whom she had been rude. Her subsequent thoughts were as follows : Miss D. did not resent the rudeness, which is like harming a dead person ; her grandmother is ill and cannot live long ; some idea of injuring her (the patient's) mother. When pressed to recall this injury, she became suddenly nauseated and had to lie down. Continuing in her efforts, she recovered a vague idea of doing something to her mother, who was dying : there was a picture in her mind of a low ceilinged-room, fire-light, and her mother sitting up in bed. She has taken something which her mother ought to have, perhaps food, perhaps medicine. Somehow her grand-mother was connected with all this. Each effort to remember more, led to a spasm of nausea, and she asked piteously to be helped to remember, but, of course, no suggestions were given her. Then, suddenly, after a spasm of nausea, she fell into a deep sleep, her body relaxing and her breathing becoming deep and regular. It soon appeared that this was a state of deep somnambulism in which she   answered   all   questions   in   a   monotonous,   inflexible voice. Apparently each question produced a vision of the events, about which inquiries were made, for she answered always in the present tense. She was asked what she was dreaming of and at once said she was in the dining room eating soup : her mother was upstairs in bed. Somebody, perhaps her aunt, tells her she should not eat the soup for it is her mother's.

" What happens then ? "

" I go to bed."

" And after that ? "

" In the morning my mother is asleep. They show me my mother and tell me she has gone away and is not coming back. I think she has gone away because she could not have the soup."

" Did anybody tell you that ? "

" Before I went to bed my grandmother called me to her room and told me that my mother was sick and needed the soup and I ought not to eat it. *Every day after that is sad !* "

More answers of this nature were given, which explained many of her other symptoms. A suggestion was given to the patient that she should remember all that she had said, which was so far successful that, when she was wakened, the record of her productions seemed familiar, although she could not voluntarily reproduce them. The pure childishness of this " crime " was apparent to her and her depression had completely vanished.

This episode is of great theoretic interest. It is surely plain that the depression was connected with the idea of responsibility for her mother's death—a deeply unconscious fancy which dated definitely from three years of age and had persisted as a buried memory for no less than 35 years. That this thought was tending to force its way into consciousness, that it had become a co-conscious idea, is shown by the directness with which her associations led to something closely akin to the original memory. As a last struggle the psychic organism attempted to dispose of the ugly theme by compromise, by a hysterical conversion symptom—the nausea. (During her somnambulism the patient explained this as an effort to get rid of the stolen soup.) Then as the idea, incompatible with every conscious standard of her personality, continued to rise, consciousness itself gave way. The depression, therefore, was connected with an unconscious crime, which had become co-conscious and threatened to invade consciousness itself. The second important observation is that *re*pression was obviously operating intensely. The patient felt that there was some thought which illuded her and that some force had to be overcome before this phantasm could be grasped. When the dramatic dissociation occurred and the unconscious for the time being displaced the waking, normal personality, there was no occasion for repression and the memories were reproduced without effort and in astounding detail.

The reader has probably been struck by now with the resemblance of this depression process to what we speak of as an " attack of conscience " in normal life. In each there is a conviction of sin and in each a benumbing lethargy. In depression, however, there is no conscious knowledge of the immorality which occasions the trouble, at best only a trumped-up excuse for the feeling of wickedness inadequate to explain the reaction. At the same time, in ignorance of the true cause, no remedy is in sight and expiation is unthinkable. The patient is, in a sense, justified in complaining of having committed " the unpardonable sin ". An unconscious and therefore unknown sin cannot be condoned. On the other hand, the conscience-stricken man knows when he has erred, is proportionately disturbed in mind and, as a rule, combines with his remorse some alleviation for his distress in resolves of reparation or reformation.

CHAPTER XXXIV

CASES OF DEPRESSION WITH ONSET OF INFANTILE IDEAS

WE shall now quote some cases illustrating the appearance of depression as a reaction to infantile ideas which are the first evidence of an abnormal state, be these produced in the waking state or in dreams. It will be noted that neither these dreams nor delusions appear in a setting of equanimity.

CASE 49. The patient *Millie B.* was 40 years of age at the time of the psychosis. She had been married for 20 years and had had five children, two of whom had died. She had had a depression lasting for six months after the birth of her second baby. Three years before, a little girl had died, after which she was depressed for two weeks but then recovered completely.

Eight or nine months before admission, while the patient was pregnant, although she had not yet discovered it, she heard that her favourite brother, who had been operated on in a hospital, was likely to die. At once she became very anxious, thinking that if he died the shock would kill her mother. When questioned on this point, she insisted that her apprehensiveness was much more for her mother than for her brother. That night she had a dream in which she saw her brother lying dead. Her mother was there looking very frightened, crying and worried, and then she too seemed to be dying and under a white sheet. In the morning she felt " stiff-like " and for three days seems to have had a rather typical retarded depression. She spoke almost not at all, said she had no feeling, so that she could be cut up without knowing it. She felt no affection for her husband and children, and thought that the best thing she could do would be to kill herself so that her husband could marry again and get a good wife. We see, then, this depression was precipitated by a typical infantile idea, the death of the mother, which content disappeared in the depression, while other thoughts of an anti-social nature—the breaking up of the home—appeared in the guise of self-reproaches.

On the third day of this depression she cut her wrists, but was detected by her son and the wound dressed so that she suffered no serious physical injury. Her depression then changed rather interestingly from one of retardation and silence to a querulous, worrying state. This phenomenon will be discussed a little later with the heading of reactive depressions. She worried and talked continually about having cut her wrist and the crime that it involved. Learning of her pregnancy, she had some slight apprehensiveness about parturition, but was in general rather indifferent about this. Unconscious criminal ideas appeared in the form of injuries to her children which she worried about. For instance, she talked a great deal about the probability of the unborn child being insane and, when her small son got hold of some pills and ate them, she was convinced that he would die and dreamed of it.

During her pregnancy this worrying depressed condition gradually increased in severity and following the childbirth became so much worse that 19 days thereafter she had to be removed to the hospital.

Under observation she was found to be rather voluble in her complaints which were entirely taken up with the topics just mentioned. She cried a good deal and could, rarely, be moved to laughter although this was usually the sardonic type. On questioning she admitted feeling mixed up and stupid, and also that she had no feeling, no capacity for love, that she was incapable of happiness. Occupational therapy caused a gradual improvement in her condition, so that she was well enough to go home some seven months after admission and had entirely recovered three months later.

The psychosis of the next patient was precipitated by an event of the kind which would naturally tend to stir up unconscious ideas of a criminal nature. It was the death of her husband. If we assume that she had an unconscious longing to be freed of her domestic responsibilities, we can understand how this event would stimulate her unconscious dissatisfaction, and this was shown by the elaboration of the ideas which immediately appeared and which had no logical connection whatever with the death of her husband.

CASE 50. *Carrie D.* was 42 years of age at the time the psychosis developed. She was described as a quiet, reserved woman, who made friends slowly, but who was efficient. At the age of 25 she married an alcoholic husband, who was mostly out of employment and treated her badly. There were four children from this union.

Ten days before admission her husband died. At once she became much disturbed, said she felt dizzy, screamed, yelled, heard voices. The content of these hallucinations was that the children would be taken away, that she had killed a lot of children, that everybody was to be killed. The death of the husband appeared only as a reproach for not having called the doctor soon enough. She rolled on the floor and called for the priest.

Almost at once she became deeply depressed and was brought to the hospital in this condition. For the first five days she seemed preoccupied, spoke in a low tone and had tears in her eyes. Her retardation (with perplexity) was evident from her saying " I don't know ", or " I feel mixed up ", or " I can t get it together ", or " I have no remembrance at all ", to some questions. Some feeling of unreality was reflected in the statement. " I don't know if I am old or young ", and when asked about her feelings, and so on, she always said " I don't know." When questioned about her children and their ages, she replied " I don't know, I don't know if I am the same person or not." Perhaps related to this were some hypochondriacal complaints. She felt funny, could not swallow, felt as if she were " stopped up in the stomach." After making considerable effort it was possible to demonstrate that she was fairly well oriented. Then for the next month, although still distinctly depressed with a marked feeling of sadness and wickedness and very quiet, she was able to answer questions and then claimed that at first she did not know where she was, felt dizzy and dry. After a month more she had recovered entirely and after going home was for a short period slightly hypomanic.

Examples such as these could be duplicated indefinitely. In fact, it is surprising, considering the repressive nature of the process, that some content of this kind is found in so many cases. When one is dealing with an intelligent patient and intelligent family, and if a thorough history be taken, it is rare not to find definite evidence of some such ideas at the onset of a more or less abrupt depression. Not infrequently in reviewing old histories infantile ideas are not recorded as such, but the sequence of what content there is, as well as the reaction, can be explained by the assumption of a link in the development of the patient's imaginations which are of this nature.

CASE 51. *Eustace B.* was a married cotton broker, aged 68 at the time of the psychosis in question, which was observed 20 years ago. At the age of 56, after losing much money, he had a depression of six months which required treatment in an institution. From this he recovered perfectly and returned to business, in which he was successful. A few months before admission he again lost some money and began to worry, sleeping and eating poorly. He then attended the funeral of a good friend (sex not mentioned) and immediately his condition changed from that of an anxiety to a depression, of which the chief content was that his wife would come to want. If one assumes that in his unstable condition the death of his friend suggested the idea of the death of his wife, we would supply a typical ideational cause for the depression in which this abhorrent idea would be repressed and reappear as the worry that she would become destitute.

The depression becoming more marked, he tried to commit suicide and was then removed to a hospital. He was found to be physically normal, in spite of his age, and presented essentially a retardation with constant complaints of lack of ambition and about the effort it required to do anything. It was found that his intellectual defect was entirely subjective. After eight weeks he began to improve somewhat and some four months later was discharged as recovered. He remained well for a year and then had another attack of depression in which he committed suicide.

An exception to what we have frequently stated as to the malignancy of infantile ideas appearing frankly in consciousness is found in some cases with compulsive thoughts where quite anti-social infantile ideas may appear as obsessions without deterioration and, in fact, with spontaneous recovery. Such cases, however, are apt to show a depressive reaction when the imperative ideas assume an anti-social form. For instance, the patient with the somnambulism quoted above, had many depressions with this type of onset. She would become irritable and quarrel with some woman associate. Then the thought would come to her that she must go to look for her baby (she was a virgin). Next would appear compulsively the idea that she had murdered some child and with this a depression would set in which often completely obliterated the compulsive ideas. During the subsequent somnambulic state these ideas were psychologically explained. In her early childhood she had two opposed fancies which persisted unconsciously and determined many symptoms. One was that a younger brother was her child and a second that this child had no business to usurp her place in the home and should be destroyed. In after life all children that she came in contact with enjoyed or suffered from their assuming to her unconscious mind the status of this younger brother, so that they were either cherished or became the object of compulsive ideas of murder. It should be added that she never injured any child actually but was merely tormented by such thoughts.

The next case illustrates somewhat the same process. The patient began with compulsive ideas and then developed a retardation, when these took on a criminal form. As the retardation lifted, compulsive behaviour reappeared.

CASE 52. *Peter V.* was single, a woodworker, aged 27, at the time when he was observed, some 20 years ago. He was described as a young man of very even temper. He had had two previous attacks. The first was a three-months depression following the deaths of his brother and fiancée.

The second, which lasted for five months, occurred two and a half years before admission, and was characterized by insomnia, seclusiveness and compulsive behaviour. A year later a similar condition developed. He had stomach trouble, and complained that his mind was givings way' probably on account of his compulsive actions. He had to comb his hair in certain ways, wash his hands frequently, move his chair in certain positions, and so on. Then appeared phobias of committing suicide or killing his sister, which even went to the point of his once suddenly attacking his sister, and sometimes he tried to bite people suddenly. On top of this a marked slowness in his movements appeared.

On admission he seemed very depressed, was consistently slow in all his movements, and never spoke spontaneously. In reply to questions he answered slowly and in a low tone, and was able to perform simple tests only with great difficulty. After a few days he showed some anxiety, having apparently a fear of being killed or injured, and with this it was noted that there was less retardation. After a few days the anxiety passed away, and he was found to be much freer in his movements and in his speech. He remained in the hospital ten months more, during which time he suffered from a typical severe obsessional neurosis that interfered with practically everything that he did. His *folie de doute* prevented even simple arithmetical calculations being performed readily. In this state there were no antisocial ideas forcing themselves on the patient's mind, but often a compulsive *déja vu*. When he heard a remark made, he would feel certain he had heard it before, and be compelled to recall the first instance under pain of great discomfort. It is interesting that he said that his mind was practically a blank for that period, during which he had been markedly retarded, which suggests the action of repression most strongly. A year after admission he was discharged while still in this condition, being transferred to another hospital. There he recovered entirely, but died of tuberculosis some months later.

The next case shows some interesting psychological mechanisms in connection with frankly infantile compulsive ideas.

CASE 53. *Sarah T..A.* was a single woman, aged 37, and a teacher at the time of her psychosis. During the winter term, prior to her breakdown, she had some hopes of getting married which were overthrown. She found herself unusually tired by the close of the school year, and soon sleeplessness began as well as a tight feeling about her head, whenever she applied her mind. These symptoms were associated, as it later developed, with compulsive ideas. About six weeks before admission the idea came to her that she might injure her mother. She became depressed at once. She then went into the country, where the idea of injuring her mother apparently disappeared, or, rather, was transformed into a fear of striking her friends. She also thought that she could not resume her work as a teacher lest the desire to strike her scholars should overpower her. A week before admission she was so troubled that she attempted suicide.

On admission it was found that she slept rather poorly, but was able to make a fairly natural impression, although it could be seen that she was despondent. She complained at first merely of the tight band about her head and of her sleep, but an account of her compulsive ideas was soon given. She mentioned that she was all the time afraid of injuring " that old lady " (pointing to another patient). She said these ideas were sometimes like visible shapes of fiends or goblins jibing at her, and she complained of a mental picture of a man in her neighbourhood who had hung himself—" this picture in my mind seems to take that man's likeness and to be jeering and laughing at me, and telling me I shall come to something quite as horrible ". All these symptoms were more marked in the mornings, and as their persistence diminished during the day she would also become less depressed. After a month's stay in the hospital she began to improve, and in a month more seemed quite well, and was discharged as recovered.

It seems that in this case the compulsive idea of injuring her mother led to a depression, in which this idea was repressed, and the only imperative thoughts which remained were of injuring strangers.

Her recovery was but temporary, and in the relapse another mechanism appeared. Shortly after her return home the impulses reappeared, and this time she was not so appreciative of their reprehensible nature, and did not seem to feel so much stirring of conscience about them. On one occasion she was said to have tried to smother her aunt with a soft pillow, but it was not stated how energetic this attempt was. Three months after her discharge she was readmitted. She seemed much more disturbed than on a previous occasion, having less control over her emotions. She cried a good deal, bit her nails, and made no attempt to occupy herself. A certain acceptance of the infantile ideas was confessed, for she said that the idea of killing her mother and aunt was becoming less and less horrible. This was associated with another idea which we have often observed in such conditions, particularly in involution states, namely, that of the patient's own death. (It seems as if these unfortunates compound for their imaginary sins with their own lives, as it were. We have seen ideas of killing the parent of the same sex appear with equally obsessive notions of self-destruction—all this in a quite benign psychosis. We have not seen such a murderous fancy accepted in any degree without being accompanied by self-death ideas, except in dementia praecox). Although she was restless, the patient seemed more depressed than before. She soon recognized the pure compulsiveness of her thoughts, and with this gained control over her conduct to such an extent that she was able to make a natural impression. At the same time she remained subjectively depressed and discouraged. After being in the hospital for seven months her mother took her home, where she soon recovered entirely. Two years later she was seen again, and was, as she apparently had been in the interval, quite well and cheerful.

CHAPTER XXXV

THE MENTAL MAKE-UP OF DEPRESSIVE PATIENTS

IN this research as to the psychological causes of depression the first questions have been answered more or less satisfactorily. The manifest symptoms of the psychosis may be attributed to repression acting against a push from the unconscious, which is formulated in an anti-social idea. The evidence—to us at least—seems to justify this assumption. But other difficulties arise at once. The whole trend of psychoanalytic psychology (which receives support from study of the psychoses) goes to show that such tendencies are universal and, almost as universal, is their repression. This however, is usually successful, and the submerged idea is transformed into some related concept that can escape censorship and gain conscious freedom. Plainly then, in depression, three differences from the normal process must be present : *the pathogenic thought must remain in the co-conscious,* as repression is continuing to operate ; *a certain mental rigidity must exist which prevents the warping of the idea into a more ethically acceptable form :* and *the bulk of the patient's energy, his potential interest, must be concentrated in this criminal co-conscious fancy.* Of course no question beginning with " why " can ever be completely and finally answered, but we can often carry the " why "back several steps towards the first cause. In this sense, if the question, " What causes these differences from normal mental processes ? " be answered, we would have begun to answer the " why " of depression.

There are two great types of variations in mental operations : the same individual reacts differently in different situations and, as individuals, our reactions differ to the same situations. Specifically we all know that certain accidents are likely to make anyone sad, while certain people are liable to be saddened by almost any accident. If we study, then, the nature of the events which precipitate depression and the types of personality prone to depression and the inter-action of these external and internal factors, we may, perhaps, gain some hint as to the cause of depression. Let us begin with the make-up of depressive patients.

I am indebted to the late Dr. Hoch for some statistics on this subject which are of particular interest, since they were compiled many years ago before psychological researches of the present kind were thought of. In this investigation he classified the personalities into five groups : hypomanic (exuberance of activity and emotionalism), cheerful, normal, quiet and " depressive ". In studying the incidence of these different types in the different kinds of emotional insanity, he found there was a marked tendency for hypomanic individuals to develop maniacal rather than depressive psychoses, for the cheerful, normal and quiet people to go equally one way or another, while the depressive personalities produced depressive reactions preponderantly. Being now interested in depression we shall consider the figures for that group alone. In 76 cases where reliable data were secured the personalities were as follows : hypomanic 6.6 per cent., cheerful 22. per cent., normal 6.6 per cent., quiet 18. per. cent.. " depressive " 46. per cent. Considering the fact that social life tends to the inhibition of aberrant emotions to such an extent that the essential character of a man often eludes the detection of either introspection or astute observation, these figures   are   striking :   64.   per cent.   or,   roughly,   two-thirds of individuals with pure depressions have foreshadowed their psychoses with noteworthy reactions or certain characteristics which we shall immediately examine.   It should be borne in mind that these figures refer to all cases, not merely those whose breakdowns had occurred independently of depressing circumstances.

On the other hand, this kind of make-up seems to lead, almost exclusively, to depressive psychoses. It appeared in the following proportions in the different clinical groups : manic o. per cent., circular, predominantly manic, o. per cent., equal circular 17. per cent., depressive circular 26. per cent., depression 46. per cent., involution melancholia 47. per cent.

Obviously this personality type is worth studying. In Dr. Hoch's manuscript there appear the descriptions of 22 cases in which some 18 traits are mentioned 57 times altogether. " Among the pure depressions we find the following descriptions : fussy, inclined to fight battles over again, tendency to blue spells ; active, sensitive, prone to worry, rather exacting ; bright, energetic, nervous, easily fretted ; good judgment, active, but worries over trifles and somewhat hypochondriacal ; never natural, buoyant but inclined to fret over trifles, shy, vacillating, hard to take responsibilities ;   easily   discouraged ;   always   borrowed   trouble ; always inclined to worry, especially in premenstruum ; sensitive, over-anxious ; apt to worry and without self-confidence ; depressive make-up ; inclined to worry and never very robust ; despondent, fussy and dissatisfied ; quiet and inclined to worry but sociable and amiable ; quiet and at times moody ; easily worried ; extremely conscientious, diffident, retiring and very unselfish ; energetic but apt to be dissatisfied with any choice, conscientious ; delicate and undecided ; stolid, inclined to worry about health ; timid and without self-confidence ; diffident, dependent and disposed to worry over trifles and look on the dark side of life. The following cases are among the few in which a definite ability is marked. One patient is described as enthusiastic, emotional, sensitive, apt to be extravagant in her statements but worrisome ; happy, active, enjoying company but inclined to blue spells; highly strung, quick-tempered, up and down in spirit, easily discouraged ; active, either way up or way down. Two cases described are sensitive and of nervous temperament ; one as active, nervous and inclined to bilious spells ; and one nervous and with a tendency to phobias." To gather any significance from the above, these characteristics should be grouped and analysed. We find that worry is mentioned ten times ; blue spells or moodiness seven times (in three instances as part of a tendency to mood swings) ; activity seven times (but never in a relatively pure form as with hypomanic personalities, four times it was associated with worry, once with vacillation and twice as part of mood swings) ; lack of confidence six times ; anxiety five times ; sensitiveness five times ; hypochondria four times ; shyness three times ; quietness or stolidity three times ; fretfulness three times ; mood swings three times ; fussiness twice ; discontent twice ; over-conscientiousness twice ; unselfishness once ; slowness in assumption of responsibility once ; exactingness once ; and " fighting battles over again " once.

One would expect, â priori, either that the personality of the depressed individual would be found to represent a diluted depressive reaction—" moodiness " and blue spells—or that it would reflect a general instability with no tendency for a definite personality type. But neither expectation is justified. Blue spells were reported only six times out of fifty-seven. But in three of them it was the only abnormality, in the other three part of a tendency to mood swings. In six out of twenty-two cases, therefore, the make-up of the patient represented a diluted depressive or circular psychosis. This is a surprisingly small proportion. The other sixteen showed fourteen characteristics which are interesting. They can readily be divided into three groups : anxiety twenty-four times ; egoism twenty-five times ; and unclassified five times.

The anxiety group comprises worry, anxiety, hypochondria, fretfulness and fighting battles over again, all of which characteristics can be seen to be closely related. What does it mean, psychologically, for a person to be of this anxious, unhappy type ? In the light of what we have been explaining in the previous chapters, it would seem that the patient's unconscious energy is always being embodied in painful co-conscious ideas instead of thoughts (like those of the manic) that can lead to activity and outlet. The individuals who habitually have this tendency, must suffer from a mental rigidity or inelasticity, which prevents unconscious reformulation of unpleasant ideas. As the co-conscious fearful idea represents a deep-lying unconscious striving, as we have seen in the last chapter, the latter accounts for the energy which lies back of this symptomatic habit of worry. An anxious make-up, therefore, provides occasion for the assumptions made above as to depression depending on mental rigidity and the concentration of energy in the co-conscious, anti-social fancy.

The egoistic characteristics are quite as important. Everyone acknowledges the instinct of self-preservation and that each person has, naturally, a strong interest in himself. Psychoanalytic research has enlarged the importance of this tendency by showing how it works unconsciously in the production of behaviour apparently directly opposed to it. We are all familiar with the manifestations of exaggerated, conscious self-interest; there is conceit, high ambition, selfishness, demand for recognition, indifference to the interest or feelings of others and supreme self-confidence. The germs of this behaviour are in us all, being particularly evident in childhood. With natural development and education, social proclivities increase and the child learns the folly of emotional isolation. Pure egoism is therefore repressed. In an individual who is naturally slow in adaptation or whose training is faulty, these tendencies persist longer and more exclusively dominate the personality. Finally, however, they are repressed—except in those persons in whom we recognize the adult life as egotistic and selfish. With this late repression a more potent force is kept in abeyance that requires every possible device for its subjugation. A conscious personality is therefore developed which seems to be the opposite of the ego type. This is the process known in psycho-analysis as *reaction formation*. Two purposes are served by reaction formation. A conscious repugnance for egotistic tendencies is built up, which aids in repression, while, on the other hand, the subject has the conscious satisfaction of feeling that of this—for him the unforgivable sin—he is guiltless.

The most prominent characteristic of this spurious conscious elaboration is a feeling of inferiority. With the unconscious demanding achievement and recognition proper only to a superman, the actual accomplishment and status of such an individual falls so far short of the ideal as to be judged as failure. All the characteristics cited above as evidences of unconscious egoism appear as their opposites. For conceit, there is humbleness ; for ambition and self-confidence, a feeling of incompetence and shyness ; in place of demands for recognition, an expectation of adverse criticism ; for selfishness and lack of sympathy, an apparent and often real altruism. In so far as the unselfish qualities become genuine, adaptation is favoured, although often interest in others is more a matter of protestation and self-deception than a working, durable altruism. On the other hand, shyness and expectation of failure are assets neither to the individual nor his associates.

Out of the fifty-seven characteristics noted in the depressive make-up, the following, which we regard as evidence of the ambivalent egoism and inferiority, appeared altogether twenty-five times : lack of confidence, shyness, sensitiveness, discontent, over-conscientiousness, slowness in assuming responsibility, unselfishness, and exactingness. As will be noted, the only characteristic cited here which could be of value is unselfishness, which was mentioned only once. It is therefore the maladaptive exhibitions of unconscious egoism, which appear in those individuals prone to depression.   It is not hard to understand how these traits facilitate depression. They lead inevitably to dissatisfaction, the prime cause of regression with its inflation of unconscious tendencies. As egoism favours crudity of infantile formulations and altruism is a necessary component of a socially acceptable formulation, this type of individual finds it hard to distort crude infantile longing into acceptable ideas, so that repression must continue. Also, since this infantile urge is the vehicle for expression of an overweening and dominant egoism, a large part of the patient's energy is bound up in it. We can see, therefore, that the inferiority make-up, like the anxious, supplies the same factors assumed above as necessary for the establishment of depression, namely, mental rigidity and concentration of libido in the repressed unconscious idea.

Another important point in the relationship of unconscious egoism to depression is the feeling of incompetence, to which we shall have to return later. This is really the same as one of the symptoms of depression, the feeling of blocking, of impotence. As a matter of fact, the commonest cause of everyday " blues " is personal disappointment—a snub, a slight, a lack of expected recognition, and so on. The probability is that the six cases in this series who suffered abnormally from " moodiness " were all, or most of them, of this type. Of the twenty-two individuals cited, fourteen had these ego characteristics, six others were given to blue spells, so that it seems probable that most people liable to severe depression suffer from the contradiction between unconscious ambition and conscious achievement. A characteristic grouped with anxiety also belongs here as well. Hypochondria is, in one of its aspects, a demand for attention, a pathological form of self-advertisement.

To summarize these words about constitutional factors, we may say that, in so far as depressions result from mental habits, it is because these habits evidence failure to get satisfaction from life, a consequent regression, and repeated failure to reformulate the repressed unconscious libido in ideas acceptable to consciousness and applicable to adaptation in real life. The commonest cause of this failure is unconscious egotism which out-distances the supply of energy or intellectual endowment of the subject. What does appear in consciousness are anxious thoughts or attitudes that are significant of repression and a sense of inferiority alike. These habits mean mental rigidity and a concentration of energy in primitive unconscious ideas—factors which favour the maintenance of anti-social co-conscious images. Such ideas are constantly being repressed and with this process come *the symptoms* of depression.

I am thus describing in heavy psychopathological terms certain principles, which might, with equal accuracy, be expressed in terms of moral deficiency. Perennial truths return, no matter what outward form they assume. So it is not surprising to find that there is nothing new in this interpretation of depression. For more than a thousand years (roughly from 500 A.D. onward) the Christian Church was much exercised over what was known as " Accidie "[1]. The layman, too, knew of it, for Dante and Chaucer have much to say about its deadliness. " Accidie " has been translated inadequately by " sloth ", but it seems to me from reading a number of descriptions of it that it included not only what we would call depression but also just those selfish habits which appear in Hoch's personality studies of patients who develop depressions. In this connection it is interesting to find that Aquinas makes of the *tendency* a venial weakness, but the acceptance by consciousness of a depressive outlook a deadly sin. In other words an actual depression is a triumph of evil. For centuries accidie was held to be a mortal sin, but, gradually, it became more and more of a disease, until now the psychological insight regenerated by Freud detects the anti-social nature of disease-producing thoughts. The only students of psychology who have dealt first hand with human problems are the moral theologians of long ago and the present-day psychopathologists. A thousand years ago preconceptions availed the confessor as little as they do the twentieth century physician, both seeking to bring peace to a troubled mind. Both have had to forget how the mind is supposed to work and to find out what really does activate it. Both have dealt with real people and both have come to the same conclusion, expressed by one in theological language and by the other in psychopathological terminology.

Accidie seems to have been a state of sluggishness in which the favour of God is no longer a vivid reality and in which the performance of duties, either religious or secular, is burdensome. This is a theological formulation ; but the descriptions of the state leave little doubt as to the clinical condition of him who suffered from accidie in its acute form. One of these, from the pen of St. John of Damascus, has already been quoted (p. 343). But, psychologically, we are more interested in what the authors had to say about the traits characteristic of it as cause or effect. They were unanimous in delineating these as anti-social tendencies. St. Thomas Aquinas, for instance, correlates accidie with hate and envy. He quotes Gregory I. as saying that it leads to six daughter vices : malice, spite, faint-heartedness (*pusillanimites*), despair, indifference to the commandments (*torpor circa praecepta*), and dalliance of the mind with forbidden things (*evagatio mentis circa illicita*). Dante describes how, in the Fifth Circle of the Inferno, were found in a stinking bog the souls of those whom anger had brought to destruction. Beside them, submerged in the filth, were those who had given way to

---

[1] For a fascinating study of this subject see the Introductory Essay in Paget's *The Spirit of Discipline*, which contains a wealth of references to pertinent literature, and which has been, essentially, the source of my information.

accidie—" Fixed in the slime they say, ' Gloomy were we in the sweet air, that is gladdened by the sun, carrying sullen, lazy smoke within our hearts ; now lie we *gloomy* here in the black mire'.   This hymn they gurgle in their throats, for they cannot speak it in full words."

CHAPTER XXXVI

PRECIPITATING MENTAL CAUSES OF DEPRESSION

THE next task is to examine the nature of those external events which precipitate depressions. They may be divided into four groups. In a series of fifty-three cases observed twenty years ago no cause was noted in twenty cases ; deprivations of one kind or another in thirteen, unconscious wish-fulfilments in fifteen, while five were not classified.

The first category is a negative one. It is important to realize that depressions begin, more frequently than any other type of manic-depressive insanity, without any history of an incident which upsets the patient. Such events are often not dramatic accidents but happenings of purely personal significance. To learn of them, therefore, one has to apply to the patient himself, who is often unable to recall the upsetting factor, which, in my experience, is sometimes a dream. Special psychological technique, such as hypnotism or psycho-analysis, may be successful in recovering the painful memory. When this is done, the existence of repression is proved. The fact that depressions occur without ascertainable cause in a disproportionately large number of cases suggests repression. We see it operating not infrequently in the course of the psychosis. The following case illustrates the forgetting of an idea which precipitated a psychosis ; it also is a good example of a depression as a direct result of an anti-social fancy.

CASE 54. *Mary P.* was a married Irish woman, aged 33, when she came under observation during her first attack. The family history showed nothing of interest. The patient was described as being efficient as a domestic servant for many years, not considered peculiar, but was quiet, and went about very little socially. Two years before admission she married a man at the insistence of her family, after being acquainted with him for only a month.

According to the patient's subsequent statement she began to feel " heavy " a short time after her marriage, although she denied unpleasantness in this relation. Eleven months before admission she became pregnant, and after this the heaviness increased. She felt difficulty in doing her housework but continued at it. She claimed that she did not feel depressed, but merely " heavy ". Ten days before the childbirth she got up one morning (after a dream ?), and said without any foundation that her husband was ill. She wanted to call a doctor, and was afraid something would happen to him. Once she remarked, " There is a sword waiting for you ". With these purely fanciful ideas of injury to her husband she became genuinely depressed. After recovery, when her memory was excellent for all external events of this period, she could recall absolutely nothing of these delusions.

366

For the next ten days she was depressed, and, in this condition, presented no evidence of having emotional contact with her actual environment. The day after these ideas of her husband had appeared she took a photograph of a woman for whom she had worked many years before her marriage, and looked admiringly at it in silence. When her husband questioned her she was mute. This suggests a regression from her married life formulated in a less objectionable form than in the thought of her husband's death. The childbirth was easy, and there was no fever, but she became even more depressed after this. " She did not seem to realize that she had a child, and appeared as if in a dream." Although she nursed the baby when it was b ought to her, she paid no further attention to it.

When she came *under observation*, she presented a picture of simple retardation sometimes amounting to mutism. When she did speak, it was usually to say, " I don't know," in answer to questions. It was discovered, however, that she was subjectively aware of the retardation, having a feeling of difficulty, feeling heavy, and so on. At times she cried, and occasionally picked her fingers, with some restlessness. Her behaviour in other respects was co-operative, and she seemed appreciative of attentions given her. Three months after admission the baby died, but this event seemed to make no impression on her.

For the next six months, in a general setting of reduced activity and inaccessibility, she smiled or laughed occasionally, also indulging in occasional pranks. Then for a year she was mildly hypomanic, and during this state denied absolutely that she had ever had a baby. Her husband died during this year, and she then was rather naturally saddened by the news. At the end of this period she recovered completely, but was then unable to explain her symptoms beyond say ng that she had felt unable to speak, that there was " like a lump of grief in her throat," and that she felt lonely and nervous. She had also completely forgotten her denial during the hypomanic state of ever having had a baby.

The second group is that of disappointments and deprivations. Every normal activity we enjoy, every person or thing we love, is an outlet for our libido. When fate robs us of such an outlet or we lose the physical energy to enjoy it, the interest returns to its source, the unconscious ; regression takes place. A girl who began to masturbate following the death of her father is a good example of regression of outlet. This principle has been dealt with in the discussion of Involution Melancholia, so needs no further discussion here. It is in such circumstances that those with a " depressive make-up " are hardest hit. But we are all unconsciously egoists. (Where we differ is in our ability to give this ego impulse a social application.) Consequently a deprivation or disappointment is always depressing. A normal man with normal resistance suffers briefly and lightly from an ordinary mischance. But a sufficiently grand tragedy will depress any individual quite thoroughly. There are only two factors to be considered, the amount of libido which is torn from its habitual application, and the capacity of the unfortunate to reconstruct his interests. The unstable individual is liable to suffer in both ways. He commonly is narrower in his interests than his normal fellow—he has all his eggs in one basket —and so accident is more likely to loosen his bonds with reality and cast his unconscious interest adrift. Secondly, he lacks the capacity to sublimate this detached libido readily. Naturally, poor physical health renders sublimation difficult. This accounts in considerable measure for the increased frequency of depression and anxiety with advancing years, as well as for similar psychoses in the puerperium.

In the 13 cases of our series where depressions were initiated by disappointment, five of these were business reverses. Three were women upset by the menopause. (Physically this may be a shock, but its essential virulence is probably psychological. To lose fertility is to lose a large part of life for any woman. It necessitates a revision of emotional outlook and the development of indirect application of the maternal instinct.) Two men were cast down by physical disease ; one woman by an operation for ovariectomy which was presumably unsuccessful, for she menstruated for a year after it, while under observation. One woman was jilted and became psychotically dejected by the loss of her lover.

Examples of business reverses, loss of friends or sudden physical incapacity precipitating depression are too notorious to justify citation here. Not only psychiatrists, but most laymen have seen them. One case may be quoted, however, as it exposes the mechanism of regression quite nicely.

CASE 55. *Sara S.* was a single school teacher, aged 29 at the time of her psychosis. Her father from his 30th year on had attacks of depression every three or four years. No abnormality is mentioned in the brief account of her personality.

Four years before admission the patient was disappointed in love, and was slightly and continuously depressed after this event, although she continued her work as teacher. During three and a half years she was apparently suffering from a loss of this type of emotional outlet. Rather suddenly, six months before admission, she gave evidence of regression with imaginary restitution of her loss. She surprised her family by saying she was afraid she was pregnant, that a certain man who was engaged to another woman had taken liberties with her. She at once became markedly depressed, occupied herself but little, sat about or walked restlessly around picking her fingers. As a rule she slept poorly, but sometimes had a good night, which was then followed by a day of greater depression. (This highly significant symptom of depression suggests strongly a regression in dreams which brings anti-social thoughts more poignantly into consciousness or co-consciousness). During this time she spoke frequently in regard to this fear of pregnancy, saying that she had committed a great crime, and, at times, became agitated when talking of it.

When brought to the hospital she was quite retarded, and spoke much of her wickedness. Particularly at night she was apt to moan loudly. Her face was peculiarly immobile. Her depression was probably not associated so much with the delusion of pregnancy as it was with still more regressive thoughts. The fact that she had picked the fiancé of another woman as the imaginary aggressor against her virginity suggests that back of this delusion the Oedipus complex was operating. An evidence of this appeared in a statement that she thought such " horrible things " about her mother, no further explanation of which was secured. A year following her admission she gave an excellent summary of her condition in a letter in which she said that the crime of her pregnancy was true, that she was not ill and had not been, but that she was wicked beyond human experience, that she had the most terrible thoughts that any one had ever had, the most sacrilegious, the most irreverent, that her whole spiritual and moral nature was wrecked. She also described well her feeling of emotional anæsthesia which blocked out love, joy, pleasure, pain, sorrow or repentance. This feeling was all due to her wickedness, which she could not get rid of, and consequently there was no hope for her.

Shortly after this she began to impiove. Her depression was always worse in the morning, and the cheerful periods towards night came on earlier and earlier. Two years after the onset of her psychosis she was discharged, although not quite well, but complete recovery supervened shortly after her return home.

The third group is that of infantile wish-fulfilments. When fate ordains that a deeply lying unconscious wish shall reach fulfilment by no act of the subject himself, this naturally inflates the unconscious. There are four possible reactions that are thereby induced. The first is the normal one. The event is accepted more or less at its face value (painful though it always is, for we hate most what we yearn most keenly for in the unconscious), and the stimulus received leads to further sublimation. A second is to deny the existence of what has happened. This is the hysterical mechanism. The literature of psychopathology is full of such instances, where an extensive amnesia wipes out all memory of the event and even of its attendant circumstances. Thirdly, the infantile fantasies may be accepted, which is the mechanism of dementia praecox. Frequently in such cases there is an initial depression ; for example, I once saw a girl of markedly seclusive make-up who lost her older sister. For two days she was retarded and sad, then a chronic hebephrenic state appeared.

If no one of these three things happens, the stimulated unconscious cravings must be repressed until such time as sublimation occurs, or dementia praecox or hysteria develops. While this repression is operating the patient is depressed In this connection one thinks of the greater frequency with which the death of the parent, siblings or friends of the same sex or of the married partner leads to depression, than the death of those of the opposite sex. Such events are fulfilments of an infantile, criminal order. It is particularly difficult to sublimate ideas of injury to others, and this is probably the reason why such trend, as we do obtain in depressions, is antisocial in its nature. There is, perhaps, a fifth solution, although it is so rare as hardly deserving classification. This is a psychoanalytic comprehension of the situation, thorough enough to protect the patient against his unconscious.

The 15 cases (out of 53 depressions) who broke down as a result of unconscious wish-fulfilments give fair examples of what these accidents are like. They fall into two groups. In the first they refer to the removal of infantile rivals or their surrogates—parents, siblings or friends of the same sex—which removal is actual, as by death, or suggested, by sickness or injury. Six of the 16 were of this order. In the second type the unconscious wish is for the solution of the marriage bond, when some incident such as sickness or death implies separation, or when something occurs to strengthen the union or increase its responsibility. There were 8 cases connected with marriage. Two of these began with the ceremony itself ; one with engagement ; two when the patients broke engagements ; three with death, sickness or injury to the partner. This series did not happen to contain cases of puerperal depression. In these, psychological study usually shows that the mental cause comes from the revulsion against the added responsibility of additional children. Strictly speaking, incidents which increase the weight of domestic responsibility are not unconscious wish-fulfilments but the exact reverse. We mention them here, however, because they stimulate the unconscious to rebellion at once. In one case the prospective marriage of her daughter upset a mother—an echo of childish rivalry.

Before citing the histories of some cases illustrative of infantile wish-fulfilments, it may be well to dispose of the five cases in our series which are classified as miscellaneous. All of these with some interpretation can be placed in the infantile or the deprivation group, but we have not so arranged them because they do not fall into these categories at the first glance. Three patients broke down at the prospect of a business change with worry about their ability to meet the new responsibilities. Psychologically this is the same situation as that of losing a business, except that the separation is voluntary. In each case an established outlet is removed, be it taken away by external agency or the choice of the patient. The same problem arises of re-attaching the libido to the new occupation, and this is the problem which proves too much for the depressive individual as we have seen. One housewife broke down as a result of moving from one house to another. We have seen many such cases. It seems that, to married women at least, this change of abode stimulates the unconscious notion of abandoning domestic responsibilities, for in the subsequent psychoses such ideas appear prominently. So " moving " may be an infantile cause. The fifth case was unusual in the nature of the precipitating circumstances. A man discovered that he had unwittingly proceeded illegally in the administration of his mother's estate (although not dishonestly). He worried unduly about this and then became depressed. If we presume that this situation symbolized the unconscious idea of illicit possession of his mother's affection (what she had to give), and therefore stimulated it, we would be justified in placing this with the infantile wish-fulfilment group.

With a little psychological interpretation, therefore, it seems that the classification of the precipitating causes of depression contains only three groups : cause unknown, deprivations or disappointments, and events which stimulate directly anti-social unconscious trends.

We may now illustrate the last type with brief descriptions of some cases. A good example was the case of Carrie D., quoted above, whose psychosis was precipitated by the death of her husband, immediately after which she developed ideas of her having destroyed her children and then became depressed.   The sequence of events in this case was interesting.   There was, first, the death of a bad husband, of whom she would naturally be glad to be rid, then an anxiety state in which antisocial ideas reached free expression, then distinct blocking, and finally simple retarded depression with no content whatever.

CASE 56.   *Charles D.* was a business man, aged 47, who had three previous attacks of depression.

Five months before admission his wife was ill and he began to complain of difficulty in doing his work and of loss of strength.   His business did not go well.   Four months before admission his wife died and he failed in business. He then became more depressed, languid, saying little and inhibited from doing almost anything.   He explained his inadequacy by saying that he could not get his mind off the death of his wife.   Then appeared self-reproach ; he said he was a scoundrel, the worst criminal that ever lived.   On admission he showed a rather typical retardation and considerable inadequacy.   His feeling of moral obliquity he justified by a belief that he had defaulted money, that people now knew his real character, so that there was no hope for him. After three weeks he began to improve, and nine months after the onset of his psychosis he was entirely well.

CASE 57.   *Edward P.* was a married farmer, aged 46.   An uncle had committed suicide, a nephew was insane, one brother epileptic.   The patient was a hard working man who was frequently troubled by mild depressions, but they never entirely incapacitated him.

About six months before admission his brother, who farmed with him, was taken ill.   He did a rather peculiar thing, in that, although his work was doubled, owing to his brother's illness, he enlarged the farm.   Three months later his brother died.   The patient then became grieved and discouraged, sold his property, pottered around without accomplishing anything, and had a marked feeling of inadequacy.   The regression with an idea of injury to his wife and children was hinted at by the statement that his family were going to come to want.   On admission he was markedly retarded with a great feeling of inadequacy.   There was a strong tendency to borrow trouble without this crystalizing into definite ideas.   He always insisted on ascribing his condition to the death of his brother which " broke him all up."   He left the hospital shortly after improvement had begun and recovered completely some fifteen months after the onset of the psychosis.

In connection with precipitating causes, or rather with the onset of depressions, a group of cases should be considered in which worries provide a setting for the psychosis.   These worries are not concerned with imaginary troubles, but the stress laid on them becomes morbid.   The worry produces an instability in which an untoward event is capable of producing a psychosis.   When this comes, the painful ideas are apt to be reflections both of the initial worry and of the precipitating cause.   The psychotic elaborations of the worries suggest that the earlier concentration of the patient's attention on the difficulties was due to regression, to the stimulation of unconscious ideas which found representation in the real situation.   All worry is probably of this order, its content, like the trumped-up petty sins of the depression, being a mere excuse for the obsessive foreboding.   The origin of the mood is in the unconscious, probably a co-conscious image of some untoward event. The case of Eustace B. quoted above is an example in point. He lost money and began to worry over this. Then on the death of a friend he developed both death and pecuniary embarrassment into the idea of his wife coming to want. This led to depression in which all such thoughts disappeared and his only talk was of his inadequacy.

CASE 58. The depression of Mary W. was of somewhat the same order. She was a widow, aged 51, whose mother was given to periods of depression. She herself was described as quiet, amiable and sociable, but always inclined to worry and had had no former attacks. Six years before admission her husband died and following that she had a rather chronic worry occasioned by the reckless expenditure of money on the part of one of her sons. Six months before admission her regular menstruation ceased. This probably was somewhat of a shock to her. About the same time she went to visit her son in a distant city and found conditions very unfavourable, inasmuch as he was not only continuing in his extravagance, but showed ingratitude to her. In the train on her return trip (as she afterwards explained) she was frightened by something and held the curtain of her berth tightly closed. When she arrived home she seemed somewhat depressed, no longer cared to meet people, spoke of her son's ingratitude and worried over the fact that her other son was not getting his share of the property. A month before admission some hypochondriacal ideas appeared and with them restlessness suggestive of an involution state. She occasionally spoke of dying, but more often of various pains, heart disease, of her throat closing up. She did not wish to go out of the house because something might happen to her, and when brought to the hospital thought she would never get away, would be put in a strait-jacket and locked up in a small room.

On admission she was found to be unoccupied most of the time, although frequently restless in an aimless way. All that could be got out of her in relation to her condition were hypochondriacal ideas which showed an interesting development. First she spoke of constipation and distress and a sinking feeling in her stomach, and then of a fear that there was something wrong there. When pressed she admitted a fear of cancer or pernicious anaemia. She blamed her condition on the trouble with her son and added, " I could not seem to be bright ; everything looked burdensome to me ; I feel now as if I were in a state of thinking nothing ; I seem as if my mind was all gone, exhaustion is nothing compared with it." After the physicians left she called them back and said she was pregnant, but would at this time give no further details. A day or so later she explained this last statement by saying that she had been assaulted on the train at the time of her fright. It is interesting to note that with this appearance of the pregnancy delusion her recovery began. First she could be easily reassured and was less restless. In two weeks she had become contented and cheerful with no apprehension and good insight, and this improvement continued except for a few brief periods of apprehension. After recovery she told of her fright on the train and explained her delusion of the assault and pregnancy on that basis. She could remember having said such a thing, although she was surprised at her ever having thought of it.

The sequence of symptoms in this case are of psychological interest. She began with worry about a real situation. Then at the first warning of the menopause she received a fright which apparently produced an *unconscious* idea of assault and pregnancy. The latter appeared as hypochondriacal notions of there being something wrong. A delusion of cancer is such a common symbol of pregnancy that this was probably a direct representation of the unconscious idea. Marked regression probably took place at this time, which was evidenced in her objective condition by an increase of the worry, symptoms of depression, together with the new symptom of hypochondria. The pressure from the unconscious demanded repression and with this came the depressive symptoms, which began to leave so soon as the plain idea of pregnancy appeared. When this came into consciousness it could (as during psychoanalysis) be consciously criticized and she speedily recovered

Such cases occur so frequently and are so much of a routine experience with the psychiatrist that no further examples would be profitable.

CHAPTER XXXVII

REACTIVE DEPRESSIONS

W E have mentioned above that a depressed patient gives the impression of not knowing the cause of his sorrow. A group which must now be considered is exceptional in this and other respects. This is the group of " Reactive Depressions." In them the patients worries excessively over some trouble and with the worry is the feeling of hopelessness and sorrow distinctive of depression. It is further characteristic of these quasi-depressions that retardation is objectively not witnessed and a feeling of inadequacy only sometimes referred to by the patient. Feelings of unreality are also in the background. On the other hand, instead of the inactive soddenness of the typical depression, there is an abnormal emotionality with tears and wailing.

The psychological explanations of these phenomena seem to be that repression is not so extensive here as in ordinary depressions. It is present more as a tendency. After some painful event which blocks a normal outlet, repression takes place, but the distressful circumstance, being capable of serving as a symbol of an unconscious wish, becomes fixed in the patient's attention, engrossing his thoughts. Consequently contact with reality is not lost, as in more profound depressions ; repression operates only against the infantile potentialities of the situation and emotions are exhibited, nay, exaggerated. As has been suggested before, frank emotional expression is evidence of contact with the environment and the frequent weeping of the reactive depression is probably to be looked on as an instinctive appeal for sympathy. In many cases, certainly, there are dramatic prayers for help. In this connection the reader may recall the case of Millie B. cited above. She began with a typical retarded depression and then cut her wrist in a suicidal effort. This gave her something real to think of and the clinical picture changed. She was no longer retarded but fussy, complaining constantly of her crime of cutting her wrist.

A word should be said about painful happenings serving as unconscious wish-fulfilments. With certain examples such as death of a loved one who is also a responsibility, divided feelings are comprehensible and many instances of " wishes " for death of husband, children, and so on, have been cited in this book. Desire for failure in personal activities is not so readily understood. It occurs primarily with those of a highly egoistic make-up, who seem

374

prone to expend great energy so long as they are successful, but to prefer no effort whatever if outstripped by others. They are in common speech " quitters." The " all or none " principle of instinctive reactions is nowhere better exemplified than in our unconscious egoistic trends. In epilepsy,[1] where egoism plays such an important rôle, failure leads inevitably to loss of interest so intense that it may paralyse all but the most primitive psychic powers and result in a profound dementia. In the " depressive " individual, however, (*vide supra*) the desire to " quit " reaches symptomatic expression in fascination with the thought of failure and behaviour that is unwittingly calculated to result in failure. This explains how business reverses (like the death of marital partners) may really be wish-fulfilments at an unconscious level.

Reactive depressions, then, are psychoses in which the patients' minds are fixed on distressing events with exaggerated attention and emotional response. Strictly speaking these events are real, but psychologically and psychiatrically analagous conditions arise when painful delusions are manufactured to which this type of reactive depression is a response. This is particularly true of the involution period when delusions of poverty often precipitate such a psychosis. As a rule, of course, other symptoms soon enter in and a typical involution melancholia is developed. The mental state of marked hypochondria is distinctly of this order. An unconscious lust for illness (which may be variously determined) leads to a focussing of the attention on real or imaginary ills with a marked emotional reaction thereto and many appeals for sympathy. In many retarded depressions a similar thing happens. After being simply depressed, sodden and dejected, the attention of the patient turns to his feelings of inadequacy and unreality and the clinical picture changes to a querulous state with much plaintive harping on the mental condition.

In the examples that follow it will be seen how usual it is for some evidence of regression to appear and therefore how superficial is the view which regards these depressions as wholly the product of unfortunate events. Although dominating the patient's consciousness, they are really only precipitating causes. The dynamic causes lie behind in the make-up and in the unconscious of the individual. Normal people throw off their troubles and turn to happier thoughts, but troubles are magnets for the psychopath. But while conscious attention is confined to the untoward circumstances precipitating the psychosis, a strong tendency exists for the stimulated unconscious to erupt. Against this is operating repression, and, in so far as the energy of the patient is thereby dammed up, to that extent is the individual depressed in the strict clinical sense of the term.

[1] MacCurdy, " A Clinical Study of Epileptic Deterioration ", *Psychiatric Bulletin*, April, 1916.

The first case illustrates how dominating ideas of failure may characterize and determine the reactive depression.

CASE 59. *Winifred B.* was a single physician, aged 53 at the time of his psychosis. He had always been sound physically and intellectually, and became a capable physician with a good practice. Temperamentally, he was shy and slow at making friends throughout life. He stated that after leaving home he missed his parents a great deal and that he had felt lonesome for the rest of his life. He also had a pessimistic tendency, although he had never been psychotically depressed prior to this time.

The patient was a visiting physician to a prison and six months before he came to the hospital a former inmate of the prison brought suit against him, apparently quite unjustifiably, on the grounds of malpractice. The patient at once began to worry over this, becoming more and more hopeless as to a favourable verdict. Soon his appetite began to fail and for two weeks prior to admission he had been restless and sleeping poorly. In this unstable condition unconscious desires for failure probably were beginning to affect his conduct, for two weeks before admission he left a patient while she was in labour, which he regarded soon after as a mistake in judgment. The subsequent delivery was difficult and the child developed meningitis several days after its birth. This affair added greatly to his worry and he became preoccupied and forgetful, betraying his depression and agitation to patients and friends alike, for he was so far affected as to neglect his duties. Two nights before admission he got so low in brooding over the lawsuit that he concluded to end it all. The next morning he went some sixty miles into the country, took with him the records of the case concerning which he was accused of malpractice and morphia with which to commit suicide. Having burned the documents his better nature prevailed and he returned home without attempting suicide. It seems difficult to believe that there was not an unconscious wish that he should be convicted of malpractice and therefore forced to give up medicine. This rather deliberate destruction of the evidence in his favour must surely have had a definite relationship to the fundamental cause of his worry. The fact that his condition was so far relieved as to allow him to drop the idea of suicide suggests that by this destruction of his records the unconscious pressure was reduced. As soon as he got home he went to see the child with meningitis, but it had died during the day.

A professional friend persuaded him to come to the hospital and this he did. For a few days he was quite depressed, kept mostly to himself, but to the physician repeated all the worries outlined above and protested that nothing was going to come out right. It was noted that the clinical picture was made up entirely of these ideas and his reaction to them, there being no evidence of inadequacy or of retardation. After a few days the depression began to lift, and in two weeks he was well enough to return to his practice.

In the next case the regression appeared mainly in distressing dreams. We have quoted earlier in this chapter the case of a woman who after the loss of her lover developed the idea of an illicit pregnancy and became genuinely depressed. In the following case the attention of the patient was focussed on her loss with a reactive depression, while a somewhat similar regression appeared in her dreams.

CASE 60. *Christine B.* was a single domestic servant aged 34. She was efficient, but her employer stated that she was quiet, sensitive and easily offended, although not depressive. She had been in this country for twelve years. On her arrival she had been very homesick with a good deal of crying, having dreams of going home or of her father and mother being dead. From this we may gather that she was an individual with whom transference of affective interest was a difficult matter.

Six months before admission some girls told her that a man, who was paying her attention and probably engaged to her, was not good. She told him about this and a quarrel resulted, in which he said that he would not see her again. She at once became downhearted, cried, beat her breast, pulled her hair and said she wanted to die. Her employer found her kneeling in her room and praying with the photograph of her lover pressed to her bosom. Although she kept on working and tried to appear cheerful, she stated afterward that her work was much harder, " It seemed to take me such a long time and I did not seem to know how to do it." During these months, so she told her sister, she had frequent dreams of a regressive order, in which she was usually the object of aggression. For instance, she dreamed that someone had stuck a knife into her heart, that people wanted to kill her, and there were many dreams of snakes. She would be eaten by snakes, and she spoke of a woman snake eater, she had seen some years before, and said that she represented this woman. The phallic significance of snakes is too notorious to deserve comment. There were also dreams of her lover, but in these she was unable to talk to him and in one of them he was drunk. After some improvement the family left the city, whereupon she got gradually worse until commitment was necessary.

Under observation she was highly emotional, at first crying nearly all the time, but later only when questioned. The content of her depression was constantly the loss of her lover. There were no self-accusations and no objective retardation, although she complained of feelings of inadequacy. The dreams did not recur. She gained weight and recovered entirely, although it took nine months. Six years later when seen again she was entirely well and had been so in the interval.

In the next case there was some slight evidence of regression which appeared in the form of worry about the patient's wife. Thoughts of injury to a wife are, as we have seen, frequent in typical retarded depressions.

CASE 61. *Adam F.* was a married business man, aged 43. He was described as always being over-ambitious. Even when vacations were granted him he would not rest, but often work even more strenuously. He had been married for seven years. Three months before admission there was a change of management in the business where he was employed, and as a result he was discharged. He began at once to worry about this, sleeping poorly and losing his weight and appetite. About six weeks later he invested a small sum of money in a commission business ; but it did not turn out well at all, and he abandoned the project after two weeks. This incident suggests that he was unconsciously courting failure, as it seems unlikely that an experienced business man would invest his money in an unpromising venture or would throw it up after such a short period as two weeks. After this he became still more depressed, seclusive, feeling that there was no more hope for him, and that he had lost all his business ability. Ten days before admission he was somewhat better and indulged in hard physical work (shovelling snow). This tired him, he had a " chill ", became agitated, could not be controlled. He walked the floor, rolling his head, wringing his hands and crying, talking continuously about his loss of money, his uselessness and incapacity.

By the time he reached the hospital, the trend of his ideas had changed somewhat, inasmuch as the fate of his wife seemed uppermost in his mind. He not only thought that she was coming to want financially, but believed that his entrance into the hospital would cause her death. In talking of his troubles, when he approached the imagined sufferings of his wife, he became very nervous, sometimes so much so that he was unable to speak. Six weeks after admission he began to improve, until he presented ordinarily quite a normal appearance. He continued, however, to have periods of relapse, which would last only a few hours, when he would walk about, moaning, wringing his hands and repeating over and over again his pessimistic thoughts.

Once during such a period there was a hint of his harbouring some thoughts of crime. When he was asked if any member of his family had had melancholia, he said, " Is that the charge against me ? " wanted to examine the doctor's notebook and insisted on knowing if any derogatory reports had been received about him. It was possible, however, to reassure him. As his improvement continued the relapses became more infrequent. Finally they occurred only when his wife visited him. After seven months, however, he was well enough to return home and resume business.

The last case of reactive depression which we shall quote illustrates a number of the points discussed above. The patient lost his position, then showed regression in his behaviour in connection with his love affairs, then had a psycholeptic crisis and following this a reactive depression, the content of which was concerned not merely with his loss of position but also with his mental state. Finally there were occasional self-accusations of the kind which are met with in ordinary depressions.

CASE 62. *Walter F.* was a single man aged 30, a librarian by occupation. His mother was a nervous woman and his father had locomotor ataxia, while a brother suffered for years from " neuritis." The patient himself was delicate as a child, never played with other boys, was effeminate and morbid all his life. He changed his occupation several times and finally became a librarian. At the age of 17 he had a mild attack of depression, in regard to which little information was obtainable.

Seven months before admission the patient was not reappointed in his position as he had expected. This was a shock to him. He became at once rather despondent, and made only ineffectual efforts to obtain other work. Nevertheless he was not gravely incapacitated until two months before admission, when he went to a sanitorium. Before going there he had fallen in love with a young woman. At the sanitorium he became infatuated with another one, and spent so much time with her that it caused considerable comment. The gossip worried him, and, in addition, he was much troubled over his unfaithfulness to the first girl. This is the type of situation which is characteristic of a maladapted individual, and, as we have seen, a not unusual cause for the ordinary type of depression. He did become more depressed, so much so that, when an excellent position was offered him, he could not even answer the letter. This caused him still more worry. He now felt that he had lost his last chance and disgraced his family. A short time before admission he had a sudden feeling that something had given away in his head, and following that the conviction that his brain was gone. He made a determined suicidal attempt, and in consequence of that was sent to the hospital.

In general his condition was typical of a reactive depression, in that there was much crying, moaning and craving for sympathy. He wanted to talk to the doctor all the time. When he secured an audience he would speak of his worthlessness, and, to accentuate this, would dwell on his superior social position and of the former virtues and gifts which he had enjoyed. With this, however, there were also many hypochondriacal complainings about something having burst in his brain, as a result of which his sexual feeling and desire were lost and gone for good. In addition he was prone to accuse himself a great deal after the manner of a retarded depression, the main accusation being that the family money was lost because he had not made a report in the capacity of executor of his father's will. This was the only idea he had which was concerned with injury to others, but he was given to blaming himself for lifelong selfishness, dishonesty, laziness and pleasure seeking, so that a feeling of immorality was prominent. After four months a decided improvement began, and ten months after admission he was discharged perfectly well, and had remained so for six years when he was again seen.

If one accepts the view that reactive depressions are compromises, in which complete regression is prevented by an obsessive pre-occupation with a painful situation, real or imaginary—one can then understand why the clinical pictures in involution melancholia are often so confused. So long as the regressive tendency is satisfied, so to speak, by obsessive thinking about poverty, physical disease or death, the mood is essentially one of anxiety or distress. But when regression tends to go further and awaken frank infantile sexuality, repression must intervene or a chronic psychosis appear. This accounts for the colouring of true depression, which is so often seen in involution melancholia. The case of Mary B., described in Chapter 17, illustrates this mechanism nicely. As will be recalled she worried about the illness of her husband and became gradually depressed with retardation. In this state she hinted at suspicions of her husband's infidelity (a rationalization of the unconscious desire for his death, which was suggested by his illness, and was probably the occasion of the regression). Then punishment ideas appeared, which began to engage her attention more and more. With this the repression lifted, as her mood became more and more one of anxiety, and the delusion of her husband's, and later of her sister's, death came to open expression, coupled with fears of her own death as punishment for these murders.

CHAPTER XXXVIII

DEPRESSION AND IMPOTENCE

IT must have struck readers who have studied the mental reactions of patients suffering from psychic impotence or fear
of it, that the inhibitions of depression are similar to, or
identical with the hopeless inertia of the impotent. The man
who feels himself incompetent in this supreme test of virility has no
courage for other activities and may, therefore, become genuinely
depressed.

To understand the relationship of these two clinical conditions
we must consider what psychoanalysis usually reveals in the unconscious mechanism of impotence. It is found that affection
has been centred on the mother so continuously and fixedly that
transference of love to another woman is incomplete or impossible.
Consequently, whatever purely sex instinct there may be in the
individual has been unconsciously attached to the mother. Any
obviously sexual act awakens the Oedipus complex and tends to
bring it into consciousness as such. To prevent this there is an
automatic inhibition of the copulating function which constitutes
impotence.[1] In the normal man emotional elasticity exists which
enables him to transfer his libido, gain conscious satisfaction in
union with a permissible mate, and, at the same time, satisfy the
unconscious craving symbolically.

This problem arises at puberty, as a rule, when the problems of
adult sexuality are first presented. In boys the conflict is commonly symbolized in a conscious mental turmoil occasioned by
masturbation. Bad advice and misinformation tend to accentuate
the morbid aspects of this habit and facilitate the development of
sexual neurasthenia with its fears of impotence and hypochondriacal complaints of headache, occipital pressure, loss of memory,
weak back, etc. The physical symptoms are all symbols of injury
to the male organs ; indeed, I have seen quite sane and otherwise
intelligent patients who believed that the penis was a continuation
of the spinal cord and semen a secretion of the brain. Belief in
impotence is often precipitated by an experience of ejaculatio
praecox, but neither this nor masturbation is essential to the picture.

[1] It is true that other and important factors such as " castration complexes " enter in as a rule. They do not need to be considered here, however,
since (in my view) they are secondary and contributory and, moreover,
confined to one sex.

In fact I have seen all the classical symptoms of this condition appear after the first nocturnal emission in an extremely seclusive boy, whose first conscious knowledge of sex had been secured at a cheap burlesque theatre to which he had been dragged the night before. Whether "sexual neurasthenia" can arise purely on a basis of physical exhaustion of the sex organs as Freud originally claimed, I do not know. I have never seen a case which was not demonstrably psychogenic.

If this neurosis, built around the concept of impotence, is fundamentally the result of repression, it belongs to the depressive group. The reason why plain retarded depression does not develop is that the libido escapes repression by means of conversion into what is, psychologically, an hysterical symptom—impotence. The repression then is focussed on a physical function and mental functions escape. As a matter of fact, this is only a theoretic case[1]. In actual practice we find that the conversion is not completely successful, and varying amounts of other unconscious energy is being repressed. Impotence is always accompanied by a setting of general depression. In this way a rather distinct clinical picture results which is characterized by depression of spirits, hypochondria and absorption in frankly sexual or closely allied problems. When such depressions are considered alone (and they are very frequent in non-institutional practice) it is easy to investigate them from the standpoint of this sex content and be led astray as to the mechanism of depression in general. Individual factors determining the specific sex problems naturally appear in the foreground and, in a small series of cases, may be sufficiently alike to suggest that they cause depression. Abraham's[2] cases seem all to be of this type.

Impotence, of course, is confined to males; yet women have similar parental attachments and must therefore suffer from analogous repressions when confronted with the adult sex problem. The differences are these: The same mechanism which produces impotence leads to frigidity, "anæsthesia" in women. This, however, is not as devastating a disability, since the rôle of the female is passive. It does not prevent fertility as impotence does procreation. In consequence the woman suffers from a lack of satisfaction (of a craving which may not be consciously felt), but the man is harrowed by a knowledge of incompetence in a most important rôle. The woman, therefore, is protected against her unconscious by a mild symptom which occasions little mental distress, while the man is protected only by a torturing disease, capable of much elaboration and further symbolic appearance in other symptoms. In other respects the conditions are the same and both live in the same aura of depression. In the woman's case there is shame about masturbation or its analogue sexual fantasy, and

---

[1] Since writing this, however, I have studied an adult case that does fulfil these conditions.

[2] *Vide supra.*

a feeling of inferiority based on social and emotional incapacity. Prudery and excessive shyness are analogues of the mental traits of the psychically impotent man. The social fear of the sexually undeveloped woman is a translation into feminine terms of the feeling of unworthiness of the impotent man. Prudery is a feeble bluff which the woman, who is, or was, subject to sex fantasies, makes in an effort to persuade herself and others that her mind is pure. For " clear-eyed chastity," she substitutes a myopic, prurient criticism. Prudery is capable of no lovely development, but its counterpart in the adolescent male, the " Galahad complex," although it does not mean a sturdy morality, may, at least, be graceful.

Such depressions are so frequently seen in youth of both sexes that the term " Adolescent depression " would not be out of place. But they occur whenever the adult sex problem becomes acute, for instance, following engagement of marriage. They are never pure depressions because the repression is never complete. Symbolic outlets, representing unconscious solutions of the problem, carry off much of the libido and only what is left, which tends to appear in the form of crude infantilism, is repressed. There are, therefore, many anxieties and worries and much hypochrondria, with only a general background of depression.

PART VIII

PERPLEXITY STATES

" Our dreams drench us in sense, and sense steeps us again in dreams."
—A. B. Alcott.

CHAPTER XXXIX

DESCRIPTION OF PERPLEXITY STATES

IN the discussion of manic states the suspicion emerged that free associational thinking had much to do with the various symptom pictures grouped under that heading. We shall now see that another reaction type is, apparently, determined by similar mechanisms.

Psychiatry has suffered greatly at the hands of such of its devotees as have allowed their ambition for originality in classification to outrun their discretion. Justification for the proposal of a new clinical group is therefore demanded by a critical reader. A taxonomic entity is not established by the discovery of previously unrecognized symptoms in the alleged group, unless these symptoms can be shown to have a direct bearing on prognosis, or unless they stand in the centre of the clinical picture, producing psychoses that seem anomalous and confusing from a descriptive standpoint. We would, perhaps, go further than this, now that we are dealing with reaction types, and demand that the bizarre form of mental disease should be demonstrated as the product of a peculiar kind of psychic process. In the present chapter we are chiefly engaged with this last problem.

Since the perplexity type of manic depressive insanity is little known, it is probably wise to postpone discussion of its psychology in order that the *raison d'être* of the new clinical grouping may be first established.

Perplexity as a *symptom* has already been brought to the attention of the reader of the foregoing chapters, but it may be well to collect some of the examples in order that the nature of the phenomenon may be appreciated. Among the stupor cases Charlotte W. (Case 3)

383

showed at times an expression of bewilderment or perplexity. After such periods, when referring to her subjective state, she spoke of things looking queer, as, for example, pictures on the wall looking like saints, actual people seeming to be dead relations, and so on. She also complained of things seeming to have a mist over them. Around this time her orientation was usually good, but she would frequently become absorbed and drift off into an hallucinatory state. Hoch says in his book on Benign Stupors, p. 164 : " Not infrequently we see exhibitions of this tendency in what are otherwise typical stupors. For example, Mary F. . . . showed for a few days after admission a condition where she was essentially somewhat restless in a deliberate aimless way. At the same time she looked dazed or dreamy. With this restlessness she appeared at times ' a little apprehensive '. Although she spoke slowly, with initial difficult,y she answered quite a number of questions. Her larval perplexity was evidenced by the doubt in a good many of her utterances, such as, ' Have I done something ? ' ' Do people want something ? ' ' I have done damage to the city, didn't I ? ' When asked what she had done, she said, ' I don't know '. She asked the physician, ' Are you my brother ? ' And when questioned for her orientation said, ' Is not this a hospital ? ' The atmosphere of perplexity also coloured the information which she did recall correctly ; for instance, when asked her address, she said, ' Didn't I live at—— ? ' then giving the address correctly."

A certain amount of perplexity is not uncommon in involution melancholia, but among the cases quoted in Chapter 7 no evidence of it is given except perhaps in that of Cora O. (Case 7). It may be recalled that she complained of not being able to grasp her thoughts properly and of her having someone with her, who put answers into her mind (for instance, answers to simple arithmetical questions). We shall see that this is a frequent type of complaint in perplexity cases.

When we turn to the manic states quite a number of instances are encountered. The first of these is in the account of Celia C. (Case 35). In her first attack[1] she passed from a depression into a state of confusion, without a great deal of subjective perplexity, in which she had ideas of guilt, of having destroyed her honour, of being a prostitute and of her mother being dead. In this psychosis a manic tendency showed itself episodically, while in her second attack five years later (which is described above) she was definitely manic but only for a few weeks. The second psychosis was ushered in and terminated by a perplexed state in which both manic and depressive episodes occurred. She spoke of being mixed up and also said such things as, " I wish I knew what was happening. It is so long since I was in the city, I forget all about myself ; I don't know whether I am coming or going." Frank C. (Case 32) was quite interesting. He was usually well oriented but he frequently became confused

---

[1] Described in Hoch's *Benign Stupors*, p. 155.

when his thoughts got on to certain topics ; a process which he well described : " Lots of things seem to run through my mind and I don't know where I stand," or, again, " I took up this book and that made me think of my uncle and that of Boston and the old man. I had—well, that makes me think of the village down here and so lots of things go through my head." Isabel U. (Case 33) when in a quiet phase would look natural one minute and then assume a blank expression.   At such times she would give the impression of having great trouble in gathering her thoughts, looking abstracted and sometimes making such a remark as " I can't say anything more. This is over-taxing my mind."   Often when speaking clearly she would seem to become side-tracked in her thoughts and thus confused. For instance, after demonstrating a clear orientation, she suddenly mixed up the hospital with places where she worked.   Blocking in her train of thought was frequent.   Frank S. (Case 36) showed a great lack of consecutiveness in his speech and recognized it in such statements as, " The various sounds that distract me and those which I have said and done ", or, " I don't know what I am talking about, I am blurred ".   Ruth C. (Case 37) had many episodes of confusion in spite of fair orientation.   She explained the former by saying she could not tell whether it was real life or the play, and went on : " Everything is mixed.   Is that the door I came in ? Then everything is turned around.   O yes, this is the stage.   My brain goes just like a tram car.   How would you like to be in a room that goes 'round and 'round ?   This room is not the same place all the time.   It mixes you up.   I don't know where I am.   They make it go around so I am in Hades."

Among the cases quoted in the discussion of depression only one showed definite elements of perplexity.   This was Carrie D. (Case 50).   She came into the hospital in a state of retardation, seemed preoccupied and had tears in her eyes.   To some questions she made replies like the following :   " I don't know ", " I feel mixed up ", " I can't get it together " or " I have no remembrance at all ". When asked about the ages of her children she said, " I don't know, I don't know if I am the same person or not ".   She was, nevertheless, oriented.

The cases chosen for description in the foregoing chapters were picked out because they were typical and presented a minimum of atypical features (with the exception of those illustrating absorbed mental states).   It is for this reason that perplexity symptoms have been described so infrequently.   As a matter of fact many case histories were eliminated although they contained strikingly pertinent material, simply because at some period of the psychosis the clinical picture was obscured by the presence of perplexity symptoms. They are really quite common.   In fact, if one tries to view cases of manic-depressive insanity from the descriptive standpoint of Kraepelin, and tries to interpret the symptoms observed as belonging to classical mania or depression, it is these perplexity features which most often refuse to fit into the picture. We shall see later that the adoption of perplexity as a manic-depressive type of reaction obviates the necessity of fabricating " mixed conditions " as Kraepelin has done, an invention which involves serious theoretic difficulties.

The occasional, or frequent, observation of fleeting perplexity, would not justify us in erecting a reaction type on the foundation of such evidence. The problem of accounting for symptoms becomes acute, and the justification for a separate group more evident, when one meets with cases showing none of the classical manic-depressive symptoms but consisting merely of the perplexity syndrome. The following is an example in point.

CASE 63. *Mary E. P.* was an unmarried woman 20 years of age when she came under observation twenty years ago.

F.H. Information is confined to the statement that there were a number of cases of manic depressive insanity in her father's family.

P.H. Her disposition was claimed to have been normal ; she was the daughter of a clergyman.

The psychosis : For about five months her conduct had been occasionally peculiar, although, unfortunately, her oddities were not described. About a month before admission she became absent-minded, refused food, and sometimes did most unexpected things. For instance, she attempted to jump out of the window, saying, " I must do my duty ". Several times she suddenly leaped from her bed and began to turn somersaults on the floor, this queer behaviour being unaccompanied by any elation. Occasionally she asked, " Where have I been ; have I been dead ? "

Under observation : Examination failed to reveal any indication of somatic disease. The psychosis lasted for only six weeks, during which time there were no marked variations in her condition until recovery took place. She usually sat quietly about the ward, unoccupied, but occasionally varied this monotony with such queer behaviour as stuffing pieces of paper into her mouth or suddenly walking to a table and naming aloud all the objects on it. When examined she was extremely reticent, and seemed absorbed in thought. Although she could be induced to answer some simple questions relevantly, her replies seemed often to be the product of her independent ruminations. She was apparently clear as to her immediate surroundings, but always uncertain about time relations. For instance, a few days after admission, she claimed to have been in the hospital for weeks, and that she had seen the doctor " ages ago ". But with this there were remarks such as, " There isn't any date," or " There isn't any time ".

The last statements were probably merely indications of what was the most prominent feature of her psychosis, namely, a marked subjective perplexity unaccompanied by well defined affect. For instance, she said such things as, " Things change every second " ; " I don't feel the same for two minutes " ; " It seems different from one moment to the next " ; " It all seems strange " ; " It is mixed " ; or " It is like a dream ". Sometimes the perplexity came out in the form of a doubtful projection of her uncertainty as suspicion that other minds were working on hers. This, however, was accompanied by an attitude of passivity not resentment. For example, she once said, " Anyone can make anything of me they choose ". She was at once asked if anyone had done anything to her. Her reply was, " Have I been doing it myself ? I am all mixed up ". Again she would make such remarks as, " I think you can make me believe whatever you like," or " It seems as if everyone knew what I think ".

The physician who examined her felt constantly that many more false ideas than these were present, and that it was probable there were even hallucinations. But no admission of this could be secured, for the patient became more than ever reticent when questioned about such matters. However there were random and irrelevant remarks which pointed towards some, at least, of her thoughts having a sexual colouring. Questions of the most matter of fact and impersonal order would lead to such replies as these : " I think I ought to go away ; I came here to be courted." " How can I be modest and answer your questions ? " (Quite irrelevantly). " What do you want to know about my monthly sickness ? " " I thought you wanted me, but I don't know whether you are the man I love or not." Possibly the following remark represented a variant of these sexual ideas : " Sometimes the idea of a surgical operation comes into my mind."

After recovery she made an impression of immaturity, but had absolutely no psychotic symptoms remaining. As to the experiences through which she had passed, she could not, or would not, say more than that it all seemed like a dream in retrospect. Four years later it was learned that her mental balance had been well maintained.

A little scrutiny shows the impossibility of fitting such a case into one of the customary diagnostic pigeon-holes. The history would make dementia praecox extremely unlikely. By exclusion, therefore, and in the absence of somatic disease, we would be safe in classifying the psychosis as belonging to the manic-depressive group ; but in which sub-group ? The absence of sadness, remorse, anxiety or apathy would eliminate a diagnosis of depression, anxiety or stupor. The only affect present was the peculiar distress that goes with subjective perplexity. One might attempt to fit the symptoms into the picture of absorbed mania, but against this it should be noted that there were no little outbursts of elation, mischievousness, erotic behaviour or self decoration. It is true there was, as is common in manic states, a paranoid tendency, but here again we are at a loss for the suspiciousness was not a matter of behaviour but merely of words. Had she been a manic patient she should have been irritable or at least querulous. Moreover, a manic, absorbed to this extent, would probably have been less well oriented.

Repeated embarrassment with this problem led Hoch and Kirby in 1919 to describe such cases as a definite reaction type[1]. Their conclusions were that the chief peculiarity of the group was a subjective perplexity, tending to be projected on the environment. They used the term " subjective " because the complaint of confusion was not justified by proportionate failure of comprehension. The affect they described as one of distress, associated with the perplexity, while the latter in turn was correlated with a peculiar train of thought. In all their cases there was a feeling, or delusion, of guilt, which, they considered, was an integral part of the whole reaction. Finally they pointed out that the perplexity picture could be seen with toxic states and in dementia praecox (like manic and stupor symptoms) but that their cases occurred with mental precipitating causes and had demonstrable affiliation with the manic-depressive groups.

[1] August Hoch and George H. Kirby, " A Clinical Study of Psychoses Characterized by Distressed Perplexity ", *Archives of Neurology and Psychiatry*, Vol. I, p. 415.

Shortly after the publication of this paper, I went over a large mass of clinical material with Dr. Hoch. We found many more cases of perplexity than he and Dr. Kirby had taken account of. This more extensive survey confirmed the published claims, except in one particular. Guilt was found not to be essential to the existence of a perplexity state, but merely the most frequent form of expression for a paranoid tendency to assume.

The *symptoms*, then, of the perplexity reaction, are as follows : In the fore-front, of course, stands the *subjective perplexity* itself. It becomeš evident from a study of the patient's expression, listening to his direct complaint and from observation of his train of thought. As to the first, he looks puzzled. This is not the blank expression of one who is bewildered and fails to grasp the environment, but of one who cannot understand what he does see and hear. There is usually a frown about the eyes and a slight stare to the eyes . . . but all facial expressions are better described in terms of the effect on the beholder than in analysis of features. The subjective perplexity is referred to directly by most of the patients. They say they feel mixed-up, puzzled, " twisted ", can't get their thoughts together and so on. A typical remark is, " Sometimes I am myself, sometimes I am not. " Occasionally this is referred to bodily perceptions with particularly frequent reference to the eyes and distorted vision. For instance, one of the cases described by Hoch and Kirby said, " They tell me I have glass eyes all over ". After recovery she explained this : she had felt confused, nothing looked natural, everyone looked alike, so she thought she could not see right. The discordance of the patient's thoughts is perhaps accountable for the delusion, which is strangely frequent, of the two sides of the body being different.

Almost always the perplexity is projected on to the environment. There are innumerable complaints of things not looking right, and of time and space relations being wrong. For instance, the hospital looks like home but is not, and the present seems to be a past occasion. This is probably the best category in which to place the feeling of *déjà vu* (a vivid feeling of " having been there before ") which is surprisingly common in these psychoses. Perplexity as to the environment is continually being expressed in questions as to the reality or nature of common articles or occurrences. For example the patient says, " Is that a pencil ? " " Are you writing ? " (to a physician making notes), and may at one interview produce very little beyond such interrogations. The false ideas, too, are equally questioned and their vagueness accentuated. A thought is ascribed to another person and immediately after admitted as the patient's own. The loose proprietorship of one's own thoughts, so to speak, is often reflected in delusions of hypnotism or of being forced to think certain things. Or, again, the patient may claim that his spirit is in the body of another whom he sees in the environment. Finally ideas of reference are asserted and denied in the same breath, or accusations are alleged and protested against, although it may be impossible to elicit the actual charge. One of Hoch's and Kirby's patients summed this up in the statement : " I am innocent of something and I don't know what it is ! "

With this apparent confusion one would expect to find gross *disorientation* as in all states of clouding of consciousness. Difficulties in arithmetic calculation, &c., are often present, but, when one analyses the clinical picture, it is surprising to find how relatively accurate the orientation is. A quotation from Hoch and Kirby will show this anomaly well ; the case was highly typical. " It is obvious that with the pronounced tenseness which we have described it was difficult to get the patient to concentrate. Therefore, orientation questions were sometimes not answered at all. She simply went on talking in the manner described, or quite often answered that she did not know. At other times she seemed to give a little more attention and then quite often gave answers which looked as if she were disoriented. She said she did not know how she got here and later that " it was all like a trance." But in the same interview, for instance, in which she said she did not know where she was and claimed not to know what the physician was, she begged him to ' do something for her head ', and later also spoke of the place being a hospital, though she added that it was a queer hospital. Moreover, when her husband came, during this period in which she appeared superficially to be so confused, she gave him a detailed account of where to find certain things in the home. Or on one occasion, when asked who the nurse and stenographer were, she claimed not to know, but later in appealing to them called both by name. At one time when asked for her husband's address she said, " He lives with me here ", and then denied knowing her own address, yet later during the same visit gave it correctly. At the third interview with one particular physician she was asked whether she knew that the doctor had talked to her before ; she said, ' Yes, but it is all dim '." One can see in this account suggestions of " rousing ", such as occurs in organic deliria ; *i.e.*, variations in the acuity of consciousness, as a result of special stimulation, such that the patient becomes able, temporarily, to grasp the nature of the environment but then sinks back into preoccupations with delirious thoughts. Rousing, in its typical form, is rarely seen in perplexity states, but a reaction suggestive of it is quite common and, in fact, perplexity is a common feature in organic delirium. We shall see later that the discrepancies between objective and subjective confusion are of prime importance in understanding the perplexity reaction psychologically.

The anomalies of *affect* noted in perplexity states contribute not a little to the difficulty of diagnosing or understanding these cases. There is only one emotional reaction at all constant in these conditions, a peculiar distress that is felt by the patient in his unsuccessful effort to control his thoughts and to understand them and the environment. It is the painful aspect of the perplexity itself and cannot be further described. Most people have experienced it, however, at times when they have attempted to wake themselves up and find that they cannot discriminate between external impressions and persisting dream thoughts. Or one may have this feeling running through a long series of dreams, particularly when one is suffering from fatigue or some form of intoxication. In our patients this distress is betrayed in facial expression or direct complaint. Sometimes it leads to extensive motor restlessness but more often the patients are quiet.

This part of the clinical picture is easily recognized and understood, but what does obscure the clinical picture is the frequent interruptions of this mood. A patient may become markedly blocked in speech, and apparently in thought, showing, for the time being, symptoms indistinguishable from those of retarded depression. Similarly there may be intervals of apparent apathy and stupor-like inactivity (this is quite common) ; or elation or more or less isolated manic symptoms may appear ; or anxiety may show itself for a brief period. It is these interruptions which make diagnosis so often a difficult matter. One mood reaction, not essential to the clinical picture but extremely common, is a marked feeling of guilt. This is not the same as the feeling of wickedness in depression for the patient has not so much a conviction of sin as of shame. That is, he feels that other people regard him as wicked and is assured there is some reason for this, although he cannot accept as justified the accusations he believes are made against him. In short, one can see that the feeling of guilt is one of sin, to which perplexity has been added, making it uncertain and introducing an element of protesting innocence that is never found in depression. We shall see presently that this guilt is connected with the tendency towards projection and paranoid developments.

When we turn to examine the *false ideas* expressed in perplexity states, we do not find a consistent content such as one meets in the other manic-depressive reaction types. These ideas, however, have rather peculiar modes of appearance. Hallucinations seem common. Not only do the patients speak frequently of what " the voices " say but they appear to be gazing at what is invisible to others. Illusions of auditory and visual impressions are, probably, constant phenomena, for references are always being made to misinterpretations of the environment. Delusions do not seem to be elaborated but come to expression in jerky, recurrent phrases or sentences rather than in well formulated and persistent false ideas. The utterances of many patients are confined to a mere beginning of sentences, interrupted by sudden and long pauses, after which there is a change of subject—an apparent blocking of the conscious mental processes. It is not unnatural, therefore, that we should frequently hear the complaint that there are many thoughts, which cannot be told in spite of a considerable talkativeness.

The delusions are, as a rule, cast into a paranoid form. " They say " so and so is the usual statement. Whereas the depressive patient may say, " I am a bad woman ", the perplexed one says, " They say I am a bad woman ". Or, it is not, " I am going to be killed " but, " They say I am going to be killed ". This goes with the general confusion between what the patient and what others think, which often leads to delusions of thought control or hypnotism, or of other people thinking the patient's thoughts. But the paranoid tendency goes further than this, for even non-human environmental phenomena, such as boat or train whistles, are felt in some peculiar way to have some personal relationships with the patient. Perhaps it is because so many ideas are cast into a paranoid form that they are almost always spontaneously questioned or denied by the patient himself.

As has been said, there is no uniform *ideational content*. In fact one can find, often in one case, ideas belonging to any other manic depressive reaction. Perhaps the most frequent are those having a depressive colouring. We have mentioned the prominence of guilt. Without the conviction of sin found in depressions, there are complaints that others accuse the patient of prostitution, stealing, murder, and so on. But even the denial of these charges has the same dubiousness as the report of them. Regression is manifest from the crudity of the delusional content, from frequent masturbation, which is often shamelessly practised, as well as in a negativistic attitude that sometimes occurs. It may be the presence of infantile reactions that produces the depressive atmosphere in which so many patients live ; it is at least certain that blocking can be correlated with a sudden regression. A tendency to self blame appears occasionally in the complaint that the patient is held responsible for some catastrophe such as the burning down of a house. Sometimes there are ideas reminiscent of stupor or anxiety, as a fear of immanent death or a vision of dead bodies, or incarceration and punishment are predicted. Hypochondriacal fancies are also common, but these are peculiar in that disturbance or loss of function is alleged, rather than pains. The patient, for instance, says he is dumb or blind, can't feel right in his skin, can't breath properly and so on. Complaints as to trouble in the head are, of course, the commonest. These are usually references to poor thinking capacity but are often expressed in terms of physical symptoms such as dizziness. Finally we sometimes meet with definitely expansive or erotic ideas like those of manic states. The patient has wealth, is God, or has many lovers. Rarely, however, do such fancies give him any satisfaction for they are usually put into the *on dit* form and immediately ridiculed.

If the general claim of this study be correct, that there is a correlation between ideational content and reaction, then we should expect to find the perplexity psychosis an unstable one. It is. When ideas of these different orders appear tentatively, there is apt to be a variability of emotion, with little episodes of sadness, anxiety, apathy or elation. Most often from this general matrix there emerges one dominating type of delusion and then the reaction ceases to be perplexity and becomes depression, anxiety (or involution melancholia), stupor or mania. Perplexity in the sense of a consistent psychosis tends, therefore, to be a brief reaction—a few weeks or months ; it is often merely a brief interlude or transitory state and is commonest of all during the onsets of manic-depressive attacks. Relatives describe the perplexity syndrome with great frequency when they tell how the psychosis began.

One more point and this description is completed. Retrospectively the patients usually speak of what they have been through as like a dream and accentuate the queerness which the environment had. They are particularly prone to say that the hospital seemed to be both the hospital and a more familiar place such as home or workshop, the nurses and doctors having the same dual character.

CHAPTER XL

HAVING these symptoms before us, it may be as well to give in outline the psychological speculations designed to explain the clinical picture. It will be remembered that, in discussing absorbed manic states and the phenomena we termed distraction of thought, it was pointed out that certain consequences—the symptoms—followed from the turning of attention from the external world to the flux of free associations which constitutes our inner (and, normally, largely unconscious) mental life. The theory of perplexity involves the same kind of reasoning. If one assumes that attention is divided, that it goes both towards inner thinking and observation of the environment, then one can see how this splitting of attention would cause symptoms such as we have described, provided the instinctive tendency to retain a grasp of objective reality were retained.

The essence of any functional psychotic state is the greater or less autonomy of free associational thinking. This process always tends to lead to the activization of unconscious ideas, and, if the process goes far enough the thoughts become infantile in content, and imaginal, rather than verbal, in form. As we shall see later, this is the kind of thinking found in dreams. Apparently this happens in perplexity states and accounts for the delusions and hallucinations which appear in brief and changing form. We shall shortly quote specimens of utterances that look like free associations. In the distraction of thought occurring in mania when the free associational process becomes intense, there is loss of regard for the environment and consequent disorientation. In the perplexity cases, however, we have free associations and an orientation that is always surprising to the examiner, who expects to find a loss of knowledge for the environment in one seemingly absorbed in inner thought and complaining of confusion. This may give us a hint. We may be dealing with a condition where the patient is making a fight against the tendency to become absorbed and is trying with doubtful success to keep contact with the world around.

In proportion as we turn our attention to our inner thoughts they tend to become " real " to us, as, for instance, in states of drowsiness or when we are falling asleep. But, if we are trying to keep awake, we maintain sufficient objectivity to criticize our wandering thoughts and know that they are only thoughts and not sensory impressions.

393

This double direction of attention would account for the constant denials made by the perplexed patient of his delusions. The normal person may, while drowsy, begin to think his thoughts are " real ", but when he wakes up, he pulls himself up short, grasps the environment accurately, and recognizes his late thoughts as pure fantasy. The perplexed patient attempts this but the pressure from the unconscious is too strong for the feeling of reality attached to the false idea to be totally dispelled. Hence they are both alleged and denied in one breath.

An analogous event is occurring with external impressions. Any environmental stimulus is recognized as such but at once sets up a train of free associations, and the latter are clothed with a feeling of reality. For example, the hospital, with its beds, &c., makes the patient think of his home and, at once, he is in two environments at once, the actual one and his habitual, but now an imaginary, one. No wonder he is perplexed, complains of thoughts flying through his head which he cannot control, and so on ! We can also understand " rousing " in terms of this mechanism. If the patient's attention is forcibly externalized—by repeated questioning, for example— he tends to think in a more normal way, and, for the time being, to grasp the environment more accurately.

A splitting of attention may, then, be assumed as the mechanistic basis of subjective perplexity. But it has also its dynamical explanation, which is equally important. The instinctive urge towards free-associational thinking is a matter to which many references have already been made. Mere free-associational thinking with splitting attention produces dementia praecox, as we shall see. In order that perplexity may result there must also be present the normal, instinctive tendency to maintain contact with external realities. The probable origin of this last will be discussed in Chapter XLIII.

A paranoid tendency, such as is common in perplexity states, may be deduced from the above. It will be recalled that this paranoid reaction has certain peculiarities. The ideas are not fixed ; the same ones may recur again and again but are not constantly present as a rule. Even when the same thought is often repeated it is apt to be as often denied, or when a patient is questioned about an idea of reference, he may say that it is really just his thought. The delusions are never elaborated as in paranoia or true paranoid states ; they are not rationalized, no attempt is made to bolster them up logically, they just unexplainably " are ". Finally a reaction of suspiciousness or irritability is highly unusual.

All this would make one suspect that this is not a true paranoid reaction but some kind of externalization of thoughts. What we regard as having objective reality is that of which we have knowledge by perceptions, visual, auditory, &c. Hence, if our thoughts appear in objectified images, as in dreams, we consider them to have reality so long as our attention is given to what appears to be a perception, rather than to the cause of the perception. When free associations become sufficiently vivid, they become hallucinations (which are very common in perplexity states). But there is another way in which ideas may come to us ; they may be acquired by listening to the words, or observing the actions, of others. A vivid internal thought may then be held to originate from someone else, just as well as it may appear as an hallucination. When the patient is aware of his poor control of associations, he may either assign this defect to himself (complaints of mental incompetence) or he may externalize it as thought-control or hypnotism. Sometimes a kind of compromise is reached, when the patient says he is, or feels as if he were, two people.

The frequency of guilt is now explicable psychologically. An unbridled free associational process tends to arrive at a crude, infantile level. As we have seen this results in a depressive reaction, with inhibition and a conviction of sin. This accounts for the blocking and strongly depressive tendency of perplexity states. But the perplexed patient is one who is dividing his attention between the environment and his surging thoughts. He compromises by allocating the ideas to others, which then take the form of accusations. Such critical judgment, as is retained, rejects these accusations as false, but as they are at the same time, in actuality, ideas of the patient himself, there is a feeling that there must be some justification for them. Hence we see perplexity and a feeling of guilt. The latter, it must be remembered, is always to be differentiated from a feeling of sin, in the fact that the former is, broadly speaking, a legal term. That is, guilt is a recognition of disapprobation on the part of a critical community. On the other hand one may have a conviction of sin and at the same time recognize that society honours him.

We may sum up this theory of the paranoid and guilt tendencies by saying that they represent primitive and tentative efforts to rationalize the false ideas appearing in the consciousness of the perplexity patient with obsessive and convincing vividness. It is a type of thinking found among primitive people, who do not discriminate as we do between internal and external origins for thoughts. The savage is not perplexed because he does not attempt the discrimination. But when one of us finds himself confusing memory and perceptual images, he is perplexed.

CHAPTER XLI

CASES ILLUSTRATIVE OF PERPLEXITY

WITH this introduction we can now turn to examine a few case histories in order to see how this theory may explain the reactions observed. A number of excellent cases have been recorded by Hoch and Kirby, and the reader is urged to study these as well if he wishes to get a comprehensive survey of this clinical group.

CASE 64. *Catherine M*[1]. Age : 24. Admitted to the Psychiatric Institute, November 10th, 1913.

F.H. Information as to the family is confined to the two parents. The mother, who was frequently seen, seemed to be a natural, sensible woman. The father, on the other hand, had been alcoholic all his life, had had two convulsions while drinking, and won little respect from any member of the family, including the patient.

P.H. The patient was said always to have been healthy, from a physical standpoint, although never robust. She got on well at school, and then worked, first as a stock girl, and later as clerk in a department store, where her work was efficient, and she advanced steadily. When a child she played freely with other girls, but little with boys. As she grew older she moved about socially a bit more, made the acquaintance of men as well as of girls, but never cared much for the former, and had no love affairs until she met her husband. She was never demonstrative, but always rather quiet and modest. Occasionally she spoke of thinking that people talked about her, but the informant doubted if she brooded over this, because she was not of a worrying disposition. Considering the ideas which appeared in her psychosis, it is striking that in her normal life she was rather antagonistic toward her father on account of his alcoholism and the cruelty of his speech and manners.

When she met her husband she liked him from the first, although she at no time became really demonstrative. They were engaged for a year, during which time she agreed to a postponement of three months for the marriage, which was suggested by her mother. For some time before this event she was working harder than usual, and seemed a bit worn out. She ceased working a month before marriage and improved physically, although she became rather nervous, that is, she was more easily startled, an accentuation of what had been a characteristic for some years. Her husband stated that at this time she became fearful of the approaching marriage relations, and asked him to be kind to her in this respect. She was married a year before admission. For two and a half months she refused intercourse, and visited her mother's home a great deal. She finally submitted. She was quite frigid, but became pregnant at once. Her abnormality then became apparent. She kept the fact of her pregnancy to herself for several months, and, when she told her mother, wanted to have an abortion performed. Neurotic symptoms appeared. She became sensitive with her husband, correcting his English,

[1] This case was reported by Hoch in his " Benign Stupors " in order to compare the stupor and perplexity reactions. The following account is largely a verbatim quotation from this book.

and cried easily. She also began to be anxious about the approaching child-birth, and with this became more religious.

For the first few days after the delivery, she was fussy with the nurse so that two in succession had to be discharged. On the fifth day she woke up, and seeing her nurse lying on the couch beside her bed thought the latter was coloured. On the seventh day she had a dream in which she thought she " nearly died in childbirth ". Then she began to talk of dying for her baby or of having two babies, of dying herself and rising again after Easter Sunday. She became antagonistic to her husband, and, with this, excited and confused, so that she was taken to the Observation Pavilion.

On admission she looked pale and exhausted, had a slight temporary fever and a coated tongue. Her orientation was usually vague, but sometimes she gave fair answers. Her verbal productions were rather fragmentary, and with the exception of some repetitions there did not seem to be any special topics which dominated her train of thought.

For some days the great weakness and the slight fever continued, and then, as it gradually cleared up, there came a change in her mental condition that settled into the state which characterized the rest of her psychosis. She talked less and was often quite inactive, frequently lying with her eyes closed for long periods, or sat or stood about. Such movements as she made were slow and languid. Her expression was either blank, absorbed, or gave the appearance of peculiar perplexity. This last was not infrequently associated with a rather sheepish smile. She was never resistive, and always ate and slept well. With rare exceptions she did not soil herself.

The most interesting feature of her mood reaction was that in a general setting of a slight perplexity there appeared at times, and evidently associated with definite ideas, changes in her emotional state. Sometimes this was a matter of distress or of mild ecstasy, sometimes she became markedly blocked. There was at no time any frank elation, but often an appropriate smile, that is, appropriate to the situation and to the thought to which she was giving expression at the time. Then, rarely, there were sudden bursts of peculiar conduct, such as throwing herself on the floor or running down the hall. When questioned as to her motive for these acts, she would flush, look perplexed and apparently be unable to explain them.

This perplexity was not merely a deduction from objective observation ; she herself frequently complained of it and always in connection with the inconsistency of the ideas which puzzled her. For instance, in speaking to the doctor she said, " I think of you as Bill (her husband's name) sometimes— I get confused thinking of Bill as God, doctor, lawyer, priest." Again, referring to her husband, she made these curious statements : " They seemed to speak of him as being in the wrong—the right—it seems that the right devil is the wrong one for me—they say he is not the right one for me ; they say he went wrong from the time we were married." Again, she said that she did not know who her father was, and went on : " It puzzles me, this father business, I knew my father at home and my father in Heaven." Again, ' Which God do you mean ? Did you say God or father ? " A hint as to how this subjective confusion made the environment seem uncertain comes from the statement, " You looked like the devil and yet you were God." Occasionally she referred directly to the perverted nature of her mental processes, as when she said : " My mind is always wandering back and forth ", or, " If only I could keep at one thing, I wander so ! " Such statements are as close as a layman could well come to speaking of free associations. Once she correlated her objective and subjective confusion in the remark, " I thought I was called Mary [eldest sister] ; I used to answer to any name ; now things are all twisted to me, I can think back too. . . ."

Her verbal productions dealt with a rather limited range of topics which can be briefly summarized. Many of her thoughts seemed to be centered round her husband. She always knew him when he visited her, but in her thoughts there was a constant change as to his personality. She persistently confused him with the physicians, with her father, and with God, and one remark is typical, " I thought he was God, priest, doctor, lawyer—well, I wanted to go to Heaven ; I thought he would still be my husband ; I always hoped that I would be home in Heaven." Not unnaturally with this confusion there were doubts about her marriage. People said her marriage was wrong and her husband bad. Frequently she thought he was dead, or voices informed her that she was not married to him, or that he was the devil in Hell. In this connection she also said that people called her a whore, or it seemed as if she were accused of not being married.

As prominently as appeared the ideas of the invalidity or impossibility of her marriage, to the same extent did her father assume an important rôle for her. As a rule he appeared in religious guise as God—" I knew my father at home and my father in Heaven ; which God do you mean ? Did you say God or father ? " At times she spoke of being in Heaven and that God seemed to be God, doctor or priest. In this connection there were ideas of being under the power of someone, God, devil or father.

As is usually the case where strong interest is expressed in the father, ideas of the mother being dead occurred, although in the frankest form she reported them as dreams ; for instance, one night she woke up screaming, said that she had dreamed that her mother was dead and her sister dying. That, in the psycho-analytic sense, this represented a removal of a rival, making union with her father easy, appeared in the statement that her father was dead, but that she had dreamed he had come to life again for someone else. When asked what she meant, the question had to be repeated several times, then she said : " My mother died, my father and mother had a quarrel." There is more than a suggestion here of a difference in the significance of death, in so far as it concerned the two parents. The mother dies and remains dead, that is, she is gotten rid of. The father dies, but takes on a spiritual existence and comes to life again, a frequent method in psychoses for legitimizing the idea of union with the parent by elimination of the grossly physical.

There were strikingly few allusions to the plainly sexual. She spoke of being married to the doctor, and even went so far as to say that they belonged together in bed. On another occasion she called him " darling." Once she reported that it was said that she was going to have babies and babies and babies. These references were, however, quite isolated, so that the erotic formed a very small part of her productions.

Delusions of death in this case were present, but distinctly in the background. She spoke quite frequently of being in Heaven. She also talked of being crucified. Once she said : " I died, but I came back again." This last utterance was rather significant in that frankly accepted ideas of death were unusual ; for instance, she would say sometimes, " I think I am in Heaven, again not. It confuses me, but I know I am in Heaven."

In general, then, her ideas were, on the whole, not at all typical of any one manic-depressive reaction. Correlated with this was an unusual mood picture. The quietness and apparent apathy of the patient were interrupted by little bursts of emotion, and throughout the psychosis there was a colouring of perplexity. Distress and anxiety appeared not infrequently and always appropriately. The distress was usually occasioned by an idea of injury to others, as when she cried over the fancied accusations of drowning her husband and mother ; or in connection with accusations of herself, such as when she reported " They called me a whore ". As has been stated, there was never any frank elation, but an element of pleasurable expansive emotion was frequently present in connection with her religious utterances. This came particularly when she spoke of union with her father as God. She seemed to swell with ecstatic emotion. It was especially well marked once when she threw herself on the floor, and when asked what she was trying to do replied, " I want to do what God wants me to do, drop dead or anything at all ".

Perhaps the most unusual emotional reaction was a blocking, which occurred when certain topics appeared. One got the impression that ideas tended to come into this patient's mind which were painful enough to disturb her capacity for connected thought.   A good example of this reaction was when she was speaking of her father having died and coming to life again. On being asked what she meant, she became quite blocked, and the question had to be repeated several times, when finally the apparently unrelated statements appeared : " I dreamed my mother died—they had a quarrel ". Who had a quarrel ? she was asked, and replied, " My mother and father ". Apparently her thinking about her father coming to life for someone not her mother stimulated deeply unconscious ideas concerning the separation of her mother and father, and her taking the mother's place, and these ideas were sufficiently revolutionary to upset her capacity of speech for the time being.

She recovered completely about six and a half months after her admission.

This brief summary gives an inadequate outline of a most interesting case.   One could profitably repeat many pages of her productions to illustrate the kind of ideas which appear in manic depressive insanity, but enough of such material has probably been presented already in the earlier chapters.   What interests us more at this point is the study of the mental processes which brought the ideas to expression.   She gave many fine examples of free associational thinking and a number of these are worthy of quotation.

The first is from an interview some six weeks after her admission. It will be seen that her mind wandered from the topic of hospital clothes to her own clothing, home, the people at home, father, God, a dream of the doctor as God and Devil, and at this point the image becomes real so that she speaks of it as an hallucination.   After much broken and inaudible talk she was urged to speak up, and began :

" Last night I got dressed up in these clothes . . . then . . . [Begins to laugh in a distinctly perplexed manner and fumbles with a magazine she holds in her hand]—I always thought that everybody that could, had their own [clothes]—I know I was not insane always —and then I can remember so much from home.   Then it comes back to you.   I was in Heaven ; I called you father."

(Who am I ?)

She makes a continual effort to speak ; fidgets, trembles all over, swallows, looks from one examiner to the other, jerks her hands spasmodically, but after some inaudible words begins : " In my dream I thought of you ; I could see you look in the window with a smile.   And it was like God and the Devil to see you smile, and you laughed in the window.   That was some time ago you seemed like the Devil, and when I came back you called . . .   In the window you looked and you smiled to me and you said, ' You cannot fool the Devil'.   I always saw your face . . . and then you came back again.   From the time you looked in the window I could see your face before me.   You looked like the Devil and yet you were God."

The next illustration does not show the free associational processes in such extended form, but is introduced to demonstrate how a perplexed patient can be both oriented and disoriented at the same time, thanks to the double direction of attention.   This is a fragment of an examination by Dr. G. E. Myers of the Institute staff.   It was three weeks after admission and the morning of a Saturday—one of the visiting days at Manhattan State Hospital—which the patient knew.

" I know I am in Heaven and with one God—three devout persons, the Father, Son, and Holy Ghost ; but there is one God. It confuses me up, but I know I'm in Heaven and there is one God. And Bill was to come to-day to tell me if I was well. [Her husband had promised to come and fetch her home when she had recovered.] This morning I'd shake hands when it was all over—with Bill [extending hand]. I knew Bill before Dr. Murray [her physician in New York] that we're in Heaven, I knew it first. I know I'm in Heaven now, and everybody seems to be God—is God. God's will is to be done and that's the way I know it is the same God— doctor, priest and all. I know that is when I lose my mind and get it back again. At the same time it is always one person. When I had that vision I used to think different about vice versa Margaret and me. Margaret [sister] was married before me, but this woman here [a patient named Margaret] looks like Margaret M. [patient's married name]."

" I thought you haunted me, but then that was along with the vision. I feel I am speaking to God now."

(Who am I ?)

" God."

(What is my real name ?)

" As I know you to be now ? "

(Yes.)

" Well, I feel that I am in Heaven and you're God—the name was Hawkey [Hoch ? who also examined her] this morning. In that office there I met you. It was all clear to me this morning, but I'm in Heaven now."

(What is the name of this place ?)

" Well, I have a letter addressed here to the Manhattan Hospital, but the letter wouldn't make any difference, I still believe the same. I know it is the same person all the way through, but Thy will be done."

(Is this the Manhattan State Hospital ?)

" I don't think it is ; I feel I am in Heaven even though letters are addressed here."

(Why do you think you are in Heaven ?)

" Because when I was here first in my right mind I asked everything of God. Dr. Murray sent me here."

(What year is it ?)

" 1914, I think, by now." [November 30th, 1913].

(What month ?)

" Well, the latter part of November or the first of December. November 29th [looking at the date on the envelope]—but I think I'm in Heaven."

(What day of the week ?)

" Well, Bill said he'd be here on Wednesday. Well, I wished for Bill, and you came in and went out again and then came back." [Correct].

(What day is it ?)

" Wednesday."

(What is my name ?)

" Bill M., so far as I know."

(Do I look like him ?)

" Well, no, you don't. I know Bill when I see him, but still there is only God ; Dr. Myers comes in it."

(Who is he ?)

" Well, I shouldn't say ' Doctor ', for there is only one God."

(Am I Dr. Myers ?)

" Well, Dr. Myers ", nodding her head in the affirmative.

(Am I anybody other than Dr. Myers ?)

" Well, God comes first—I get confused with Dr. Myers . . . well, Dr. Myers, Dr. Murray, and Bill . . . priest and lawyer and one God."

A good example of how even her own identity seemed to depend on associated thoughts occurred two months after admission, when she was asked what her name was. She replied that on her arrival she was strapped down to the floor (she was brought in on a stretcher) and that a nurse took down her name as " Miss Catherine D." She was then asked what her real name was, to which she responded, " When I think of New York, it is Mrs. M."

Some four months after admission the patient had a birthday, she received a letter and some flowers and immediately became upset. She threw up her arms, screamed and once rolled on the floor, kicking her feet in the air. Even after being put to bed the disturbance did not entirely disappear, for she would scream at intervals, and often tried to leave the bed. At this stage of her psychosis she was still distressfully perplexed but had more memory and knowledge of her thoughts. So she was able, when quieter the next day, to explain this attack. As will be seen, the flowers reminded her of the events and her thoughts shortly after the birth of her baby, which, included, of course, her removal from home to the hospital. As she told of it in her wandering way the memories became vivid enough to upset her emotionally and renew to some extent the confusion between hospital and home.

(Why were you so upset yesterday ?)

" The time the baby was born the girls brought me in flowers and they put them into vases just as Mrs. H. [a fellow patient] was doing yesterday."

(Is that what upset you ?)

" Yesterday was my birthday and I remembered when I got the flowers, when the baby was born. I saw all the different roses, and I thought I would have liked American Beauties."

(Go on !)

2 D

" I let them lie on the box, and Florence [fellow patient] fixed them for me."

(Were you afraid ?)

" I thought of Kathleen, Bill's sister. She stood over me that time, that made me cry."

(When?)

" That was yesterday when I cried."

(When did she stand over you ?)

" The time the baby was born." She cries. " It reminded me of that time yesterday."

(Why did you get fussed up then ?)

" I always thought I could get the baby back ; that I could go home again ; I never thought the baby died."

(Who said you did ?)

" I used to wonder if I was the baby. Bill said one day that I was his baby."

(Who said you thought the baby died ?)

" I don't remember leaving the baby behind me. I must have walked out in a dream. I didn't know where I was going."

(Who said you thought the baby died ?)

" I used to think it did. die."

The receipt of the flowers therefore, made her free associations turn to her puerperal period ; she lived over in imagination the distress of leaving home, being separated from the baby, and believing that the latter was dead.

When she had been in the hospital for nearly five months the most marked symptoms of her psychosis had disappeared. She no longer looked constantly perplexed and distressed, but went quietly about, often with a dreamy expression, but occupying herself in a docile way. She never did any work spontaneously. Sudden blocking was frequent. The last citation to be made from the record of her case shows how the perplexity would return when old false ideas were enquired after. It also gives an example of a common phenomenon, the persistence of a train of thought, in spite of irrelevant remarks or answers to questions.

On this occasion she was being asked for the names and ages of the different members of her family. Her answers were fairly accurate. Finally she gave her mother's name and age. The examination proceeded :

(Is she well ?)

" Not that I know of."

(What is the matter ?)

" I don't know where my mother is."

(Is she sick ?)

" She may be ; I don't know."

(Is she living or dead ?)

" She was here a few days ago to see me."

(You once thought she was dead ?)

" My mother ? I don't think so." This was said languidly.

(What is your father's name ?)

" Thomas."

(How is he ?)

" I don't know."

(Where is he ?)

" He may be still at home."

She then gave correctly the name of the hospital, of the one who was examining her, and of another doctor who saw her frequently.

(Do you know now that I am not your father ?)

" My own father is at home."

(Do you know I am not God ?)

" I doubt it," with considerable uncertainty in her voice and expression.

(Doubt what ?)

With this she became blocked but finally managed to say, " That you are not God ".

(Do you mean to say that you still think that I might be God ?)

" Yes," she replied with her old expression of perplexity.

(How is your husband ?)

" I don't know."

(When have you seen him ?)

" A few days ago ", which was correct.

She was then asked repeatedly as to how her husband was. She could only reply " I don't know," but finally added, " I felt very distant about him ". This recollection of her feelings at the interview with her husband evidently had been engrossing her attention too much for her to answer the questions as to his health. This preoccupation continued.

(Do you worry at all ?)

" I think so many different ways ". She could not be induced to explain further but finally smiled, remarking, " When I sat on the couch with Bill, something seemed to hold me back ". Having finally told of this, she was able to answer the next question quite prompt and pertinently.

(Do you worry about anything ?)

" I have worried so much about everything. I have given up home. At times I try to forget all."

(Forget what ?) No answer. She was told that she was awfully slow, to which she responded, " I am unable to speak right ".

(Well, how is your mind ?)

" It is always wandering."

The next case illustrates perplexity on a background of depression, occurring with unformulated paranoid ideas, and appearing particularly when the patient's attention was not focussed on a concrete task.

CASE 65. *Bridget B.* Aged 45, widowed. Admitted to the Psychiatric Institute, December 30th, 1911.

F.H. One sister was suffering from a chronic psychosis and one brother was alcoholic. In a large family (17 or 18) these and the patient were the only ones showing any abnormality. Both parents were living and well.

P.H. The patient was born in Ireland, and received primary school education there. At the age of 19 she came to the United States, and worked efficiently as a domestic servant until she was married in her 29th year. She was industrious, " free in speech " and a trifle hasty. In the intervals between attacks she gave the impression to her physicians of being a particularly level-headed woman. She bore nine children, six of whom survived.

First attack. When about 35 years of age she began to complain occasionally of numbness in her forehead when exposed to the sun or the heat of a stove. When 38, a sister married a drunkard. The patient, on one occasion, interfered in a quarrel between this couple and knocked the man down. Immediately she became odd, did not treat visitors properly, and once announced that the President's wife was coming for supper, and heard people outside shouting " Three cheers for Teddy ! " [Roosevelt]. Four days after the fracas with her brother-in-law she passed into a partial stupor in which condition she was removed to Manhattan State Hospital. Her attack lasted altogether for nearly a year. At first she was stuporous with much resistiveness, the latter being associated with complaints of perplexity. From this she gradually recovered, but before she was well had a sudden rise of temperature and a delirium-like episode lasting for a week.

Second attack. Two years later, and nine days after childbirth, an aunt, who had been looking after her, suddenly left. She became confused, and for two weeks was suspicious of those about her, thinking visitors were detectives and so on.

Present attack. Two years before admission the patient's husband died. After that she had to work very hard as a laundress in order to suppot her children. She also had a great worry with one son, who would not work and was delinquent. Three months before admission he had been sent to a reformatory. About this time she began again to complain of her head, and say, " Oh, if I could only rest for a couple of weeks ". She also was having difficulty in thinking, and believed she could not see well with her right eye. A couple of days before Christmas her younger sister told her of a story that was going around. Some girls had written to her parents that she (the sister) was not making the wages she pretended to earn. For some reason this disturbed the patient greatly. That night she dreamed that she went to talk to the p-iest about her delinquent son ; he was so angry that he took a broom and swept her out of his room. She awoke vomitting, and sat up in a chair for the remainder of the night.

The next morning something snapped in her head. She was restless and began to hallucinate. She fancied she was being watched, and saw two detectives in an opposite house dressed in the uniform of Rough Riders [a reminiscence of Roosevelt in the first attack ?]. She had a large picture of the Virgin, which seemed to be turned with the face to the wall and to have Roman numerals written on the back. This she took for a sign that she was cut off from God. The next day (Christmas) her daughter brought her a rosary ; when she saw the beads this reminded her of the reversed picture, she had a chill, and felt that her prayers would not be answered. A doctor was summoned, but her jaws were set, and she could not speak. He asked where her boy was, and when she did not reply said, " Why don't you obey me ? " After recovery she told how she misinterpreted this question, thinking he said, " Why didn't you make that boy obey you and you wouldn't have any trouble ".

For the next couple of days she suffered from many, apparently continuous, misinterpretations of the environment. She thought, when they came to see her, that her daughter and sister had lost their positions ; all visitors seemed to be making fun of her ; her children were screaming because they were being beaten ; she saw two long objects in shape like long squashes, tan coloured ; these were fighting together, and, as she watched them, she thought this was a spiritual manifestation. Any parcel sent to her or her daughter she imagined was sent to test her honesty ; if she kept it, she would be arrested for stealing. This she fancied was a result of her boy being sent to a reformatory. Her hands and body felt heavy, as if melted lead were poured into them ; her brain felt as if she were going into another world, " as if I passed into Eternity ". She made up her mind to go to the Observation Pavilion, and did so.

From these symptoms, gathered largely from the patient's retrospective account, it seems that her thoughts were in such a flux as to produce a semi-delirous condition. When she arrived at the Observation Pavilion, she was slow in her movements, looked depressed, expressed ideas of reference, and seemed to have hallucinations.

On admission, nothing noteworthy was found on physical examination. She was fairly well oriented, being sometimes a day or so out in gi.ing the date, and, except for slowness and difficulty in keeping her attention on the problem, was able to perform the usual intellectual tests. The emotional and ideational features were the prominent ones in her psychosis. At first she was depressed and inconsistently retarded. When asked why she was sad, she said that something like a cloud seemed to press on her head for half an hour and then go away. She was usually slow at the beginning of an interview, but would brighten up a little as she talked. On the other hand when asked about the events leading up to her break-down she was apt to block and become more depressed. She told in a fragmentary way of the false ideas and misinterpretations from which she had been suffering, seeming to have glimpses, at times, of their psychotic nature.

An examination made four days after admission produced, apparently, a curious effect. She was more than usually depressed. When questioned about what had caused her trouble, what she had been worrying about, she admitted something had happened which disturbed her greatly, but which she was unwilling to tell. After a good deal of arguing she said it was something that had been said, but was without foundation. Her sister had said something about a man and a woman, and it had annoyed her because she had not wanted to hear it. When urged to tell what it was, she said, " I don't know ; I feel my head is all mixed up again ". A few days later it was noted that this patient was objectively perplexed.

Retrospectively she dated her perplexity from this interview, and threw an interesting light on her mental processes. It will be recalled that what actually occurred was that her sister had told her of gossip to the effect that her wages were less than she alleged them to be. By some curious elaboration this was transformed into the statement quoted above to the effect that her sister had said something about a man and a woman. Retrospectively she claimed that the examiner had asked her if her sister had done anything with this man, and that she had replied, " Yes ". There were probably thoughts she had at this interview which she did not express, and which caused her confusion. She said that at this point she felt she had done wrong, had " given scandal " to a sister who had been kind to her. This depressed her greatly—" I felt as if I had been struck by a sledge hammer ". She became mixed up, and remained so for ten weeks. She thought all the people around knew what she had said about her sister, so she was unable to trust them and was afraid of them.

For the next ten weeks the patient remained in bed, often with a vacant, abstracted expression, and sometimes resisting passive movements. When examined she would become perplexed, and, if questions were directed toward discovery of the occasion of her breakdown, would usually become blocked. She was spoon-fed. She said nothing spontaneously, but after initial hesitation would answer questions about her current thoughts. She thought that those in the ward controlled her brain, they talked about her in signs saying that she was a burglar, that she was sleeping in another patient's bed, that she had deserted her children. The patients also controlled the weather, bringing on snow, hail or rain. By various movements they could control her thoughts and movements. Every event, even such a trifling thing as the window rattling, was a sign ; everything seemed to refer to her. For instance, she heard the words " Dead woman " and knew that, " They mean when I was here eight years ago I thought I was dead and in another world ; they mean I was dead and my body was returned again ". She could not think about her children for quite a while, couldn't bring them to mind at all, but had no difficulty in thinking about the events on the ward. She explained that there was so much going on that it took everything else out of her mind. Everything was queer ; if a patient brought her some chocolates they would appear white, when handed to her, or an apple would turn into an orange. An evidence of the lack of elaboration of her paranoid ideas appeared in her denial of the patients' having any enmity towards her, in spite of her constantly hearing accusations made against her honesty. As she spoke of these things she was occasionally tearful, again seemed slightly apprehensive, but was always perplexed. She was invariably oriented.

After recovery she gave a fuller account of her thoughts at this time, telling of such continuous misinterpretations as to suggest a delirium. If one nurse had a red pencil, and another a yellow one, that was a sign made for her. Every word spoken in the waid referred to her. One patient (whose bed she thought she was occupying) controlled her particularly. She had to turn over on her left side whenever this patient appeared. The patients were always making faces at her. She was only entitled to eat a small amount, because the food belonged to other patients, and she could never eat anything red like strawberries because that was the blood of Christ, which meant she was rejected by God. A coloured woman in a near-by bed seemed to be a man. It seemed as if all around were moving pictures. She also explained her perplexity. She said that every word was a sign, but what it meant she could not divine. Once she heard one patient call another a " bum " and a thief. She thought this referred to her, but could not understand the basis of these accusations. One must remember that while these false ideas were rushing through her head, she was all the time well oriented.

For the next three and a half months the patient was up and about the ward, but initiated very little activity. When set at it, she would polish the floor, but often ceased working with a far away, puzzled expression. When actively doing something, or when talking with a physician, she could free herself from her imaginings but at other times was lost in misinterpretations. Natural objects seemed queer. For instance, trees seen from the window looked to be close at hand. The water of the river seemed once to be divided in two, like two banks of sand, and boats looked as if made of sand ; people approaching her seemed to be coming through a snowstorm. One of the doctors looked like a picture of a detective she had seen in a newspaper. She complained very often of feeling dizzy in her head. Her vision constantly troubled her, and concerning this she made an interesting remark : " My sight is not clear . . . when the right is clear the left one is cloudy, and when the left is clear the right is cloudy ". Since tests showed no abnormality of vision one might be tempted to suppose that this belief of altered sight was dependent on her attention being given to reality and fantasy at the same time. That is, she saw things both accurately and inaccurately, and incorporated this abnormality in the feeling of seeing properly with only one eye and obscurely with the other. She explained that these perversions of visions, and all her false ideas occurred only when she was alone.

About six weeks after she left her bed she had an acute spell of hopelessness. She felt a constriction in her chest, cried a good deal, and wished to die because people were all against her and thought her a bad woman. This lasted for only three days and then she began, almost imperceptibly, to improve. When her psychosis had run for about six months, the physician told her that if she recovered she could go back to Ireland. She at once determined to get well, and forthwith began to occupy herself as much as possible, greatly to her advantage. Then one Sunday, as she started on the way to church, things suddenly looked natural, people no longer seemed to be making faces at her, the candles in church burned brightly and naturally, flames no longer stretching out into prongs as they had before. Although it was raining, everything was so bright that it seemed as if the sun were shining in the windows. For the first time in a year she could read her prayer book. Her sight was restored in both eyes. Within a few days she had entirely recovered with excellent insight, no longer wanted to go back to Ireland, but made up her mind to stay with her children. She left the hospital seven and a half months after the onset of the psychosis.

The next case is interesting from several standpoints. For years she had been neurotic, even psychotic in tendency, and after her psychosis became much more normal. It began as a partial stupor but soon turned into a perplexity reaction. Her confusion seems to have been occasioned by two main trends : first, that she was or had been dead (which disturbed her orientation), and second, a regression (like that of many manics) to the adolescent phase of her life just prior to marriage. These ideas were for a long time insistent, but they never dominated her attention so exclusively as to blot out recognition of the environment completely. Even when her orientation seemed most defective, she was apt to show her relatively good memory for the recent past, thus proving that she did not entirely lose herself in fantasy. Another interesting point is that, when otherwise apparently well, a few questions as to her false ideas would cause a re-appearance of her subjective confusion.

CASE 66. *Anna L.*[1] Age 24, married. Admitted to the Psychiatric Institute, August 21st, 1916.

F.H. Maternal grandmother temporarily insane during illegitimate pregnancy, thereafter a little odd. Mother high strung and emotional. Father high strung, impulsive and irritable.

P.H. As a child she was quick tempered, quite a spit-fire and given to tantrums. At the age of 14 she became a vaudeville actress in Cleveland, which was the home of her childhood. When 17 she married a Jew, although she was herself a Catholic. Her husband noted that she was fretful, sensitive, resentful, and quick-tempered, although apt to recover quickly from her rages. Previously healthy, neurotic symptoms began with marriage, taking the form of stomach trouble and a tendency to fatigue. Shortly after marriage an abortion was induced. After being married for two years she had a quarrel with, and separated from, her husband. They were reconciled later, but in the meantime she had been having relations with another man. When 20 an abdominal operation was performed in the hope of relieving her gastric symptoms, but no improvement occurred. The patient after recovery stated that she continued to be nervous, shaky and dizzy, at times trembling when going to bed at night. Two years later, however, she took up Christian Science, and showed objectively some improvement in her health, although, according to her later accounts, she continued to feel somewhat nervous and fatiguable. Her husband stated that at this time she also began to ponder much about such questions as the difference between life and death, what " matter " was, and also studied " grammar " and " etiquette ". According to the patient some five or six months before admission she began to have

[1] This case was described in Hoch's *Benign Stupors* to illustrate the relationship between stupor and perplexity.

peculiar sensations following intercourse—a feeling of bulging in the arms, legs and back of the neck. One evening after an automobile ride there were peculiar sensations in her right side like " electricity " or as if she were inhaling an anaesthetic. She gasped and thought she was dying. Two months before her admission she went with her husband to a summer resort, Bradley Beach, where she felt increasingly what had always been a trouble to her, namely, the nagging of his family.

Just before her breakdown, because she went daily to the Christian Science rooms in order to avoid the family, they suspected her of immorality, and accused her of going to meet other men. Even her husband began to question her motive. Retrospectively the patient herself said that she now felt she was losing her mind, and did not wish to talk to any one. At the time she told her husband that she felt confused, and as if she were guilty of something and being condemned. Repeatedly she said she knew she was going to get the family into a lot of trouble. Once she spoke of suicide, and for a while felt as if she were dying. Finally she became excited and shouted so much that she was taken to the Observation Pavilion, where she was described as being restless and noisy, thinking that she was to be burned up, and that she had been in a fire and was afraid to go back.

On admission she looked weary and seemed drowsy. Questions had to be repeated impressively before replies could be obtained, when she would rouse herself out of this drowsy state. She seemed placid and apathetic. She said that nothing was the matter, but soon admitted that she had not been well, first saying that her trouble was physical, and then agreeing that it had been mental. When asked whether she was happy or sad, she said " happy " but gave objectively no evidence of elation. Her orientation was defective. She spoke of being in New York and on Blackwell's Island, but could not describe what sort of place she was in, saying merely that it was " a good place ", or " a nice country place ", again " a good city ". Once when immediately after her name L. had been spoken, and she was asked what the place was, she said " The L." She knew that she had arrived in the hospital that day, but said that she had come from Cleveland, and to further questions, that she had come by train, but she could not tell how she reached the Island. She claimed not to know what the month was, and guessed that the season was either spring or autumn (August). She gave the year as 1917, called the doctor ' a mentalist ", and the stenographer " a tapper ", or " mental tapper ". She twice said she was single. When asked directly who took care of her, said " Mr. Marconi ", who, she claimed at another time, had brought her to the hospital. To the question, who is he ? she replied, " Wireless ", and could not be made to explain further. That night she urinated in her bed, and later lay quite limp, again held her legs very tense.

For five days she remained lying quietly in bed for the most part, although once she called out " Come in, I am here, Jimmie, Jimmie " (her husband's name). Several times she threw her bed-clothes off. Otherwise she made no attempt to speak and took insufficient food unless spoon-fed. At one examination she looked up rather dreamily, but did not answer. When shaken she breathed more quickly, and seemed about to cry, but made no effort to speak. When left to herself she closed her eyes, and did not stir when told she could go back to the ward. She was then lifted out of her chair and took a step or two and stopped. Such urging had to be repeated, as she would continue to remain standing, looking about dreamily, although finally when taken hold of she whimpered. When she got to the dining-table she put her hand in the soup, and then looked at it.

So far there is nothing in this case atypical of what we would call a partial stupor. The cardinal symptoms of apathy, inactivity, with a thinking disorder, are all present and dominate the clinical picture. There is, further, the history of a delusion of death during the onset of the psychosis.

Five days after admission, however, a change was noted in her condition. She became restless, distressed, and announced that she wished to talk to the physician. During the interview which followed, she continued to act in a distressed way, whimpered, complained constantly of her subjective per-perplexity, and sometimes cried about it. Apparently this change in her clinical condition was coincident with a re-appearance of some interest in the real world, for her first remark was to say that she wanted to see her people, " my mother and everybody ". She often went at once to the crux of her difficulties : " I don't know what it is all about ; I know you are a doctor, that is all. I don't know whether I passed out and came back again or what—I don't know what to make of it." Every question brought out similar perplexities. For instance, when asked about her marriage, she said, " That is where all the mix up is. I was married when I. was 16 ". (You once said you were single). " I am single." (Where is your husband ?) " He must be dead."

After recovery she explained that at this period she thought she had been dead a long time, and, in fact, was not sure whether she was really alive or not. This naturally affected her orientation, for at times she realized her environment in a way, but again would lose herself in her delusions, as was epitomized in an answer to an orientation question some days later. Her reply was : " This is the world, isn't it ? " When asked what the place was, she answered, " Hospital for crazy people, I think ". She remembered coming to the hospital on a boat, being interviewed on admission in another ward, and also some of the questions which she was then asked. On the other hand, when she was asked when she came, she replied : " Don't go so fast, doctor ; I know that it's years and years ago ; I know that when I was supposed to go I was 26 years old ". (Go where ?) " To die." She then said something about being married. (What about being married ?) " That's where all the mix up is ; I was married when I was 16. I know I got here yesterday, and it was all so strange to me, I was like underneath something." (Did you come yesterday ?) " I remember coming into a different office of yours, on a different side, quite a while ago." After speaking of being dead for a long time, she was asked how old she was. Her answer was, " I don't know ; according to that I must be awful old ".

The puzzling elusiveness of her thoughts comes out in the following : The discrepancy between her statements of being married and being single was pointed out to her, and she was asked where her husband was. To this she replied, " He must be dead ". (When did he die ?) " Wait a minute, doctor, I'll straighten it all out. If you could tell me what year this is, I would be able to tell you something." (What year does it seem to be ?) Seeing the date on the case record she said, " I can read the date on the book ; that was the year I was on earth ". (What year is it ?) " Isn't it 1917, doctor ? " [1916]. (Where were you when you died ?) " I don't know whether I died or not ; that's what is puzzling me."

A distraction by free association seems to appear in the next example. The thought of death apparently suggested to her mind the attack like elec-tricity, when she thought she was dying ; but the electricity appears as a therapeutic measure. She had been speaking of her career as an actress, and claimed both to have been off the stage and acting before her breakdown. When challenged with this discrepancy, she said, " Wait a minute, I'll straighten it out ; wait till it comes back to me, it's back too far ". (What ?) " Well, I know that before I passed out I was in Bradley Beach, New Jersey, we were down there for the usual summer vacation. That was a year ago, doctor, in 19 . . . [looks puzzled] just a minute now . . . Didn't someone try to do something for me with electricity ? " (What do you mean ?) " I don't know, I'm just like this [pointing to her stomach and holding out her hands] I'm shaky. I do not know that Mr. L. is my husband, whether he is dead or not."

This condition persisted for some two and a half months, there being no essential change except for a somewhat increased emotionality in latter part of this period. Her orientation also improved slightly. As to this last she said after recovery that some six weeks after admission she saw " Manhattan State Hospital " printed on a telephone card, and that from then on she knew where she was ; but as a matter of fact she frequently gave the name of the Hospital correctly before this time. She gradually learned the names of the doctors and nurses. Even when giving the year wrong (a result of her delusion of having been dead a long time) she usually could say with fair accuracy how long she had been in the hospital, when the last interview with the physician had taken place, and so on. For the first month of her admission she remained quietly in bed, but, when she got up and dressed, it made no conspicuous difference in her condition. She simply sat around, often biting her finger nails, and usually only mildly distressed in countenance until she was questioned, when an expression of pained bewilderment would appear, sometimes associated with restlessness, tears or, rarely, smiles. One striking feature in her case was the inactivity and apathy which existed when she was left undisturbed. Considering the obvious stupor symptoms at the beginning of the psychosis, it does not seem unreasonable to suppose that a background of stupor persisted, and that any stimulus aroused her, not to normality, but to a preoccupation with psychotic thoughts that were latent in the intervals. Then came the perplexity and emotional reactions appropriate to the coincident thought.

During this time there was a comparatively small compass to her ideas. The most frequent was that she was, or had been, dead. Sometimes she thought the other patients lying in bed were dead too. The next commonest delusions had to do with her marital condition. She rarely could be induced to admit that she was married, and usually gave her maiden name. Sometimes this was elaborated with the statement that she was living with her mother in Cleveland (her home before marriage). Not infrequently a compromise was reached by imagining that Jimmie (her husband) was her fiancé. This, of course, is the kind of content one finds in a manic state, so it was not inappropriate that such statements should be accompanied by smiles and associated with identification of the doctor with Jimmie (a rare symptom in this case). For instance, during an interview four weeks after admission, her husband's name was mentioned, and she promptly cried. She was then asked who she was, and gave her maiden name. (Who is James L. and what is he to you ?) " He is everything to me . . . he is my sweetheart." Then, smiling, and with the attitude of greeting a stranger, she asked, " Aren't you Jimmie ? " No amount of leading questions would induce her to admit that he was her husband. She would often say, " He is my . . ." and then block. The nearest she got to it was " He is my sweetheart ; we are going to be married ". Retrospectively she told of thinking a great deal about the time when she was 16 years old.

Associated with this annulment of her marriage, so to speak, were ideas of her husband's death or injury, and these were always accompanied by sorrow or alarm. When he interviewed the physician, the patient was convinced that the doctor had put something in his ears. When he left after a visit, she feared an assault would be made upon him. Once at such a time, hearing a sudden noise, she was convinced that he had just been shot. On one occasion only did she imagine he might be married to someone else.

An idea that occurred fairly often was that her mother had been put into a box. This was apparently some rather vividly hallucinated experience, for she once added details about hearing the men laugh and the remarks they made. As we have seen, such a delusion is highly typical of depression. Ordinarily this patient had little to say in the way of self blame, but once a feeling of wickedness came out as a free association, as it were, to this idea. This was ten days after admission, when she remarked quite irrelevantly, " I am not my mother ; my mother was here with a blue dress on " [correct]. I remember they took her into a back room and put her into a box. " (What did they do to her ?) " Oh, I don't know [repression ?] I have just been so unhappy." (How ?) " I have done so many wrong things." (What things ?) " It seems as if I lay in bed [said rather penitently]. I don't know what to make of it." (What wrong things ?) " Why I don't know— then it comes back to me I didn't do wrong. It seems as if I got all mixed up here.".

There was no record of her father appearing in her autistic thoughts, except perhaps by implication. She once said that her mother had come to her several times, and said, " I am a widow. "

Finally, there were some curious ideas as to the patient's identity. These were probably to be explained both by her delusion of death and as an expression of her perplexity. She spoke of herself as a spirit, but also of there being several of her around. This was also associated with a confusion about her name, as when she said (more than once) " It seems as if everything got mixed up between the L.s [married name] and the G.s [maiden name] ". Three weeks after admission she remarked irrelevantly, " Another girl comes in at night ; she looks like me. I think she is a spirit ". A week before this she was asked how long she had been in hospital. For answer she pointed to the window, and said, " I remember walking in there. They said I was a spirit ". The question was repeated, but all she could say was, " A long while ". Then quite abruptly : " There are two other girls here that look like me . . . You asked me if I was Mrs. G. [mother], and I said I was ". (Why did you say so ?) " Because you had all Anne L s, and I knew they were not all."

Her recovery began rather suddenly. She herself ascribed it to the influence of a fellow patient, a girl about her own age. She had begun to think more of her husband, and was worried enough about his not coming to see her, to have a crying spell. This girl then told her to cheer up, that the doctor would soon let her go home. This made her think much more of her home, awakening a desire to get well and leave the hospital. One of her first moves was to ask the nurse questions about the hospital, how long she had been there, and so on. Then she talked to the physician about her false ideas. She told of having had a feeling of being dead, and walking around, and wanted to know how this could be. She also asked to have other false ideas rectified. A little talk about them, however, threw her back into her old confusion, and she began to cry. But this lasted only for a day or so, after which she could discuss her whole psychosis intelligently and without bad reaction. Her recovery was, apparently, complete. In fact her husband insisted that she was better than for years.

In connection with this case it would be well for the reader to refer to a somewhat similar one also described by Hoch[1]. This is the case of Celia H. She too began with a stupor-like reaction, the atmosphere of which persisted throughout the psychosis. Perplexity was present in a mild degree, but the complication of the stupor picture seemed to be more in the direction of absorption.

The next case, which we shall describe more briefly, is interesting as demonstrating the relationship of perplexity to absorbed manic states. It would have been a typical absorbed mania had it not been for the coincidence of a strong tendency to distraction of thought with good orientation. This incompatibility produced, as it should according to our theory, the added symptom of perplexity. The psychosis began with a rather pure reaction of absorption complicated only by episodes of blind excitement. Then contact with reality was attempted and the perplexity picture appeared. In this her verbal productions were singularly like manic flight of ideas, including comments on the environment, with an obviously free associational quality. In this " flight " she made many references to her subjective confusion and to delusions as to her identity. In this flux, erotic ideas, complaints of accusations made against her, and, more rarely, fearful pre-

1 " Benign Stupors," p. 167.

sentiments were expressed-   There were naturally changes in her emotional reaction with these variations.

CASE 67. *Rose E.* Age 18, unmarried. Admitted to the Psychiatri[c] Institute, January 14th, 1908.

F.H. The father was an insane criminal, and the mother died when the patient was a baby. Otherwise there were no pertinent data about the family.

P.H. The patient was brought up by an aunt in Troy, N.Y., from whom this information was secured, which is supplemented by the retrospective account of the patient herself after recovery. She was never good at school, wasted her time, could not work up interest in any of her studies, and was rather cranky and sneaky. From examination made after recovery it seemed probable that she was somewhat defective intellectually. She was, however, sociable. After leaving school she got a position, but not succeeding, soon gave it up, and remained idle in her aunt's home. About a year before admission she entered into sexual relations with two men. Six months before admission her aunt sent her out of the house, and she came to New York. Here again her virtue did not seem to be impregnable. She obtained work, but did not get along very well. In fact her employer described her as " giddy and without depth, simple, fidgetty and rather too fond of young men ". She was homesick for Troy, and wanted to return to her aunt. Then for two months she was a servant in a clergyman's house, who complained of her that " she was not capable and wanted to go out nights ".

Onset of Psychosis. About Christmas, 1907, that is, about three weeks before admission, she was discharged, and celebrated her release by having intercourse with two men that night. But she then became depressed and stared silently in company. Nine days before admission she was informed that her aunt would have nothing more to do with her, which worried her greatly. A few days later she wrote a letter to her aunt in which she said she had done her wrong. The next day she went to church where a mission was in progress. A sermon was preached on goodness and purity ; she cried and felt lonesome. Then she began to pray a good deal, and spoke of having fallen and sinned. A young man came to see her, and talked about her wrong-doing, which produced what she retrospectively described as a " fit ". She shivered as she sat on a chair. That night she had a vision of a cousin, Mary H., who died while pregnant. There were also visions of God, Christ, the Devil and of her mother. She was taken to a general hospital, and from there to the Observation Pavilion, where she was described as " depressed " and " confused ". She remained there for three days. After recovery she could remember the trip to the general hospital, and the transfer to the Observation Pavilion, but had no more recollection of her stay there or of her being taken to the Manhattan State Hospital.

On admission the patient had a coated tongue, pulse of 110, but a normal temperature. She was at first dull, moaning, and sometimes weeping, apparently absorbed in thought. She did not react to pin pricks, and often showed marked resistance when interfered with. As a rule she would not answer questions except with gross irrelevance, or she might show that she heard merely by repeating automatically now and then a word that had been spoken. Naturally her orientation could not be established, but it seemed as if she knew she was in a hospital. Her scanty verbal productions, which were given entirely in whispers, had that fragmentary quality noted in some cases of absorbed mania where the thoughts are rarely expressed in sentences, but represented more often by detached, and therefore incomprehensible, words or phrases. The following is an example : " Cry L., what on the side . . . sister, French, T., too . . . right on the T. She did shiver and shake on the blue sea [shivers] . . . be a good girl to St. Joseph three times . . . sitting on the chair . . . I left her on the cold . . . she did . . . I did speak out . . . G.A. . . . A.H. . . . H.A.S. . . . type she said . . . turn your back." The word " black " often occurred.

This state lasted for a week, but during this time she sometimes had periods of blind excitement, accompanied by slight fever and a mouth so dry that it was difficult to get her to swallow. In this coarse excitement she threw herself about, often spitting, or biting at her tongue, or even trying to pull it out with such violence that the nurses had to hold her. She seemed dazed, and usually presented no definite emotional reaction beyond the crude excitement, except for an occasional appearance of fear. At the end of the week she seemed suddenly to awake, asked where she was, and explained that she thought she had been in the Tombs prison accused of killing her father, and that she was going to be thrown out. A brief relapse of absorption occurred, and then she entered the chief and last phase of her psychosis.

This was a condition which lasted for three months, of clear orientation but accompanied by a state of perplexed uneasiness and delirium-like talk. Emotionally, she had as a rule the distressed uneasiness so common in perplexity states, but this was often interrupted with whimpering, sometimes with smiling, and, rarely, with anxiety. She often peered about her with a puzzled expression. After recovery she gave some account of the different false ideas that had been engrossing her attention, and it may help the reader to understand her verbal productions if these be stated before giving examples of her speech. She said that, when she was at the Observation Pavilion and when she first came to the hospital, her mind left her ; she wanted to go to Troy. She thought that she was in the Tombs for killing her father ; again, her father wanted to take her out, but she did not want to go with him, but rather with Eddie (one of her lovers). Her main purpose was to go to Troy. Eddie was in the hospital, he was on an adjoining bed. She knew no one else ; but, again, the nurses seemed to be relatives, and another patient, Jennie, resembled her cousin Mary H. who died while pregnant. Sometimes she thought she was dying (episodes of fear). At the beginning of her perplexed phase she spoke of a vision, but, after recovery, could not recall it, and denied any vivid hallucinations.

As has been stated, her train of thought was like manic flight ; there were frequent sound, as well as sense, associations and comments on the environment were intruded. The most prominent topic to which she referred was her perplexity. This appeared in three forms, direct complaint, delusions as to her spirit or individuality, and, in a more obscure way, in remarks about two halves of her body. This last would be meaningless were it not that so many perplexed patients express themselves in this way, so that it seems reasonable to suppose that such statements represent vague and symbolic reference to the splitting of interest or attention between inner thoughts and outer events. In quoting her words we shall italicize the perplexity utterances. The second most prominent theme was the erotic, associated sometimes with infantile ideas. Finally there were a number of scattered remarks that could only have been understood had more extensive collection and collation of her verbal productions been attempted.

She frequently stated that she was " *twisted* ". " *I cannot think clearly* ; *my mind seems to go away.*" " *I am afraid I am lost in the scrape, twisted in the scrape.*" A great many occurrences in the environment were referred to herself. " *I am mixed up with Mrs. C.* [another patient]. " I am Dr. K.'s [ward physician] wife . . . *I am supposed to be dead on one side* [pointing to a case with hemiplegia] . . . I wish Mrs. Newman—new red man—I put blood on the *wrong side* . . . Mrs. H. was transferred [correct] . . . they say *I am inside of her and she is inside of me.*" Like the sound association from " Newman " to " new red man " was this : " Miss Hartnet—the net from her hair ". The following productions were typical : " A lot of flowers, red roses on the outside ; I wanted to be one too. I stood by you ; *I don't want to be in two.* That wind is coming in so cold [correct]. *You see I am blind if I go back that way* ; *I want to go forward to-night.*" (What hospital did you come from ?). " I thought I was swallowed down quick, it's over the 'phone [foam ?] that I came here." " *Nobody seems to know who I am* ; you [addressing the doctor] are that lady's husband ; *this is an awful puzzle.*" When a nurse urged another patient to go out she said, " Let me go out on the ship. A woman's drawers, there's a miscarriage in it. Someway nobody cares for me . . . that woman there annoys me ; *I think she is a spirit of mine* ". " They call me a rat from Troy. I must have had hydrophobia ; I thought I had it. At first I spit froth from my mouth [during coarse excitement ?] ; I am a murderer now."

Although she was always oriented she made many remarks, which taken alone, would have indicated that she did not comprehend the environment. For instance, she said, " This is a hospital for infants, for child-birth, for sore fingers ". Or she said she was there " for womb trouble ". She frequently mentioned the actions of those about her with the comment that she did not know what they meant. The patients looked at her as if she were " a street-walker or a street cleaner " ; they laughed at her and all they said referred to her. " I guess all the other patients are married women. I was married in my bed ; I should have a nice clean bed." There was some misidentifcation of persons, but this was largely associated with the feeling that those about her signified something which she could not understand.

Connected with her thoughts of dying there was apparently some fantasy of mutual death. She once said : " Nobody cares where I live—I don't know whether my father is dead [living] ; I know my mother is." Speaking retrospectively of her father's imagined death, she made it appear that this was connected with thoughts of her own death and of the fancy that her father wanted to take her out of the hospital or prison. There were two settings of this idea. One was that she and her father were both dead or going to die. The other was that her father would remove her from the institution. Against the latter she struggled, as she wanted to join Eddie. This is interesting, because it seems that when reunion with a real person (actual father, not a spirit) was the formulation her thoughts turned to a more natural object of adult interest, namely her lover. A melodramatic formulation of the death idea occurred in a letter the patient wrote to her aunt at this time. She begged repeatedly that her aunt should come and take her out of the hospital, saying that she might be dead before her aunt came, that she might be cut in pieces.

Some remarks about Jennie, the patient that resembled her cousin that died in pregnancy, illustrate beautifully the type of thinking in a sufferer from perplexity. She said : " I must be cursed by my people. Jennie came to my bed—she died in the family way. I thought she was some kind of a saint," or, as she put it on another occasion, " She appeared from the dead ". Now, since she was oriented, she recognized Jennie as a real person and as a fellow patient ; in fact, she called her " Jennie " not " Mary H." Her actual sexual experiences were enough to suggest the idea of pregnancy, and her remarks about child-birth and miscarriages (v. supra) show that this thought was in her mind. This accounts for the statement " Jennie came to my bed ", i.e., she was identified with Jennie, because the latter looked like somebody who had been pregnant. A normal person having similar free associations would think : " Jennie looks like Mary H. The later died when pregnant. I wonder if I am pregnant. Jennie looks like a re-incarnation of Mary H.". An absorbed patient would misidentify Jennie altogether, and see only Mary H., believing that the latter had come to life (or was haunting her) because the patient was pregnant. The perplexed patient combines these two modes of thinking. Free associations to the death of Mary H. and her own pregnancy are set going by the sight of Jennie. The free associations then have enough feeling of reality to them to make Jennie appear to be somebody else, and to be in the patient's bed, although she still remains Jennie. This is naturally a puzzling business.

About three and a half months after admission her condition improved greatly, but she still complained of feeling confused. Within a week or two, however, her recovery was complete. Her intelligence was then tested and found to be definitely defective. After her discharge she wrote the doctor a natural letter, expressing gratitude, but with gross mistakes in spelling.

The chief interest in the next case lies in the patient's having had for some months brief spells of being "dazed" and that, when such attacks became prolonged into a real psychosis, her confusion seemed to be definitely associated with a vaguely formulated paranoid tendency.

CASE 68. *Grace P.* Age 40, married. Admitted, January 3rd, 1905.

F.H. One paternal aunt and one maternal uncle had each a psychosis. with recovery. Otherwise all hereditary taint was denied.

P.H. It was claimed that the patient had had a rather cheerful disposition. Before marriage she filled a responsible position. She was married at 26, but never had any children. This was probably the result of an ovarian tumor and an operation to remove it, which took place after marriage, and after which she never menstruated again. For four or five years she had had fairly frequent tantrums, "hysterical attacks", when anything went wrong. She would then make scenes, growing more and more excited until, with exhaustion, she would become "almost powerless". No clouding of consciousness was observed, however.

The onset of the psychosis was gradual and without ascertainable cause. Three months before admission she one day felt confused on the street, not knowing in which direction to turn for home, but this lasted only for a few minutes. Similar spells returned, however. Five weeks before admission she became depressed, sat idly about, and cried at times. A week later she thought people were talking about her, that a friend of her husband was a detective, that her husband was going to have her arrested or otherwise injure her. She wrote a sentimental letter to her physician and later woke her husband up in the middle of the night to ask him if, after all, it would be right for her to go with the doctor. Three weeks before admission she woke him again, and asked him if he were ill. She often complained of being dazed and also of a headache. Towards the end of her psychosis she described this headache as a pressure behind her forehead, but also as a kind of dazed feeling, which prevented her from thinking well. So it was probably not a usual type of pain. At about the same time as these complaints appeared, she one night said to her husband, "Come, let's end it all, let's take chloroform". In spite of looking confused, she nevertheless continued to do some work about the house.

After recovery she gave the following account of the onset : The confused spells consisted in a peculiar feeling that she could not see well, not in the sense that objects appeared blurred but that somehow things went away from her. Her eyes felt big, and she thought that they appeared big to others, and that she looked funny. This was projected as well, for she claimed that for a few days she saw double, people looked funny, their eyes stuck out. They also acted peculiarly, and seemed to be talking about her. She felt that she was followed by men who wanted something from her. Later she was convinced that she was wicked, and was going to be sent to gaol, for her husband wanted to get rid of her.

On admission nothing significant was discovered in physical examination. For three months she appeared subdued and inactive, although not specially slow in many of her answers. On the other hand, when her feelings and troubles were enquired into, she had to be urged a good deal to answer. There was no doubt that she was downhearted, and sometimes said she wished she were dead. She was easily startled. But, above all, she looked puzzled and was constantly speaking of her perplexity. Thus, when she was asked why she worried, she was apt to say, "I don't understand the situation," "I can't realize anything," "I don't know what is right or wrong," or "I can't understand it". Then, too, she complained of not being able to see well, but when questioned as to her meaning she replied, "Perhaps I should say that I couldn't think". She claimed that she could not read, but denied blurring in vision ; it was rather, "I can't put my mind to it".

As to her false ideas, she had only one dominant one, and that was that her husband wanted to get rid of her. Other current delusions were remarkably vague, and expressed only after much urging. She was more communicative about past experiences. She told of being given medicine at home from a bottle with no label ; after taking it, her head felt like wood and the blood rushed up and down in her body. It had seemed as if someone had always followed her around, and, when she spoke, she felt herself to be a prisoner. For some time she had not been able to correlate events. For example, once when she told a woman that she was nervous, the latter replied that she was nervous too ; " It was as if she said exactly the same things which I said, and as if I were answering to other people ". (This is like the phenomenon of *déjà vu*, which we shall be discussing presently). Again, someone came up to her on the street and greeted her as aunt. Such stories were not further elaborated, and she usually added, " But I can't understand the situation ". Once she warned her nurse not to open her trunk when it came to the hospital, as it contained incriminating evidence, and added that she had had an abortion performed when she was 18. She also referred to incidents that had occurred since her residence in the hospital ; why did her husband, when he called with a friend, talk about Nan Patterson before her, and why did he say that she should be happy ? (Nan Patterson was an actress who killed her lover).

There seemed to be a definite connection between the lack of formulation in these delusions and her perplexity. The patient who elaborates ideas of reference into anything like a logical system has no doubt about them, in fact, they become clearer in his mind than anything else. They are rationalized in their systematization. It is when this elaboration is lacking that a patient is puzzled by the discrepancy between the delusions and actual experience. Thus she said, " There seems to be a conspiracy," but when asked to explain could only reply, " I don't know myself ; I have thought and thought, but I don't know. I don't understand the situation ". On another occasion she remarked, " I believe my husband has been paid to down me ." Such an explanation, if accepted, would, of course, clarify the problem. But she added immediately, " But I have no right to make statements, I am so confused. I can't tell, I can't think ". Another time she commented, " I have tried to understand it, but I can't ". She explained her dilemma more than once. She felt that her husband did not like her, and that he wanted to get rid of her, yet he was spending a lot of money to keep her in the hospital, and he surely would not make this sacrifice were he indifferent to her. Then there were many statements like the following : " I have had letters from him begging me to try and understand the situation, but I don't understand it. He says he is working hard to keep me here, but he knows I never wanted him to work hard like that, I always tried to help some myself . . . If my husband liked me, why on Christmas Eve did he and a friend of his talk about Nan Patterson and a whole lot of absurd things before me. And why, when the friend left did he tell me that I ought to be happy on Christmas Eve instead of so blue ? " Her failure to elaborate this paranoid tendency was shown in her never being suspicious about anyone around her. Once she attempted a rationalization of her husband's antagonism in a half-hearted way. She confided to the nurse that perhaps some money might have been left to her, and that he wanted her destroyed in order that he might obtain it. The only basis she could offer for this fancy was that he had often said he hoped to get a fortune some day. This feeble effort at systematization was tentative and isolated.

Her orientation was always quite good for place and persons, and aproximately correct for day and date. Invariably she was able to give a good account of recent events. When asked for data of her early life that had no emotional significance, her replies were full and accurate. But, if enquiry were made about such events as her marriage, she had difficulty in collecting her memories. As is so frequent in perplexity cases, she had trouble in performing any but the simplest arithmetic calculations, and was apt to speak of her poor mental efficiency. This was patently due to deficient concentration of attention, a natural accompaniment of a tendency to free associational thinking.

About two and a half months after admission she began to occupy herself more with little tasks, and even in talking with other patients.   At the same time she ceased spontaneous reference to her false ideas.   A couple of weeks later she received a reassuring letter from a relative, and then began to think that perhaps she was wrong in feeling that her husband wanted to be rid of her.   When he visited her shortly after this, " It all lifted suddenly ". An interesting thing was that she claimed that with her mental improvement her headache, which had been absent throughout the psychosis, returned. She added that during the bulk of her illness she had not felt pain nor cold, and had not had any feeling for anything or anybody.   She then made a rapid and complete recovery.

The next case had a prominent paranoid tendency but an equally strong depressive reaction. The latter seemed to have two effects : he was down-hearted in the extreme, while the repression, which we have seen to characterize depression, affected his train of thoughr, preventing him from reaching, consciously, any definite formulation of his ideas. They remained more intangible " feelings " of reference than actual delusions. Another interesting point is that his conviction of moral failure was associated with memories of masturbation. Now the adolescent, who is struggling with onanism is very apt to have a paranoid tendency like that of the perplexed patient. He is constantly thinking of his secret sin and its effects upon him so that the glances and words of those about him seem to refer to himself and his trouble. If a false interpretation can be put on any remark, it is made, because, of all possible interpretations, that which fits in with his obsessing thoughts, is chosen. But like the paranoid tendency in the perplexity case this does not go on to any systemization. It remains more of a " feeling ".

CASE 69. *Henry R.* Age 39. Admitted, October 28th, 1904.

F.H. A paternal first cousin was feeble-minded. Otherwise exhaustive enquiry failed to reveal any mental taint. The patient's mother died when he was nine months old, and his father remarried.

P.H. The patient was said to be a natural, healthy child up to his twelfth year. He then had an attack of measles which left him with a slight throat trouble. Fearing that this might be a warning of the tuberculosis, from which his wife had died, the father then instituted a system of coddling. The boy was guarded against all possible exposure, encouraged to avoid exertion, either mental or physical, and in general badly pampered. As a natural result he grew up introspective and hypochondriacal. Nevertheless he did well in his studies, and even attended a University for one term. Then his health was ·thought to be failing, so his further education was abandoned, and he was sent down South to spend two years in idleness. On his return he began to work in his father's business, but for a year or two gave it most desultory attention, this being encouraged by his father. Then, however, his industry increased, although he retained a tendency to shirk responsibility.

Previous attack. When 37 years of age he had an attack of depression, lasting about three months, which came on and subsided gradually. First he could not concentrate his mind, and wanted to be left alone ; then he accused himself of sin, and wanted to be killed in punishment for the suffering he caused his family ; next he thought he had a disease which he might communicate to others, and finally he went into a kind of stupor, refusing to eat, and passing his urine and faeces involuntarily. After recovery he did not seem to realize the gravity of the symptoms he had exhibited, and tended to laugh at the whole affair.

He then improved physically a good deal, and began to play games, which he had never done before. After being idle for a year he went into the photography business, which was not successful. This led to periods of depression which he managed to shake off until about six weeks before admission.

Onset of psychosis : He gradually lost interest and became inactive. Then three weeks before admission he showed another stupor-like reaction, refusing to eat or speak. This lasted for two days, after which he got out of bed, sat by the window, and told his nurse that he had been " imagining things different from what they really are ". He went on to speak of the awful sin he had committed, bringing his family into disgrace and making people talk about him. For this he thought he ought to be punished. Again, he had the delusion of suffering from a loathsome, contagious disease, and thought his hands smelled badly. There were also ideas unusual in a depression. He spoke of being in the centre of the earth, and that it would crush in on him or the Tower of Babel would fall, saying to the nurse, " You'd better get away ; you'd better get away ! " with an anxious expression. He several times tried, with violence, to hurt or kill himself. He became slow in speech, although not in movement, and for a week had declined to eat, taking only a little liquid nourishment when urged. For three weeks he had no sleep except when drugged.

On admission, physical examination showed no abnormality beyond a heavily coated tongue and foul breath. He made at once an impression of depression and confusion, that was confirmed in all he said. He made several energetic attempts at self-injury. At first he refused to do anything asked of him, but his resistance was short-lived ; he would soon comply, uttering continuous complaints. For instance, when asked to eat, he would say, " This isn't right, I do not understand ; everything I take only makes it worse ". His face was not immobile, but had a perplexed, troubled expression, and, rarely, a smile would pass over it. Thus, when asked to shake hands, he drew his hand away, saying, " This is not right, I ought not to do it ; what shall I do ? " but, when his hand was grasped, a smile played momentarily over his features. Then the same troubled expression re-appeared, and he went on, " Everything I do is wrong, everything I do makes it worse. I can't do anything right . . . It was right but it isn't right now ". (Why ?) " I didn't tell the truth originally, and it's all wrong now." (I think not). " I know it is, I didn't tell my Heavenly Father the truth ". (In regard to what ?) " Oh, I don't know ." (What did you do ?) " I sold my whole body and soul [meaning he masturbated] ; it was too late ; I did not tell my father. That was wrong . . . I have done everything to preserve my own life—I have deceived others. I ought to be punished for selling my body and soul as cheaply as I did."

He gave a fragmentary account of his past life, his former attacks, and of the onset of this psychosis. It was drawn out of him piece-meal, in slow words and with a nervous shifting about in his chair. He was constantly punctuating his utterances with such statements as, " This isn't right, it's all wrong, I don't belong here. I ought to be punished ". He knew that he was in a hospital, and that he was talking to a doctor, and gave the year correctly, but even his correct answers he would supplement with, " That is not right—it's all wrong ". Simple calculations he performed well, but more complicated ones were abandoned with such explanations as, " This isn't right ; I don't understand," or " I can't think connectedly of anything ". (Is it hard for you ?) " It is hard to think of anything but myself, and that is wrong."

It was only for a few days that it was impossible to tell whether he was disoriented or not. Then it became evident that he knew where he was, the names of those around him and the day and date. But, for three weeks his complaints of not understanding things were incessant. There was a constant difficulty in arriving anywhere in his talk ; he would begin sentences and not finish them or become side-tracked. This was not the product of any evasiveness, for he seemed anxious to impart his trouble, in fact he would follow the physician at the end of an unsatisfactory interview, but be incapable of explaining himself when he re-opened the conversat.on.

After about three weeks residence in the hospital he became a little freer, dressed himself of his own accord, was more co-operative, yet for a week or two more his confusion of thought and depression of spirit troubled him a great deal. During this period efforts at digging out his painful ideas were a little more successful. A frequent remark was " I don't understand the system " by which he meant the significance of the hospital. When urged to elaborate this difficulty he replied :

" I have thought I was to go away. Of course I know I was upset physically . . . if I had to go to a place of rest, I thought everything ; that is what I can't account for—why there should be so much confusion . . . whether everybody is taking a cure or . . . I don't know how to express it." Then he went on : " I don't know how to express it exactly. I am here shut up in a room, and forty or fifty people are going through various evolutions and hollering and all sorts of things. It does not seem to be conducive to rest exactly. I don't see why it should have any bearing on me ".

He spoke of many strange ideas he had had when first coming to the hospital, although it seemed clear that he had not full insight into the fantastical nature of these thoughts. " I had lots of imaginations ; I worked out things which happened in my life." " If I am accountable for the strange ideas I had, then, of course, I am to blame ! " Every thing had seemed unnatural, and he imagined he had got into another world. His people were no longer alive. There was something very wrong about his having a picture of his father and stepmother—something entirely wrong about that. " I haven't come here with any scheme." Again, " If there is anything I have done before I came and that ought to be known, I am glad to tell it ".

Everything in his environment, animate or inanimate, was suggestive of some meaning beyond its obvious significance. Apparently what he saw or heard set up a train of free associations, the meaning or feeling of which was attached to the original stimulus. Sometimes this produced a *déjà vu*, a feeling of unnatural familiarity. For instance, everything that was done reminded him of things at home. This led him to believe that he was being prompted to do as his father wanted. When his clothes closet was locked, he thought it was his duty to get inside of it. He thought it was his duty not to eat. This was partly because he had no appetite, but food seemed to be connected, as well, with religion and a sacrament.

This tendency to ascribe meaning to the environment came out most strongly in the interpretation of the actions of those about him. He was forever speaking of the bearing on him of all that was done. People seemed to have an eye on him ; he could not understand why they chased around so ; they seemed to think he was guilty of something. People made suggestions to him by their actions, as if everything that he saw was an object lesson to him. " It was as if they wanted me to do something I couldn't get a hold of." When asked for examples, he mentioned the way they walked about, or a hat being left in a certain place, which seemed to indicate that a change was expected, someone was to take the place of someone else. Once he went so far as to say, " I don't know whether it was mind reading or not ". When carefully questioned about this he said, " I am afraid they thought there was something malicious in my thoughts, and they seemed to try to find out what I was thinking ". He added that they seemed to find out little that was true ; it was mostly erroneous. (Hence the perplexity. If he had accepted these suspicions as being well-founded, there would have been no discrepancy between his thoughts and his knowledge and, so, no confusion).

Although he spoke at this time mainly in the past tense, he was constantly slipping into the present, showing that the paranoid tendency had not disappeared. For instance, hs spoke of his still being watched, and made many references to his failure in understanding the ". atmosphere ".   Yet he would at the same time, intrude his knowledge of the real nature of things.   Thus he said, " It doesn't seem as if these people are sick—the patients, if they are patients ".   Or, again, " I don't know what bearing it has on me, but it seems as if there was some purpose in this walking about . . . if it's for exercise it's all right ".

Then his condition improved markedly.   He became helpful in the ward, dusting, making beds, and so on.   He even began to play games, and expressed a desire to go skating.   In fact his activity became a little abnormal a couple of months after admission, and merited a cautionary word from his physician.   His reaction to this showed a lingering trace of his earlier difficulties.   He protested that this was his normal disposition, and then began to bother himself with speculation as to why he should have been warned. Moreover he had a tendency to be stubborn and morose in the mornings. This phase was quite brief, however, and after three months of hospital residence his recovery was complete.   Retrospectively, he could offer no further explanation of his perplexity : " It seemed to me as if I ought to do something, yet I did not know what to do ; and, if I did do something, it seemed the wrong thing, and that is the way it was."

CHAPTER XLII

RELATIONSHIP OF PERPLEXITY TO OTHER PSYCHOSES

FROM these cases, typical of the forms which perplexity psychoses assume, it is hoped that the reader may be able to envisage this reaction. We must now consider a few generalities of a psychiatric and psychological nature. The first of these has to do with the analogy between the kind of thinking that occurs in dreams with that in the mental derangement we have been studying. In an earlier chapter it was suggested that absorbed mania is probably very like dreaming. Here again we find such a similarity. As Freud has shown, we do not think in abstract terms when we dream, but parade our strivings, opinions and judgments before us in images, mainly visual. Very aptly he compares this type of expression with the conduct of political argument in the form of cartoons. The patient suffering from perplexity seems to be thinking in this way, at the same time that he is endeavouring to maintain a waking contact with the environment. He is dreaming dreams and seeing visions although he is not asleep. This accounts for the great frequency of hallucinations and also for the bizarre nature of some of the delusions, which investigation shows are expressionless in images of abstract ideas. The reader will recall, for instance, a curious complaint of one of the patients studied by Hoch and Kirby. She said, " What do they mean by saying I turn into two girls ? " and also, " They tell me I have glass eyes all over." She later explained these peculiar sayings by the statement that she felt confused, nothing looked natural, everything looked alike, and she thought she could not see right. These are typical dream expressions. Things not seeming right suggest poor vision, and poor vision, glass eyes. Since everything seems queer, the glass eyes are all over her. Similarly her being two girls is characteristic of dream " language ". Her mental life was split in two directions, an absorption in inner thoughts and coincident recognition of the environment. Such opposed tendencies are often represented in dreams by two persons, who act separately.

The paranoid tendency is a corollary of this. In sleep we are quite out of touch with the environment, so that the imagery of our dreams is derived wholly from within. But the perplexed patient is trying to keep in contact with the world around. A compromise is reached in the paranoid idea. Anything—inanimate object, person or action—which the patient observes may be used as the image to express the thought that surges up, provided only some free associational relationship can be established between that which is seen or heard and the idea that is coming to birth. This idea is like a spirit seeking incarnation. It takes up its abode in the most suitable body it can find. For instance, Rose E. was troubled with fears of pregnancy and death. These ideas are combined in the fate of her cousin Mary H., who died while pregnant. Then Jennie looks like Mary H., so it is all fastened on to her, becoming a paranoid idea. So Jennie comes to the patient's bed (dramatizing the identity of situations between the patient and Mary H.) and also haunts her as a spirit from the dead.

The psychological relationship between the thinking processes of dementia praecox and perplexity is of no small theoretic importance. In speaking of dementia praecox I refer particularly to that type in which scattered speech occurs, although the same generalizations will hold for other types where the reaction is merely more dilute, or less frequent. As has been remarked earlier in this book, scattered speech is really a free associational process. Its peculiarity lies in the fact that the patient regards each element in the series as having equal validity, equal claim to reality. Each association is, so to speak, a symbol; that is its function is to express some unconscious idea or trend, its "meaning" lies not in its obvious connotation but in the emotional value attached to it. The dementia praecox patient, having lost his normal sense of reality, regards these symbols as having the same validity as his perceptions of environmental data. An example may make this plainer. A girl suffering from dementia praecox once explained to me that practically everything she saw or heard had two meanings. It had the meaning given to it by others and a symbolical significance as well, the latter being almost always sexual. The second meaning to her was more "real" than the first. For instance, she said, when a waiter poured out coffee from a pot with a long spout he was urinating for her benefit, an exhibitionistic performance. She went on to say that other people around looked on the act merely as serving coffee, but *he* knew and *she* knew that it was really urination.

Now, if our theory of perplexity be sound, the patient in this unhappy state sees just this dichotomy of meaning in his own thoughts and in events going on around him, with this great difference. He had not abandoned his habit of applying the conventional critique of reality, so that the two meanings puzzle him. The girl quoted above felt no sense of confusion; she accepted the double meaning and felt no inconsistency although she saw it. Had her's been a perplexity case, however, she would have been greatly worried by the action of the waiter, which was two inconsistent things at once. When the consecutive thoughts, in free association, of a patient seem to have equivalent meanings for him, although the manifest meaning is changing, he either accepts this unquestioningly and has *ipso facto* dementia praecox, or else he tries to reconcile the irreconcilable and is perplexed. Naturally, before the sense of reality is wholly lost, a patient may suffer from this kind of thinking and be puzzled until such time as the effort to be logical is relaxed. Hence we may find—and often do—the symptom of perplexity appearing in the earlier stages of dementia praecox. The differential diagnosis then rests on an inconsistency of effort—the occasional acceptance of the incompatible; and on the type of ideational content which is expressed. This latter criterion has already been discussed in connection with the differentiation of manic reactions in manic-depressive insanity and in dementia praecox.

The relationship of perplexity to other clinical conditions also deserves comment. We may consider absorbed manic reactions first. We have seen that in some cases an absorbed mania merges over into a perplexity reaction. This transition can now be explained. In discussing the former conditions, evidence was adduced to justify the view that free associational thinking had progressed to a point where the thoughts were no longer incorporated in appropriate words but in images of symbolic meaning. This is the kind of thinking in dreams and between it and normal mentation there is a wide gap. If a patient thinking in this way should make an effort to put his thoughts into words he has to leap this gap and take his ideas with him. This is a hard task; so soon as he begins to think in words, the images begin to slip from his grasp. He is left with certain verbal formulations that have only a symbolic relationship to the original ideas, although the *feeling* of the latter persists. Hence his verbalized thoughts have an obvious meaning but feel as if they meant something else. Hence perplexity, similarly determined, may appear in the transition from dreaming to waking thought.

Apart from the presence of a feeling of mental confusion, perplexity cases differ from absorbed manias in that the former maintain a fair or perfect orientation. This bespeaks contact with the environment—a *sine qua non* of perplexity. The manic patient abandons himself to the flux of his thoughts and lives in this imaginary environment. If, in such a condition, an effort is made to re-establish contact with the world around, that is a move towards recovery. The patient who has been absorbed and becomes perplexed is therefore beginning to get well. This enables us to understand, as well, why perplexity reactions tend to have a short duration. They are compromises between conflicting tendencies, adaptation to a real world and withdrawal to a life of fantasy. Such a compromise is unstable; one tendency or the other gains the upperhand; there is recovery or a change to another type of manic depressive reaction.

Mention has already been made of the stupor or anxiety episodes that may occur in the course of a perplexity psychosis, when the ideational content tends to appear in the form of death or injury. Further comment on these developments is unnecessary. Of greater theoretic interest is the occurrence of depression. A state of perplexity is not a happy one, so this reaction is apt to be accompanied with despondency. But a more specific relationship exists. Free associations tend to reach a goal in psychological infantilism. As we have seen, crude infantile formulations appear in dementia praecox, but their emergence in manic-depressive insanity is prevented by inhibition—repression. Hence, as the flux of thought in perplexity states tends in this direction, we are apt to see blocking as a frequent symptom ; and each example of blocking is a miniature depression.

But perplexity does not occur in functional psychoses alone. It is a frequent accompaniment of organic delirium. Here we get normal thinking interrupted not by pressure from the unconscious but as a result of the disintegration of the higher mental functions associated with consciousness, thus liberating the more primitive forms of thinking. In delirium free associations engross the attention of the patient and, moreover, these associations are extremely apt to assume the form of hallucinations, that is, of images mainly visual and auditory. If the deliriant tries to maintain contact with the environment, perplexity results. I remember well a delirium from which I suffered in a prolonged attack of typhoid fever at the age of ten. Few of the hallucinatory or delusional experiences through which I passed were in the slightest degree unpleasant in themselves, in fact, some of them were a re-enactment of quite pleasant experiences. Yet the whole business was distressing, because the nurse, the doctor and members of the family seemed to insist on being other people as well as themselves. Even furniture seemed to participate in this mazing play. I spent weeks in a wearied, futile effort to solve these problems. Then the effort itself became the subject of delirium, when I sought in vain to find a needle in a haystack, and even asked my nurse to help me find it. This presentation of a psychological difficulty in dramatized, symbolic form is quite common in delirium.

Another condition in which perplexity appears is in the psychosis accompanying Basedow's (Grave's) disease. Although psychiatrists do not describe it in their text books, perplexity is quite a common symptom in this condition. Bonhoeffer[1], however, does speak of dreams intruding themselves on waking consciousness and producing disorientation. The determining factors of perplexity are present in Basedow's disease. There is a lowering of normal critique, thanks to the toxic interference with the higher mental functions ; while, at the same time, the general facilitation of all reactions of the nervous system characteristic of hyperthyroidism produces an abnormal activity of thought. These are just the factors which would produce thinking of the free associational type, and, until such time as the toxic state is severe enough to cause disorientation, perplexity occurs.

[1] *Die Symptomatischen Psychosen*, Deuticke, Leipzig, 1910, page 115,

CHAPTER XLIII

" DÉJÀ VU "

THE phenomena of perplexity states and of what is called " *déjà vu* " illuminate each other reciprocally. The latter is a peculiar experience occurring in many normal people—one writer claims in 30 per cent. of adults. It is still more frequent among children and adolescents. Some actual perception, usually visual or auditory, is suddenly felt to have been experienced before, although its previous occurrence cannot be explicitly remembered. The affective accompaniment is its most distinctive characteristic, thus differentiating it from the normal recognition of the familiar, or from the ordinary confabulated memories of the insane. The subject strives to recall the earlier incident, cannot do so, and feels particularly and unpleasantly at sea. This painful and tantalizing emotional state may so far engross the attention that the perception which has occasioned it, may pass out of mind leaving only the affective state behind. Many terms have been applied to this phenomenon. Kraepelin called it paramnesia, while French writers have employed such labels as *fausse reconnaissance, déjà acoute, déjà éprouvé, déjà raconté,* and so on.

Occurring as it does with highly intelligent people, it has been the occasion for much speculation, one of the earliest to discuss it being Pythagoras. In it St. Augustine saw the origin for the belief in reincarnation. The earlier speculators found here proof of a previous existence. In modern days some " scientific " explanations have had no more justification, as, for example, the hypothesis that the two halves of the brain do not act simultaneously, thus " doubling " a perception. A great deal has been written on the subject by psychologists in the last thirty-years, the most important contributors being Leroy, Grasset, Freud, Dugas, Janet, Bergson and Havelock Ellis. The last brings together the essential contributions up to 1911[1]. This is not the place for any exhaustive discussion of this problem, and I must content myself with mere mention of the two types of solution offered.

Most of the French psychologists have sought an explanation in some disorder of attention, some disturbance of apperception

The World of Dreams, 1911.

at the moment that *déjà vu* is experienced. Havelock Ellis being the most recent exponent of such a view, we may regard his hypothesis as typical and criticize it. He claims that a paramnesia exists in the hypnogogic (or hypnopompic) period between dreaming and full wakefulness, because there may be at this time a persisting belief in the reality of the remembered dream images. This, he says, is a species of illusion. In an ordinary illusion one kind of external impression is mistaken for an external impression of another kind. In the hypnagogic paramnesia there is a false belief, in that a centrally excited image of one order (dream) is mistaken for a centrally excited image of another order (memory). He then adduces evidence to show that *déjà vu* is apt to appear in conditions of fatigue, under the influence of mild general anaesthesia, in toxic states and so on. Then, assuming such an abnormal background always to exist, he concludes : " It seems as if externally aroused sensations in such cases are received by the exhausted cortical centres in so blurred a form that an illusion takes place, and they are mistaken for internally excited sensations, for memories."

Several criticisms may be directed against such a hypothesis. The most serious one is that it is questionable whether he is speaking of true *déjà vu* at all. As Grasset[1] has pointed out (following other authors) an essential feature of this peculiar mental state is the painful affect which accompanies it. From Havelock Ellis's description one cannot see that there is any such unpleasant emotional reaction in his " hypnagogic paramnesia ". He seems rather to be writing of the usual hazy grasp of reality that exists in the dozing state. He does not mention any unsuccessful effort to discriminate between the dream images and memories such as is a *sine qua non* for true *déjà vu*. It is true that this phenomenon may occur before one is fully awake, but it is not a regular event, far from it. Similarly, his diurnal *déjà vu* seems to be merely false recognition, which often occurs without exciting discomfort ; in fact, it is usually unaccompanied by any emotional reaction whatever. What characterizes real *déjà vu* is that there is first a recognition of " having been there before " and then a compulsive and *unsuccessful* effort to resuscitate the details and setting of the original experience. It is the failure to do this, together with the internal urge to keep at the problem, which produces the unpleasant effect.

Secondly, Havelock Ellis is right enough in saying that the phenomenon is apt to occur in fatigue or toxic states, but, if his hypothesis is to hold, cerebral embarrassment should be demonstrable in all cases. Unfortunately, for this view, those who have studied the matter statistically claim that, although an

[1] Grasset, " La Sensation de ' déjà vu' ", *Journal de Psychologie, norm. et path.*, Tome I, 1904.

extra-psychic factor is usual, there are a number of instances recorded when it may be fully excluded. There is, however, a third objection which eliminates the necessity of considering this last argument. He says that the actual sensations [does he not mean perceptions ?] are received in a blurred condition by the exhausted brain. Now, it is characteristic of *déjà vu* that attention is riveted on that which seems to have been experienced before, each detail stands out sharply, and each detail, as it is remarked, seems to add to the feeling of familiarity.

It must not be thought that this hypothesis is in any sense identical with or modelled on earlier ones of the French psychologists. (A digest of these may be found in Havelock Ellis's book). It has merely been selected for certain criticisms because it is the latest known to me and because it is similar to all the others in seeking the explanation in some failure to grasp the immediate stimulus in the normal manner. Similar criticisms may be made of all such hypotheses for the simple reason that the facts do not seem to bear out the basic assumption. There never is a failure to understand the actual situation ; it is the intrusion of some other influence which produces the peculiar reaction we are discussing.

Grasset was the first to offer anything like an adequate explanation. He derived the unpleasant affect from the *unsuccessful* effort of the subject to recall what the earlier experience was, to correct the contradiction of recognizing something as familiar although the first experience of it cannot be recalled. Whence comes this intrusive element that is really not remembered but only felt ? Grasset then made use of the concept of the unconscious as it had been elaborated by Janet. He said the explanation lay in the *unconscious* existence of a memory. This memory might be of something which actually happened, identical with the current, real experience, or it might be of a similar dreamed experience. Such a hypothesis seems much more adequate to account for the phenomena. If the real experience coincides with the image in one's mind of an earlier experience, it will be recognized as familiar although the memory of the first experience cannot be recovered (being unconscious) but only appears as a feeling. This view fails, however, to explain the persistent and compulsive intrusion of the unconscious memory, that makes one strive to resuscitate the setting of the unconscious experience. This lack is met by psycho-analytic investigations, which also show that the unconscious element may (and usually does) only resemble the actual event. Actual identity between the two sets of images is not necessary and is, in fact, rare.

Independently of Grasset, although three years later, Freud[1] explained a case of *déjà vu* in one of his patients as due to a recog-

---

[1] *Psychopathologie des Altagslebens*, Zweite Auflage, 1907.

nition in a new environment of an element common both to this environment and to an unconscious fantasy. Briefly, the situation was this. His patient at the age of 12 had had an unconscious fantasy (and therefore " wish ") that her brother, who was ill, should die. He recovered, but a few months later she visited a girl friend, whose brother was very ill. On coming to the house every detail seemed tantalizingly familiar, so much so that the patient remembered the experience clearly when analysed sixteen years later. In this instance only one detail in a complex experience was identical with the unconscious fantasy—the illness of a brother. But the activity of this unconscious complex spread the feeling of identity over every room in the house. In other words, wherever she was she had a feeling of familiarity, and this was attached to each new detail of the really strange environment. An excellent example of displacement of affect ! In the third edition of this book (1910) Freud[1] adds to the discussion a footnote, in which he reports the experience of Ferenczi. The latter found *déjà vu* occasioned not merely by day dreams but by the unconscious activity of the memory of true dreams as well.

In 1913 Pfister published an excellent case with an overdetermined unconscious causation. A girl of 14, pregnant, visited a gynecological clinic and was seized with the feeling of *déjà vu*, which she knew was unreasonable but which nevertheless persisted. Her free associations led from the woman's clinic to another she had visited two years before and where she had feared she might be infected by a man who was swollen (as she was when pregnant). Further associations related the afflicted man to the one who was responsible for her pregnancy. The similarity of the two experiences lay not in the similarity of the two clinics but in the unconscious identity of the ideas of infection and pregnancy. That is, in the first experience, the conscious fear of infection was probably represented by an unconscious idea of impregnation. When she finds herself in a clinic and pregnant, a situation, which had previously existed only in the unconscious, is duplicated. But the analysis went further. When asked when the *déjà vu* had first appeared she recalled that it was when she sat on a bench. Association from this led to a bench she sat on when five years old and when she indulged in a day dream of marriage. The erotic idea therefore appeared as a day dream when five, as a fear when twelve, and produced the feeling of *déjà vu* at the age of fourteen.

In 1914 Freud[2] continued his discussion of this interesting problem, drawing attention to a particular form of false recognition that occurs during the course of psycho-analytic treatment. The patient, in the course of free association, mentions some incident

---

[1] *Die Psychoanalytische Methode,* translated by Payne, Moffat, Yard & Co., New York, 1917.
[2] " Ueber *fausse reconnaissance (déjà raconté)* während der psychoanalytischen Arbeit," *Internal. Zeitschr. f. Aerztliche Psychoanalyse,* II, 1914.

or fancy of the past and then adds, " But I've told you that before."
Since the communication is often of crucial importance in the
analysis, the physician feels justified in believing that the material
is really new, but often fails to convince the patient of this. Freud
in this article explains the basis of the false memory in one instance.
The patient told of having had the delusion as a child that he had
cut off one of his fingers, but insisted at once that he had divulged
this before. On investigation it was found that what he had previously spoken of was getting a knife as a present. The latter
turned out to be a " Deckerinnerung ", that is a memory of a
trivial circumstance remembered since early childhood, because
there lay behind it, unconsciously, an emotionally important idea
(in this case of mutilation and, eventually, castration). Freud
therefore adds to the list of unconscious memories, which may
excite a false sense of familiarity, the significant incident (or fantasy)
which is represented in consciousness by a substituted memory.
The list would then be : day dreams, night dreams and fears or
" wishes " (Pfister), which, operating unconsciously, produce
déjà vu when an actual experience bears some similarity to the
unconscious element. To these may be added : an original unconscious thought which, when it appears in consciousness, seems
to have been recited before, because its substituted memory has
already been retailed. It should be pointed out that the particular
form of *déjà raconté* discussed by Freud may not really be classifiable
with *déjà vu* in the proper sense of the term because the unpleasant
affect is lacking. The patient has a calm conviction that he has
told his secret before and feels no compulsion to recall the occasion
unless he be convinced by the analyst that he has made a mis-
statement. The phenomenon is much more a simple false
recognition. Nevertheless, there seems no reason to exclude
" Deckerinnerungen " from the list because one can see how their
analysis might easily lead to the emotionalized form of false
recognition.

How essential the affective element is in the formation of true
déjà vu appears in the following example—a personal experience.
On getting out of bed one morning I caught sight of my walking
stick, hanging on a bookcase across the room. At once, I began
to say to myself, " I have seen that stick before. I have seen it
hanging there. When did I see it there ? " etc. The ridiculousness
of these speculations was immediately apparent, because I knew
that I *always* hung my stick in that place and, of course, I had
seen it precisely there a hundred times. Nevertheless, the peculiar
feeling of *déjà vu* persisted. Then I tried to solve the problem by
associating freely from " walking stick ". Almost at once there
came to mind memory of a complicated dream of the night before,
several incidents of which had centred around the stick. Immediately the *déjà vu* disappeared. There are two important
conclusions to be drawn from this example. The peculiar emotional

reaction may be entirely independent of the question as to whether the memory of previous experience is accurate or inaccurate. In this case the correctness of the recognition was not open to doubt. *Déjà vu* is really the form which recognition of something unconscious assumes, when the thought itself cannot appear as such, because it remains unconscious and is not available for conscious inspection. The second deduction is that the unconscious thought is active before the *déjà vu* is precipitated by some externally derived stimulus.

A moment's consideration would show that this last claim could hardly be gainsaid on *a prioristic* grounds. The ideas represented in the unconscious are legion ; moreover they are constructed from experiences that are, roughly, identical with the data of present conscious experience. We see the same kind of people and animals, eat the same food and so on. In other words, the building blocks out of which unconscious and conscious thoughts are constructed are identical. Consequently it is probable that we rarely receive a conscious external impression that is not like some unconscious memory. If this resemblance were all that was necessary to produce *déjà vu*, we should be experiencing it constantly. A normal man may have had—and who has not ?—some terrifying experience as a child with a dog or horse, the memory of which has survived in the unconscious. Yet every time, as an adult, that he sees a dog or horse he does not feel fear or *déjà vu*. Before the presentation of some common object can excite such a reaction, something must have happened to activate the potentialities of the latent unconscious memory. In other words, it must have become co-conscious.

A wealth of psycho-analytic experience—as well as innumerable experiments with word-association tests where mediate associations occur—has shown that free associations may proceed without the awareness of the subject. In fact, where any consciously received impression awakens a reaction from the unconscious, it seems that this must be the mechanism of activization. It has been demonstrated time and again that these extraconscious associations can take place with extreme speed.

With this in mind, we are in a position at last to formulate the probable course of events when *déjà vu* takes place.

Every sensory impression calls up instantaneously and automatically a host of associations. In fact this is the way in which we understand the environment ; the immediate stimulus is correlated with similar ones of the past, eliciting an habitual reaction appropriate to such stimuli. These associations tend to extend to truly unconscious as well as fore-conscious memories. If such associations reach a goal in a co-conscious image that is similar to the original perception, the co-conscious image is further activated and tends to become conscious. But repression tends to keep it beyond the range of awareness. This is the general situation in which data of conscious experience take on values derived from the unconscious[1]. The energy of the activated co-conscious idea is transferred to the conscious image ; the latter becomes supernaturally real and vivid, amazingly familiar. The conscious image is now performing two functions : it is a normal perception, and it is at the same time a symbol-like representation of something that is unconscious. Hence its peculiar doubling. The active co-conscious idea appears in consciousness directly only as an affect, as a feeling of familiarity, but this latter is rationalized in the belief that an experience is being re-lived. So long as the emotional reaction persists, the rationalization continues. Hence every detail of the actual experience seems to duplicate some earlier one. This in turn only increases the conviction of the subject that he is re-living an incident of the past ; but it brings him no nearer to the resuscitation of the memory of the alleged previous experience, so his painful mystification is increased. If one were to view the whole story teleologically, one would say that by making the actual experience a symbolic representation, the unconscious has succeeded in expressing itself and at the same time in distracting attention away from the unconscious image by producing a compulsive preoccupation with the details of the environment.

This discussion of *déjà vu* may seem a tedious irrelevance to our main problem, but its psychology is closely related to that of the clinical group we have been studying and we shall later on see that it has an important bearing on our final theoretic conclusions as to the mechanisms of emotions. Psychiatrists are apt to mention this phenomenon as occuring " sometimes " in the course of psychoses, specifying only epilepsy.[2] For instance, Kraepelin says, " This disturbance is observed here and there in pathological conditions, particularly among epileptics in association with their attacks ". No one, so far as I know, has noted it in manic depressive insanity, yet many perplexed patients complain of just this kind of familiarity in the environment which they cannot account for. For instance, Bridget B., in her first attack said, " All my people are imitated here ; there is not a scrap of clothing I ever had which there is not a sample of . . . " Henry R. somewhat similarly complained that everything in the hospital reminded him of things at home.

A pretty example of false familiarity appeared in the incubation period of the manic psychosis of Ruth B. (Case 18). Regression had begun, stimulated in part by the reading of a novel the action of which paralleled many of her own experiences. It ended with the heroine going off on a journey. The patient had already so far identified herself with the heroine as to imagine that she too was going to travel. Then her sister took her to stay with a friend in

---

[1] As, for example, the attachment of fear to a harmless object, i.e., a phobia. The perception of an innocuous object activates a co-conscious image of something that is dangerous.

[2] Hughlings Jackson was the first to note *déjà vu* in epilepsy : *On a particular Variety of Epilepsy, &c.* Brain, 1889, vol. XI, p. 179.

the country. To quote from Chapter 20 : " On the train marked symptoms appeared. She felt as if she were walking in a dream, everything looked queer and funny, old-fashioned, yet familiar. From then on till her recovery her ideas came thick and fast." First they were day dreams, then she began to misidentify people. The latter is interesting. The same mental process which produced the feeling of familiarity went on developing until false identification appeared.

It must be admitted, of course, that such statements do not represent accurate descriptions of *déjà vu* in the narrow sense. The analogy lies more in the perplexity psychosis as a whole. The patient is perturbed by just that kind of doubling in meaning of the environment, which we have seen to be essential to *déjà vu*. In the psychosis the feeling of there being a second meaning to things, which cannot be understood, seems to be paralleled in *déjà vu*, by the unsuccessful search for the earlier experience which seems to be duplicated in the present one. The pathological state seems, then, to be an extension of what appears in miniature in the normal person's paramnesia. Theoretically the important point to realize is that psychoanalysts have elaborated an hypothesis to account for *déjà vu*, which is identical, essentially, with what we have found, by direct observation of his mental processes, to be the abnormality of the perplexed patient. Hypothesis is less necessary in the latter instance because we can see the free associational thinking in progress, we can see how the thoughts of internal origin gained a prominence which we are forced to assume for the unconscious train of associations in *déjà vu*.

CHAPTER XLIV

THE AFFECT IN PERPLEXITY

THE last problem with which we are concerned is the *raison d'être* of the peculiar stress which seems to be associated with perplexity—the distress which separates it off from the purely intellectual reaction of objective confusion, such as is seen in clouding of consciousness. The most popular current view as to emotions is that they are somehow connected with instincts. Our problem is, what instinct is at work? Is there any instinct for normal clear thinking?

The following case, which we shall present very briefly, may suggest an answer to our question. The patient began his psychosis with a reaction essentially that of involution melancholia. Then with improvement in orientation, perplexity appeared and what had been fear for his life seemed to change into a distress about his name, about his identity.

CASE 70. *George H.* Age 44, Married salesman. Admitted, April 28th, 1903.

F.H. The patient's father was said to be rather worthless, otherwise enquiries elicited no information of hereditary taint.

P.H. A meagre history stated that the patient had been normal in disposition, although suffering from heart disease for some years. There was some question as to whether there had been previous mental attacks, for the patient himself said he had been depressed before, although never forced to cease working.

The Psychosis. Two months before admission he lost some money, became depressed and slept poorly. For three weeks he had not been working, and was reduced to wringing his hands, claiming that his ruin was complete.

On admission he was found to have signs of somatic arteriosclerosis with enlargement of the heart to the left. He ate poorly, and was very restless, wringing his hands, sighing and moaning over and over, " Oh, my poor wife ! " He claimed that she was in the hospital, for he heard her voice. He also spoke of being scared of everything, but could not, or would not, say what terrified him specifically. He was well oriented.

Within four days his agitation had much increased, unstable delusions had appeared, and his orientation was grossly defective. He was very restless, often showed fear and spoke only between moans. He said he had signed papers, which would sign away the whole United States ; when some people walked out of the building, he vowed he had opened all the asylums in the country ; some blood on his hands showed that he had killed his wife ; she was downstairs, chopped up into pieces. A man in the room was going to kill him, or the register was an instrument for his destruction. Yet when interviewed, he admitted that these ideas were all nonsense, although he could not get them out of his head.

This state lasted for a week or two, after which his condition improved, but soon there was a relapse into the state which interests us now. His

433

agitation was intense, with continuous, aimless fumbling of his hands ; he was fearful.   Now, however, he was well oriented, and, with this, perplexed. His ideas still contained an element of danger to his life, but most of his jerky statements referred to perplexity about his ideas and, particularly, about his name and identity.   The following remarks were typical :
    " This [sigh] . . . this [sigh] . . . this [sigh] . . . Harry W. . . . its . . . something terrible."   He had just seen Harry W. enter the ward.   (What ?) " This W. business . . . I don't know what it will all mean . . . this Harry W. will tear me all to pieces . . . I don't know what it is . . . It may be a name I picked up myself, and, if I have, I have, killed myself, and that's where it comes in ; and I have killed myself [with an air of resignation]. I've mixed that up with some other name I've mentioned . . . I've done a terrible thing, when I said that . . . about that Harry W. business.   I don't know as it's . . . anything may be under an assumed name . . . and, if it is, I may be a ruined man."   Or, again, " I'm not George H.   I ought to be him, but I've taken these names along when I've seen them in the yard . . . They've been in my mind . . . I'm in the soup ".   (Why ?)   " I've thought of such ones and called them such names.   I've made myself as G. . . . I've been here as George H., and have a home in X. . . . Not I but George H. has a home in X. as George H."   (Why are you not George H. ?)   " I've made myself a different one.   I'm all mixed up.   I'm weak."
    As the weeks went on his condition became worse.   He spent all his time sitting, bent forward, rocking in his chair, moaning and whispering in broken sentences, " It's all a mistake, I'm all mixed up.   I am not Mr. H.   All gone now ".   Such statements were repeated over and over ; in fact, instead of answering questions, he would simply repeat these plaints.   He had to be tube fed.
    Two and a half months after admission he was transferred to another hospital, and there died (tube-feeding accident), three days after arrival. An autopsy failed to reveal any abnormalities in his brain.

One would, of course, have liked to follow this case further before making a positive diagnosis.   The repetitious, monotonous complaints of his last days would make one guarded as to the prognosis. Yet, from a psychological standpoint, the case is important.   A psychosis developed in which great distress, and an element of fear, were centred around subjective perplexity and a delusion of lost identity.

This may give us a hint as to the origin or basis of the affective element in perplexity.   In civilized adults the ideas are closely allied of life, in the biological sense of a living organism, and of maintained consciousness of personal identity.   We are interested in preserving our psychic existence, just as we are in keeping our bodies from mortal harm.   The former, in fact, is apt to be a matter of greater concern than the latter—consciously at least.   Instinctively, of course (when we behave as animals do) we react more violently to a threat against physical dissolution than we do against the thought of mental annihilation.   It is only when we indulge in abstract speculations that we hold *psyche* to be superior to *soma*.

In our emotional life it seems as if mental existence and stability represent organic viability in a dilute and quasi-symbolic way.   The instinct of self-preservation operates directly and violently when the body is threatened, but we have transferred some of this tendency to the maintenance of a mental *status quo*.   This is probably the instinctive basis of our distress at the thought of a loss or change of personality, which is represented as well in any disorder of conscious mental function. The religious person may feel terror for the loss of his soul ; the epileptic fears a loss of consciousness ; the insomniac fights restlessly against sleep[1] ; the deliriant or perplexed patient is distressed by loss of control over his thoughts—all these probably are but different and progressively more dilute reactions of self preservation. In *déjà vu* we suffer from the same apprehension : the prime function of consciousness—control of one's thoughts — has failed ; we feel we must make every effort to localize the elusive original experience, because, if we fail, it means that we are no longer captains of our souls. In fact, this emotion is probably to be identified in a much commoner phenomenon, a lapse of memory for some word or name that is familiar and ought to be recalled instantly. The fuss we can get ourselves into over such a failure, is often ridiculously disproportionate to the practical importance of having the memory available. But it stands for integrity of our mental processes as a whole and hence we are disturbed.

---

[1] *Vide supra*, the discussion of insomnia in connection with Involution Melancholia, chapter XVIII.

PART IX

PSYCHIATRIC
CONCLUSIONS

CHAPTER XLV

TREATMENT

THE object of the clinical researches which are reported in
this book, was to gather data from which deductions might
be drawn as to mental mechanisms resulting in the symptoms of manic-depressive insanity. A complete study of
symptoms would involve, of course, an understanding of the way
in which they subsided, as well as the method of their growth, but
it was deliberately neglected. Therapeutic imvestigations and
experiments to be anything more than random gropings must be
based on hypotheses, which, in turn, are developed logically from a
theory of the conditions to be remedied. Our attention was therefore directed solely to the problems of psychogenesis. If symptoms
be understood, it is conceivable that the disease which they manifest
may also be grasped, and it is only on knowledge of a disease as a
whole that rational therapy can be based.

On the other hand it was inevitable that striking variations in
the direction of recovery should have been noted, as well as any
changes in external situation, which was coincident with improvement or cessation of the psychotic reaction. These are, perhaps,
worthy of record. At the same time, since some general theory of
the disease as a whole has been arrived at, the bearing of this on
therapeutic experiment should be stated. Frankly, however, this
chapter is inserted more to round out the account of manic-depressive
insanity in the conventional way, than to liberate opinions coloured
with that conviction which forces publication. The following
conclusions are drawn from scattered observations and are tentative
in the extreme.

437

The only generalization we arrived at is a negative one. Any special psychological technique, such as suggestion or psycho-analysis, is of no value whatever, except in certain special conditions.

The original view as to the nature of psycho-analytic cure was that, when unconscious strivings reached expression in consciousness, they were shorn of their pathogenic power. The latter depended on their gaining indirect and symbolic expression in symptoms. Experience with the psychoses, however, has demonstrated this view to be untenable. In dementia praecox, for example, infantile ideas reach expression spontaneously and in no other condition is "analysis" so easy. A few free associations may produce an avalanche of the ordinarily tabooed thoughts. This does not improve the patient's condition; if anything, it makes it worse. The reason for this is soon obvious. Repression is weak, or at least relatively weak, when compared with the pressure exerted from the direction of the unconscious. The normal functions of consciousness are consequently disturbed by this irruption of unconscious material. An important function of consciousness is the distinction between fact and fancy. When a psychoneurotic is analysed, the buried "wishes" which are exhumed are recognised as fantastic, consciousness is able to estimate their importance. But, when unconscious elements appear as delusions, consciousness has, *ipso facto*, lost this discrimination. Consequently, the exorcizing of more ideas from this underworld merely tends to enlarge the list of false beliefs. When they come they are accepted as facts. The same principle, although to a lesser degree, seems to hold in manic depressive insanity. When judgment is already weak or absent, psycho-analytic procedure seems to be fruitless or pernicious.

Suggestion seems to rest on somewhat similar mechanisms. It consists in a re-orientation of consciousness towards all cognitive material, no matter whether that have its origin in the outer world or be endopsychic. Consciousness must, therefore, be relatively intact, if suggestion is to relieve symptoms, and, as it is disturbed in manic depressive insanity we should not expect relief from this source[1].

There is one exception to this generalization. In depression the content of consciousness is often normal except for the pathological affect. Interestingly enough this seems to be the one condition in which special psychological technique seems ever to be effective. This group will shortly be discussed.

These conclusions do not extend, of course, to the application of special psychological measures in prophyllaxis. The consciousness of a manic depressive patient, who has recovered, is in no wise different from that of a normal man, so long as no psychotic manifestations are evident. His later abnormality is therefore capable of modification, when his attack is over—theoretically at least.

[1] I have discussed the problems of psychoanalytic and suggestion therapy more extensively in *Problems in Dynamic Psychology*, Part II.

Practically, however, difficulties arise. These are three in number and may be discussed separately.

The first is the question of insight. Hospital physicians are accustomed to complete the history of a manic-depressive attack with the statement that the patient has recovered with insight. Yet this is often a superficial judgment or the careless acceptance of the patient's statement. As a matter of fact, when one begins to search more closely, it is surprising to find how flimsy the alleged insight may be[1].

With perfect insight there is recognition of the abnormality through which the patient has passed. Very often he says, " I have been crazy " and means no more than that he finds himself in what is without a doubt a hospital for crazy people and thinks he must therefore have been considered insane by those who put him there. When such a patient is then asked (as the physician frequently neglects to do), " What do you think about X now ? " he is apt to say, " I know he is my enemy ". The false idea may still persist although it has lost its insistence ; it is no longer in the centre of the patient's attention. Or, if he say that X is his friend, he may deny that he ever thought otherwise. Mary S. is a case in point. She not only failed to recognize, after cessation of symptoms, sayings of hers read to her from the record, but even went so far as to insist that mistakes must have been made—*she* could never have said such things. A patient who recovers with this degress of repression of his psychotic thoughts is a poor subject for analytic treatment. Although he may recognize clearly that he has, and is likely to have, many terms of hospital residence, each attack seems like some visitation of external influence. Lacking any memory of actual abnormalities, the psychosis cannot be demonstrated to him to be a product of his abnormality ; he cannot feel that his actions or thoughts are being discussed, they seem to belong to somebody else. Perfect insight is therefore a requisite for analytic treatment.

The second difficulty has to do with the make-up of the manic-depressive patient. As we have seen time and again, it is an individual who is already abnormal that breaks down. Prognosis, with psychological treatment, depends on two variable factors— the degree of latent and constitutional abnormality and the skill of the therapist. Comparing as groups the psychoneurotics, manic-depressive patients and dementia praecox subjects, there is an increasing degree of maladaptability observed. The mental health of the individual depends on his adaptation to the environment in which he is placed. A poorly adaptable person can only remain normal in an environment that is artificially adjusted to his needs. Analytic treatment frequently enables the psychoneurotic to adjust himself to the problems which confront him in everyday life ; this

---

[1] We gained the impression that defective insight was commonest among cases with frequently recurrent attacks, but never investigated the problem sufficiently to gather statistics in confirmation of the impression.

is possible less often with manic-depressive subjects, while those who suffer from dementia praecox are practically never capable of maintaining their equilibrium in any but an artificial environment. This is the reason why in every institution there are inmates to be discovered who seem to be sane. Repeated experiment has shown that serious symptoms arise whenever these unfortunates are permitted to return to their families.

The third difficulty has to do with external factors. In actual practice the hospital patient is found to have real problems. He may suffer from the *res augustae domi*, that may or may not be the product of his inefficiency. He may never have been able to attain to a business or professional position that suits his taste, and therefore feels that he has a real grievance. Most important of all, he is often unhappy in his domestic life. This may be the result of mischance, but more often it is part of his unhappy fate. Like not only likes like, but like breeds like. Hence the abnormal, " neurotic" person is frequently either living with parents or siblings that are also " neurotic ", or has married a wife who also has her peculiarities. One exclaims to oneself so often, when trying to help some psychotic man to get and stay on his feet, " If only his wife would give him half a chance ! "

A number of these difficulties are observable in the record of William A. W., a hypomaniac patient with recurrent attacks, in whose case some therapeutic experiments were made. It will be recalled that he had many recurrent attacks, each one inaugurated by his leaving the service of others to go into business for himself. As time went on it seemed more and more probable that his lust for independence and affluence was an expression of an early ambition to make a fortune for his mother. Although she had died, successors had been found in the persons of his two daughters, one married and the other a little child. This is a normal enough kind of development, or would have been, had he been capable of transferring his idealization from his mother to his wife. Unfortunately this was beyond him, partly, perhaps, because of the efficient selfishness of the woman he had chosen for his mate. The result of going into business for himself was therefore to activate his Oedipus complex, and this, demanding directer outlet, involved antagonism to his wife. So, when he attempted to build up a new sublimation, he destroyed an old, essential, one. It seemed reasonably certain that this was the mechanism of his psychosis.

His intelligence made the hope justifiable that such a simple mechanism could be understood and his knowledge of it enable him to order his life more sanely. The first difficulty encountered was his lack of insight. When he had become " normal " efforts were made day by day to get him to realize the irrationality of his previous behaviour and boasts. They were unavailing until his wife visited him one day and treated him kindly. Apparently this stirred up his desire to be at home again and may have been the only reason he had for listening docilely to our words. At any rate he learned to say his " peccavi " with some show of sincerity. But about this time his wife informed him of her decision to leave him for ever ; she had sold the furniture and put their little daughter in an orphanage. This news threw him into a depression for some weeks, but, at the end of it, he professed a willingness to make a new start. The mechanism of his symptoms was explained to him patiently ; he listened as patiently and with apparent sympathy. He agreed to use some money that was advanced to him to start into business, to make no effort to see his wife or daughter, and to report to his physicians every day. As soon as he left the hospital he broke each one of these promises. He took his daughter out of the orphanage, spent his money and time on her and tried to recover the furniture by litigation. In five days he was back in the hospital with querulous manic symptoms.

In retrospect it was not difficult to see the two main factors responsible for this *débâcle*. The more important was his inherent weakness of character. It was betrayed in his life-long failure to build up any one workable sublimation, and in his moral lapse when he was given a reasonable chance to do so. But there are many folk, no stronger, who seem to drift through life without falling victims to either criminal or psychotic tendencies. These more fortunate ones have stronger people to support them. And this is where the second factor appears. His wife, who has always made his home unlovely, betrayed him in an emergency that was the turning point in his life. What could any psychological insight do in the face of these difficulties ? It is merely a weapon, and to wield it one must have courage and strength.[1] As a matter of fact it is doubtful whether he ever gave more than verbal assent to the analysis of his symptoms.

The object of special psychological techniques is to modify abnormal thinking by frontal attack. Another method of combatting the evil is to change the environment of the patient. If maladaptive trains of thought have been produced in any given situation, it is surely unwise to leave the victim exposed to the same stimuli (unless one can teach him psychologically to neglect these stimuli or to react to them normally). As it may require nothing short of divination to discover the specific elements in any environment that are causing the mischief, the easiest way to meet the problem is to transfer the sufferer to a special institution. It is often thought that " custodial treatment " simply means proper medical nursing and the application of such restraint as is necessary to prevent self-injury and avoid danger to others. As a matter of fact, these factors, although essential, are not the only ones involved.

[1] This is a principle of wide reference in therapeutics. If a man have courage he may learn to triumph over almost any mental abnormality, with the aid of psychological knowledge. Without it, his only hope lies in his environment being altered to suit his weakness.

In hospital, entirely apart from what he may get in the way of expert psychopathological handling, the patient enjoys a change in environmental influence that is highly beneficial. These changes may be introduced into an environment that is not institutional, but they are most easily applied intramurally and so only the principles seen operating in this highly artificial life need be discussed.

The first of these is absence of relatives. If any one observation in these clinical studies stands out above the rest, it is the universality with which manic-depressive patients develope false attitudes and beliefs concerning their relatives. Moreover these distortions are seen to be intimately associated with the whole delusional system. If a tendency exists towards the production of a perverse train of thought, it ought to be obvious that abnormality would be fostered by the continued presence of that stimulus. Nevertheless relatives are continually fearing the effects of removal of patients from their care, apprehending "loneliness" in a person separated from those who love him and whom he loves. Moreover, patients themselves, when sufficiently rational to talk of such matters, will protest that they could never stand this isolation, nor the horror of being with crazy people. Such arguments are based on the assumption that the subject is normal. But he is not, and is even exhibiting his abnormality most strikingly in such connections. The truth is that he is wrapped up in himself and cares too little for others either to miss them or to be horrified by their actions. A woman, for instance, whose child or husband dies, while she is in a psychotic state, almost always shows little evidence of being affected by this loss.

In so far as the patient's interest is turned on himself the nature of his environment is, psychologically, a matter of indifference. It is when response is made to external situations that his surroundings are important. If relatives are the excitants, maladaptive trains of thought are set up and the psychosis is only aggravated. This is well shown in the effect of visitors in any hospital for the insane, ·as every institutional psychiatrist knows. Until recovery is well under way (and, indeed, even then) a visit from relatives is extremely apt to be followed by an accentuation of symptoms. The curve of frequency of excitements in a hospital for the insane rises regularly on days when visitors are allowed. We may quote a paragraph here from a paper on "The Management of Disturbed and Excited Patients"[1]:

"The number of disturbed patients will vary with the frequency of visits by relatives. This cause operates most at the Manhattan State Hospital, where it is not infrequent to receive 1,200 visitors in one day. It is here a matter of common experience that on Sunday and Monday [visiting days are Saturday, Sunday and Monday] the daily average of disturbed patients is much higher than towards the latter part of the week. Moreover, during the recent

[1] Poate, Ernest M., *The State Hospital Quarterly*, vol. II, No. 2, February, 1917, Utica, N.Y., The State Hospital Press.

quarantine of this hospital the number of disturbed patients, of minor accidents and injuries, etc. [and also the consumption of sedative drugs], decreased to an extent which has been the occasion of general remark among the ward physicians."

The second environmental factor is, psychologically, intimately connected with the first. The less one is in contact with reality, the less accurately consciousness is working, the more does intuition play a rôle. In so far as a patient does not respond to his environment, therefore, he tends to be more influenced by the emotional attitude of his attendants than by their overt actions and words. Again, in so far as psychotic behaviour strives for effect, the more successful it is the more it will be persisted in. No one unfamiliar with insanity can remain unmoved by psychotic exhibitions. Try as he will a layman is affected by it. This effect the patient intuits, if he does not wittingly observe it, and it therefore aggravates his symptoms. The mere indifference of *blasé* attendants to absurd complaints and outbursts has a sedative effect, just as indifference may quell a savage dog. Only an institution can furnish this indifference. So, for these two reasons, even a bad institution is often a better environment than his home for a manic-depressive patient.

The two factors so far discussed are negative. The third is positive, is definitely therapeutic, and the extent to which it is present is a measure of the virtue of any institution. I refer to re-education, to occupational therapy. So long as a patient's thoughts are turned in upon his own imaginings, his own condition, he is in an unhealthy state. Normality can only be achieved by a re-direction of his interest to things outside of himself. It is a risky business to excite emotional contact with other people too soon, for human attachments are prone to be woven into the delusional fabric, as we have seen so often in the identification of the doctor or nurse with father or mother. An interest in something inanimate is a safer road to follow ; every road in the end leads to some habitation.

From a psychological standpoint, the direction of occupational therapy requires a knowledge and utilization of two simple principles. The first is that a person who is mentally diseased is, *ipso facto*, unlikely to have spontaneous interests in any activity. Consequently his work or play will not be spontaneously undertaken but must be suggested to him. Nay, it may even have to be forced on him more or less. On the other hand any occupation that remains artificial will never make a bridge over to normal interests. It must be something which represents, and can be allied with, a natural interest. We are prone to assume that all other people have, or ought to have, and, therefore, should be made to have the same interests as ourselves. Every little girl ought to be fond of dolls and every boy of toy guns and fire engines. But the fact is that this often is not the case. A woman, well or ill, is often bored into rebellion by domestic employment or a man outraged by carpentering or gardening. Another problem arises when improvement in a patient's condition has produced more capacity for expression of interest than a simple task affords. It follows, therefore, that, when improvement does not occur or is temporary, the reason is lack of pressure in keeping him at his job, innate aversion for what is offered him in the way of employment, or insufficient facilities in the institution for exciting progressive interest. Under these circumstances any hospital which aims at being more than custodial must have a staff specialized in individual supervision of employment and able to offer varied occupations to its inmates.

These are the general considerations to be borne in mind in the treatment of manic-depressive insanity as a whole. In addition the separate groups should be discussed separately. A few points have emerged from our studies that may have suggestive value.

Only under exceptional circumstances can stuporous paitents be looked after in their homes, were it only for their obvious need of specialized nursing care. This is particularly true of the suicidal cases. When we consider the psychological nature of their disease, it becomes apparent that the treatment of stupor must be different from that of most manic-depressive conditions. Hoch says[1] : " If the stupor reaction be a regression, which is essentially a withdrawal of interest and energy rather than a fixation on a false object, then excitement is desirable and interest must be re-awakened . . . .

" Consequently, although trying to those in charge, persistent attention should be given the patient. Feeding and hygienic measures probably have considerable value in this work. As soon as it is at all possible the patients should be got out of bed and dressed. When up, efforts should be directed towards making them do something, even if it be as simple as pushing a floor polisher. On account of their lack of enthusiasm the stupor cases are often omitted from the list of those given occupation and amusement. Even if they go through the motions of work or play with no sign of interest, such exercises should not be allowed to lapse. Then, too, the environment should be changed when practicable. A patient may improve on being removed to another building.

" Perhaps the most potent stimulus that we have observed is that of family visits. In most manic-depressive psychoses visits of relatives have a bad effect. . . . But the stupor needs excitement, and an habitual emotional interest is more apt to arouse him than an artificial one. As a rule manic-depressive patients have delusional ideas of attitudes in connexion with their nearest of kin, so that contact with them stirs up trouble. The stupor regression, going beneath the level of such attachments, leaves family relationships relatively undisturbed. Hence, while the visit of a husband is likely to produce nothing but vituperation or blows from a manic wife, the

[1] *Benign Stupors*, p. 231, seq.

stuporous woman may greet him affectionately and regain thereby some contact with the world.

" So many cases begin recovery in this manner that it cannot be mere chance. One patient's improvement, for instance, dated definitely from the day a nurse persuaded her to write a letter home. It is striking, too, how quickly a patient, while somewhat dull and slow, will brighten up when allowed to return home. . . . Such experiences make one wonder whether perhaps these alone of all our insane patients would not recover more quickly at home than in hospitals, provided nursing care could be given them."

The treatment of involution melancholia from a psychological standpoint must be a matter of delicate, individual adjustment on account of the differing symptom complexes exhibited in this disease. We find in this group—and even sometimes in the same case—anxiety, hypochondria, perverse conduct, and a tendency towards apathy. Any rule-of-thumb course of treatment could be designed only for combatting one of these. There can, then, be no conventionalized treatment for the disorder as a whole, therapy must be adapted to the special case and, further, modified as the clinical picture changes.

For the hypochondriacal, querulous type there is nothing more useful than interning in a special hospital. In no other manic depressive group does one see such striking results of hospitalization. For instance I recall the case of a hypochondriac who had been tyrannizing over her terrorized household for more than three years. Her family were finally persuaded to the " desperate remedy " of putting her in a hospital for the insane. Within two months she was well enough to go home and in another month had become a placidly efficient mother. The reason for such a change is not far to seek. Hypochondria battens on misplaced sympathy. If sympathy be denied the patient feels that his querulousness is justified ; if sorrow is expressed for his sufferings, the hypochondria is, so to speak, paying dividends. The secret of treatment is that sympathy be given the patient (who *is* suffering) but entirely withheld from the symptoms. In other words, he must be comforted as one suffering from mental but not physical disease. This is an attitude which is extremely difficult for the layman to cultivate. If he decides that the disabilities of his companion have no, or an insufficient basis, he says not that the basis is imaginary but that the whole trouble is imaginary. If there be no trouble, no sympathy is required. This is, of course, false logic, which the patient knows, for the reason, obvious to him, that he *does* suffer.

All pain is subjective, because it is something which can be felt and, as pain, has no existence before it is felt. There may, or may not, be an adequate physical stimulus for it. If my head aches no one can persuade me that it does not ; all he may do is to persuade me that the occasion for feeling the pain exists in my thoughts and not in anything physical. I may be induced to listen to the latter argument but the former will only enrage me.   We can thus see why the home environment is bad for the hypochondriac.   His family either sympathize with his sufferings and so aggravate them, or argue that his torments being imaginary are non-existent and so have no sympathy for him.   Since an inner craving for sympathy is one of the chief motivating forces back of hypochondria, this last situation only aggravates the patient's maladaptation, even though it may silence his complaints.   In a good hospital, however, the complaints are neglected but not the patient ; hence, other things being equal, recovery takes place.

Involution melancholies often succeed in having their own way at home by flying into tantrums when crossed.   The treatment for such exhibitions must be discipline, as in the analogous case of the fractious child.   In an institution these patients can be disciplined by removal to the disturbed ward, cessation of special privileges, and so on.   In practice one cannot go further than this through fear of brutality developing on the part of attendants, or, at least, its being charged against the hospital.   Yet one often feels that a little corporal punishment would do these people good.   They behave like very naughty children and should be treated as such. The bad child is functioning on a level where physical pleasure and pain are the only things he cares about, and many involution melancholies regress to just this primitive state.

As to the treatment of the dramatic anxiety so often seen in this group, our observations have given us no clue.   It is certainly idle to argue about the baselessness of their fears.   If isolation is found to aggravate the panic, such patients should, obviously, not be left alone.   One can advise nothing further than trial and error in this and similar problems.

A psychological understanding of the apathetic, deteriorating tendency is of value, however.   As we have seen, this type of regression is the same as that in stupor and the same rules apply. Stimulation, even emotional stimulation, is strongly indicated. And, again, we find that recovery, once it has already begun, proceeds much more quickly when the patient has returned to his home.   In reviewing about a hundred cases from this standpoint, it was astonishing to observe how infrequently complete recovery occurred in the hospital.   The involution melancholic is at an age when it is comfortable and easy to remain in an environment that calls for little exertion and practically no self direction.   Hence it is easy for him to become institutionalized and maintain just enough of his symptoms to keep him a " patient ".   This mistake is more apt to be made of retaining him too long, than of returning him to his normal environment too soon.   Naturally, however, home conditions have to be considered.

When we turn to manic states, we find quite different mechanisms in operation—at least in typical cases.   The problem here is one of avoiding exciting agencies.   Either a hypomanic or a manic patient is definitely stimulated by talking about anything in which he is interested, particularly about his psychotic ideas. The case of Alfred J. gives excellent examples of this. These patients should therefore be isolated as far as possible from all exciting contacts. A mild hypomanic may become quite manic as the result of an argument or a talk with some sympathetic listener, ready to hear his opinions. A florid manic, however, will often rouse himself to a high pitch of excitement on merely catching sight of a new person, who might listen to his oratory. For the latter complete isolation is desirable. The padded cell, now so generally abandoned in America, has, I believe, its usefulness in treating such cases. Occupations of a routine, uninspiring order may be helpful in bringing a patient back to earth ; while others of greater interest may be of value later on in renewing contact with reality.

Artificial sedation and restraint furnish many problems for the conscientious and thoughtful psychiatrist. No hard and fast rules can be laid down, treatment must always be experimental. In rare cases manual restraint may be useful, but only if the patient feels overawed by the superiority of the force opposed to his. Naturally, overawing is difficult to achieve without brutality, hence its great danger. If a patient be not cowed at once, his pugnacity is aroused and rage is hardly to be regarded as a quieting influence. If restraint is obligatory, inanimate bonds, such as a comfortable restraining sheet, are much less exciting. The continuous tub is often extraordinarily effective in quieting even a florid manic, but may have no such influence at all. The sedative effect of warm packs, when it occurs, is to be similarly explained.

The relative ineffectiveness of drugs in allaying manic excitement is a fact calling for some psychological comment. A powerful sedative like hyoscine is often effectual in quieting excitement in organic conditions such as that of paresis but may have little or only a temporary influence on a florid manic. If temporary, its repeated use involves great and obvious dangers. To explain this contrast one has to think of the psychological effect of such drugs and of the difference in the psychological mechanisms of the two diseases which lead to what is apparently the same result. A sedative operates by reducing, somehow, the irritability of nervous tissue. Its first effects are on the higher, more elaborate, functions which we call mental. Of these the least stable are the discriminative functions of consciousness and the inhibitions allied therewith. Hence the initial effects (or the only effects with a mild dose) are to abolish inhibition and produce clouding. In paresis an organically unstable nervous system facilitates an over-reaction to environmental stimuli. Hyoscine makes the patient less acutely aware of the environment and reduces the irritability of the nervous system. Both the excitement and its cause are thus abolished. In mania, on the other hand, the nervous system is not organically unstable (so far as we can judge) but a relative weakness already exists of the inhibitive forces as compared with the creative, unconscious impulses. The initial result of sedation is, therefore, to weaken inhibition still further and thus to increase the excitement. If the drug be pushed to the point where torpor appears, the patient is naturally quiet ; but when he recovers from this intoxication, the more primitive, unconscious forces reassert themselves before the more susceptible inhibitory ones. Excitement therefore reappears so soon as the torpor has worn off. Sedative drugs with mania are useful, therefore, only in real emergencies.

Stimulation by employment or emotional contact seems likely to be useful only in such cases of manic stupor as have become thoroughly dull. But our observations do not give us empiric ground for this, which is merely a theoretic opinion.

The psychological mechanism of recovery in manic states seems to be that a sublimation is elaborated which brings the patient in contact once more with reality. This was prettily illustrated in the case of Elizabeth K. When we know much more than we do now of the psychology of manic depressive insanity, it is to be hoped that psychiatrists may be able, by occupational therapy or otherwise, to facilitate the development of such sublimations and thus shorten the course of an attack.

All that has been said about the value of institutional care is specificably applicable in the treatment of depression. If a depression be severe the mere nursing and custodial needs of the patient make it advisable to have him interned. Then, too, the home environment, at this stage, is apt to set up those trains of unconscious thought which result in the depressive reaction. Treatment, to be psychologically sound, must aim at either re-establishment of interest or lifting of repression or, best of all, at both. A hospital with facilities for varied occupations gives the best opportunity for re-directing interest to the real world. At the same time more can be done there in the way of forcing activity. In all but the severest depressions the state of the patient is better as the day wears on, and this seems to be due to a summation of environmental stimuli that have a cumulatively greater effect. This gives a hint for treatment. The patient should not be allowed to lie abed in the morning ; he should be got up and dressed. A cold bath often assists in the waking-up process. When about, he should not be suffered to sit idly, but should be forced into activity, even if it be only walking. Once recovery has begun his normal environment may furnish him with more effective stimulus than the institution ; when the psychotic reaction has begun to wear itself out the presence of relatives is more apt to cause revival of interest, than unconscious elaboration of unwholesome thoughts. Hence we find that many a depression (like stupor or involution melancholia) disappears entirely only after return home. To tell just when the turning point in response to emotional stimuli has been reached is, naturally, a difficult matter, and one in which mistakes are bound to be made. Yet I believe that, on the whole, more good than harm would result from liberating patients earlier than is customary, providing reasonably intelligent and continuous observation can be secured in their homes. To send a depressed patient back to a family that considered him well, would be, of course, to encourage suicides and other disasters.

The problem of breaking up repression is one calling for much knowledge, delicacy and the application of special technique. In the course of treatment of psychoneurotics minor depressions (such as those resulting from dreams) are easily and dramatically exorcized. In the discussion of the mechanism of depression instances are cited of such cures. With hypnosis the repression may be so effective that the disturbing thought is driven out of co-consciousness into the limbo of the deep unconscious. With psychoanalytic technique the offending idea is dragged into the light of common day in spite of repression, which is thus robbed of its prey and ceases its frantic efforts at keeping all doors locked lest one should open. But we must remember that in these minor depressions, we are concerned with one idea only, or one circumscribed complex of ideas. In the severe retarded depression, the most basic unconscious ideas seem to be activated, viz., the Oedipus complex with many of the elaborations. If these were liberated dementia praecox would, or might, appear. In fact, it sometimes does, as we have seen. Such being the case, it would be a risky thing to lift the repression suddenly even if we could.

After a retarded repression has endured for some weeks or months it seems as if the clinical picture were remaining unaltered, not so much, perhaps, because repression and expression are so deadlocked as because the equilibrium has resulted in an inertia not unrelated to stupor. The problem here is one of producing a reaction somehow or other. In this connection some experiments with bromide intoxication have considerable theoretic interest. In 1916 Ulrich[1] reported his observation on the treatment of depressions with sedobrol given in conjunction with a salt-free diet. The basis for these experiments was the production of euphoria in normal people when bromide intoxication had been achieved. In ten cases of severe depression he broke up the psychosis within a few months by the induction of bromide intoxication, either once or repeatedly (the latter when the first euphoria did not subside into normality but a recurrence of the depression). Such experiments are not without danger and halogen excretion has to be followed with great care. Perhaps it is for this reason that others have not repeated his experiments—at least I have not been able to find further references to this mode of treatment. In well-equipped hospitals the work ought to be reasonably safe and should repay repetition.

---

[1] Ulrich, A. " Ueber psychische Wirkungen der Broms und die wirksame Behandlung melancholischer Zustaende mit Sedebrol ", *Korrespondenz, f. Schweizer Aerzte*, XLVI, 641. Abstracted in *Zeitschr. f. d. gesamte Neurologie v. Psychiatrie*, XIII, 126.

In the light of our theory the mechanism can be understood psycho-physiologically. The substraction of chlorine from the nervous system abolishes or weakens inhibition and thus increases the native irritability. A condition roughly analogous to that of paresis is thus produced.

We have nothing to say in regard to the handling of pure anxiety states or perplexity. They are almost always temporary reactions and we observed nothing in them to suggest special lines of treatment.

CHAPTER XLVI

THE NATURE OF MANIC-DEPRESSIVE INSANITY

IN the psychiatric introduction to this book several problems were proposed for solution and it is now time to see what conclusions may be drawn from the material, as studied by our method of psychological investigation and interpretation. First a word as to the broad question of psychogenesis, that is, the theory that symptoms in constitutional psychoses may be shown to have a psychological history and interrelation rather than to be the direct expression of somatic disturbances. If the reader is still unconvinced that this is a workable hypothesis, it would seem idle at this stage to indulge in any argument. The clinical material either demonstrates it, or it does not ; further attempts to prove it would be waste of time. In the following discussion I shall therefore assume that psychogenesis, in so far as it may affect manic-depressive insanity, is a valid assumption.

A question more fruitful to discuss is the unity of the so-called manic-depressive psychoses. Kraepelin has put them all in one group for reasons that have been already fully explained (pp. 2-4). Prominent in his argument are the features of periodicity, or recurrence, of attacks in a given patient which may be of one kind in one attack and of another in another ; and the frequent presence of transitions in a single attack from one type to another. These are unquestioned facts and their use makes his argument strong, although not final. The difficulty is that neither phenomenon is universal. A patient may have only one attack in his life, the symptoms of which bespeak typical mania or depression. Or such an attack may remain mania or depression showing no tendency to abnormality of another type. Moreover, there are fine gradations between manic-depressive psychoses and dementia praecox, and the latter disease may be periodic. Should one therefore say that manic-depressive insanity and dementia praecox are one disease with a variable prognosis ?

A medical analogy may make this point clearer. A person with predisposition may have several attacks of pleurisy ; an attack of pleurisy may merge into phthisis. This is not held sufficient reason for making pleurisy and phthisis different exhibitions of the same disease. It is only in cases where the " predisposition " is demonstrably tubercular that physicians feel justified in regarding the attacks of pleurisy as exacerbations of a tubercular process and, even then, more conservative ones will demand further evidence before being certain that the pleurisy may not be due to some other organism than the bacillus of Koch.　In other words, conditions that are clinically different cannot be more than tentatively grouped together for any reason except the demonstration of a common pathology.

Now Kraepelin's pathology of manic-depressive insanity is a highly hypothetical somatic disease state, or process, which is invented—in so far as it is claimed to be specific—simply to give the required unity to these psychoses.　It is therefore tautological and, so long as the *raison d'être* of the manic-depressive group is dependent on the data and arguments which Kraepelin puts forward, its stability is precarious.　But our studies would seem to promise the desired unifying elements, provided one is willing to accept a pathology expressed in functional rather than anatomical terms.　We can demonstrate common psychological processes which may be held responsible for the wide range of symptoms observed in manic-depressive insanity.

According to practically all modern schools of psycho-pathology, the basis of the psychoneuroses is the activation of unconscious complexes which, operating unconsciously, produce the symptoms by their indirect conscious reverberations.　This type of thinking that the patient consciously pursues is not materially different from normal thought.　But in manic-depressive insanity we see a kind of thinking, characteristic of unconscious mentation, not only appearing in consciousness but even dominating it ; this is free-associational thinking.　Integrally connected therewith is a deflection of interest and attention from the environment (" reality "), and from normal pursuits to more primitive interests and fantasies.　This is regression of interest, just as free associational thinking is a regression in mentation.　The two run hand in hand.　When attention is wholly given to regressive thoughts, the latter become " reality ", that is they seem real to the patient, who then has delusions or hallucinations.　The emotional reactions of the patients to these imaginary elements constitute the moods of manic-depressive insanity ; there is, apparently, nothing abnormal in these emotions *per se :* anyone would behave similarly if placed in the position in which the patient believes himself to be.

One cannot classify nor understand the false ideas which appear without knowing Freud's scheme of psycho-sexuality, with its emphasis on " infantile sexuality " as the foundation on which adults reactions are built.　In manic-depressive insanity regression activates these fundamental processes, but they are either limited in their conscious exhibition (sexless union with the parent, simple autoerotic practices), or else they are reformulated (attachment to parental surrogates, hypochondria).　Historically the different aspects of infantile sexuality are interrelated.　It is therefore only natural that the free associational process should produce different aspects and different formulations of it. When these variations occur different clinical pictures appear just as the behaviour of a normal man will vary from one situation to another. And, just as this is the same man throughout, so the patient is always manic-depressive, because it is the manic-depressive process which is changing his environment. The fundamental regression characteristic of all the psychoses in this group may take a number of different paths : each one of these constitutes a reaction type and so we have mania, depression, anxiety, and so on.

Having thus stated the general psychopathology of manic-depressive insanity an exception must be admitted. When the stupor psychosis is reduced to its simplest, and purely stupor, elements, neither free association nor infantile sexual complex is encountered. No ideas whatever may be expressed nor betrayed in behaviour. That the stupor process is regressive has already been claimed, so there is nothing to be gained by rehearsing the arguments. The questions now to be ventilated are, what is the nature of the regression and what is its relationship to manic-depressive insanity.

Every regression involves leaving the present, the world as it is, and most of them involve flight to another environment, the past as remembered or a future conjured up in fantasy. Stupor in its simplest form represents only the initial step in regression, the escape from things as they are. Because this is true of all psychopathic reactions it may be said to be the most basic of all regressions and not specific for manic-depressive insanity. If we are to found our grouping of psychoses on common psychopathological processes, we should ally stupor more with epilepsy, of which the *sine qua non* is a break with the environment, than with psychoses characterized by the appearance of ideas suggesting alternative outlets for interest or " libido ". If we are to use only such psychologic principles in our classification as are applicable to the actual psychosis, we must logically deny stupor a right to a place in the manic-depressive group.

But, even if our bias be psychological, there are still good reasons for including this psychosis as we have done. It is a rare stupor that runs its entire course without the appearance of false ideas or without some evidence of infantile reactions. Particularly in the incubation period, the psychosis may look like any kind of a manic-depressive picture. Again, when other reactions are present, free associations may present ideas of death and stupor features appear, even though as a temporary phase. Further, the tendency to apathy, a central characteristic of stupor, may co-exist with other manic-depressive reactions and so tone down the latter. Finally, and most of all, we must take account of the relationship of stupor to the whole life of the patient. As we have seen so often in thoroughly investigated cases, psychosis and personality cannot, psychologically, be treated as two different things. Stupor behaves exactly as do other manic-depressive reactions as an expression of defects in adaptation. The psychological difference between stupor and epilepsy rests not on difference between the basic mechanism of symptom production, but on markedly contrasting " normal " reactions. The epileptic patient is, after all, an epileptic ; the stupor patient has a manic-depressive make-up. This is not merely a verbal discrimination. The epileptic type of personality defect makes loss or clouding of consciousness psychologically inevitable. The abnormality of the stupor patient, however, is expressible in any kind of emotional disturbance.

The intimate relationship of stupor to manic-depressive insanity may be explained in this way. Before a manic-depressive reaction can be established (free associational thinking on an infantile theme), contact must be lost with the normal environment and interests. If the mere break alone be accentuated, as in the case in preoccupation with the theme of death, stupor results. The wheels of the mental machine slow down, may even seem to stop ; if they pick up again it is because new interests are established, either normal ones or those inciting the other manic-depressive reactions.

Mania, depression, anxiety, involution melancholia and perplexity all fall more easily into our scheme. In mania the symptom of flight of ideas is a prominent one and it has been demonstrated to the satisfaction of the reader, I trust, that flight is a vocalized and swiftly moving free associational process. Moreover, an attempt has been made to show how the different clinical pictures in mania can all be correlated by assuming that this type of thinking is more or less dominant. In mania the patient seems to abandon himself to free associations and the reckless way in which this is done is probably to be explained by the ideational content. The associations play variations on the theme of sublimations, taking that term in its widest sense. Sublimations in normal life are vehicles for energy expression, so it is only natural that manic states should be the ones characterized by the greatest activity.

Psychologically, perplexity is closely allied to mania, although clinical resemblance appears only in some phases of the manic reaction. Free-associational thinking seems again to be the key to the symptoms, but here the ideas do not consistently incorporate thoughts that are welcome to the conscious personality, even in its psychotic state, as they do in mania. So the unconscious type of thinking overwhelms the unwilling consciousness and a conflict results in which both environmental data and the flux of verbal and imaginal thoughts seem to have equal validity. Hence the peculiar subjective perplexity. But one kind of content seems in manic-depressive insanity to tend to assume dominance ; hence perplexity states are liable to pass quickly over into other more commonly recognized psychoses.

Anxiety states are also easily understood by the adoption of our psychological principle. Here the free associations lead to presentations of sexual outlet in aggressive form. These are easily symbolized as attacks on the patient to which he responds in the normal way, that is by fear. This holds either for the episodes of anxiety seen in ordinary manic-depressive attacks or for the more protracted states of apprehension characteristic of involution melancholia. In the latter, however, a deviation in the goal regression is to be detected. Infantilism tends to avoid the Oedipus complexes, remaining a simple negation of living—that is, as in stupor, a preoccupation with death—or it resuscitates early autoerotic practices and interests. The latter produce the hypochondriacal delusions which torment these unfortunates and plague their listeners.

The applicability of our principles to depression is less obvious, so that more interpretation is necessary in their demonstration. The patient who is silent and in a state of profound inhibition can hardly be used to exemplify free-associational thinking. Yet when one studies the onsets of depressions this kind of mental process is seen to be in operation and there is evidence, particularly in perplexity states, of the depressive reaction occurring when free associations introduce ideas, so incompatible with the basic trends of the personality, that they must be repressed lest the personality be disrupted. The repression becomes wholesale and contributes the inhibition which can explain and correlate so many of the symptoms. It is observable, however, that few depressions are consistently without content. There is something as a rule in consciousness that rationalizes the patient's unhappy state to himself. If these complaints, or confessions of sin, be examined they can be seen to represent distorted and emasculate symbolizations of a crude infantile content, which inference has led us to think is the pathognomic excitant of depression, even though these ideas may be operating from levels of the mind inaccessible to the patient's introspection. Depression is not a condition without thoughts as is stupor.

These, then, are the major reaction types which we have identified in manic-depressive insanity. But one difficulty must be admitted at once. The very phrase " reaction type " implies some consistency, some stability, some definite path that thoughts are following. Yet the essence of free associations would seem to be their kaleidoscope character. It is true that Freud has shown the connection between the elements in an apparently lawless sequence to be an unchanging theme, represented in varying symbols of quite different conscious significance. It is just this kind of consistency which we are claiming for the manic-depressive group as a whole. But why the relative permanence and consistency in one given reaction type ? Why should the basic theme for weeks and months be presented in one kind of symbolization ? It is true that careful observation will usually show that no psychosis is " typical " in this sense : little episodes occur in which other ideas and other reactions appear temporarily, often to the discomfiture of a teacher who expects to demonstrate a typical case. But, on the whole, one reaction type or another does tend to persist for long periods of time, even though the purity of its form be only relative.

Quite frankly we have no satisfactory solution to this problem. All that can be done is to point out that it is part of a much larger, and a general, psychological problem. It might just as well be required of us to explain why any normal individual behaves in a consistently different way from his companion in the same environment, having enjoyed (roughly) the same experiences in the past. In other words, this is the problem of personality. It will be answered only in that day when psychology can adequately account for habit and instinct and probably by that time psychology and metaphysics will meet. It will be a long time hence! Meanwhile all we can do in answer to this psychopathological problem is to suggest that in manic-depressive insanity the personality of the patient is not abolished but merely altered : that the peculiar factor in it which gives it its consistency and essence is still there. A mental structure which is normally hidden from consciousness is exposed and, for the time being, constitutes the personality. In the normal periods of the patient's life this structure is probably also present and may be just that which, operating unconsciously, so guides his interests as to give consistency to his conscious reactions. In fact, some such view as this must be held if one is to account for the continuity between mental make-up and psychosis.

A corollary of this hypothesis should be mentioned. Although personality has stability it is not absolutely permanent ; it changes slowly under the pressure of changing environment and advancing age. The outlook of the adolescent, adult and senile man is a different one although the same personality may be obvious throughout. If the manic depressive reaction be expressing the unconscious contribution of the patient it should change as life goes on. And this is statistically demonstrable. Stupor is a reaction of adolescence and early manhood, mania occurs in young adults preponderantly and diminishes in frequency as middle and advanced age creep on, while the depressive reactions preponderate in the involution and senile periods.

A question which the reader has probably been asking is, " Are Kraepelin's ' mixed conditions ' not reaction types ? " Undoubtedly they are—of a kind. He too has been unable to fit all manic-depressive psychoses into the two pigeon holes of mania and depression and so has invented other categories. But this method is diametrically opposed to ours. His analysis of the clinical syndrome is into separate symptoms which, he maintains, have independent existence and value and hence can be combined into different groups. This is a relic of the old faculty psychology which represented the mind as being a mechanical mixture of separable elements, and not a combination of integrated elements, as the present day psychology would have it. An analogy may make this clearer. The old psychology looked on the various mental elements as if they were building blocks of simple geometric design which could be put together to form different structures. Modern psychology considers that mental elements are more like pieces in a puzzle picture. Each piece is of peculiar shape ; it will not combine with any other piece but has meaning or value only when it is placed in such combination as will produce a picture or design. Symptoms, according to our view, have no meaning or value, except as they are inter-related and their inter-relation constitutes an integration which we call a reaction type. We hold that our reaction types have some *raison d'être*, while Kraepelin's " mixed conditions " are artificial.

If our view be sound, no mere chance or mathematical system of formulation can account for the grouping of symptoms as they occur in the different forms of manic-depressive insanity. There must be inter-relation and correlation of symptoms. By making the basis of clinical grouping a psychological reaction type, we are able to correlate symptoms not by chance but in virtue of the operation of principles of wider reference than mere psychiatric expedience. This is perhaps most easily and most thoroughly demonstrated in the manic states. Here the deflection of interest and attention from adaptive regard of the environment to indulgence in fancies, which we have termed " Distraction of thought " (producing delusions and hallucinations), induces free-associational thinking (flight of ideas) ; conventional restraints are inevitably withdrawn as indifference to the environment proceeds and this leads to excitement and emotional display (mood symptoms) ; as the process advances further, externalized activities are reduced (reduction of emotion and inactivity of manic stupor), while intellectual capacity progressively diminishes (disorientation) ; finally a condition is reached in which the patient, although seemingly awake is apparently dreaming. No symptom fails to fall into place in this scheme and, further, it seems to account for the paradoxical variations in the observable phenomena of manic states.

Kraepelin's theory of the mixed conditions has a seductive simplicity but even this could not recommend it alone. It must surely have some relevance to clinical observations, and we ought to be able to account for this relevance. It is probable that such applicability to clinical problems, as his system enjoys, can be explained in two ways. The first is that a patient may exhibit during a protracted period symptoms which, when put together, do constitute a mixture in Kraepelin's sense. As I have argued in the Introduction this method of description if applied to the observed behaviour of a normal man might depict an incongruous series of reactions. But we deny the legitimacy of this method and insist that, in a disease of which transition is a basic phenomenon, description should be confined to the symptoms appearing during one unit of time ; and, that when this is done, mixtures are not observable. In other words, we claim that symptoms of mania and depression do not coincide although they may be consecutive. This principle is well demonstrated in the case of Mary S. (q.v.). The second explanation is, that a renaming or reinterpretation of the symptoms he describes, may show that some of his mixed conditions resemble reaction types we have postulated, in addition to those of simple mania and retarded depression. For instance, if one regards mere quietness and inactivity as depressive symptoms it is obvious that a mixture in Kraepelin's sense would exist in a case where inactivity coincides with evident elation.

It may be well to run over his different mixed conditions in order to see how far this re-interpretation would identify his groups with ours. But at once a difficulty presents itself. Kraepelin does not give us any case histories : he merely states the symptoms to be found in his different groups, with only an occasional reference to actual clinical data such as, " One of my patients said so and so " or " One of my patients did so and so ". In order, therefore, to discover what the clinical states actually were, it is necessary to reconstruct in our imagination the psychoses which he describes *en masse* in general terms. This process is so unreliable as to be dangerous. It is one of the great vices of conventional descriptive psychiatry that it tends to portray phenomena in set terms that have shades of meaning varying from school to school and from psychiatrist to psychiatrist. The best we can do is to see how far his descriptions *might* cover the material with which we are familiar—such cases as have been presented in this book.

His first group is *Depressive* or *Anxious Mania,* of which the cardinal symptoms are flight, excitement and anxiety. The patients are distractable, talk about everything in the environment, catch up words and are talkative, losing the thread of their discourse. They are somewhat unclear about the environment. There are depressive ideas of sin, of being persecuted, or of a hypochondriacal nature. Emotionally they are fearful, with various forms of restlessness, or may be hopeless.

There seems to be nothing in this description that would not cover cases of involution melancholia in which free associations are prominent.

The second group is *Excited Depression,* which has the same structure as the first with the substitution for flight of an inhibition of thought. They are restless and talkative but unproductive of real ideas, for their complaints have much sameness. They are well oriented. There is anxiety, surliness or tears, which may be mixed with self-irony. Occasionally they may make sharp, witty remarks. Delusions are frequent but are less fantastic than in depressive mania.

It is difficult to reconstruct the living patient from this outline, but one might suspect that the man with these symptoms is an involution melancholic in whom many normal reactions are retained. He would be a person who has not abandoned himself to free association, his delusions are not so urgent as to absorb his whole attention but, at the same time, he is not fighting to maintain his sanity. Like many involution cases, he has given up the struggle and finds it easier to use his intelligence in defending his false views wittily than in spurring on his insight. One would expect a longduration to the attack. Kraepelin says nothing about the age of these patients but I would suspect that they are mostly beyond middle age.

His third group is *Unproductive Mania*, a quite common condition. These patients take in the environment or questions slowly and inaccurately ; they are inattentive and apt to give wrong and often evasive answers. Their verbal productions are empty and the same jocose remark may be repeated many times ; often they appear as if demented. But there may be fluctuations so that, sporadically, their replies are good. Emotionally, they seem to be elated, laughing much, although sometimes irritable. Motor excitement is confined to grimacing, self decoration, throwing things about and occasional dancing. Often they may sit about silently but then suddenly begin to laugh. Or they may be pottering about and, without warning, commit an impulsive act.

These cases we can identify without much difficulty as those manics in whom distraction of thought has proceeded to such a point that the life of the patient is essentially concerned with inner events but has not lost contact with the environment completely. The latter is represented by brief, perfunctory utterances, the relevance of which does not interest the patient, or by sporadic bodily actions. The stage is not yet reached of total indifference to the real world and hence emotional expression persists. It is this partial externalization of mental processes that differentiates the condition from the complete absorption of manic stupor.

The fourth group is *Manic Stupor* characterized by retardation, irresolution and elation. The patients seem to take no interest in the environment, are inaccessible and make no answers, at best mumbling to themselves. They smile without appreciable cause, fuss with their bedding or may decorate themselves, but all this is done without any evidence of excitement. Catalepsy is not unusual. Sometimes there are occasional delusions. Orientation is usually good. This condition is liable to interruptions, when excitement may appear, with running about, removal of clothing, or assaultiveness. Or there may be normal episodes. Other inconsistencies with the general tendency to inactivity, are walking about without talking but with erotic behaviour, or sudden pert remarks. After recovery they have a good recollection of the attack but are unable to explain their conduct. Kraepelin says that not infrequently this condition of manic stupor may be the transitional state between depressive stupor (close to what we call simply stupor) and mania.

" Manic stupor " is pretty plainly our absorbed mania and it is characterized by just those interruptions which we expect with the process of distraction of thought. Kraepelin says that it was study of this group which first led to the investigation of mixed conditions.   It is therefore interesting to see how he has succeeded in establishing a " mixture ".   Text book depression, he says, consists of retardation of thought and action, but nevertheless good orientation, and emotional changes associated with sadness.   If, for the last, elation be substituted, it is claimed that manic stupor will result. It is therefore necessary to demonstrate in this psychosis retardation of thought and action, good orientation, and elation.   We may accept the evidence for elation as being sufficient.   But how about the other symptoms ?   If a patient makes no answer and is indifferent to the environment how can one deduce anything as to the nature of the mental processes that may or may not be present ? In a case of organic dementia, when no response to question or environmental stimulus is discernible, it is usually assumed that mentation is absent or defective, rather than merely inhibited. Might not the manic stupor, when inactive, be failing in mental operations ?   Kraepelin would reply that at times the patient does answer and then intellectual processes may be shown to be competent.   But this is doing just what we have alleged Kraepelin to have done in fabricating his mixed conditions, that is, combining observations of different periods, when the psychotic reactions were different, into one picture.   The manic stupor patient who talks is no longer exhibiting the symptom of inactivity which is the *sine qua non* of stupor.   In other words, for the time being, another clinical state is present.   Now the type of argument which Kraepelin uses here is unreliable, if not dishonest, because he selects the symptoms out of the interlude, which suit his purpose and neglects others.   Why does he not recognize the episodes of excitement in his theoretic fabrication of the clinical picture ?   Plainly because that would make the wrong kind of mixture ; inactivity is essential, and, for his ideal symptomatology, inactivity must remain. The reader will doubtless recall that in our more careful clinical studies it was often possible to demonstrate in such cases that mental competence was correlated with activity so that, when the patient was active, orientation and so on were present.

   The next group is *Depression with Flight*.   Whatever these patients see or hear stimulates a train of thought ; they read much and watch everything going on about them with interest and comprehension. In spite of a depressive mood facetious remarks may be made. Some of the patients can write.   During the attack, but more after recovery, they complain of not having been able to control the train of thought and the appearance of ideas they never thought of before. This looks like an internal flight of ideas in support of which is the added description some patients make of these unspoken thoughts being determined by sound associations.   This psychosis not seldom merges over into manic excitement.

   We would take this to be an inaccurate and incomplete description of what we call perplexity states—at least the latter would fall into no other group that Kraepelin gives.   There is at least one curious inconsistency in this account.   How could a patient who is capable of controlling his thoughts read with sufficient intelligence as to have interest in it, or, indeed, be accurately cognizant of what is going on about him ?   Such an inconsistency makes one suspect that here again Kraepelin is mixing the symptoms of different periods in a varying psychosis.   Another point should be noted. Kraepelin has here admitted the existence of a flight of ideas not appearing in spoken words.   If this be permissible (and we believe it to be), why could it not be used to account for many of the symptoms of such a condition as manic stupor ?   But, if there were an internal flight of ideas producing occasional smiles, erotic behaviour, and so on, what would become of the inhibition of thinking ?

The last group is *Inhibited Mania*, which is composed of elation, flight and motor retardation.   The patients are elated, sometimes showing irritability, distractable, tend to make jokes, and are easily led into flighty talk with many sound associations.   But, as a rule, they lie quietly in bed only occasionally making a remark or laughing. It seems that a strong inner tension exists, " since the patients may suddenly become very violent (gewalttätig)".

We have no difficulty in recognizing these cases.   They are those that, in the process of distraction of thought, have just passed from florid mania into an absorbed state but, with wild inner or outer stimulation, return to the florid manic state.   Kraepelin is here confessedly speaking of a varying, not a constant, clinical picture, and again he selects from the episodes only those features which suit his scheme.   If he chose to reckon with the motor excitement that occurs when the patients become " violent ", what would become of his motor inhibition ?   He says that formerly he used to group these cases with manic stupor but now classes them separately on account of the flight of ideas.   The flight of ideas that appear only (according to his description) when the motor retardation has also disappeared !   If he had said " In some cases of manic stupor the inhibition is less constant, so that the patients sporadically become typically manic ", we would have less quarrel with him.

These, then, are the famous " mixed conditions ", fabrications which, as he once told Dr. Hoch, were the great achievement of Kraepelin's psychiatric career.   We think better of him than that. The separation of the dementia praecox and manic-depressive groups from all the pre-existing welter of constitutional psychoses took courage and a *flair* for psychiatric classification approaching genius.   But the theory that Kraepelin built up to rationalize his work was based on a fossilized psychology, that fitted normal behaviour ill, and is meaningless when applied to abnormal reactions. Nourished on this theory and spurred on by the national frenzy for new diseases, he has produced in his " mixed conditions " a series of groups which are so artificial that they can only be maintained by the selection of symptoms from poorly observed cases.   If I have succeeded in nothing else I hope the reader will at least be convinced that patients with manic-depressive insanity are still human beings. And the mind of a human being is not like a case of pigeon-holes, one of which may be filled or emptied without affecting the contents of the other spaces.

The discussion of reaction types in manic-depressive insanity must not be concluded without a confession. Kraepelin has been criticized for basing a clinical classification on a purely psychological scheme. But our reaction type grouping errs probably in the other direction. If constitutional psychoses are to be divided on the basis of differing psychologic processes there should probably be more of them. Analysis of clinical pictures reveals more reaction types than we have used in our classification of manic-depressive insanity, and the only reasons we have had for restricting the list has been clinical expedience and, perhaps as well, a fear of being too unconventional, of getting too far away from current classificatory terms. It is possible, however, that the future may see the general adoption of methods such as we have employed and, if that come about, there will certainly be more reaction types used in describing these cases.

As an example of the way in which clinical expedience has curtailed our procedure, I may mention the depressive groups. Involution melancholia, for instance, includes at least three different reaction tendencies, as distinct as others which we have differentiated. These psychoses would probably be more easily understood if we spoke of hypochondriacal depression, death-anxiety reaction and indifference reaction. The fact that in many a case all three tendencies may appear at different times or even, to some extent, be combined, is not, theoretically, any reason for putting them all together. Such arguments, if valid, would mean the abandonment of the whole reaction type method. In the future we may very well see some such division of the depressive psychoses as this : Retarded Depression, Unreality Depression, Reactive Depression, Agitated Depression (when the patient reacts to ideas of hopelessness with panic), Hypochondriacal Depression, Death Anxiety (including fear of poverty, etc.), Simple Anxiety (fear of sexual assault and bodily harm), Listless Depression (when the patient responds to depressive ideas with effortless resignation).

There might be practical as well as theoretic advantage in such a grouping for the clinical behaviour of these different groups varies a good deal. This has not been worked out as yet, but I may mention that the situations (including age period) in which these reactions occur may be sharply contrasted. For instance, Death Anxiety and Listless Depressions are rare outside the involution period. The others appear mainly between the years of twenty and forty. Reactive Depressions always have some real foundation and Hypochondriacal Depressions usually have. Real cause is totally absent from Unreality reactions, and most frequently from Retarded Depressions. The outcome as well is often different. Listless

Depressions have a long course and may easily become chronic. Unreality cases clear up, objectively, in the average time for a manic-depressive attack, but freedom from subjective symptoms is often attained only after years of apparent normality.   Similarly recovery from a Hypochondriacal Depression is apt to be merely an attenuation of the symptoms.   On the other hand, when a patient with Retarded Depression, Agitated Depression, or either of the Anxieties recovers, there is a real freedom from symptoms. Retarded Depressions often pass into manic states ; so may Agitated Depressions or Simple Anxieties.   The other types rarely do.   It might well be argued that these all represent distinct disease processes.

In completing discussion of our psychiatric problems the relationship of manic-depressive insanity to dementia praecox should be included.   Clinically, the symptoms of insufficient or inappropriate emotional reaction and scattering of speech, when plainly observable, serve adequately to differentiate the cases with a bad prognosis. But, when these symptoms cannot be identified with certainty, difficulties in diagnosis often arise.   We feel that our clinical studies, as well as our psychological theory, have reduced the number of these cases.

If mental reaction types are constituted by the integration of component elements or functions, which can be rearranged to form other combinations, it follows that transitions are to be expected between different reaction types.   Yet, when clearly established, the differences between such reaction types as produce a chronic or deteriorating disease or one with recovery must be marked, unless psychological studies have little practical value.   The psychiatrist, *qua* psychiatrist, is not going to have much interest in an explanation of conditions which will explain other, and quite different, conditions as well.   He wants specific explanations for specific differences. The master key to all constitutional psychoses is regression ; special keys are specific kinds of regression.

In the psychological introduction it was pointed out that there are two chief aspects of regression, return to earlier interests or objects of attachment, and return to more primitive kinds of thinking. The reactions we know as dementia praecox and manic depressive insanity may be differentiated in both directions, that is, both as to ideational content and as to mental mechanisms.   Both regressions tend always to proceed hand in hand, probably because they both represent manifestations of the same, as yet undiscovered, fundamental tendency.

The tendency in dementia praecox is to return to undisguised infantile sexuality.   Specifically we find the Oedipus complex coming to literal expression in the patient's delusions.   The parent is represented not merely as an object of affection but as an unequivocally sexual object.   In manic depressive insanity, on the other hand, the parent is seen as an object of sexless attachment and, when sexual interests are plainly spoken of, the act is portrayed as taking place with one who is not a blood relation. (That this sexual partner can be identified as a father or mother surrogate has been shown repeatedly in our cases).

If one is to label this manic-depressive regression in terms of a development period, I think it can best be called a puberty regression. But in so doing, it should be borne in mind that this means psychological, not physiological puberty. I have elsewhere discussed this discrimination[1]. During psychological puberty the subject is becoming conscious of his or her sexual destiny. This implies, on the one hand, sophistication as to the phenomena of generation and development of the primacy of the genital region, and, on the other, a growth of social interests paralleled by an unconscious elaboration of the Oedipus complex that gives it its specifically genital aspects. It follows from the latter pair of developments that this is the time during which surrogates are being found to represent the earlier nursery objects of affection. In psychological puberty, therefore, repression of the sexual potentialities of infantile attachments has taken place, while, since psycho-sexual development is still incomplete, fantasy is the outlet for such libido as is not autoerotic nor narcissistic. The ideational content of manic-depressive insanity expresses just such processes. The Oedipus complex is more powerful, appears more nearly in its original form, than in normal adolescence or adult life : the chief objects of affection are the members of the family ; and auto-erotism is but weakly repressed. In the fantasies of mania we have a repetition of the indulgence in ambitious thoughts that is characteristic of late puberty and adolescence. So the regression is not merely to a puberty phase. This is hardly to be expected, since there are varying degrees of severity in manic depressive insanity and therefore presumably of regression, and, on the other hand, the stages in development are artificial reconstructions. In actual cases the transition from infantilism to puberty and from puberty to adolescence shows imperceptible gradations. In milder manic-depressive reactions the regression is much more to adolescence, more accurately, to any earlier phase. For instance, the married woman who denies her marriage and revels in delusions as to the presence of suitors she had before marriage, is not necessarily going so far backwards as even to adolescence.

The essential point, psychiatrically, is that the manic-depressive reaction is never, literally, infantile. Having convinced ourselves of this point from study of many cases, we began to examine the content in cases that had seemed to be symptomatically manic-depressive but had deteriorated. In some of them we found literal infantile sexuality and were then able to see this symptom prognostically as has been described (Chapter XXIX). What had been a

---

[1] *Problems in Dynamic Psychology*, p. 304, seq.

matter of psychological interest became a fact of clinical importance. This extends the range of symptomatology. No matter what psychopathological theory he may hold, the psychiatrist of the future will not be able to afford the neglect of ideational content in the psychoses which he observes. We suspect, it may be added, that psychiatrists of long clinical experience have often used this principle unwittingly. When they said that they could give a reason but they knew that the patient was not going to recover, they were possibly impressed by infantile sexuality without being consciously aware of it.

The other aspect of regression is type of thinking. *Pari passu* with the development of interest in the outside world is the growth of the sense of reality. This is formed by the associated factors of independent observation of, and reasoning about, the environment, and of adoption of what people say about the things there are in the world. In this way knowledge is categorized ; things are abstract or concrete, real or imaginary, past, present or future, we have bodies, souls and spirits, and so on. When this development is complete the categories are kept separate. We do not confuse a thing and the idea of a thing. This is one of the functions of consciousness : it tells us which elements in the mental content are perceptions of the environment and which are thoughts. But this capacity for discrimination is a much more unstable specialization than we are accustomed to admit. Notoriously, when we lose consciousness in sleep, dream thoughts take on the value of environmental realities. This loss of discrimination is normally accompanied by other intellectual deficiencies, reasoning is faulty, the environment is poorly grasped or not noted at all, the past and future seem the present and so on. Many "faculties" are thus weakened or abolished together and this is because our minds are highly complicated integrations that do not operate in independent functions.

But it was not ever thus. The integration is a product of individual evolution from a stage in which one function might exceed another in development or operate in relative independence of others. The integration is established together with consciousness. Now the little child cannot be said to have consciousness in the adult sense of the word ; it has a mass of poorly combined, and relatively independent, reaction tendencies. The mental behaviour of the infant is produced mainly by two factors, stimulus and a pattern reaction. (This pattern is either racial or individual habit or both). Into nearly all reactions of later periods a third factor is introduced, the controlling influence of personality, which gives the response an individual quality. This is like the incorporation of mass reflexes into voluntary movements in neurological development. It follows from this that a characteristic of regression to infantile type of thinking would be a relative independence of different kinds of mental processes. This dissociation of functions is the " splitting "

of dementia praecox which Blenler has signalized in his term
" Schizophrenia ".

Observe a child who puts a row of chairs together and calls them
a train. He knows a chair for a chair yet there is more than mere
" make believe " in the train. There is real belief if one can judge
by his behaviour. The chairs have become railway carriages for
the time being, and woe betide the infidel adult who thinks otherwise !
Now this is just what the dementia praecox patient does. He knows
the accepted meaning of a given object or a given word as well as
any of us, but he has a private meaning for it as well and this second
meaning is just as important as if it had universal validity. Scattering of speech is thus easily understood. The dementia praecox
patient connects words together as a result of his private interpretations of their meanings as well as in virtue of their dictionary
associations. Hence what seems utter nonsense to us appears in his
talk. His arguments, his beliefs, his delusions and his behaviour
are similarly determined. It is because the process is half rational
that it seems so utterly insane to us.

An example may make this clearer. A patient of mine had an
acute psychosis that was highly typical of dementia praecox and
then " recovered ". That is he became well enough to perform his
duties in a fairly responsible position with apparent competence.
But in all his private thinking, so to speak, meanings were given
to words and ideas in a peculiarly arbitrary way. For instance he
wrote me at the beginning of the War that France ought to have
Alsace because that meant All Sauce and all sauces were French !
A manic patient might produce such a statement as a joke (although,
as symptoms, outrageous puns are much commoner in dementia
praecox and always suspicious), but my patient was in deadly
earnest about this. He spent hours every day with speculations of
similar merit and believed he was solving world problems.

In studying the correlation of symptoms in manic depressive
psychoses, particularly manic states, we were struck by the fact
that, when one mental function was disturbed, others were as well.
For instance, when a patient became absorbed by the interests
reflected in delusions and hallucinations, sense of reality was
weakened in other directions as well : he was no longer properly
oriented and could no longer perform simple intellectual tests. The
integration of mental process therefore continued, although functioning at a lower level. And this furnished us with our second new
diagnostic criterion. If a patient is so absorbed in his delusional
thinking as to talk nonsense, or if he seems to be living essentially
in a world of his own making but nevertheless is well oriented and
can perform the usual intellectual tests, that patient is suffering from
dementia praecox[1]. This principle may frequently be of use in
arriving at a diagnosis early, for many a manic patient may produce

---

[1] Credit is due to Dr. Hoch for this discovery.

what is apparently nonsense in the course of his flight, nonsense that it is hard to distinguish from scattered speech. Moreover, the manic who talks nonsense may be so distracted in thought that he is not exhibiting the typical emotional behaviour of a manic. If such a patient be disoriented, watch him further before making a diagnosis. But, if he be clear as to the environment and, on testing, show intellectual competence, he may safely be called dementia praecox.

PART X

DATA FOR A THEORY
OF EMOTIONS

CHAPTER XLVII

MATERIAL DERIVED FROM THE PSYCHOGENIC PSYCHOSES

IN Chapter XI (*q.v*) a tentative theory of emotions was advanced but left for further discussion till our clinical observations should be presented. It is now time to gather the pertinent data together. It was at that time stated that information should be gathered in order to settle three points. The first was the question as to whether emotions *qua* emotions are pathological or not, that is, whether it is the emotion or the stimulus which sets it off that is abnormal The second was the presence or absence of inhibition as a factor in the production of emotions. The third was the search for the psychological mechanism which produces the effective stimulus to one emotion or another.

The first point may be dismissed with brevity. A pathological emotion, according to some authors, would be one that occurs without adequate and appropriate mental stimulus, in other words, the expression of a physiologic process A number of psycho-pathologists have demonstrated in neurotic cases with apparent abnormal emotions the operation of unconscious ideas to which the emotions are a response. Morton Prince has called these ideas " co-conscious ". If nothing else has been proved it will surely be granted that in our manic-depressive cases ideas have been found to which the recorded emotions would be appropriate reactions. We will therefore take it as demonstrated that in these psychoses the emotions are mental products. It must be admitted, of course, that there are many clinical notes which refer to emotional disturbance without demonstration at that interview of ideas being present to which the emotion might be a response. But to demand that the cause and effect should always appear together would be to ask much more than we do of introspection in normal people. A disappointment may cast a man down ; he knows just what has disturbed him and the mood will persist after he has ceased to think of the occasion. He may be focussing all his attention on some task, consciously thinking of nothing else, but ask him why he is sad and he can call to mind the cause of his despondency at once. It has remained in the fringes of consciousness.

The same thing is true of our psychotic patients in all probability. The emotion persists as a mood ; with their weakened control of mental processes they may be unable to supply the disturbing thought on demand, but that does not prove its non-existence. In some cases the offending idea may have really disappeared from potential awareness and be co-conscious, but in most cases this is unlikely since the essence of a psychosis is a breaking down of the barriers between consciousness and co-consciousness. The latter becomes the fringe of consciousness, or the fore-conscious, to use Freud's term. In cases where the emotion producing thought is really co-conscious (as in the attenuated hypomanic states, for instance), it is probable that we are dealing with the same factors as in normal moods, for these mild psychoses cannot be clinically discriminated from normal reactions, unless they follow or precede more violent mental disturbance of which they are judged to be a phase.

In discussing the second and third points of investigation it may be well to review briefly our conclusions as to the different psychoses in order to see what each may contribute.

In stupor the evidence is more suggestive than compelling. Since there is great poverty of thought it is difficult to detect what mental mechanisms there may be in operation. But the material, nevertheless, is not without value. We have found the following correlations in stupor : when no ideas are expressed and inactivity is complete there is no emotional reaction, and this holds as well when a certain amount of motor activity is present ; if ideas of death as simple nullity appear, emotion is still absent, but, as soon as death in other aspects (danger, translation to heaven and so on) is mentioned emotion begins. The affective reaction increases in intensity in proportion to the degree in which the other aspects are consciously elaborated. Indeed, if this elaboration becomes more prominent than the primary death idea the whole reaction will change (usually in a manic direction) and a remission in the stupor takes place. Again, when the thinking disorder is at its height, there is no emotion and, with the lifting of the former, the emotional reaction increases. These correlations suggest that *emotion is a product of thinking* and that associational processes (that is, specifically directed sequences of ideas) have much to do with it, for it is presumably an associational process that evokes ideas elaborating the secondary aspects of death.

The rôle of regression is also suggested in stupor reactions. The regression has been seen to be to a preconscious phase of development with its accentuation of death as an abolition of the present environment, with the tantrum behaviour or resistiveness in partial stupors and with the autoerotism that often occurs. When this regression is complete, or even relatively complete, no emotion appears.

We may therefore conclude that consciousness is essential to emotion. Now consciousness is associated in development with repression and it would be difficult to imagine consciousness that was not demonstrated in virtue of a selectivity of stimuli. Selection implies repression, so we may assume that without repression there would be no emotion. This argument is far from conclusive, it must be admitted, but I have introduced it simply to show that a principle appearing more plainly in the other psychoses is not unrepresented in stupor.

When we come to consider the involution melancholias the factor of repression comes more plainly to view. Many psychiatrists regard the group as having a variable prognosis and we have found it expedient to divide the cases broadly into those related to dementia praecox and those classifiable with manic-depressive insanity. We have further learned that a bad prognosis may be determined by detecting any one of four symptoms, although two, three, or even all four are often seen together. These are insufficient emotional response, extremely ridiculous delusions (usually hypochondriacal), grossly infantile sexual behaviour or delusions, and excessive irritability. The insufficient emotional response to ideas that ought to be fearful or distressing is always present when any one or more of the other symptoms is well marked. It has been argued that the grave loss of sense of reality which ridiculous delusions imply, infantile sexuality and irritability all represent an infantile regression. Such tendencies are present in the cases with a good prognosis (as they are indeed in normal people) but they do not come ot open expression. They must therefore be repressed. When this repression is lifted the regression goes further and emotional reaction is impoverished. This may be taken as one bit of evidence for the view that repression plays a role in the mental processes leading to emotion.

A prominent symptom in the anxious involution cases is the facility with which a fear reaction is elicited by apparently innocuous environmental events. The fear is a response to a delusion and the latter is transparently the result of an associational process. A typical example is this : a patient is in a panic because he is going to be boiled alive and he explains that he knows this because he heard somebody say " Lobster ". This is, on the mechanistic side, like distractibility in a patient with flight of ideas. The word " Lobster " excites associations, one of these is of the animal being boiled alive, next comes the generalization, " violent death ". This is something which fits in with the general trend of the patient's thoughts, so suddenly the delusion of his being boiled alive appears. Until he heard the word he may have been tense perhaps, but not in a state of dramatic fear. A chance word has excited a train of thought which results in a delusion and the delusion precipitates an emotional reaction. As has been said in the preceding chapter, if we could explain why the associations go toward this particular goal we could explain personality as well as psychosis.

Parenthetically we may revert for a moment to the point discussed above as to the existence of abnormal emotions. States of fear are often held by psychiatrists to produce delusions, and the fear of involution patients is often alleged to create delusions of death. That the sequence is the reverse of this can be claimed for four reasons. First, there is good ground for believing that ideas of death are a natural product of the involution situation. Second, impulsive suicide is common, which could hardly be the outcome of a primary fear state. Third, the emotional reaction may fade away and leave the delusion of oncoming death. Fourth, stupor episodes (another reaction to death) may occur.

The data derivable from simple anxiety cases are of the same nature as from involution melancholia. The transition to dementia praecox shows the relationship of repression to emotion very nicely. A patient with the chronic psychosis may have a delusion that he is going to be assaulted and show no fear ; he may even smile as if he liked the prospect. In this instance the lifting of repression has permitted a grave regression (usually evidenced by infantile content as well as by the infantile thinking the " splitting "—which gives assault a pleasant meaning) and the appropriate emotional reaction no longer appears.

When we turn to depression the evidence for repression is well-nigh overwhelming. Superficial analysis reveals it in practically all the symptoms, while the central one, that of retardation itself, is nothing but inhibition. For our theory of emotions this is important because, although emotional expression may be so reduced as to be imperceptible, the affect is particularly strong. " I had the power, if I could raise myself to will it ; and yet again had not the power, for the weight of twenty Atlantics was upon me, or the oppression of inexpiable guilt." As matters of pure feeling, paralysis in fear and the impotence of depression probably have more poignancy than any other affects, and in each case it is surely correlated with the blocking of activity. That is why, psychologically, there is a gulf between the quietness of apathy and that of sadness.

Although the demonstration of inhibition is the more important contribution from the study of depression, the association factor may also be discerned. A depressive patient who is able to talk freely enough about impersonal matters is liable to sudden blocking, a sudden aggravation of all the symptoms, if certain topics are mentioned. In many cases any personal matter whatever will precipitate this reaction. It seems inconceivable that this is not due to associations echoing off into the unconscious regions of the mind and thus activating processes which must be repressed if the personality is to preserve its integrity.   One sees more of this process in perplexity, where the sudden appearance of depressive symptoms is a common occurrence.   Or, in studying onsets to depressions the same observation may be made.   The rambling thoughts of the patient trespass on forbidden ground ; then repression sets in and the psychosis is established.

Both from clinical and psychological points of view the manic states are of greatest interest and that is why so much space has been given to them.   They abound in paradoxes.   Elation is the typical mood but many cases show little of it, as, for instance, the querulous manics.   Or, if we allege free emotional expression to be the central symptom, then we are confronted with the fact that in many cases the emotional reaction diminishes although the patient is not recovering, for the mental abnormality is greater rather than less. Again, verbal and bodily activity seem to be the essence of manic excitement, but all excitement may go.   Quick wit is a characteristic of the manic but he may become so slow and stupid as to seem demented.   All these apparent contradictions can be shown to be the expression of a single principle operating in opposition to such factors as make normality.   This is the principle of distraction of thought, the abandonment of normal critique for indulgence in free-associational thinking.   Here and in perplexity states the emotional reaction can be seen to depend on the nature of the ideas that turn up in the course of free associations and then tend, we have seen, to assume more and more an imaginal, even an hallucinatory form, as absorption increases.   It is true that emotional expression diminishes *pari passu*, but images that merge into hallucinations must have vividness, and subjective feeling is not absent in absorbed mania. Retrospectively they do not describe their psychotic state as a blank as do the equally quiet stupor patients ; they say, generally, that it seemed as if they were in a dream.   According to our general theory, as instinctive behaviour and emotional expression decrease, affect should increase in intensity.   Depressive patients whose expression betrays little complain of the intensity of their feelings, but equally quiescent absorbed manics do not, and we may therefore assume that the subjective aspect of emotion is not strong among the latter.   Before allowing this to upset our theory, we should see what rôle repression plays in their conditions.

At first blush it would seem as if the rollicking manic with his crude jests and erotic behaviour was hardly practising repression ; and, indeed, in comparison with depression repression would seem to be absent.   But we should remember that, if our whole psychogenic structure be sound, all the symptoms in manic-depressive insanity must depend on an incomplete regression.   We see everywhere a tendency to infantile content that never gets full expression.   Presumably it is being hampered by something, that is, there must be repression. This is true even in the boisterous manic states. It is doubtful if this conclusion would ever be reached were it not for the occurrence of cases in which the regression does go farther. In such cases actual infantilism is reached, dementia praecox results, and with this more complete regression—this is an all-important point— the emotional reaction deteriorates. When the inconspicuous barrier falls, emotion fails as well ; apparently the latter really depends on repression.

How may we understand this ? We must remember that what we observe in manic patients is, broadly, their behaviour. We presume they are happy (that is have pleasurable affect) because they laugh and joke. In this presumption we are often confirmed by current or retrospective statement from the patient. But this subjective elation is rarely emphasized when activity is at its height. In fact, if one keep in mind the discrimination between affect and emotional expression when observing manics, it is astonishing how little one needs to assume subjective feeling to understand the psychosis. Compare it with depression, for instance. Subtract from the picture of depression what the patient says about his feelings and there is little left to record that is not purely negative. But take this element out of mania and the psychosis seems to have lost nothing essential. In other words, mania is a condition in which the objective aspects of emotion preponderate. The patient's reactions are turned outward not inward ; it is not a state of intro-spection but of expression, verbal and physical. At least this is true of those cases where absorption has not taken place ; the latter we will consider in a moment. Now studies of the process of distraction of thought teach us that outward expression is correlated with interest in and grasp of the environment. When contact with the environment is defective, expression is weakened or irrelevant. This is dementia praecox ; when regression to infantile thinking occurs the environment loses its meaning, and expression, both verbal and emotional, either lapses or becomes inappropriate. In manic states this regression is prevented by a repression. The free associational processes liberate instinctive reactions referring to the outer world and appropriate behaviour appears, a large part of which we call emotional. In dementia praecox free associations call up similar instinctive reactions, but, actual and fancied environment having commingled, the instinctive reaction that ought to have external expression may complete itself in fancy and so produce little that we can describe as emotion. Sufficient contact with the environment has been maintained, however, for us to see that the patient has registered stimuli to which response ought to be made in emotional expression.

The same principles will explain the absorbed cases. The ideas called up by free associations gain more and more attention from the patient, while less is being given to the environment. This is like dementia praecox except in one all-important point. The process in manic states is consistent, so that the environment of fantasy is substituted for the external world not confused with it. As in dementia praecox emotional expression becomes less marked and less frequent because the instinctive reactions are being carried out in imagination, not in relation with an outer world.   But then, different from dementia praecox, stimuli from without are no longer registered.   Just as reactions are imaginal, so are the stimuli images. In dementia praecox imaginal reactions are given to outer stimuli. In both cases emotional behaviour is reduced or absent, but in the chronic psychosis this is due to absence of repression of infantile thinking.   In absorbed manic states we have no reason to believe there is anything more than withdrawal of attention from the environment and its direction towards an inner world.   This is a regressive mechanism if you will, but it is merely the mechanism of reverie, not that of infantile thinking.

Now, according to our theory of emotions, when emotional expression diminishes affect should increase.   Are we therefore bound to assume that the subjective feeling state of an absorbed mania is intense ?   As we have seen there is no warrant for this in the statement of the patients, and we have no right to assume the existence of symptoms which cannot be clinically demonstrated.   The discrepancy may be accounted for easily.   The statement of our theory just given is incomplete.   It is when instinctive reactions are stimulated that do not gain expression either in conduct, emotional expression, or fantasy, that the affect is intense.   It is the prevention of expression of instinct either in behaviour or conscious thought that leads to intense affect.   In other words the energy of the organism, activating an instinct process, must be blocked by repression before poignant feeling is excited.   Now the passivity of an absorbed manic is not the result of repression—there is not a shred of evidence for that.   In fact, evidence all points towards a free indulgence of instinct processes in fantasy.   Clinically, then, the absorbed manic states really confirm our theory of the psychology of emotions.   There is no expression of emotion because instinct reactions are directed into fantastic outlets not toward the environment, while the affect is not intense because instinctively activated thoughts are allowed admission to consciousness.

The phenomena derived from study of all these different manic depressive reaction types can all be duplicated in observations of perplexity states, for these are characterized by kaleidoscopic emotions.   The dependence of different emotions on the appearance of ideas which stimulate specific emotional reactions can be shown nicely, as manic, anxious, or depressive episodes appear.   Again, the effects of distraction of thought are displayed exquisitely, particularly in one manifestation, namely, the splitting of attention between inner events and the environment.   This is a mechanism which, given free play, produces dementia praecox, and the reason for perplexity remaining a manic-depressive psychosis goes right to the root of the theory of emotions. Any tendency when activated will gain dominance in the mind unless it is displaced by an alternative reaction or unless it is blocked by some inhibition. Both these fates are discernible in perplexity. When alternative reactions appear, different clinical pictures result (episodes of mania, depression or anxiety). According to the theory here advanced, when inhibition alone is preventing free expression, an emotional reaction must occur, and this is just what happens. So long as there is a struggle against the tendency to live in two worlds at once, a peculiar distress is present, colouring—in part contributing to—the subjective bewilderment that is the *sine qua non* of a perplexity state.

This sounds as if the repression were actuated by a specific revulsion for a special kind of mental abnormality, because, as stated, the claim implies a horror of a peculiar type of psychologic aberration, viz., dementia praecox. But many of these patients are simple, untutored folk in whom one could hardly expect to find psychological, let alone psychiatric, sophistication. Our theory demands for the appearance of emotion the operation of instinct. Are we postulating an instinct for dementia praecox and a counter instinct against it ? It seems more likely that the instincts involved are of a much simpler order. Regressions such as we have been describing produce a disintegration of thought processes whose nature is determined by the integration we call normality. In other words dementia praecox owes its phenomena not to a specific instinct but to the constitution of the factors which bring it about, that is the regression and the normal mind. On the repression side the instinct is probably that of self preservation which is attached, in beings with self awareness, to the concept of self, the personality. Personality, as each of us knows his own, is an apparently self-regulating consciousness. When control of consciousness over thoughts is imperfect we feel that *we* are suffering dissolution. Hence the discomfort of losing consciousness under an anæsthetic, the fear of an epileptic for his seizure (he knows nothing of the convulsion except by hearsay) and the distress felt by a perplexed patient because he cannot control his thoughts. In this interpretation we are not therefore assuming the existence of an intellectual judgment with instinctive force. It is a very primitive instinct (self-preservation) which produces one symptom that is essentially an epiphenomenon—the dynamic cause of the whole reaction is the regression which produces all the queer thinking.

A final word should be said about the nature of the elements in free associations. The investigations of Morton Prince tend to show that co-conscious thoughts which produce emotional reactions take the form of images or tend to do so. That an emotion is more likely to be excited by an image than by an abstract thought, we can readily understand. I can think of an abstract lion in an abstract jungle and not feel the slightest suggestion of timidity. But if I imagine the lion before me and the jungle around me, some fearful excitement is apt to occur.   Instincts are patterns of reactions to real situations, fundamentally, and simple instinctive reactions are most likely to be set up by stimuli, which are environmental, or imaginal reproductions thereof.   Any abstract thought I regard as my thought, but every image I tend to project on to the environment. If free associations awaken emotions we should therefore expect them to be imaginal.   This expectation is amply fulfilled in studying manic depressive insanity.   The greater the abandonment to free-associational thinking the greater is the vividness of the presentation, the more is it projected on to the environment.   So true is this that actual hallucinations result.

CHAPTER XLVIII

DREAMS AND EMOTIONS[1]

IN order to test out our theory of emotions an extended description and discussion of manic-depressive insanity have been given. Clinical material seems to justify the theory, so now we turn to normal phenomena in order to see if its applicability is also demonstrable there. Introspection deals essentially with the narrow range of highly specialized mental processes which are conscious. Emotional reactions are obtruded into consciousness, and do not seem to originate there. Hence introspection is apt to yield mere description of affective phenomena or, at most, rationalization of emotions. Nevertheless, Dewey was able from observation of such material to claim that inhibition was essential in the production. But, when he attempted to describe the processes which were inhibited, he lost himself in a maze of tautological physiology and psychology. Introspection alone cannot carry us very far in this quest. The behaviourist method compliments it, but, since it aims at the exclusion of consciousness, its material is also incomplete. Such a combination of these two methods as is represented in our psychopathological procedure would seem to be a better way of studying emotions. But with what material should we work? Our method seems to be applicable to study of the psychoses, but have we any analogous material in normal people?

We have seen that a manic-depressive psychosis brings to light mental processes that were active during the normal life of the patient, although then unconscious, and that the same processes may be seen to affect reactions after recovery. But for the ideas and type of thinking portrayed in the attack, we should not know of these deep-lying currents of thought. Precisely the same statements may now be made about dreams in normal people, thanks to the work of Freud. Few discoveries are totally new and never hinted at before the publication to which credit for originality is given. In this sense Freud's theories were not new. But, to an unusual degree, his work was independent, and previous theories were such random guesses and airy speculations as to be scientifically valueless. We owe our knowledge of dream psychology to Freud alone. It was

---

[1] The main argument of this chapter was presented to the American Psychoanalytic Association in 1916 under the title *The Embryology of Dreams*. As " *The Metamorphosis of Dreams* " it was published in *Problems of Personality. Essays in honour of Morton Prince.* (Kegan Paul & Co.).
The present chapter is largely a transcript of this paper.

Freud who showed that a dream brings to light unconscious thinking that pre-existed and continues to flow on.

It will now be my task to show that, in addition to the identity in general principle, more than an analogy of detail exists between dreams and psychoses. This is why the material is so valuable in studying emotions. It may seem to some readers that the conclusions arrived at are quite different from Freud's. In minor details this is true : occasionally, I am bound to admit, I find I must reject a formulation of the founder of psychoanalysis. But in general the difference is one of point of view which does not imply fundamental variance in interpretation of the phenomena which both are considering. The aim of psychoanalysis is mainly to discover the ideas that are expressed in dreams ; my aim (at present) is mainly to discover the ways in which these ideas are expressed.

The importance of this discrimination may be detected in considering what would be observed in manic-depressive insanity from these two points of view. The Freudian would see—in looking for fundamental ideas—little more than the Oedipus and other such complexes. We, who are interested in how this complex may be expressed, have discovered that the different disguises it assumes produce different people, as it were, that is, different psychoses. As to the likelihood of finding infantile sexual thoughts at the bottom of dreams I am entirely in agreement with Freud ; and, if one is seeking to cure a patient through dream analysis, the discovery of these ideas is the all-important quest, one that should absorb the attention of the therapeutist. If, on the other hand, one's interest is primarily in psychological mechanisms (which it never should be during treatment), other phenomena of dreams come into the limelight, and these are to be correlated with similar processes observable in clinical material. An architect, a builder and an economist, may all look at the same building but see different things there. They see different things because their interests relate what is observable to different fields of experience.

Now the psychoanalyst rarely has an opportunity to study directly the mechanisms producing symptoms. He detects underlying tendencies and infers the mechanisms connecting them with the symptoms. The hypnotist, on the other hand, can study the mechanisms directly but gets little light on the fundamental instinct drives that are pushing in wrong directions. The psychopathologist dealing with the insane has the advantages of both methods, although he has less control of his material than either of the others, for experimentation is limited. If, however, one works both with the dreams of neurotic (or normal) people and observes the psychoses, as I have done, he sees the identity of underlying tendencies but gains a new light on mechanisms. In studying the transformation of unconscious idea into conscious reaction, he has the advantage of seeing the process more or less exposed in the psychoses ; he is not confined to mere inference. It has therefore been possible for me to pursue studies in these two fields side by side. How much each study has contributed to the other it is impossible to say. But it is my belief that, when I differ from Freud, I have been forced to that difference by consideration of material with which his experience is small. But, let me repeat again. I believe that there is much less variance than appears superficially ; it is the architect and economist saying different things about the same building.

In what follows I shall be treating dreams in the same way as we have the symptoms of manic-depressive insanity. I am going to regard them as little, recurrent psychoses that expose from time to time processes of thought, otherwise unconscious, that have been operating unseen before and will continue to do so again. Two questions will naurally be prominent. What is the relationship of emotional reaction to the form of dream thought, and what are the mechanisms that produce the differing forms ?

At the outset one objection to dream investigation must be met, a criticism heard frequently. The critic says that one has no right to draw inferences from the dreams of neurotics and apply them to normal psychology. There are two answers to this, a practical and a theoretic. First, it may be stated categorically, that no one who has ever investigated the dreams of neurotics and of normal people has ever been able to detect any difference in kind between them. Secondly, we can see why this should be so on theory. The neurotic differs from the normal person in the possession of symptoms. A symptom is something that interferes with normal living. But do healthy people not have similar difficulties ? We have noted that Janet groups all emotions with psychopathological processes : whenever anyone of us is emotionally stirred he is experiencing something that is identical in kind with the symptom of a neurotic. That is, it is an irruption into conscious life of something that is not consciously willed. Dreams represent such anomalies developed to a degree of absurdity (from a conscious standpoint) that neurotic symptoms never obtain. Between the thoughts and thought processes of a dream (in either a normal or neurotic subject) and the symptoms of a neurotic there is a much wider gap than between the thought processes of a normal and of a neurotic. We use dreams to study processes that belong to the abnormal order, not to explain ordinary conscious mentation. The processes involved in my transferring these ideas to paper are not likely to be illuminated by studying my dreams. But scrutiny of my dreams might expose something about where the ideas come from and how I happen to be interested in them, neither of which can be learned by any direct introspection, no matter how concentrated that may be. Emotions, neurotic symptoms, delusions and dreams are all products of thinking hidden from normal awareness. Not one of them can be understood alone ; each has to be studied separately but in the light of what is learned from the others ; and, when we come to general psychological theory, all must be interpreted together.

The statement that dreams are like insanity has been made so often that the mere resemblance needs no further mention. We are more interested in identity of process. In this connection the dependence of symptoms on dreams is more important. Wernicke has mentioned that confabulations in the insane may be the direct product of dreams and speculates timidly about the possibility of dreaming having the same abnormalities of thinking in it as are observed in the psychoses. Kraepelin speaks of the transitions from mania to depression (or vice versa) often occurring suddenly, and says that the change always takes place during the night. The patient wakes up in quite a different clinical state from that in which he went to sleep. This would suggest that dreams had changed the ideational content.

To us this would be no surprise, because our patients so often tell of being profoundly influenced by a dream during the incubation period of a psychosis. Two typical instances may be mentioned. The first was a woman of nineteen years of age, who, on marriage, began to show signs of instability. Six weeks later she suddenly awoke in a panic, saying that her mother was dead and that she had seen her ghost. She went on to say that she had seen her father's ghost as well and that she herself was dying. For nearly three months following she had an hysterical neurosis in which she complained of symptoms, suggesting mortal disease. Treatment was ineffective and eventually she believed that she was dying. Then a psychosis appeared in which the dominant topic was her being with her father in heaven. Her mother was also dead ; sometimes she was the only one of the family to reach heaven while the others went to hell.

A second example is the case of Catherine M. (case 64). It will be recalled that she reacted poorly to marriage, developed fear of childbirth and, when that came, became definitely psychotic. While quite disturbed a dream occurred in which she " nearly died in childbirth ". At once she began to talk of dying for her baby and was soon launched into a perplexity state with ideas centering around her being in heaven and the identification of her father with God. In both of these cases a dream introduces ideas which are elaborated and made real, so to speak, in the delusions of the psychosis.

If this intimate relationship may exist between a dream and subsequent symptoms, one might reasonably expect the dream of a normal person to affect the waking state which follows in what is the normal analogue of symptoms, namely emotion. And this will be shown to occur. Again, if the principles we deduced from manic-depressive insanity have any wider reference, the emotion in the normal man ought to be correlated with the form in which the unconscious trend is expressed, that is, the manifest content of the dream, to follow Freudian nomenclature. Similarly free-associational mechanisms ought to be detectable in the building-up of the manifest dream. These latter expectations will also be fulfilled.

And what of the so-called day-dream experiences, of the influence of events in the waking state that are reflected in dreams ? Opponents of psychoanalysis are prone, in criticizing Freud, to offer alternative interpretations of dreams, alleging that the thoughts of sleep are either distorted memories of recent experiences or responses to somatic stimuli, which, of course, continue in sleep. They trace all the dream thinking to influences playing *on* the mind of the dreamer ; the Freudians talk mostly of what is going on *in* the mind of the dreamer. The two views need not be mutually exclusive and are not so regarded by intelligent psychoanalysts, who say that the dreaming mind is not totally immune from stimulation during sleep but that the stimuli, be they mental processes still active from waking life or stimuli impinging from the body or environment on the dreaming consciousness, are woven into a dream structure that has its own *raison d'être*. This structure is essentially the product of a latent " wish " and of certain mechanisms called by Freud the " dream-work ". Really, then, each school is stressing one set of factors and tending to eliminate the other. When the opponents, for instance, admit that memories of the day are not accurately reproduced in the dream, they fail to account for the distortion. It is just this distortion in which Freud and his followers are interested, and they show that in many cases the distorting factor may be so powerful as to make the day-dream experience difficult of detection or even impossible of discovery.

It is my opinion that, from a psychological point of view, both sides have lost something of value (although the psychoanalysts may have lost little or nothing therapeutically). Any biased investigation is likely to be limited. An example may make this clearer. A patient may dream of a cathedral spire, a May-pole, a sword or a snake. The opponent finds a recent experience to determine each picture and is satisfied with that. The psychoanalyst applies his technique, finds each to be a phallic symbol, and says they are all the same, tending to regard the manifest differences as largely or entirely accidental. If, however, we approach the dream problem as we have the psychiatric one, a double enquiry will be prosecuted. First we want to find what the unconscious drive was, which produced any kind of a symbol, and would thus detect an unconscious erotic preoccupation, and then we look to see what specific meaning each phallic symbol has for the dreamer. The emotional reactions excited by these various dreams will probably differ widely. Each will correspond to a different psychosis, as it were. This method, I believe, will give us a broader understanding of dreams.

When one considers how closely analogous dreams are to delusions or hallucinations, it is tempting to see how far our psychiatric principles may be applied to dreams. I may say that by following such methods I have been able, with few exceptions, to predict the emotional state of the patient during the day following a dream, when once that dream has been revealed. It is, therefore, immediately evident that the manifest content of the dream has a profound significance for the patient. In fact, one might even claim that it determines his waking health and happiness.

There is another problem bound up with this. As has been stated, much attention has been given to the waking thoughts that determine the content of a subsequent dream, but little has been written about the fate of these fantastic ideas. Not a few neurotic symptoms have been traced to dreams[1], it is true, and Jones has given us an example of " The Influence of Dreams on Waking Life ", but no attempt has been made as far as I know to trace the mechanism by which our dream thoughts pass over into our waking activities. Yet this is bound to be a matter of theoretic importance, once dreams are viewed as psychological rather than spiritistic phenomena.

The problem is necessarily a somewhat speculative one for reasons which will be immediately obvious. We have to rely almost entirely on subjective, introspective data, and it is a peculiarity of such material that it is almost necessarily incomplete. We dream, of course, infinitely more than we remember ; our nocturnal adventures are forgotten with all possible speed ; in fact, the instantaneousness with which an elaborate memory of dream experiences can be wiped out of consciousness is one of the most astounding phenomena of mental life. As a rule our attention is fixed with sufficient intensity to register in waking consciousness only one or a small group of many dreams which we have had. This applies to true dreams. There is also a drowsy state of half sleep when dreams seem partly true and the real environment is also grasped in part. For this period we also tend to be amnesic. If we attend to this, then the previous incidents—the real dreams—are lost to consciousness. Now for our present problems we need to have succinct memories, not only of our dreams proper, of our thoughts in the twilight state, but also of what we think and do when fully awake. Naturally we cannot hope to obtain this full sequence frequently. More often we can get fragments that enable us to reconstruct the gradual transition from sleeping to waking thoughts, which our amnesias have made to seem abrupt.

It has long been a commonplace of psychoanalysis that the same theme tends to run through all the dreams of any given night. Sometimes a careful noting of all details immediately on waking may enable one to demonstrate the latent content in such a sequence by the mere principle of equivalents. That is, details may vary

---

[1] Prince, for instance, tells of a patient with a phobia of cats who all day long, after dreaming of stepping on cats, was in continual apprehension lest she should step on something unpleasant. Prince says in this connection : " Such phenomena would seem to compel the conclusion that the same process which had produced the dream content continued to function subconsciously during the waking state . . ." " Co-conscious Images ", *Journal of Abnormal Psychology*. Vol. XII, p. 298.

so little from one act to another of the drama that the patient can see for himself the meaning of the symbols. A condensed example may make this plainer. A young woman has three dreams of which these are the central incidents : First, she sees a bull and a cow mating in a barn yard—she is disgusted but morbidly attracted to the spectacle ; second, she spies on a boy and girl cousin who are flirting ; third, she watches her father with much interest pouring gasoline into a motor. In all three curiosity is expressed. The transition from the crude to the innocent sexuality and from that to the pure symbol is evident. This much the patient could see for herself. The analysis showed by definite associations a specific curiosity, which was the common latent content of all three dreams. The important point for us to note here is that the manifest content is changing, as she comes nearer to waking, so that the reaction to it is more comfortable. The first dream is grossly unpleasant ; in the second (she complained) she felt *de trop.* in the third she is comfortably interested. It could never disturb her peace of mind to see her father put gasoline in a car in waking life. This familiar type of sequence is still in the pure dream stage.

The next example gives us the birth of the dream into waking thoughts and actions. The patient is a physician whose father died, while the patient was still a young boy, of a lingering illness. He has specialized in the treatment of tuberculosis and is head of a hospital where many incipient cases are successfully treated. He appeared for analysis one day very depressed, apparently as a result of a dream where the latent content of eliminating his father from the family was not sufficiently distorted to be comfortable. This is typical of a depressive dream, as we have seen it to be in psychotic depressions ; an anti-social tendency comes to consciousness in a form which represents something repugnant to the patient's normal standards of conduct. The analysis obliterated the depression. The next day he appeared elated and reported an extremely active, successful day's work. His first thought on waking was the problem of telling an older married man that he had a serious tubercular infection. Next he recalled that he had to examine several cases which were suspected of early tuberculosis. He looked forward to this and when the time came made unusually good examinations and was able to satisfy himself that his suspicions were correct. This buoyant efficiency lasted through the day. When asked for his dream, however, he had to make a confession. On rising, he had jotted down a few headings but on looking at them later in the day they were meaningless to him. The dream was gone. Fortunately a few associations from his notes led to the discovery of it.

His chief friend at college had died from tuberculosis after some years of unhygienic life during which he had been in ignorance of his disease. The patient had felt that if only a diagnosis had been made earlier he would never have succumbed. The dream accomplished this : He was back at a house party where they had been fellow guests some years before (at the time when the friend's symptoms first developed only to be disregarded). The patient examined the latter's chest, discovered the lesion and turned him over to the head nurse of his hospital for treatment. A brief analysis made the whole sequence transparent. His father dying of a wasting disease had created the patient's interest in tuberculosis. It was a sublimation of the idea of death in connection with his father. Both his friend in the dream and the old married man who was doomed in real life were successive father-surrogates. What had been the night before a depressing theme was changed to a sublimation—it gave an outlet to the underlying wish in a form that met the approval of the patient's every standard.

The fact that this dream was forgotten deserves some comment. It was not of an unpleasant nature, in fact, it remained in consciousness long enough to allow the patient to make notes of it. Moreover it was revived by a few associations. For this lapse of memory one probably does not need to presume such a desire to forget as is necessary in most cases. Entirely apart from dynamic reasons we tend to remember best what is connected with our daily life, simply because it is more in our waking consciousness, is more associated with our waking activities. This probably is one factor accounting for the topical memory of stages leading from pure dream thoughts to pure waking ones. One object of the process is to give a form to the latent thought that is adaptive to our waking needs. Each of a series of successive formulations is a substitute for the preceding one, and so there is always a tendency to remember only the last. This accounts merely for such amnesia as is here described ; the effectual, hysterical type, which dissociates the dream from consciousness in spite of effort to retain it, is obviously not adaptive and can be explained only on dynamic grounds.

The next example from the same patient shows a less extended sequence but again illustrates the transition from dream to waking life. He was a man of 36 years, superficially normal, but suffering from enough inhibition to have adopted the belief that he was not " a marrying sort ". He had resigned himself comfortably to the idea of celibacy until suddenly an ejaculation, while examining a boy patient, startled and depressed him. He recognized at once a homosexual tendency of which he had been previously totally unconscious. The resulting depression impaired his efficiency seriously and finally he applied for psychoanalytic treatment. The results were rapid and before long hopes of marriage filled his mind. There were two not unimportant difficulties in the way : there was no one in whom he felt sufficient interest to begin a courtship and his income was hardly large enough to support a family in the same comfort that he enjoyed as a bachelor. In a more or less conscious effort to surmount the first obstacle he began to indulge much more in social activities than had been his wont, which caused considerable comment among gossips.

It was at this period that he awoke one morning with the thought which he could not identify with certainty either as a dream or as an actual experience at a dance the previous evening. It was this. He was watching one of his patients dancing with the latter's fiancée and wondering how they could get married, as the man had little money. This was all he could recall till on his way to the analysis, when he remembered a real dream : " I was in a doorway of the ballroom. Toward me came a patient who has owed me money for some years. He and his wife began talking to me about this bill, which embarrassed me very much, as all the other guests were looking at us. He shouted at me that he would pay it soon—next month." In his associations, the embarrassment led to his sensitiveness, to the gossip about him, as it was said he was looking for a wife. The public promise to pay led to the idea of his demanding the money, which he needed for marriage. This shows at once the significance of his drowsy thought. The problem was transferred from his own to another's shoulders, it was then a real situation, not a dream imagination, and, moreover, its contemplation gave him no discomfort.

Part of the following dream sequence was reported by me ten years ago[1] to exemplify the mechanism by which a day-dream experience precipitates a dream. At that time I spoke of the waking distortion as an example of what Freud has termed " secondary elaboration ", but on more mature consideration I feel that Freud does not intend to include such complete metamorphoses under that term. The following account is quoted, in part, from this previous article.

This dream was produced on the seventh day of the analysis of a woman suffering from morbid anxiety. From the very beginning a strong " transference " to the physician was evident from her dreams, which had been readily understood by her as an expression of confidence, reliance and gratitude. Then came, as soon as the analysis began to touch her vitality, the opposite feelings of hate and distrust, coming to consciousness during associations as an expression of the fear that the analyst would abuse his privilege as a physician, a feeling that he was exposing her life history for his own gratification, that he was " outraging her innocence ". These ideas came relentlessly to expression, and for several days were regularly accompanied by harrowing attacks of anxiety that interfered temporarily with the analysis. The underlying craving for erotic satisfaction—an idea repugnant and foreign to her conscious personality—had remained unconscious however. But one day she read in the newspaper about some deal that J. P. Morgan had put through by unfair means, or so it seemed to her. The following night she had this dream, which I quote from her written record of it :

" This dream is really too vague to tell. *I feel it has changed its*

---

[1] " A Psychological Feature of the Precipitating Causes in the Psychoses,' *Journal of Abnormal Psychology*, vol. ix, p. 297.

form at least three times before I finally got it into my mind. This is it : There was a financial deal to be put through. Several people were going to do it, but at the last they were afraid, and Morgan went in alone and managed the thing. An element of indignation and scorn on Morgan's part. *Before the dream changed to Morgan, it was something about the wheat pit, with a feeling that I was connected with it. Before that it was something about myself.* [My italics.] I awoke with the impression that someone was knocking at the door. Somehow a vague thought in my mind of something—then the word ' modesty '. There was no connection between the knocking and the thought in my mind. I seemed to pick up this vague thought when I realized that no one was knocking."

Associations showed, with multiple over-determination, that Morgan represented the physician, who scorned her " virtue ", and who abused his medical privilege to seduce her. The scorn was, of course, in turn, a projection of her hatred of the analysis, consciously, and unconsciously, her opposition to seduction.

Now, how did this dream come into being ? Reading of the financial operations of Morgan, who " betrayed a confidence ", touched off the unconscious " wish " to be betrayed. She said, that, while waking, she had the feeling that she must record the dream, and knew that it concerned herself ; but, while thinking of it, it turned, like the Old Man of the Sea, into the dream of the wheat pit, with which she was somehow identified. To the wheat pit she associated directly the " lambs " who are ruined, and her own innocency. Already there is here the staging of the financial world, but the wish was not sufficiently distorted to be acceptable to the waking consciousness, so it again underwent a complete metamorphosis and became the final Morgan dream. The loathsome caterpillar had changed into the butterfly and she was witness of the change.

The same latent idea is carried over into the semi-waking stage of consciousness with the hallucination of someone knocking on her door (attempting entrance to her bedroom) and the apparently irrelevant word " Modesty ". The truly unusual feature of the sequence is, of course, that the patient was herself conscious that the three dream formulations were somehow all one.

I once had an opportunity to confirm this theory experimentally. The patient (the same one whose somnambulism was mentioned in Chapter XXXIII) was an unusually competent nurse whose psychosis had been as puzzling clinically as it was baffling therapeutically. Anything like an adequate description of the case would require a fair-sized volume, but the features essential for our present purpose may be given briefly. She was at this time 36 years of age and single. In her late teens she began having attacks of depression, a number of which were severe enough to demand confinement in institutions for the insane. The attacks increased in frequency so that for the previous few years she had never had more than a month or six weeks of continuous mental comfort. What the earlier attacks were like it is impossible to state, but all the later ones were characterized by a gradual onset, with irritability towards women in her environment, followed by compulsive thoughts that she must kill or otherwise injure different people—often her fellow nurses, often a *child*, or all the children, when she had been working in a children's hospital. With these compulsive ideas there began a certain amount of clouding of consciousness. As this last increased the compulsive ideas became delusions—she had killed these people, was the wickedest criminal living, and so on. Sooner or later there was an insistent demand to go away or to kill herself. If she could not do one of these things, she felt she would lose all control of herself. In this state she usually packed a bag and left her hospital or her case, was absent for a week or several weeks, and finally returned, much better, but able to give only a meagre account of where she had been. Ordinary psychoanalytic methods failed, perhaps for the following reason. She had a rich dream life to report and these dreams led to the recovery of many important childish memories plainly related to her symptoms but, unfortunately, significant associations were always produced in a sort of twilight state for which she was largely amnesic afterwards. As a result she was never able to bring her unconscious ideas into the limelight of her fully waking and critical consciousness. Nevertheless, much was accomplished in aborting attacks although no permanent health had yet been obtained.

Once, however (as already related in Chapter XXXIII), when in an attack, she was trying to recall some ideas at my request and became dizzy and nauseated. Persisting in her effort she suddenly went fast asleep, " as though I had fainted ", she said later. This sleep was evidently a deep somnambulic condition for she answered all questions put to her in a dreamy, almost emotionless far-away voice. Subsequently the same state was produced artificially by suggestion—with ease when she was partially clouded already, and only with great difficulty when her mind was clear. Her productions in these somnambulisms were unique. It was apparently a condition in which all resistance was removed and the unconscious spoke unimpeded. She would give with ease detailed memories of significant events and of her thoughts at the age of two and three and, with as much directness, explain the meaning of contemporary symptoms in unconscious terms. In these séances she told of how her father found her little brother (two years younger than herself) in a hollow tree and brought him home to her mother. He should have given him to her, however, for her brother was really the child of her father and herself, and she often insisted " He is my baby ! " Both her parents died when she was three years old but she spoke of them in the present tense, when questions were asked referring to the period of her life when they were alive.

In one attack she had come to the point where she felt an un-

governable impulse to go away. Before doing so she came to see
me. She was too upset for ordinary advice to affect her, so an
attempt was made to hypnotize her. This produced only a mildly
dreamy state in which she said that she had had a dream the night
before of going with somebody who had a baby carriage ; that she
had had compulsions to steal children on the street ; that she had
been thinking of asking her brother (who was now married) to give
her one of his children. Finally she added, " If I could only find a
baby of my own." At this point she was told she would go to sleep
if she continued to think of this baby. A minute later she was
asked : " What else about the baby ? " Immediately came the
reply, in her typical somnambulic voice : " The baby ! My father
gave me my own baby ! " She then gave explanations of her
symptoms. She had wanted to go away to find this baby. It must
be lost. She must have her own child, she did not want to nurse
some other mother's child. After more questions, not relevant to
our present purpose, she was asked to say what she was dreaming.
Her reply was :
      " Crossing Queensborough Bridge—sky and clouds—cherubs ;
there are children in the clouds, playing. I cross the bridge and I
look at the children in this cloud. Beautiful day. I look in the
shops and buy presents for my brother's baby." (Is that all ?)
" Going to the home in the hospital—babies ; their mothers have
gone away and left them. They are my children ! The king comes
to see the children. (Is that all ?) " Yes."
      She was next asked if she would not be able to wait till the next
summer, when she could take a position as head nurse in a hospital
for children, where she had previously been ; if that would not be
better than going away at once. She agreed to this. Then she was
awakened and I asked her at once what she had been dreaming.
Her reply was :
      " Queensborough Bridge—blue and white clouds—walking home
on Queensborough Bridge—something about a hospital or home—
about children—some little boys and girls—nice place—belonged to
somebody—somebody had charge of it. Seemed like they said it
was the king—but we don't have a king. A nice man—he came to
see it—he stays there most of the time—he had charge of it. (Was
he the superintendent ?) " Yes, I think so." (What had you to
do ?) " I had charge of it—took care of the children—part of it.
Had nice things for the children." (Presents ?) " They had toys
—they belonged to the place." (You gave them any ?) " Yes, I
bought them, but not with my money, but with the money of the
place ; it was a nice place. They had lots of money and took good
care of the children. I took care of it and looked after them."
      (On waking her symptoms had totally disappeared.)
      We have, then, this sequence : A dream of going with somebody
who has a baby carriage. The next day compulsion to go away
and to steal children ; in a somnambulic state these are both

explained as the unconscious desire to gain possession of her brother as her child. Still in this sleep she has a dream representing proprietorship of children. On waking she recalls the essence of this dream with elaboration and distortion both of which adapt it to reality, making a sublimation of this wish her professional activity and, with this, her symptoms disappear.

The tendency to distort a dream so as to make it fit in better with normal activities is identical with what we have seen so often in manic-depressive psychoses, when a patient's delusions approach nearer to working sublimations as recovery proceeds. Another example of this may be added, pertinent now because it introduces a " dream ". Celia C. (case 25) in the height of her second attack, spoke constantly of death and sexuality, usually mixing them up. One would expect thoughts of death to introduce religious ideas as well. Yet rarely—she was well observed—was record made of anything suggesting this. Once she said : " Key means key to your heart, gate of St. Peter, death." Again she spoke of not wanting to suffer for her sins in Heaven but on earth. Neither of these has any unequivocal religious implication. A third time, however, she said something about a " religious fight " going on. But this was all. If she were having religious delusions or hallucinations she must have been reticent about them, which would be surprising considering many of the other remarks she did let slip.

It seems more likely that at this stage death meant little more than a queer sexual experience. But, as recovery began, she did speak of religious ideas although dating them mainly to the past. The first indication of this was her evasion of a question about a man who played a sexual role in her psychosis, with the statement : " I don't know, I forget. I am busy studying about Christ." Five days later the following was produced : (What do you mean by " dying on your own bed ? ") " I felt very sick and low." (When was that ?) " When I said that, I just felt sick and lifeless." (Did you see anything, any visions ?) " No." (Never ?) " Oh yes, dream visions when one gets together and talks all day." [This probably was her description of an absorbed state.] (What kind of visions ?) " Very pleasant ones." (Describe them.) " If I were an authoress I would, but I can't." (What were the visions ?) " Lots of angels. I suppose the patients make you think of them. They look nice before bedtime. Little children, they look like little children, in their nightgowns. I suppose that is why you dream of babies." (Do you dream of babies ?) " Oh, I think of things ; of how I would like to have things happen." [She refused to specify this.] (Did you have any religious visions ?) " I know I said things to that effect, but I did not have what you would call religious visions." (What came nearest to them ?) " O, doctor, don't talk about it." Again, " I can't think of any." (You thought you were dead ?) " Yes, I remember that."

As soon as she had begun to gain any insight this patient was very sensitive to the thought of her having been insane : she said so, and the productions just given, suggest it strongly. Some memories of her insane thoughts and experiences persisted, however, so she refused to talk about them, tried to give them a religious meaning, referred them to suggestion from the environment (the patients going to bed), or talked of dream visions. Some sixteen days later she seemed quite normal, admitted having been mentally ill, but threw no further light on her psychosis. She seemed to have repressed her psychotic experiences. But she did say one interesting thing. She had several times dreamed, so she alleged, of a cake, something like a wedding cake, and white birds were flying around it, circling about it.

This is a pretty example of the point I have been trying to make. As she turns more to reality her ideas must either be repressed or re-formulated. In this last utterance she expresses symbolically, one may presume, the gist of her delusions. The wedding cake is sexuality. Birds are angels, and angels are death. But why does she call it a dream, and, moreover, one that she had several times ? She had had many opportunities before to tell of this, but had admitted nothing but delusions. Presumably the delusion had become a dream in her mind ; it is preferable to dream, because normal people do that. And perhaps, in a way, she was right. We shall later have occasion to ask the question : Is a dream anything more than a memory of thoughts and experiences which we cannot allocate to any real situation ?

Three more examples may be given of the metamorphosis of dreams into adaptive settings. The first was given me by a colleague who had turned his attention to possible sequences in his own dreams after I had told him of the theory which I am now exposing. This dream cycle shows prettily the carrying over into the night of mental processes active in the day, their crude, ridiculous expression in earlier dreams, and their reappearance as a bit of serious scientific speculation. Retrospectively my friends could discover three experiences of the day before which seemed closely connected with the dream thoughts. First he had been planning a method of demonstrating to his children the germination and growth of seedlings. Second, he discovered himself, hours later, à propos des bottes, wondering if the stories were true about wheat grains found with mummies still being able to sprout. Third, he spent a long time in the evening telling a lay friend about the work of Stockard, Evans and others on the oestrous cycle and its relation to the implantation of the ovum in the uterus. (The point of these discoveries is that the lining of the uterus goes through a regular cycle of changes and, during one stage only, a small foreign body, if it rests on the lining of the uterus, is enclosed by a rapid growth of cells. These last form the decidua, without which normal gestation cannot proceed, and this decidual reaction is dependent on an internal secretion from the ovaries.) Several ideas appear in these closely connected topics :

the beginning of life, the development of an individual organism, and the perpetuation of potential life during a long period of time, or its possible death. The conversation about the oestrous cycle occurred before going to bed.

Apparently towards the end of his sleep he had this dream or dreams : Civilized man had evolved from his primitive state in this way. He lived in the middle of the earth and the pressure exerted there by the weight of all the mass around him affected his brain, through the centuries, and caused it to develope. It was difficult to describe the actual form of this dream, because he saw all this, or rather he knew he was a witness of what, in his waking state, he had to call a process of evolution. In the dream it was all images. Particularly vivid in his recollection was the appearance of the brain. In profile it was half like a brain without the cerebellum but flattened and lengthened so that it also looked like an embryo, the big head of the latter corresponding to the occipital and temporal lobes. Then, probably half awake, he began to see the ridiculousness of having a brain exist under such pressure. Abruptly a new version appeared : Primitive man lived in big natural gas pockets of the Devonian Period. The gas was under pressure and this affected the molecular structure of his brain, producing a higher degree of intelligence. Almost immediately after this, the dreamer awoke sufficiently to know that these had been dreams but continued to compose variations on this theme, in his still sleepy state.

These thoughts—rather than dreams proper—were all forgotten except the last of the series, which suddenly riveted his waking attention as a bit of reasonable scientific speculation. This was it : A variable time probably elapses between the extrusion of an ovum by the ovary of a woman and the appearance of a decidual reaction in the uterus. An ovum might then be fertilized and begin to divide for some time before it was implanted in the uterus, from which it derives its nourishment. If a long enough time elapsed all its yolk substance would be exhausted and the embryo would die. If death did not actually result, there might be a period of starvation in which the stamina of the new organism would be prejudiced. This might account for differences of physical and mental capacity observable in children of the same parents, for which one cannot account by heredity. Continuing to think about this, my friend next thought that mental influences in a woman might affect her fertility : the glands of internal secretion are all of them modifiable by emotional states ; if the internal secretion of the ovary were thus altered, implantation might not occur, although viable ova were produced. He remembered, then, the popular belief that love matches are the most prolific.

This sequence illustrates beautifully several important principles. That the dream thought was re-formulated several times, each bringing it more into keeping with reality, is too obvious to need comment. What does not appear at first blush, however, is that

it can be analysed in two opposite directions. The Freudian type
of analysis takes us to unmistakeable symbols of generation, the
bowels of the earth that give birth to man. No better example of
" mother-body " symbols could be found, for the later thoughts show
that to be the central thought. From the standpoint of unconscious
interest, preoccupation with pregnancy seems to have guided the
thoughts of the day before, of the night, and of the waking period.

But there is something else here, a scientific theory. What was
the mechanism by which it came into existence ? If we analyse it,
not for its motive, but to discover its parts and mechanisms, we see
that it consists of a combination of what has been learned about the
oestrous cycle with the idea of limited viability of a developing
organism. The secondary theory has to do with the combination
of the oestrous cycle phenomena with another phenomenon, the
influence of mind over body. During the day thoughts about
germination and viability of seeds and of the oestrous cycle came into
the subject's mind apparently by chance. Freudian analysis would
indicate that this was not chance but the result of unconscious
preoccupation with the theme of pregnancy. But they came singly.
Next morning they were combined in a logical theory, sufficiently
coherent to serve as the working hypothesis of investigation, if one
wished.

When did the combination occur ? Apparently it began, at
least, in the dream. There we have the idea of development (in
the dream it was conceived as of a species rather than as of an
individual) associated with external influence (pressure) and of
a time factor (centuries). As it stood, this dream was nonsense
but the germ of the theory was there. It became reasonable when
external influence was re-formulated as the oestrous cycle. But
there was another correlated theory, that of the influence of mental
factors on fertility. This too appeared in the dream for it was the
change in the brain that was going to produce the evolution in
man. Man, however, was not merely a species for the peculiar
organ called " brain " in the dream also looked like an embryo,
that is, an individual unit. Here we have the combination of the
mental factor with the procreation idea. (The profile image of
" brain-embryo " is an excellent example of condensation, by the
way). In the second formulation the mental factor may, perhaps,
be represented by the gas, an intangible agency—but this is mere
conjecture. There was no dream day experience related to account
specifically for the intrusion of the psychic element into this composite picture. But this was not necessary, for interest in the
psychological was chronic and intense with my colleague.

One might well ask whether it was mere chance that brought
these elements together in the dream or whether the theory was
already formed in the unconscious and expressed in symbols that
were nonsensical merely from the standpoint of consciousness.
In other words was the final formulation potentially present in the

first dream and merely translated into sensible language by waking consciousness ? When Freud says that the illogicality of dreams vanishes as soon as it is analysed into its latent thoughts, he is implying that unconscious thinking is logical and sensible. In this particular sequence of nocturnal experiences there is no proof either way. It may simply have been chance. But I shall shortly be quoting some dreams in which demonstration of unconscious reasoning is more compelling.

Although it is not pertinent to our present enquiry, it is tempting to consider the bearing that such a dream as this (and it is not unique) has on the problem of original thinking. An unconscious interest, it would seem, tends to activate various ideas that can serve as vehicles of expression for the interest. Possible relationships between these ideas do not appear in consciousness but rather occur in the unconscious. This is observed, occasionally, in dreams or, perhaps, it may take place co-consciously in waking life as well. This first combination may be ridiculous as it stands, but the substitution of one symbol for another that is, in the Freudian sense, equivalent, may bring about a combination that is not unreasonable. One combination after another is formulated by the unconscious and offered to consciousness. The latter rejects all but the sensible and useful one ; the earlier ones slip from attention and are so completely lost that the subject is aware only of the last.

The explanation of conscious incapacity to make new combinations is that consciousness (in mental health) is rigidly controlled by a sense of reality. The latter, as we have seen, is largely a product of conventional formulae. Thus I believe that the earth turns around while the sun stands still, in this belying the evidence of my senses ; and I hold this view rigidly, although I cannot prove it. It is part of my scheme of reality. In the unconscious, however, (as in dementia praecox with its scattered speech) there is less sense of reality, so that new combinations can be made. An original thinker would then be one who can allow new compounds to appear in his conscious mind long enough to examine them. Most of us are afraid to "let our imaginations run." Of course there is more to the problem than this. As stated, it would mean nothing more than thinking alternately like a dementia praecox patient and like a sane man. Such patients rarely produce ideas of value. There must also be some kind of unconscious interest that keeps building up accumulations of related symbols, some kind of representation in the unconscious of the problem that is in consciousness. Further than this we may not go at present, but shall continue the discussion in the next chapter.

The second dream to be cited is interesting because, at first sight, it appears to be an exception to our metamorphosis theory. As related, it seemed as if the final formulation was a less comfortable one than the first. But the very first associations to each of these dreams gave them quite different meanings from what they had when unexplained by the patient. The justification for considering immediate associations as part of a dream will be made clearer in the next chapter, but one essential point may be mentioned now. All experiences that are individual and emotionally toned derive their peculiar meaning from the attendant circumstances. To take a banal example an ardently religious person, an aggressive atheist and an architect might all dream of a church, and, knowing their different interests we would expect " church " to mean something different for each of them. But, if we know nothing whatever of the dreamer, we would be at a loss to know what " church " meant until he told us. The first association to any element in a dream does not expose really unconscious material but simply gives, as a rule, the meaning of this detail that is already in the patient's mind consciously. For the dreamer, this is really part of the dream.

The patient was an unmarried man of 35 who had never had any overt sexual experiences with women. Like many neurotics he had always rather prided himself on his purity although later events showed that his " Galahadism " was as much related to psychic impotence as it was to idealism. A mild neurosis brought him to me and after three months analysis he was near enough to being well to justify abandonment of regular treatment, although he continued to consult me when anything bothered him particularly. About this time he met a married woman of whom he grew very fond and who seemed to reciprocate his friendship warmly. Probably as a result of the relative freedom from his inhibitions that the analysis had produced, he became conscious of a definitely sexual attraction this woman had for him. In fancy he indulged the idea of leading her into adultery, although he said or did nothing to betray his guilty thoughts to her. In his fancies he believed that he could succeed in seducing her because he saw signs that, to his new sophistication, spelled sexual dissatisfaction in her marriage. As he continued to see more of her and of her husband, however, it was forced on him that she really cared infinitely more for her husband than for him and that her friendship was just friendliness and no more. Having reached this conclusion he began, of course, to feel ashamed of his earlier thoughts but comforted himself with the argument that his fancies were not really an insult to her, so long as they remained unspoken to her or anyone else. This was his state of mind when the dream occurred.

The day before it he had been telling his friend how grateful he was to her for her friendship, how much it meant to him and so on. Not unnaturally the seduction fantasies came into his mind but, of course, he said nothing about them. He awoke the next morning with no memory of any dreams and went to sleep again at once for half an hour. This did not seem, he said, to be a deep sleep, so one would expect to find that any dreams occurring in it would be so formulated as to refer fairly directly to current diurnal problems or interests. The first dream was very vague in his memory : he seemed to be telling someone he had never had sexual intercourse ; or, perhaps, he was defending himself from a charge of it. Following this there were a number of dreams, totally forgotten after waking. When almost awake he began thinking about the first dream and realized he had told a lie. He remembered all the details and circumstances of his having had intercourse with a relative of mine in my house. With this false memory there was a feeling of shame and regret, which persisted for a short time after waking. But, even when the painful affect disappeared, he still had a feeling he could not shake off that the incident had occurred, in spite of realizing the absurdity of this. Several times during the day he recalled the dream fleetingly and each time the aura of reality floated around it. So he came to tell me about it.

At first blush it seemed as if in the first dream he had had no more painful emotion than that of protesting innocence. The last, however, was surcharged with a feeling of guilt, that was far from pleasant. So it looked as if the re-formulation had been in the direction of discomfort rather than comfort—and further from reality as well, for the truth was that his protest in the first dream was justified by facts and the attack of conscience in the last dream was without foundation. This is the reverse of what the metamorphosis theory would demand. But his first associations put the cycle in a new light. We considered the last dream first.

He was reminded at once of the first dream he had had when the analysis began. In it he had been flying off in an aeroplane with this relative of mine. To his mind this had implied such an assumption of intimacy that he had been ashamed to tell me of it for several days and when he did so was astonished to find that I was not shocked by the dream elopement. Here then was a fantasy of intimacy which he had admitted and which was regarded as innocent when told. Further than this, the circumstances were such as to make this a much more permissible relationship than the imaginary affair with a married woman. My relative was a cousin of marriageable age, whom he knew socially and whom, prior to the flying dream, he had idly thought he might marry. It was far from an inconceivable match, externally. As a matter of fact the mutual liking was more a matter of social convenience than of any personal affection. But it was because he had had this fancy of marriage, which he was too shy to tell, that he had at first refused to divulge the dream. We see then that in the last dream he was confessing a manifest falsity, which, had it been true, would still be a less heinous offence than the one he had indulged in fantasy. But why any confession at all ?

The answer appeared in his first association to the first dream. He told at once of the fantasy of seducing his married friend. It is not impossible that during the night he had dreamed of actual seduction but repressed all memory of it. At any rate this was his problem. In the first remembered dream he was engaged in denying it. This would have been a satisfactory dream solution, if he had actually been guilty of an adulterous act, but his "crime" had only been committed in imagination and the dream represented this imagination as known. And this was where the rub came. The day before he had had an urgent desire to tell his friend about his fantasy, in order, so he rationalized it, to explain how pure his friendship now was. But the silliness of this had been too apparent ; he feared that it would be "misunderstood". What he now realized was that he had wanted to confess, because the intimacy such a confession would involve, would be as near a sexual outlet with her as anything short of a physical act could be. This analysis he gave himself as soon as he had told me of the interview of the day before. I demanded that he, not I, should furnish the interpretation ; and this he was able to make as soon as he was forced to think of the meaning of the dream, rather than of its superficial content.

We see then that there is here an almost complete metamorphosis that failed in its last step, which should have been a fully conscious thought, and the reason for the failure was manifest. The dreams were really about the wish to tell of his secret sin to the imaginary partner in his guilt ; to do that which he had refrained from doing the day before. In the first dream he was denying that he had such a wish, which was a ridiculous thing because the wish was actually in consciousness as such. So he makes it into a confession (what he really desired), but confesses something manifestly untrue, or, had it been true, innocent under the only circumstances in which it would have happened. Attached to this second dream was a curious feeling of reality, that was based, apparently, on the real truth, namely a desire for sexual intimacy. The dream then supplied material which consciousness might use for a decision. In fact his conclusion—the end of the cycle hours later—was reached by him with no more outside assistance than insistence that he should discover for himself the meaning of what he had been dreaming. The conclusion naturally was that he should not tell his friend of his adulterous schemes and that the desire to divulge them had been a wish for sexual intimacy. The last dream stressed the fact that confession itself would be sexual. In it a sexual fantasy was made an actuality. Had he been willing to face this fact, he would have completed the cycle before ever getting out of bed.

Decisions reached after "sleeping over" problems are possibly always arrived at in this way, although the intervening dream cycle may be totally forgotten. In the dreams, elements are so combined or re-arranged as to make a waking thought that is a feasible plan. When we worry over problems we always go over

2 K

the trying situation again and again, thinking of it each time as it actually is. Before solution of it can be reached a change in it must come about. Diurnal imagination baulks at any alteration, but in dreams elements are easily dropped out or added. Most of these are ridiculous but one may reappear that represents the situation as it might be in the power of the dreamer to change it. If one has the faculty of being half awake and half asleep, of using conscious critique while imagination is still rife—and people vary greatly in this capacity—then dream metamorphosis may be a useful means of solving problems for a person so gifted.

I have had no patients potentially incapable of this kind of thinking but many of them fail to exercise it. The dreams just cited occurred in a man of more than normal intelligence, one who, in spite of his neurosis, had a stubborn will and was accustomed to force solutions of difficulties either external or internal. He was a person who could, and did, think things through, so that he was able to utilize dream metamorphosis in solution of his problems. The next dream is from a patient of a different type. Although beset by the same kind of neurotic tendencies, he had accepted these without struggle and let himself be a creature of his environment as well. His dream sequence illustrates his passivity, for he used his native capacity for re-formulation in order to protect consciousness from painful thoughts rather than to give consciousness material for their solution.

This dream was produced after three weeks of analysis. The patient was an unmarried man of 32 who lived with, and completely under the domination of, his mother, a querulous, hypochondriacal widow. His father had died when he was five years of age and he had been brought up in the country with little masculine influence. Always seclusive in tendency he had made little effort to conquer his shyness, his few friends were older women and he excused his shunning of men's society on the ground that he had no interest in masculine activities. It is needless to say that he had had no love affairs and he even went so far as to deny, at first, that he ever thought of anything sexual. Physically he was not robust. His complaints were of vague depression and general lack of efficiency, which he hoped the magic of psychoanalysis would exorcise. As might have been expected there was some improvement under treatment but it was as ill-defined as his symptoms had been. He got somewhat better but, in the end, he was as much better as he had been ill. One cannot make a vertebrate out of a mollusc. After taking his history I explained to him that his social ineptitude and his sexual inhibitions were probably both expressions of the same fundamental difficulties, which he would have to conquer together. To this—as to all subsequent interpretations—he said " Very interesting " and gave no evidence of resistance. The first dreams led to explanations of a number of boyish experiences as potentially homosexual. Then followed a series of dreams representing, with greater and greater clearness, his father as a great and terrible sexualized creature of whom he was afraid. Nothing had been said as yet about the Oedipus complex. Then came the following dream :

1. " I seemed to have become aware of the fact that a friend of ours, an old lady, Mrs. O., was living at a certain boarding house, and also that some young woman, named H., whom I knew or wished to know was also in the same house. I accordingly went to the house (probably thinking that Mrs. O. would facilitate my seeing the young woman). I reached the house and found an American Basement house ; I went up the first flight and found the floor reached by it used as a dining room, into which the stairs directly gave. There were numerous small tables around. At one of them in a corner of the room sat Mrs. O. I went over and spoke to her. I think we then went to another table in the room and sat with the young woman, to whom Mrs. O. (I think) introduced me, or, at least, she aided me in speaking to her."

2. Just before waking. " I was in bed and hardly awake and there was brought to me for breakfast half an orange and a whole grape fruit. I thought that in a boarding house I should get only one. I seemed to enjoy them greatly and to take special pleasure in mixing the two fruits and eating them so. I felt, however, that I had not done so before."

Any experienced psychoanalyst would probably recognize the personality of the dreamer from this dream. The first dream could have been recorded, well enough for practical purposes, in these words : " Mrs. O. in boarding house. I go there, American Basement, dining-room whole first floor, small tables. She introduces me to Miss H." Instead of this he wrote out 160 words made up largely of secondary elaborations and retrospective comments. Having been told to mark all possible details in his dreams he does not rack his memory for items like peculiarity of dress etc., but writes out a description of what the scene ought to have been like, what he ought to have thought and so on.

An experienced analyst could also guess, roughly, at what his associations would be. The two characters in the first part of the dream he referred repeatedly to as relatives. Mrs. O. was his mother or grandmother. Miss H. was a cousin who looked like his grandmother etc, etc. Having breakfast in bed made him think of being in bed with his sister as a child. Mixing fruits led (an apparently illogical jump) to filling a fountain pen, and thus to a sexual act. A new experience he referred to being in love ; the lack of such an experience, I had told him, was a sign of defective emotional development.

The Freudian analysis was clear enough and, naturally, introduced an explanation of the Oedipus complex. More interesting to us now, however, is how the dream deals with his real life problem. I had told him that he was too much tied to his mother's apron strings, that he was not social enough and that a normal man of his age would long since have had some kind of a love affair. In the dream he sets about remedying these defects. First he indulges in what was for him an adventure in social promiscuity, going to a boarding house. Once there he does not discover the stenographer from his office or a pretty girl he had observed in the street, as any normal dreamer would do. He gets the plainest kind of a mother surrogate to introduce him to a girl cousin that looked like his grandmother. The curtain falls on their decorous conversation. At least, however, he has made a venture, even if he does not get very far away from home. He does meet a strange young woman and the curtain rises on his " new experience," the second act in this comedy and one with, as his associations showed, erotic symbolisms.

According to our theory the last dream before waking should show the adaptation of the dream theme to the personality of the patient. It does. The patient's capacity for vivid living was well represented by his lying in bed mixing fruits that were brought to him. In the first act he goes seeking adventure ; in the second " experience " is brought to him. That was precisely his attitude toward the world and towards treatment. The world had not furnished him with a wife ; I was going to give him health. It was chance that he had never fallen in love ; he was going to get well by no effort of his own. A purely personal association explained the symbolism of the fruit and showed how the second part of the dream was only a repetition of the first. His home was in Orange County and he always referred to his boyhood as life in Orange County. In Orange County he would have preferred to live rather than in New York. Grape fruit is, of course, first cousin to the orange, but a trifle more tart in flavour. The acidity of the grape fruit he reduces by mixing it with half an orange. Half a mother half himself, brought about the meeting with the cousin. This was the solution that really suited his personality. He could metamorphose his dreams but did not utilize this capacity to produce solutions of his problems demanding aggressive action.

I may add that at the time I did not see the full significance of this dream. It was only on going over my notes long after that I realized how the futility of his career was displayed and predicted in this sequence. From his standpoint the analysis was successful. He got his fruit salad. It is made of a large amount of sweet orange and very little grape fruit.

" MANIC-DEPRESSIVE " DREAMS

We have seen time and again in our clinical material that the emotional reaction of a patient seems to be determined by the specific formulation which an unconscious theme assumes. Analogous variations, in the formulation of basic unconscious ideas, have just been demonstrated in dreams. Naturally, then, the next enquiry would be to see whether emotional responses to dreams would follow the same general laws. They do ; so much so, in fact, that it is often possible to predict the mood that will follow from a dream, when the latter has been related.

By all odds the most notorious emotion connected with dreams is fear. Nightmares are so common and so well known that to quote any would be superfluous. That a dangerous situation is portrayed in nightmares is realized by everyone ; on the other hand, that these situations are symbolic outlets for unconscious "wishes", is not so universally recognized. But I may say that in all the dream analyses I have made (in civilian practice), I have found none, which as a class, are more reducible to plain sexual determination. Battle dreams in the anxiety of soldiers may be shown to have a similar mechanism[1] ; so they form no exception to the general rule that fear is a reaction to the specific formulation which the unconscious theme assumes. The energy of the reaction seems, however, to be traceable to the pertinacity of the unconscious impulse, for the painful affect may linger long after waking—and usually does—although recognition of the innocuousness of the actual environment is complete.

Depression dreams are less well known and hence more interesting. It has been suggested that the normal sequence of dream thoughts is their gradual metamorphosis from a direct representation of infantile cravings, into a setting which is adapted to reality and to the patient's adult ambitions. A failure of this process can be remedied only by complete amnesia for the dream or by analysis of it. If neither occurs there is an abnormal mood during the following day, usually elation or depression. We have seen that a psychological peculiarity of depression is its coincidence with the presence of an idea, ethically unwelcome, on the fringe of consciousness. That is, depression corresponds to an unsuccessful effort at repression. The repressing forces, having failed specifically, seem to become diffuse and inhibit all interest, making the patient inert, and all activity unattractive. Forel seems to have glimpsed the gaseous tail of this idea in his book on " Hypnotism and Psychotherapy " where he speaks of curing depression by suggestions of amnesia for unpleasant dreams.

These principles are well shown in the following dream. It should be borne in mind that a frequent idea of the anxious depressions in the puerperal psychosis is that of the death or injury of a child. This is a particularly painful thought because it is the last thing the mother consciously wishes. Similarly an unconscious urge towards the destruction of the foetus seems to determine many of the neurotic symptoms of pregnancy, which find a convenient vehicle for somatic expression in the unstable metabolism accompanying gestation. (Hence many difficulties in the inter-

---

[1] *i.e.* symbolic representation of a " wish," although in the latter case not sexual. See MacCurdy, *War Neuroses*, Cambridge Press, 1918.

pretation of symptoms which are really neither physical nor mental in origin but both.)

The patient in this case was a young married woman, six months pregnant. She came to me late one afternoon complaining of considerable depression which she felt was somehow connected with a dream of the night before. She confessed that although she suspected the association of her mood and the dream, she had not been able to bring herself to think of it. The dream was—omitting unessential details—that there was some trouble on the inside of her left thigh that demanded surgical attention. When asked what the trouble was she first claimed it was a sore but then remembered it was a tumour. Associations to "tumour" led almost immediately to the idea of pregnancy—another form of "new growth." When asked for a further description of the tumour, she said there was a pain in it and that the pain was like that she felt in an old appendix scar consequent on the abdominal distension of her pregnancy. When she had said this, the depression instantaneously disappeared and she remarked : "If I had only thought of that pain I would have seen the meaning of the dream immediately !" It was obviously a thinly disguised wish for an abortion —a wish that had been neither recognized nor completely repressed.

A friend of mine, a psychiatrist and thoroughly familiar with psychoanalysis, came to me one day complaining of a harrowing depression he had had all day. The night before he had been cheerful as usual. I asked him what he had dreamed and without difficulty he recalled the following : He saw the superintendent of a hospital at which he was an attending physician being supported in trying to walk across the garden of the dreamer's boyhood home. The superintendent fell. He tried to run and summon assistance but his feet were rooted to the ground ; the paralysis of movement was horrible. He awoke with this feeling and it had persisted all day. When to the obvious content of this dream is added the information that the subject's father was a hospital superintendent the motivation of the whole structure becomes plain. So poorly disguised is the idea of his father's death that, not satisfied with dramatizing the collapse of a father surrogate, the scene is laid in the garden of the actual father. It shows what repression can do, that the dreamer, although not forgetting this nocturnal experience, although familiar with dreams producing symptoms, had never been able to direct his attention to the dream till forced to do so. Of course once he thought of it, its meaning was manifest to him and the depression disappeared.

Another example of a depression dream may be cited which is also interesting as a part of a cycle of settings for the same basic idea. The patient was a Swede, aged 39, who had suffered much from an unconscious antagonism to his father, that led throughout his life to unnecessary rebellion against authority and friction with superiors. It is also necessary to state that he had a fierce antagonism to the paternalistic institutions of the "Fatherland" where he spent a number of years studying, and then practising engineering. He appeared one day—this was in 1915—depressed, and stated that the one bright spot of the day had been when he had heard one Italian labourer address his companion as "Pig of a German". The dream of the previous night was this : He was in a boat sailing out of the harbour of Stockholm for Finland with three companions of his rather riotous youth. The captain and owner of the boat had been left behind and some discussion took place as to whether they should proceed or put back for him. The dreamer urged that they keep on their course, and his argument prevailed. In this dream a crime—stealing the boat—is all but directly expressed and the patient is the chief of the thieves. Analysis revealed that the captain stood for his father, the dream as a whole representing his leaving home and using his father's money in activities, largely sexual, of which his father disapproved.

The next day he was distinctly elated. He awoke amnesic from his dream but with the picture in his mind of a painting of a Swedish artist representing two eagles sweeping regally over the surface of ihe sea. A few associations brought his dream to consciousness. He had been flying the night before in an aeroplane over the Western Front, dropping steel bolts on the German lines. Analysis was not necessary. He recognized at once a sublimation of the wish to destroy his father, now represented by the "Fatherland". The flying of the dream had been transformed into something real on awakening but the elation of the sublimation had persisted.

Of easily identifiable affects in dreams the commonest is fear. After that come depression and elation. These are the usual ones ; but subtler feelings also occur. Among these is to be found the peculiar distress associated with subjective perplexity. Manic-depressive insanity has thinking in it essentially of a normal type, because attention is turned either to the environment or to imaginations. A normal person attends to his surroundings and thinks adaptively when awake, or he loses himself in dreams. But he may find himself in a drowsy state in which both processes go on. When he knows that the images that crowd his vision (dreams usually are of visual imagery) are unreal although he cannot shake himself free of them, he is always unpleasantly affected and may be actually perplexed. Sufferers from insomnia consequent on fatigue or concussion are apt to have a long period of hypnogogic hallucinations, which they cannot dispel, much to their annoyance. Or if one has difficulty in waking up in the morning and tends to confuse the dream world with diurnal life, a true perplexity may appear. The following dream illustrates perplexity appearing as part of a dream itself.

The patient was a teacher of economics who came for treatment after the Peace Conference in 1919. During the war he had been engaged largely in looking after interned Germans. The dream in question was produced on the third night after analysis had begun. All his dreams before had turned on the problem of " Authority ". The first night he had dreamed of high and mighty Germans prostrating themselves before him. Associations led, with many over determinations, to the President of his university. The next night he was in Europe supervising new state boundaries, at times he was the arbiter, deciding where Germany should end. Associations led to the development of his interest in economics as a means of wielding superior authority. His father was a business man, but, so far, his father had not appeared directly in his dreams nor associations:

Then came the perplexity dream. He was sitting at a desk trying to sort out lists of names of people who were in front of him, or, perhaps, only their personalities were. He could not make them fit although the conditions were plain enough. It was something, he explained to me, like trying to place names correctly on a new class. Somehow the Germans were in it and it was all very puzzling. He then awoke with the puzzled feeling of the dream, the unsolved problem being in his mind. The main data of the dream were in his mind clearly enough, however, until he reached for paper on which to note them down. Then the dream suddenly faded into the vague form in which it has been given and the patient was left in a state of acute and painful perplexity.

Now this dream and the perplexity can be understood by utilizing certain principles that have been re-iterated in this book. I have repeatedly observed that patients whose analyses go quickly do not dream in any haphazard way. One theme is developed in dreams, night after night, until some analytic solution is reached. There is then a lull, and soon another theme is taken up in the same way. Formulation and re-formulation then proceed, as in the metamorphoses I have been describing, but during successive nights. This patient had begun with the theme of authority, and his jealousy of it. The problem was : Whose authority did he fear or wish to usurp ? Was it a personification of authority or was it a real person ? I had purposely made no suggestions to guide him.

In this dream he set himself the task of solving the problem, which, stated in dream terms, was the fitting of a name to a personality or person. This is an intellectual task. But he was dreaming. Therefore (as we shall see in the next chapter) his thoughts were wandering. Fitting names to people was a professional duty and, also, his last job before leaving the army had been to go over lists of interned Germans with a view to deciding their disposition. So he symbolized the problem in the plural, made different groups of people the subject matter of his effort, and, in addition, had abstract ideas turned into visual imagery. The problem, as I have said, was an intellectual one, but the material was fantastic. No wonder he was puzzled ! Then, to make matters worse, when he actually awoke, the clarity of the data vanished and he was left with a set of symbols which were manifestly different but seemed to be identical. Naturally his perplexity increased. If he had been deeply asleep during this dream the attempt at a conscious kind of effort would not have been present. He would then have combined his data with no feeling of incongruity, but, on the other hand, the material on waking might have looked like nonsense. This dream, however, was not useless ; it did present the problem that must be solved, namely, who or what was " Authority ? "

After noting down the apparently useless dream he went fast asleep again and then he dreamed the answer. A dog he had had as a boy was capering around. Suddenly it ran up into a tree, turned into father, threw apples and nuts at him, dived off it and ran down with insulting gestures. The dreamer felt fear lest his father should fall and hurt himself, then rage at being insulted. His irritability lasted till after breakfast. In the analysis explanation of the whole story was made manifest. He now told of his fear of his father as a boy, his envy of his father's physical prowess and his zeal to rise superior to him in some way. He also recounted childish fantasies on the last theme that seemed to have moulded his whole life.

There is, perhaps, a psychological moral to this tale. It is the old one of, " One thing at a time and that done well ". Imaginative and critical thinking cannot coincide in time ; they must succeed one another or alternate. The painful perplexity taught this lesson. The patient was trying to do two things at once, so he would not let himself stay decently asleep and dream proper dreams. The perplexity showed the futility of his attempt. He then gave up the effort, relaxed into deeper sleep and immediately the answer appeared. One is tempted to ask : How much intellectual sterility is due to our always making our minds work, and never play, with our problems ? There is nothing new about this. It is the main point of the admonitions against worry in the Sermon on the Mount, which culminate in the words, " Be not therefore anxious for the morrow ; for the morrow will be anxious for itself." It was, indeed, the occasion for reproof of Martha. She " worried " (μεριμνάω) over expressions of devotion while Mary, who chose the better part, just gave herself up to the feeling of devotion.

If knowledge of the psychology of manic-depressive insanity helps us to understand dreams, the obligation is in part repaid. We have seen that familiarity with the mental and bodily state of dreamers has enabled us to guess at what may be going on in an absorbed manic state. If we were ignorant, introspectively, of dreams, we should probably be unable to conceive of mental activity in a subject who was silent, motionless and expressionless.

The illumination of certain symptoms of depressions by the phenomena of dreaming and waking is quite as valuable. It is a commonplace that, when we first begin to wake, we exhibit some symptoms of typical depression—lethargy, lack of initiative and retardation. The reason for this is now clear. At this time we are repressing our crude dreams and elaborating (unconsciously) the themes of these dreams into settings adaptive to reality. When this process is complete we are " awake ". This phase in the dream metamorphosis is also responsible for the phenomenon so many of us exhibit, that unless we get our half-hour from 7.30 to 8 (or whatever it may be) we are tired all day. We seem more dependent on being allowed to have even fifteen minutes to wake up in than we do on being given a definite total number of hours of sleep. We must be allowed time to change our dream thoughts to waking thoughts. The first sign of a developing neurosis or psychosis is not infrequently an extension of this period. As we all know, a certain type of invalid makes this waking state last all day. I have had one patient who complained that in the prodromal periods of his mental attacks he would be depressed till noon, unable to apply himself to any work and never sure whether the environment or his dreams were real.

Precisely the same mechanisms may explain certain standard symptoms in psychotic depressions. We have seen that arguments on quite different grounds lead to the same conclusion ; that the depressive patient is troubled by a surging up from the unconscious of crude ideas, which he is unable, for some reason or another, to formulate in an adaptive setting. Repression or dementia praecox are his only alternations. When repression becomes effectual he can pursue his normal life but before that time he is depressed. It is

" At the midnight in the silence of the sleep-time,
When you set your fancies free. . . . . "

that unconscious mental processes tend to appear most freely. The repression, effective in the day, is withdrawn in deep sleep and the stage of the poor depressive is re-set. Had he not some peculiar defect, he would in his waking period reformulate the tabooed thoughts into an adaptive setting. But he cannot, so repression must again becloud his vision, until the horrid thoughts are really banished. This means that he is depressed in the mornings and better towards night—a regular symptom.[1] Similarly, if he sleeps lightly, regression is not apt to go so far and the task of repression will not be so great. But, if he sleeps deeply, a thorough-going regression ensues and he is worse in the morning. Thus it is that a paradoxical symptom appears : sleep, that ought to be health restoring, increases the trouble of a depressive patient, if it be a sound sleep. This penomenon, although it is of regular occurrence, is not as well known by psychiatrists as it should be. The patients know it, however.

[1] Cassion, in the fourth century, describing the state of one suffering from " accidie," noted that it was worse in the mornings, and suggested that this was the Psalmist's " Sickness that destroyeth at noonday ".

The dreams which we have so far considered are mainly those occurring a short time before waking, and it is these that we have been comparing with manic depressive insanity. But there are other kinds of dreams just as there are other kinds of psychopathtic states. May further parallels be drawn ? The question is undoubtedly speculative but none the less interesting. The phenomena of dreams and psychoses are alike, both being constructed of delusions, hallucinations and queer emotions. In both unconscious tendencies seem to be the dynamic factors. If common causes produce similar results a general parallelism ought to be found.

We know that in dementia praecox we get open expression of infantile sex wishes ; in the benign manic-depressive group these tendencies are in evidence but never with the same directness ; here they are " adultified ". As in real life the infantile object is represented by a substitute, or, if it be present as such, the outlet does not appear in its crude form. On the other hand in epilepsy we have a reaction that leads, in the *grand mal* attack, to a state where there is no content at all, presumably a regression to a period before ideas of any sort are well developed. It may be possible that in sleep we reproduce each night these different types of insanity. The depression and elation dreams I have cited are certainly closely analogous to the content of the manic depressive psychoses. But we know that people do have cruder dreams than these. As far back as Sophocles, there are reports of actual incest dreams. May not these correspond to a dementia praecox level in sleep ? I have had one patient who could distinguish in a vague way different levels in his dreams. One, which he said was very " deep ", was of his mother coming into his bed. Other dreams of the same night which had not this " deep " feeling were adultified versions of the same theme. If we go deeper we would come to a level corresponding to epilepsy, where the content is extremely vague and impalpable, or where there is no content at all, as in physiological unconsciousness, which may perhaps exist in deepest sleep[1].

If there be dreams at, or near, the level of physiological unconsciousness, one would expect the content to be of " feelings " rather than of " thoughts ", and have to do with memories of experiences antedating language or conscious thinking. That is, they would be memories expressible only in symbols, not in words of specific meaning. If something he experienced in early life, before conscious-

---

[1] The mere fact that experiments of waking people at different times have always revealed a dream is no proof of dreams being constantly present. That a dream can be manufactured instantaneously is notorious. (I have known one case where a man fell asleep between two words in a sentence, and had a long dream, although his hearer noted no pause). Now, if a person comes to life out of a deep sleep, that waking process involves some time, long enough for some dream thoughts to be elaborated. In fact, it is hard to imagine an absolutely instantaneous orientation, and if we admit any delay in these perceptions we have admitted the conditions necessary for the fabrication of a dream.

ness, language and ideas have developed, a repetition of something like the first stimulus will give to dawning consciousness a vague feeling of familiarity. The second experience thus becomes a symbol for the first and, indeed, is the only possible way of representing it. In this sense it is possible to " remember " a birth experience, or reproduce it in a dream. The various stimuli received at that time are duplicated in quality, in feeling, at later periods. Metaphorically the latter may represent the former, and it is, therefore, only in metaphors that a preconscious experience can be reproduced[1].

De Quincey seems to have done this in the dream with which he closes his " Confessions ". He has come to the point of describing his abstention from laudanum drinking and introduces it with this dream. When I first read it, it struck me as probably a birth dream, and I was then astonished to find that he followed its recital by references to death and rebirth—data as near to interpretive free associations as anything I have met in literature. It is, perhaps, worth while to quote the dream as he gives it, although the reader should bear in mind that it has probably suffered from a good deal of secondary elaboration and literary embellishment. If one thinks of how a baby would feel while being born, if it could feel, then the feeling which his metaphors give may represent those of the first passage from one world to another—an emotional rather than a critical memory.

" Then suddenly would come a dream of far different character —a tumultuous dream—commencing with a music such as I now often heard in sleep—music of preparation and awakening suspense. The undulations of fast-gathering tumults were like the opening of the Coronation Anthem ; and, like *that*, gave the feeling of infinite cavalcades filing off, and the tread of innumerable armies. The morning was come of a mighty day—a day of crisis and of hope for human nature, then suffering mysterious eclipse, and labouring in some dread extremity. Somewhere, but I knew not where— somehow, but I knew not how—by some beings, but I knew not by whom—a battle, a strife, an agony, was travelling through all its stages—was evolving itself, like the catastrophe of some mighty drama, with which my sympathy was the more insupportable, from deepening confusion as to its local scene, its cause, its nature, and its undecipherable issue. I (as is usual in dreams where, of necessity, we make ourselves central to every movement) had the power, and yet had not the power, to decide it. I had the power, if I could raise myself to will it ; and yet again had not the power, for the weight of twenty Atlantics was upon me, or the oppression of inexpiable guilt. ' Deeper than ever plummet sounded ', I lay inactive. Then, like a chorus, the passion deepened. Some greater interest was at stake, some mightier cause, than ever yet the sword had

---

[1] I have discussed this at length in the Chapter on the Origin of Symbols in *Problems in Dynamic Psychology*.

pleaded, or trumpet had proclaimed. Then came sudden alarms ; hurryings to and fro, trepidations of innumerable fugitives ; I know not whether from the good cause of the bad ; darkness and lights ; tempest and human faces ; and. at last, with the sense that all was lost, female forms, and the features that were worth all the world to me ; and but a moment allowed—and clasped hands, with heart-breaking partings, and then—everlasting farewells ! and, with a sigh such as the caves of hell sighed when the incestuous mother uttered the abhorred name of Death, the sound was reverberated—everlasting farewells ! and again, and yet again reverberated—everlasting farewells !

"And I awoke in struggles, and cried aloud, ' I will sleep no more ! ' "

He immediately proceeds to describe how necessary it was " to wean myself from opium " ; next comes his account of his painful struggles to break himself of the habit. Then he makes what seems to be the remark, interpretive of the dream :

" Lord Bacon conjectures that it may be as painful to be born as to die. That seems probable, and, during the whole period of diminishing the opium, I had the torments of a man passing out of one mode of existence into another, and liable to the mixed or the alternate pains of birth and death. The issue was not death, but a sort of physical regeneration : and, I may add, that ever since, at intervals, I have had a restoration of more than youthful spirits."

From this standpoint, we could describe the metamorphosis of the mentation in sleep as proceeding from waking thoughts, to phantasy allied to reality, to a manic-depressive phase, then a dementia praecox level and finally an epileptic stage. On waking the reverse process would take place. It is possible that the physiological repair goes on only in the epileptic period although great mental relief may be obtained from a brief flight into fantasy such as takes place in a light nap. This, however, pending rigorous investigation, is mere conjecture.

From all that has been said it is obvious that mental health is secured by a completion of this development before waking. To employ the obstetric parallel, the foetus must come to full term.[1] Our final problem is, what may produce an abortion ? A complete answer would, of course, be equivalent to a final settlement of all psychopathological problems, which is an absurd demand. Nevertheless a formulation may be given which relates this problem to others. All psychotic and psychoneurotic conditions are dependent on a lack of balance between the regressive and progressive forces. The same cause which forces regression would undoubtedly prevent elaboration of a dream thought from a crude to an adaptive setting.

But there are in this case specific disturbing influences as well. I refer to waking stimuli. These have received large attention from non-psychoanalytic investigators but have been deemed less import-

[1] *The night is pregnant ; what will to-morrow bring forth?*—Eastern proverb.

ant by psychoanalysts with good reason. Jones has given the excellent formulation that when a dream bears an obvious relationship to the waking stimulus, the latter operates as does the dream day experience in providing a setting for a latent theme. With this I agree heartily. In the light of " dream metamorphosis ", however, one may see a wider importance to this factor than has been granted it. If waking is accomplished before the development of the idea is complete, the subject faces the world with non-adaptive thoughts—which always cause trouble. Moreover, as the setting of the dream corresponds to the stimulus, development is apt to proceed to that point and no further. For example, a painful stimulus may inhibit development further than a painful setting for the dream thought. An ethical censorship may be satisfied but a comfortable, " normal " setting has not yet been reached.

It may be this mechanism which accounts for a great difference between the dreams of men and women. The former frequently remember frank, unvarnished sex experiences in their sleep, the latter rarely do. In the light of this theory a satisfactory explanation can be given. The male genitalia react to sex thoughts by erections and emissions which cause much more physical disturbance than do any analogous reactions of the female. In other words the erection or emission of the male wakes him up while the dream thoughts are still at a crude sex level of development. It is astonishing to find how " praecox " so many emission dreams are, when note is taken of them ; they are not merely sexual, but infantile sexual. In quite a similar way we can explain the nightmare after the proverbial Welsh rabbit. The gastric distress wakes the subject and provides a painful setting for an imperfectly elaborated dream thought.

To sum up : There is evidence to show that our dream life demonstrates not only regression but progression. That there is a tendency for crude ideas to be completely metamorphosed—as far as the manifest content is concerned—until a point is reached where a thought is present in the subject's consciousness that is fully adaptive to his diurnal life. At this point the individual is awake. The sequence of settings for expression of the latent content are analogous to the types of ideas seen in different types of psychoses. Mental health is dependent on the continuity and completeness of this process. If, to use the obstetric parallel, the thought is born before coming to full term, the abortion disturbs the subject and produces an abnormal mood during the day, at least until it can be repressed and a new formulation found. In this way the waking period is the crux of the whole day, if it be disturbed, the psychic processes proper to that time are carried on through the day with disastrous results. In our sleep the strain of adaptation is relieved and we regress to the primitive type and content of infantile thinking, but if we are to be normal and efficient this process must be reversed, we must have developed an adult type and content of thought before fully waking to face the world.

CHAPTER XLIX

THE NATURE OF THE THINKING IN DREAMS[1]

The vision of dreams is as this thing over against that,
The likeness of a face over against a face . . .
Divinations and soothsayings, and dreams are vain ;
And the heart fancieth, as a woman's in travail.
Ecclesiasticus, XXXIV.

IN our study of manic-depressive insanity we reached two important generalizations : that emotional reactions are responses to the specific formulations which the patients' imaginations assume, and that variations in formulation are reached by the process of free association. The first of these conclusions, as has just been indicated, may be true of dreams as well. I shall now attempt to show that the second principle is also applicable here ; in fact I believe that the structure of the dream is dependent, fundamentally, on free associations and that its final form is the result of the fitting in of free-associational with conscious thinking.

The reader is probably familiar with the chief mechanisms which Freud has postulated to account for the manufacture of the manifest content of the dream out of the latent " wish " ; so they may be dismissed with little more than mention. These processes are condensation, displacement, dramatization and secondary elaboration. There are in addition more intricate factors concerned with the shifting of the structure from unconscious to foreconscious levels, but these are not essential for an understanding of the basic principles of his " dream-work " and I have discussed

---

[1] A considerable part of the argument in this chapter is reproduced—sometimes in actual transcription— from my book *Problems in Dynamic Psychology*. When writing this I assumed that some of my views were unique. But, when the book was in press, I was delighted to find an article, just published, that echoed many of my claims. This was a paper by Kiewiet de Jonge on " Dreams as a Manifestation of Lowered Consciousness " (*Der Traum als Erscheinung erniedrigten Bewusstseins, Journ. f. Psychologie u. Neurologie*, Bd. XXVII, Heft 3.) It gives me pleasure to record my tardy appreciation of this work. With nearly everything that he says I agree. He is, however, an avowed opponent of psycho-analysis. Consequently he has failed—so it seems to me—to grasp the significance of dream thoughts although recognizing their mechanism. For instance, he claims that the train of thought in a dream is without a goal, so that actual events cannot be retold logically. This is, in general, true, but he goes on to say that it is like manic flight without conclusion nor sense. Throughout he fails to grasp the fundamental significance of unconscious thinking.

them elsewhere already.[1] *Condensation* is the representation of more than one element of the latent content in a single detail of the manifest dream. A banal example is a name, occurring in a dream, which is made up by combining parts of the names of two people ; for instance, two people, Dewar and Walker, might be represented as one man having the name " Dewkar ". By the process of *displacement* an important element of the latent content may appear to be insignificant in the manifest dream and *vice versa*.

Freud says that the affect is transferred from one element to another. I admit that this frequently seems to be the case, if one takes the dream as related at its face value ; but I cannot confirm it from my own experience after including a careful introspective account from the dreamer. Dramatic emotion may, it is true, be absent from a manifest element that analysis shows to have such unconscious significance as to be central in the final interpretation. But if at the outset one makes the dreamer pick out one element that *feels* queer, striking, or unreasonably insistent in the memory of his nocturnal experience, he will usually point to something that neither he nor the analyst thinks ought to have special significance but which analysis will show to be crucial. It is natural that my experience in this matter should be different from that of most psychoanalysts, because I have for years made a practice of studying the emotional reactions of the dreamer both during and following the dream. *Dramatization* is a term that covers all the means used in translating abstract ideas, wishes, attitudes, etc., into image elements in images of people, objects, places and actions, and these are put into a play. Essentially this is the literary method of allegory or, in the graphic arts, of caricature. Moral attributes appear as noble actions or in beautiful faces, as ignoble deeds or repulsive features, and so on. Dramatization may also involve the intrusion of many details that have no latent significance whatever but serve merely to round out the picture and give it verisimilitude—a process like that of the Homeric simile. *Secondary elaboration* is the change the dream undergoes in becoming part of the subject's conscious memory. Logically irrelevant details may be pruned off, or details, from actual waking experience of people or situations recognized in the dream, may be intruded. I should add that Freud's term, for experiences of the waking life prior to sleep, that are incorporated in the dream, is *day remnants*. He has some complicated theories about their operation that need not be gone into here.

Now when we come to study the structure of dreams an all-important point has to be kept firmly in mind, a fact that seems too obvious to mention, yet one that has been neglected by practically all who have worked in this field. It is that dreams, recognized

[1] *Problems in Dynamic Psychology.*

as such, are memories appearing in consciousness for the first time as memories. If I remember what I thought of yesterday I am recalling thoughts that had a conscious existence and were constructed on the principles of conscious thinking. But when for the first time I recall a dream of last night, I am bringing into consciousness thoughts that were not consciously elaborated. If unconscious processes are different in kind from conscious ones, and if, as all psychoanalytic experience seems to show, an unconscious thought tends to show distortion in its translation into conscious terms, then the very act of remembering a dream is likely to be a process of distortion. So, if what we have for study is only the conscious rendering of the mentation in sleep, *the " dream ", as we call it, exists only, and for the first time, when it becomes conscious.*

This may be put in another way, utilizing Freudian terminology: the latent content of the dream is a theme expressed in unconscious " language ", while the manifest content is this " language " translated again into terms of consciousness. If transition from deep sleep to full waking were a sudden matter the likelihood is that we would know of very few dreams. But, fortunately for psychology and psychopathology, waking up is apt to be a relatively protracted process. The conscious type of thinking appears gradually, so that the mental processes just prior to full waking are a mixture of the unconscious and the conscious types of thinking. At the same time, introspection is gradually being applied, resulting in criticisms of the thinking on the one hand, and memory of the earlier phases on the other.

In studying the metamorphoses of dreams, the conclusion was reached that there is a tendency towards reformulation of dream thoughts as the deepness of sleep is diminished. Dreaming, in general, is regressive in tendency and, as we have seen in the psychoses, the regressions of content and of type of thinking tend to run hand in hand. One would therefore expect that the reformulation of content would be paralleled by the adoption of conscious modes of thinking, that is, that as the dream is expressed more and more in terms of diurnal interests, it would also tend to be more logical in the arrangement of its component parts, and (as we shall see shortly) to contain more abstract thinking and less imagery.

There seem to be five ways in which dreams may appear in waking consciousness. The first is the metamorphosis of the dream into such a logical form that it seems to be really a thought occurring to the subject after he is awake, the second is the persistence of the affect belonging to nocturnal imaginings without there being any memory of the latter. Perhaps these should not be called dreams at all, for there is no realization of there having been any dreaming. The other three have to do with appearance of memories in consciousness which are labelled " dreams ". The commonest of these is the persistence, over into waking thought, of the nocturnal mental processes, still in such a relatively crude form as to appear foreign to consciousness and therefore regarded as dreams. Then there are memories of past experiences which we recognize as never having happened in reality and which we therefore assume to have dreamed. Such dreams appear as a result of association with something during the day; usually we think we dreamed them the night before, but sometimes it is only, " I must have dreamed that ". The fifth type is the result of direct effort to gather dreams either just after, or during, the waking-up period.

Examples of thoughts apparently initiated by the awakened consciousness and of persisting affect have already been given. Of the perpetuated dream thoughts nightmares are the most notorious ; there is no question in such cases of the dream having forced itself on consciousness. But exactly the same thing is true of the ordinary dream, which is told at the breakfast table by the egoist, who has no interest in dreaming as such, but fancies that his auditors will be fascinated by what he has experienced.[1] Dreams that suddenly pop into one's head are not so common, but yet everyone has experienced them. The usual introduction is, " That reminds me of a dream I had last night ". The reminder which calls up the dream may be a stimulus from the environment or some idea occurring in a train of thought, i.e., a free association. An example of the latter has already been given when discussing manic states ; the patient, during free associations to " Epson ", (a mis-spelling for " Epsom ") gave " Epsom, Epsilon, Elson, Nelson ", and then suddenly remembered a dream about a man named Nelson. Presumably this dream had been active coconsciously, when other dreams were being written and caused the mistake in spelling.

I may add another example, which is chiefly interesting in that it shows the effect on a dream of the intrusion of a conscious type of thinking. One morning I remembered several dreams when I awoke and made a mental note of them. That afternoon I walked on a path where I had not been for two months. On the former occasion I had been with a friend who shortly after died suddenly. Suddenly I thought of a dream : My friend's ghost had appeared before me in a cowl and long white robe, and he had a drooping moustache. I was frightened but managed to scrutinize the figure. Then it struck me that there were three things out of keeping with my friend as he had been. He would never have worn any kind of religious garb, in stature he was not so tall as the ghost, and in real life he had had a very short moustache. I said to myself, " This is a composite figure [condensation] therefore it is

---

[1] It is significant for Freudian interpretation that intelligent people will retail dreams, compounded of such banal symbolization as to bring blushes to the cheek of an *apache*, but do it in complete blindness of the meaning which they would see in the dream of anyone else.

a dream figure and can't be a ghost ". Abruptly the " ghost " vanished, leaving me alone and, still dreaming, rather proud of myself. I did not awake, which is important. The emotional reaction seemed to have come near enough towards waking me to activate a conscious type of thinking. This was effective in abolishing the occasion for fear and hence I could stay asleep. Had I been fully wakened, I should probably have remembered the dream. Another point is of interest : I felt that I had dreamed this the night before and not any other night. This conviction was justified by analysis. Associations from the ghost dream and the ones I had remembered on waking led to precisely the same themes. It is possible that I had activated memory of the other dreams (which were on the fringes of consciousness) and had already associated them together. This gave me the " feeling " that the dreams were all about the same topic and hence belonged to the same night.

Examples of dreams gathered by direct effort are the least common, but, for our present purposes, the most important, as they are likely to contain greatest detail and suffer least from secondary elaboration. They fall into two groups. The first are those which some patients bring for analysis. Many of those who apply for psychoanalytic treatment claim, at the outset, that they never dream, or can, at most, recall having dreamed only two or three times in their lives. If one instructs them, however, to make up their minds before going to sleep that the first waking thought will be memory of a dream, before long they will have something to report. At first there is often only one word that filters through into consciousness, or some simple scene without any action, or perhaps merely a waking thought that may be taken as the starting point for analysis. Free associations from these will lead almost always to incidents of importance in the emotional life of the patient, and frequently an actual dream will be recalled. This material becomes more and more extensive until an account of nocturnal experiences, rich in detail, is of such regular occurrence that both patient and analyst forget that there ever was a dreamless period.

How is this phenomenon to be explained ? It cannot be a matter of mere suggestion, as that term is ordinarily used, because it has been shown time and again that suggestions to be effective must be specific. If I told a patient to dream of the Eiffel Tower and he did so, that might be regarded as the result of suggestion. But, if I simply say " Dream ! " the command has produced merely a change in consciousness that makes it receptive to dreams. The latter are a spontaneous and independent production. Up to the time when these instructions are followed, a barrier has existed between sleeping and waking thought. This barrier may be broken down by attack from either side. Ordinarily dream thoughts intrude themselves into waking consciousness, but, in these cases the reverse process must take place. That is, consciousness must make itself aware of the dreaming processes before waking is complete. The dream is then associated with diurnal experiences, while the content of diurnal consciousness has come to include nocturnal as well as waking thoughts. A continuity has been established. So long as consciousness introspects only the logical thinking of the waking state, it will take no cognizance of anything formulated without reference to the environment and to the subject's standards of reality. But, if an interest be established in imaginations *qua* imaginations, the previous automatic rejection of what is " unreal " will cease.

There is an all-important corollary to this. All perception—whether it be of things or of thoughts—depends on two factors, the nature of the stimulus and the earlier experience of the observer. Further, whether a potential perception is consciously registered or not depends on its pertinence for the current interest. (Although different psychologists would stress one factor more than the other, probably all would agree to this as a general formulation). Afferent impulses become perceptions only when they serve to activate residues of past experiences ; what comes into the mind is a blending of past and present impressions. The present sensory event would be meaningless without former ones. This, at least, is held to be true of environmental perceptions. The principle can be extended to perceptions of mental events. From a conscious standpoint an isolated mental process, unrelated to other mental processes, would be a meaningless thing. What its nature may be we can never *know* directly, any more than we can know a simple " sensation ". What does appear is an image or a " thought ". Either of these has its form determined very largely by past conscious experience. Images, with which we deal consciously, are fairly accurate duplications of actual perceptions, or simple combinations thereof. For instance, it is only by an effort that I can summon the image of a rat with a bushy tail, whereas I cannot fabricate at all an image of a rat with a tail the size of an elephant's trunk. On the other hand, " thoughts " are abstract ideas of generalizations, and both are given—with most people at least— a verbal form. Language is a product of experience, so " thoughts ", too, are dependent for their conscious formulation on past experience.

Now it is probable that the process of becoming-conscious of mental elements is similar to that of simple sensory units in being built into perceptions. We see—as has been shown experimentally —what we expect to see and do not perceive the unexpected, unless it assume some startling form. A savage, a farmer and town-bred man will be aware of quite different things in walking across a field. Each becomes conscious of only a small number of all the stimuli impinging on his organs of special sense, and each, too, will exhibit a still narrower selection in his memory of what was there. It is the nature of past experience that determines both the conscious perceptions and the memories. The latter will present themselves to consciousness as images, in verbalized labels for images, or as purely abstract ideas, according to the habit of thinking. This habit governs the nature of introspectively recognized mental experience just as dominant interests have governed perceptions.

If the dream, then, be originally some kind of primitive mental process, it will tend to assume a form in conscious memory that is compatible with the subject's habit of thinking. Ordinarily we admit into consciousness, and retain there long enough to register them, only such data as are adaptive to the immediate situation or are in tune with dominant interests. Furthermore, these data must be formulated in terms such as consciousness is used to, otherwise they would be meaningless or, at least, useless in further elaboration. For instance, one who is a poor linguist may be able to think of his simple needs in a foreign language, but totally unable to think of any abstract problem in any but his native tongue. But, if one develops a strong interest in another language, he can acquire the habit of thinking in it about anything.

This brings us to our corollary. People belonging to our culture and of normal intelligence, tend to cast their thoughts in words and to deal with abstractions, ideas of relationships, judgments, and so on. As civilized adults we have passed the phase of image thinking in its crude form. Hence the primitive mental processes, of which we presume dreams to consist, are not welcome in consciousness until they have been exchanged into the legal tender, so to speak, of consciousness. The more intelligent a man is, and, therefore, the better observer he would be in ordinary investigation, the less likely he is to admit into his consciousness, and retain there, the data of sleeping mentation in their original form. But there is one way in which this difficulty may be avoided. if an interest be developed in dreams *qua* dreams, then data may be brought into consciousness in somewhat the same way as ideas may be made welcome even in a foreign tongue.

This, however, is not an easy business. Until a student gains real facility in the use of another language, he will tend to do one of several things. He may read a sample of it, fail totally in understanding it, and so remember nothing more than " It was German ", for example, which is like remembering only that one has dreamed. Or he may translate it completely into his mother tongue and remember it in that form. This is similar to recalling a dream expressed in terms of verbalized thoughts, judgments, and so on. Or again, he may translate it only partially, retaining some of the foreign words and phrases both in his thinking of it at the time and in his memory of it. This is analogous to the remembered dream that is partly formulated in words and abstract ideas and partly in images. But the latter, like words in a strange language that are totally incomprehensible, will tend to escape memory altogether.

If we pursue this analogy further, we may see how the original form of the dream thinking might be discovered. If one wished to find out in what language a man had read a certain argument, one would listen to see what foreign words, phrases, or constructions might appear in his recital of the argument. For the purpose of determining the original tongue only these imperfections would be of interest, all else would be eliminated. The wisdom or folly of the ideas themselves would be beside the point. So, if we wish to study dream thinking, there is one promising method, that might be followed. We might take a dream as remembered and substract from it everything that looks like conscious thinking and then examine the residue.

Often there would be little left over! Some patients are continually reporting dreams that seem like excerpts from their daily lives (and dull lives too!) so " conscious " in structure that, when substraction of this element is made, almost nothing remains. Incidentally, I may say, these patients in my experience gain little from analysis. They fail to extend consciousness beyond the range of thoughts that have assumed conventional form. Their " dreams " give no affront to conventional standards of morals, propriety or speech, no matter how much they really reflect an essentially dishonest cowardice. On the other hand, most people can remember a great deal more of their dreams than is their custom, when they give their minds to it. To do this with real success it is necessary to have a thorough-going psychological interest in dreams, an interest that has become well integrated with the personality.

Personality may be defined as an integration of the sum total of the reactions of an individual that are peculiar to that individual. Every mental reaction is probably initiated unconsciously, but, before it becomes conscious or is expressed in action, it tends to be modified by the peculiar integration we call personality. This is what gives consistency to the thoughts and behaviour of the subject. If the personality be strong, always selecting, rejecting or modifying reactions, we speak of a well integrated personality. If this control be weak, the personality is poorly integrated, or perhaps, disintegrated. In a poorly integrated personality control of reactions is dependent on a highly self-conscious proceeding known as exercise of will; a well integrated person, on the other hand, chooses his thoughts and guides his behaviour without much sense of effort—except in crises. Such reactions as are thoroughly integrated may function, then, without the intermediation of consciousness, or at least without vivid consciousness. The importance of this for our knowledge of dreaming can easily be seen. The interests that are integrated with the personality will intrude themselves into the waking up period, while interests that are consciously assumed will not. It follows from this that, as we have seen, *easily remembered* dreams will be formulated in terms of dominant interests and occupations, while the *extent* of apparently nonsensical material will depend on how automatic is the interest in psychological data.

I have confirmed this time and again in my practice. I have found that patients will dream in terms of almost any set of symbols the importance of which has been sufficiently impressed on them. This is the reason why the patients of one psychopathologist tend to prove his pet theories in the dream material they present to him. On the other hand, I have found the widest range of material, and the most easily analyzed dreams, in my more intelligent patients who were fascinated early in treatment by the purely psychological aspect of the analysis. (Why most easily analysed will appear immediately). One of these patients was the professor of economics with the perplexity dream quoted above. Another was a physician interested in functional cases, a third a historian, and so on. It is interesting that not one of my women patients have ever given me dreams with nice discriminations as to affect or accurate accounts of how " real " or " unreal " different elements in the dreams were. But, then, none of them developed any psychological interest in the undertaking. Consequently the dreams they (and most of my male patients) reported were usually almost as clear-cut as the first impression of an etching and as unmodifiable as the record on a photographic plate that has been developed and fixed. Yet I believe that dreams become clear and unchanging only when committed to memory or writing. Needless to say I have learned a good deal about dreaming from introspection, because it is as easy for me to think about dreams in my waking up period as it is for a banker to think about money.

And here I should insist on one discrimination being kept clearly in mind. A psychoanalytic analysis of a dream and a psychological study of dreaming may be quite different affairs. The inability of a psychoanalyst to analyse his own dream thoroughly is notorious. I would not claim to be an exception and to found any theory on analysis of my dreams would be to court discomfiture. But in studying dream thinking it is only necessary to introspect at the right time. In this latter work one is interested not so much in the latent as in the manifest content and, particularly, in gathering a great deal of the latter.

If one, during the waking up period, forces his attention back to the experiences he has just been through, he finds that the recollection of one image or set of images calls up another and another, some clear, some vague and elusive. When one is clearly focussed in attention the others seem to slip out of consciousness in a most baffling way. The dreamer seems to be in a maze of moving pictures, he feels that he has dreamed of thousands of things, but to bring them all into his waking consciousness is an impossible task, and that the effort is inexplicably difficult. Finally some items are chosen for concentrated attention, he holds them in mind as he achieves full waking consciousness. After some hours of diurnal activity, this memory may become clear and distinct ; there is no longer that penumbra of elastic elaboration which it had when he first began to think of it. All this suggests that the final remembered dream is only a highly selected fragment and that it attains definiteness only when this selection is complete.

Those who have practised themselves in the art of introspection and retrospection during the period of morning drowsiness are aware of the fact that a richness of detail can often be secured which betrays the significance of the central data of the dream. This is because more detailed memory may abolish condensation and displacement of affect. It is not difficult to see how this may come about. If the awakening, but still inefficient consciousness grasps the details incompletely of two figures, it will tend in remembering the dream to rationalize these data as belonging to one individual. If I see and identify the head of Tom but no more of him, and something striking about the clothes of Dick but no more of him, I am not going to be so silly as to say (to myself) I dreamed of Tom's head and of Dick's clothes. I make up a figure on which grows Tom's head and which wears Dick's clothes. The remembered dream will contain this actor. The associations from his features will lead to ideas about Tom and the rôle he plays in my life, while associations from the clothes will produce similar thoughts about Dick. The analyst will then say, quite truly, that the dream figure demonstrates condensation. But, had consciousness been more active when it inspected the dream process, it would have been more than Tom's head and Dick's clothes ; it would have seen Tom and seen Dick and probably, as well, have observed them engaged in separate activities—there even being two separate dreams, perhaps.

In the same way one can see how displacement of affect may arise. If Dick threatens me in the dream, I am frightened. But, if my clouded consciousness registers only a vision of Dick's neck-tie, I awake with memory of a neck-tie, with which is associated fear. Apparently I have been in my dream afraid of a neck-tie. Both condensation and displacement of affect can be explained by the same mechanism : an inefficient consciousness sees and registers only a fraction of the images parading in the dream, these alone are remembered and then rationalized as belonging together. If, therefore, the awakening consciousness observe more keenly, two dream episodes are remembered instead of one. If the material be sufficiently extensive, the mere placing side by side of the data will show the nature of the underlying unconscious trend without further analysis. An example of this was the curiosity dream cited in the last chapter. Three different dream episodes were remembered : watching the copulation of a cow and a bull, the flirting of two cousins, and her father pouring gasoline into a motor. Had the last episode only been recalled a lengthy analysis would have been necessary in order to demonstrate the symbolism of her father's act.

Not infrequently free associations during analysis will resuscitate these details, which, when secured, may complete the analysis up to a certain point: An example will make this clearer. A patient dreamed of a house with an ash can in front of it, at least that was all that he could remember in the afternoon. He felt rather depressed and knew that his mood was connected somehow with the dream, " as if my hopes were buried in that ash can ". When asked to describe the house he said it was an ordinary New York brownstone front, but his associations led quickly to a particular house in Boston. This was the home of an elderly friend of his to whom he had written only the day before. Then he recalled more of the dream. His friend had come out of the house carrying a piece of paper which he crumpled up and threw into the ash can. Analysis was easy. The patient had counted much on the friendly reception by his friend of some proposals set forth in the letter. In the dream his plans were laid to rest with the garbage. Here we have condensation of the ideas with two meagre images and displacement of the affect on to the ash can. These mechanisms were, however, not present in the dream but occurred in the repression of its memory.

This, however, was not the whole story. The patient then interjected (what the analyst had failed to note) that ash cans do not stand in front of houses in the part of Boston where his friend lived. This location of refuse made the patient think of his boyhood's home and of an incident there. As a very small boy he found in an ash can, exactly so situated, a broken toy, covered with filth, of which he had been deprived as a matter of discipline some weeks before. Elaboration of memories connected with this period gave the dream a deeper meaning. He had looked to his father for sympathy he had never been shown and from this had developed a yearning for friendship with men, combined with hostility towards them, which had gravely complicated his social and business life. Now no dream of that night was recalled which dramatized the infantile foundations of the finally remembered dream, but that does not prove that it did not occur. In fact sufficiently rigorous effort during the period between deep sleep and fully awakened consciousness will usually reveal a number of dreams with pure infantile content. From this we may infer that the incomprehensibility of dreams is largely a matter of the selectivity of memory process by which continuity is established between the imaginary experiences of the night and the real ones of the day. It is more a matter of dream destruction than of " dream-work ".

What, then, is the nature of the thinking in dreams as they actually occur ? By direct observation we can study types of thought in the psychoses and in analogous states artificially produced by hypnosis. These methods are truly objective. But mentation in normal sleep is never open to direct inspection and hence its laws must for ever remain a matter of inference. Psychoanalytic procedures may lead to valuable and practical speculations, but they can *prove* nothing. Our inferences may proceed from data derived at the two extremes of the period of sleep, and they seem to lead to the same conclusion.

When we compose ourselves for sleep we continue as a rule to think about the events or problems which have been occupying our attention throughout the day. Soon the connections between our thoughts begin to lose the logical sequence that is characteristic of diurnal, directed thinking. One may have a house in mind, then its bricks, their red colour, a red flag, a bull, bull in a china shop, and so on. These are *free associations*.

It seems that this is a natural way to think, which we normally inhibit in the waking state because it distracts our attention away from consideration of the immediate problem before us. When our minds " wander ", we indulge in free associations. We have seen that the random sequence, which is so obvious, is random only so far as it is obvious, that is, that each element in the train of thought is the conscious representation of an underlying thought or a series of thoughts which actuate the process, although the subject may be unaware of this at the time. For instance, the associations given above would become explicable if one more were added—equally fortuitous from the standpoint of conscious logic. If the series ended with " social revolution " one can see the sequence as representing the fancies of an anarchist. The house is the home of the capitalist, which should be destroyed, then by gradual transitions come the ideas of the revolutionary flag and destruction of property.

This is *undirected thinking* and has two further characteristics of importance for our present problem. First, it occurs whenever one's supply of energy is low or its application is withdrawn from conscious effort (hence the " wandering " of thought in toxic delirium and idleness) ; second, it is closely associated with one's innate desires and interests (hence the intrusion of thoughts irrelevant to the immediate situation at times of emotional stress). Since what we call the " unconscious " exhibits itself in mental disease and provides an explanation for mental operations of the emotional rather than of the intellectual order, it is surely safe to assume that unconscious thinking is of the free association type. It occurs as the first step in the change from diurnal to nocturnal thinking.

The next stage is that of hypnagogic hallucinations. In this the idea—house, bricks, flag, etc.—are not thought of as abstractions but are actually visualized. This phrase is, normally, brief, or at least seems to be. Soon we are fast asleep. Naturally it is not easy to detect this kind of mental process without abolishing it. We can hallucinate easily enough (as it seems), but to know that we are hallucinating requires a coincident recognition of reality. When attention is turned from the visions to reality, the former are apt to cease. Hypnagogic hallucinations lead immediately over, therefore, into dreams. So soon as attention is given exclusively to the hallucinations, the environment excites no interest in the dreamer unless it applies an unusually strong stimulus. We can presume, therefore, that in dreams there is a continuation and enhancement of the free association process, each item of which is hallucinated.

We have already discussed the final product of nocturnal activity as it is presented to us in remembered dreams and concluded that these were only distorted selections of an almost endless riot of hallucinations. In the period of half-waking of which we have spoken, when it is possible with effort to recall many dreams, it may be observed that one dream or dream event calls up another or merges into it. The process seems to be the same essentially as that of free association and sometimes the associated memories become vivid, they turn to visions and the observer becomes a dreamer once more. He has gone asleep.

This is regression of consciousness following a regression in ideational content and it has clinical parallels. I once studied intensively the case of a patient who had been a " drug fiend ". Forced abstinence induced a delirium with a most extensive and interesting content. When first brought to the Psychiatric Institute, this delirium was continuous ; he was living solely in his imaginary environment and was consequently completely disoriented. But after a few weeks, interruptions occurred in which he realized where he was and could give a fairly detailed history of his life. Then a curious phenomenon was observed. If he were asked about any of the delusions and hallucinations from which he had been suffering, he would begin to talk about them objectively. But, as he went along, they would become more " real " to him, remembered psychotic experiences became vivid once more, again he hallucinated, lost contact with the environment, spoke with a crooning intonation characteristic of his delirium and was, in fact, in precisely the same state as when admitted to the hospital.

Another example of this kind of regression has already been mentioned in the last chapter : this was the patient with somnambuilsms, at first spontaneous and then reproduced by suggestion. But sometimes I could not hypnotize her by direct command. If then, I told her to think of her (imaginary) lost baby, she would think herself into a condition in which the imagination became real. This was a somnambulism, different, apparently, from ordinary sleep and dreaming by her maintenance of the capacity for answering questions and in its being produced at times artificially. She had, however, showed this phenomenon long before definite somnambulism appeared. When giving free associations of real significance she was prone to speak in a dreamy voice, and I found to my discomfiture that if I attempted to interpret her dream or symptom on the basis of these associations, she was completely amnesic for the latter. A dream-like state had been induced merely by the thinking of thoughts that belonged to her sleeping and not to her waking life.

I once saw a case in which this mechanism was exhibited, apparently in a peculiar attack of " unconsciousness ". The patient was a man who complained of chronic depression but was really troubled by perverse sexual desires (to which he often yielded) and various mild compulsions in thinking and speaking. His " depression " was simply a worry about his symptoms. Years before, when he had attempted to repress his sexual impulses by strenuous effort of will, he had got himself into a condition of extreme absent-mindedness that resulted in temporary losses of orientation. A psychoanalyst who was treating him explained that a number of his symptoms were sadistic in origin. The patient realized that this was true and that it meant he had to get rid of his sexual inclinations. Then he had a dream representing almost transparently his being killed by a perverse act. The next morning he was sitting at his desk thinking about this dream when he began to feel as if he were losing consciousness under a general anaesthetic. He tried to distract his mind with different pieces of work, but could not. So he decided to go for a walk. By the time he reached the door he felt he was going to collapse, and called to an assistant. The latter made him sit down again and gave him some whisky. Soon his eyesight began to be dimmed. His assistant supported him to a sofa. He remembered lying down but nothing more for an hour. (He seemed to be in a normal sleep). On waking his eyesight was still misty, so he walked home on the arm of his assistant. Once there he half dozed for several hours and then felt relatively well. Only relatively, however, because although free from urgent sex thoughts, he was very absent-minded, forgot appointments, made *mal apropos* remarks, and so on. Physical examination failed to reveal the slightest abnormality, as was to be expected, for the whole story is typically psychogenic. Apparently he did succeed in dissociating his troubles to some extent. Then there was a dream of dying, in which he became absorbed, so that sleep of a hysteric type ensued. After that he was in a state half dissociated, half absorbed. Needless to say the patient had a highly psychopathic constitution.

The next point to consider is that there is a great difference between the content of the hypnagogic associations of hallucinations and the remembered dream visions. The former are more or less like ordinary conscious thoughts having to do with commonplace objects and events and, moreover, the superficial sense connection between any two is more or less obvious. The latter, however, may be fantastic in extreme and the pictures succeed one another in an apparently lawless manner. This difference may give us some suggestion as to what happens during sleep.

We may derive some help here from the phenomena of free associations as they appear in the course of psychoanalytic treatment. We find that the latent unconscious ideas are nearest to open expression when the transition from one association to another is superficially senseless. So long as the connection is logically sound the critique of rationality, which we normally impose on our thinking, is operating to inhibit emotionally urgent but irrelevant thought. Examples may clarify this. If John Doe associates to the word " yellow " by the words " ochre, paint, linseed oil, flax, spinning, weaving, tapestry ", etc., anyone can see the connection between the ideas expressed and they are not necessarily bound together by any emotional complex. But, if he jumps from " yellow " to " Mary ", he alone can explain the connection, which turns out to be that there were intermediate associations of " yellow dress and yellow dress of Mary ", which passed so quickly through his mind that he gave no attention to them. If numerous other words lead to similar short-circuiting to " Mary ", we presume that he has a " Mary complex " (or more correctly a " Mary sentiment " since his interest in the knowledge of her is conscious), i.e., a group of ideas about Mary that are cemented together by his interest in her. The mention of any word which represents one of her characteristics or an event with which she was connected will serve to recall Mary to John Doe's conscious attention. But he may also give a third type of association. The word " yellow " may lead abruptly to Philadelphia, a jump which neither he nor his auditor can explain. The analyst presumes some connection, unconscious if not conscious, between these two ideas. His interest in Philadelphia is inquired into. After a few perfectly reasonable opinions about that city are uttered, he begins to think of the Philadelphia dog show. He is not interested in dogs except negatively ; he dislikes them. Asked to visualize the show, he thinks of a big mastiff. Then comes a memory long absent from consciousness. When a little boy, visiting Philadelphia, he was terrified by a big yellow mastiff, the origin, apparently, of his hatred for dogs. This important discovery might never have been made had it not been for the psychoanalyst's attention being directed to an extremely illogical association.

Similar conclusions may be reached more easily and directly by examining the speech of many cases of dementia praecox. When their speech is " scattered ", there are many illogical jumps which the patients themselves will often explain on request, for it is an essential peculiarity of this disease that (as has been mentioned before) both as to content and type of thinking, unconscious mental processes are allowed relatively free of expression. For instance, a patient may say " He stuck his knife into the door and she had a baby ". Ask him what knife is and he will say without hesitation " penis " and as unreservedly explain the door as " vagina ". For him the unconscious interest in " penis " is as well expressed by the symbol as by the real word for it. The illogicality disappears so soon as a translation can be made into the ideas which are symbolized.

From such studies we assume that sequential ideas, logically unconnected, are the conscious representations of unconscious ideas, which they symbolize. The underlying ideas may be progressing in a perfectly logical way. Ideas are united then in three ways—consciously (logically), unconsciously (illogically), or both. The more potent is the unconscious connection, the less logical does the sequence appear.

Applying this principle to what is gathered by retrospection of nocturnal experience, we can see that the series of visions we call dreams are hallucinated free associations that differ from those occurring during the induction of sleep merely in that unconscious links bind them more exclusively than in the hypnagogic state. When the thoughts symbolized in these visions are dragged into the critical light of common day, we find that they are usually of a type which is unfit for conscious entertainment, they are adaptable neither to real life nor to the moral code of the dreamer. They are the kind of ideas which are repressed into the unconscious. We thus have a second reason for presuming that the basic elements of dreams are unconscious : not only are they mental processes of an unconscious type but the ideas thus elaborated are also of the unconscious order.

It will be noticed that nothing has been said about the " day-remnants ". It is questionable whether they have anything to do with dreaming as such. That experiences of the day are reflected in dreams we remember the next day is probably the most universally known phenomenon of dreams. Everyone who has given the most fleeting attention to them knows that. If our view that dreaming is simply unconscious thinking be a sound one, the latent content of the remembered dreams is dependent on the nature of the current, unconscious thoughts. It appears that the path from consciousness to unconsciousness is always open : to use an anthropomorphic figure of speech, it seems that the unconscious knows everything that consciousness does, while the reverse is far from true. Consequently any experience during the day may have enough latent significance to divert unconscious thoughts into some specific channel. When sleep comes this train of thought is continued and is dramatized in countless images, with hallucinatory vividness. On waking, as we have said, there is an effort to adjust the remembered dream with reality, so the formulation which contains elements repeating the day experiences is selected.

Theoretically then there is no a priori reason to expect an invariable appearance of day remnants in dreams. The unconscious may be working away at some train of thought started many days or even weeks before. And, indeed, experience shows this to be true. We not infrequently are given dreams by our patients from whom it is impossible to elicit any evidence of the day's experience having entered into the themes of the night's unconscious performances. When I say " any evidence ", I mean any direct and compelling evidence. During analysis the patient may refer to day thoughts symbolically related to the themes in question, but it seems simpler and more logical to relate these to the undercurrent of unconscious thought than to regard them as building blocks in the subsequent dream.

At this point of my argument it may be well to insert a dream that illustrates how the successive items in a dream may be simply free associations. The patient was a gynecologist who had been engaged to a girl for some months ; then she broke with him utterly at the insistence of her father, so he suspected. Always with a neurotic tendency, this blow resulted in a reactive depression, for which he sought treatment. One of his symptoms was a wish to die that never reached the proportions of a sturdy suicidal impulse, but was more a subject for sentimental, melancholy pre-occupations. These in turn led to his speculating in a hypochondriacal way on every little ache or pain on the one hand, and, on the other, made him anxious about accidents. A few days before the dream he had a letter from an ex-patient of his, a Miss Roberts. He had operated on her a year before and she had thereafter become insane (apparently) and had developed the delusion that he had removed her sexual organs. In her letter she threatened him with legal action, and, if that were ineffective, with physical violence. He did not wish to go into court with all its notoriety and as little to have her confined as insane, for that was as certain to mean notoriety. Therefore he was fearful of being shot, with the anxiety that all people have who desire death only in a sentimental way. I should add that in his conscious mind death meant nothing but retreat from his trouble.

At the time of the dream he was at a house-party in the house of a man named Robb. Robb's father was very ill, and, if he died, the house-party would be broken up, so this illness was in the minds of all the guests. On the day before the dream the patient had got himself into a panic when walking, over the thought that he might slip on the hill where he was and fall down. He had also a slight pain in the left side of his chest. It set him thinking of tuberculosis and how that would mean his abandonment of his practice and going South—a comfortable invalidism. That would be better than arteriosclerosis and death from heart failure. His mother had died with arteriosclerosis and he was convinced that he would end with the same disease. He awoke the next morning with the following dream :

He heard that Mrs. Robb, the mother (not the father) of his host, was dying of heart disease. Then he was with her ; she turned into his own mother, who told him it was lung trouble. (This was visualized as a lesion in behind the heart, just where his own pain was). He took her in his arms. She was fainting, so he had to support her. Then he felt his own consciousness going, and this scene ended with his feeling himself falling backwards. Next he was sitting at a table with Mr. Robb (senior) and they were discussing some peculiar note-paper that was there. (All the details of this talk were gone on waking). While seated at the table he put his hand to his head and felt it moist, as if blood were oozing from a cut in the scalp. At this point he remembered having been hit on the head earlier in the night (or rather earlier in that period of time when the dream action was going on). He knew his skull was fractured ; there was actually a hole in the bone ; brain substance was beginning to protrude. Cerebro-spinal fluid was escaping and he knew that if much more ran out he would lose consciousness. He must maintain it or he would die. People came running up and he had just strength enough to say " Get Cushing to operate ". When consciousness had almost ebbed away, he woke up.

The reader can probably analyse this dream completely when given the meaning of the note-paper. It was of a peculiar kind and the dreamer knew it only in one connection. It was what his fiancée had always used in writing to him. This symbolized the cause of all his trouble ; a letter from his fiancée really dictated by her father (represented in the dream as Robb senior). To get away from his trouble he wanted to die, and all the action of the dream concerned his death. But the really important element in the dream, psychoanalytically, was the appearance of his mother. He and she were dying together. This element of positive attraction in death had never entered his conscious mind.

Our present interest, however, is in the structure of the dream. Without one element being omitted, the various ideas could all be written out so as to represent free associations. Even the images might occur in a day dream or in the train of thought of a visualist ; their vividness alone is characteristic of dreaming proper. We could then translate the dream into these free associations : Mrs. Robb is dying of heart disease—my mother died of it—I am going to die too of my mother's disease—but I have lung trouble —perhaps my mother has—I will die with her—when I die I will lose consciousness—I want to die because my sweetheart's father made her break her engagement. One can lose consciousness from a blow on the head. Then follows a series of images (and a few abstract thoughts) that illustrate beautifully pure free associations developing the theme, " Loss of consciousness from head injury " : my scalp has been cut—I must have received a blow—my skull is fractured—there is a hole in it—brain substance and fluid are coming out—I will faint if I get no assistance—assistance is coming—but laymen are no use—a brain surgeon is the only man who can help.

This much is presumably clear, but two points deserve comment. The first is the way in which two bits of reasoning are treated in the dream structure. The thought " I want to die because I am jilted ", is dramatized as *a* father (who may interfere with other plans), showing his fiancée's paper. Then the problem, " I can't have a head injury without being hit " is solved by inventing an earlier dream in which that occurred. (The patient was totally unable to recall any other details of this allegedly separate dream). The second point is the way the waking type of thinking is intruded, withdrawn, and then reappears. Everything was imaged and without emotion up to the point when he felt himself falling with his mother. Then, so he told me, he became vividly self-conscious and rather fearful. This induced a more diurnal thought—his conscious reason for wanting to die. But, naturally, this reason led to many thoughts about his love affair, so consciousness sinks again as he is absorbed in a long dream, most of which was forgotten, and in which condensation occurs in what is remembered (confusion of the two fathers, who very well may have figured separately in the actual dreaming). Then thoughts return to death, portrayed as the result of injury to the head. Everything from there on is pure free-association and purely imaginal up to the point where the injury is (to the consciousness of a surgeon) a very serious one. This activates logical thinking, so there ensues a judgment that consciousness will lapse but can be maintained by effort and that appropriate surgical treatment must be undertaken. On awaking the patient felt his head immediately, and, finding it intact, had no fear whatever. He set about collecting the data of the dream to report to me.

In all branches of psychology one deals with two sets of factors which it is rarely possible to consider separately. They are on the one hand, the reactions of the organism to the environmental stimuli, which are too complicated to be regarded as mere reflexes ; and, on the other, the processes, purely mental, which go on in apparent independence of stimuli. One of the unique features of most dreams is that they proceed unaffected by outer events. They are—or seem to be—mental processes pure and simple. But, as everyone knows, a strong enough stimulus may wake the dreamer, and, before this occurs, it may change the flow of the images or thoughts, that are in progress. The commonest interruption of this kind is a loud sound or one for which the subject is instinctively attuned (as, for instance, the baby's cry to a mother, or the doctor's bell to the physician). Other such stimuli are flies settling on the face, too many or too few bed-clothes, or visceral disturbances. Any one of such stimuli may act in precisely the same way as a day experience in starting a train of unconscious thought and hence appear in some form in the remembered dream. Some authors (the most recent is Lydiard Horton) have laboriously " proved " that dreams are simply expressions of bodily sensations. The experience, even of the layman, is so much at variance with this view that it seems unnecessary to discuss it.

The problem of " diagnostic dreams " deserves comment at this point, however. How is it that one can dream of a somatic disturbance when it is too slight to be recognized consciously ? Nicoll and Riddoch[1] have observed, for instance, that the patient with a complete lesion of the spinal cord does not dream of being paralyzed,

---

[1] *Personal Communication.*

which the man with the partial lesion does. This difference is noticeable before there is any return of conscious sensibility in the legs. It should be noted that the afferent impulse in all such cases does not appear in the dream as it would if it were consciously recognized. It is not registered in accurate terms but symbolically as a rule. This supports the view that the threshold for definite sensations and perceptions is higher than for indefinite ones ; that a stimulus may be strong enough to be registered unconsciously and appear improperly described in consciousness but cannot be specifically recognized by consciousness until it becomes stronger. This is, of course, nothing new. Twenty-five years ago hypnotists did a great deal of work on this subject—Boris Sidis probably performed the most exhaustive experiments—and showed that the range of sensibility (like that of memory and efferent impulses as well) was much wider unconsciously than consciously. (It is to this that suggestion owes its effectiveness in therapy.)

The frequent failure in psychoanalytic treatment to resuscitate infantile memories the existence of which is repeatedly indicated in dreams may be explained by this principle. The memory is present unconsciously and may be potent there, but it does not exist in such an exact and detailed form as will enable it to enter consciousness. (It should be remembered that children are several years old before they are capable of recalling voluntarily and in detail what happened even the day before. Yet their experiences obviously make impressions and produce specific reactions. Consequently it is only to be expected that events from this period of life would be recalled as reactions rather than specific memories.)

Another corollary has to do with waking stimuli. The threshold for external sensory stimuli is certainly raised during sleep. It is possible that stimuli which would be well over the threshold in the waking state may merely give direction to unconscious mental processes until the strength of the stimulus is such as to be *accurately* registered by the sleeper. It then crosses the threshold and becomes a waking stimulus. In this sense waking is simply the accurate recognition of external stimuli. The reverse would be true of falling asleep, which could be said to take place at that point where the impinging stimuli are not recognized clearly but distorted or neglected.

There are probably three conditions that must be fulfilled before a visceral disturbance can be interpreted in dream imagery. First, it must be strong enough to produce afferent impulses that can cross the unconscious threshold. (The various processes of digestion, for instance, that certainly involve reflexes in the involuntary nervous system, do not normally affect dreams at all). Second, the stimulus must not be strong enough to cause pain. (If there be pain, which does not awaken the sleeper, it is registered as pain, and the dream imagery rationalizes it—a blow, a wound and so on—but does represent it as a pain). Third, consciousness must not be roused to the waking point.

This third condition requires discussion. Consciousness is a function that is bound up with discrimination. It may be activated but not reach the point of capacity for accurate discrimination and then curious mental states are induced. Self-awareness is present, the subject feels and knows he feels, but is unclear about what he feels. Any reader who has been operated on under a general anæsthetic will know what I mean, provided he be interested in introspecting his unusual states of mind. Under these circumstances, a persistent stimulus from the body may seem, somehow, to come from the environment, or one may be uncertain which is body and which bed. A clear consciousness is always striving to keep one actively aware of the environment, and it is essential that the feeling of self should be sharply discriminated. If consciousness be dulled, however, the discrimination between the body and its surroundings may be ill-defined. But, if there be self-awareness, there is a desire to feel oneself as an individual ; hence the personality may seem altered. This dubiousness may exist on first waking, before the process is complete. If the subject has been dreaming, he may mingle the real and imaginary environments and be disoriented. He may even think, or rather feel, that he is somebody else. Or, if there be some visceral disturbance, he may suffer from dis-orientation as to self. It must be borne in mind that visceral impulses are not localizable by consciousness and tend to be referred towards the surface of the body as pains. If less acute than pains they produce a vague unrest. The tendency to project the sensation exteriorly is probably still present, but is inhibited by conscious recognition of the actual environment and the consequent knowledge of the absence of cause for feeling anything on the surface of the body. But, if consciousness be dull, this inhibition may be lacking so that stimuli seem to come from the body, and the environment at the same time. Thus curious distortions of personal and bodily personality may result.

The following notes illustrate this well. I am indebted for them to a colleague, a psychiatrist doing laboratory work, who thought his experience might have some psychological interest and so made notes of it. I give these notes in his own words :

" Sunday, the 16th of July, ate two Frankfurter sausages and drank a glass of beer in the afternoon. Felt well, slept well all night. Got up on the 17th feeling all right. In course of forenoon, abdominal pain, with slight diarrhoea. About 10, sal hepatica. Then kept having much abdominal pain, many little movements. About noon, lay down. On getting up felt much abdominal pain, pain worse, went to have a movement, had a slight one. Now sweating, feeling of collapse, things got dark, went round and round, distinct feeling of anxiety as of impending death. Did not lose consciousness. Bowel movements all afternoon, with blood.

" Went to bed at 8.30.   Slept well.

" Woke up. not clear when.   At any rate I felt awake. Without getting out of bed, looked out of the window, recognized the sides of the house, saw the moon—but I had no consciousness of being a person—an uneven surface squirming around and spreading all over the bed—and I felt it was a terrible mix-up and I could not get straightened out in any way.   I tried to get some lines into it, some direction, but I could not get it into any lines, it was all this mixed-up, uneven muss.   I was moving, I think.   At this point I began to think of bodily delusions, and whether patients had such feelings.

" Then I got up, which quite convinced me I was fairly awake. I went back to bed.   After a while things began to get in groups or lines.   I was not so diffusely spread all over the bed, it was collections of muss rather than a diffuse muss, but I was not any-- thing yet.   Then I think I dozed off ; at any rate, I am less clear about my feelings for a while.   Then I became aware once more of my spread-out body, but I found my legs first getting into more definite shape, and soon after that I became conscious of having my usual form.   All this time no abdominal pain, except that condition which was quite distressing and bothered me considerably.

" I have no idea how long it lasted from the time I awoke until I got assembled, because I do not know how long I dozed in between. In guessing I might say that the whole thing might have occupied an hour.   No further experience like it, and intense waking up in the morning."

The last matter to be considered is the most difficult, but perhaps the most interesting of all.   It is the nature of the mental processes. which are expressed in the images recalled as dreams.   The reasoning or judgment of a conscious order, expressed (or directly expressible) in words, that occurs in the waking-up period, offers no theoretic difficulty.   We can look on it as the work of a consciousness which is awakening although not yet dominant.   But, unless all of Freud's work on dream interpretation is to be discarded, it must be admitted that there is a meaning in the apparently senseless jumble of images constituting the bulk or entirety of many dreams. It seems as if ideas or thoughts were being expressed in a " language " that was not foreign nor strange to consciousness but, rather, had an entirely different meaning from that determined by analysis.   I have frequently fallen into the temptation in these chapters of using the terms " thought " or " idea " to label what should be called merely " unconscious mental processes ", unless one is to prejudge a question with wide theoretic implications.   Another view could easily be maintained and one fitting well with my theories of dream construction.

It could be argued that the juxtaposition of different images, which have symbolic significance, might be ascribed to the mere chance of free association, and that the relationships and judgments.

thus represented appear, for the first time, when the dream is analyzed. For instance, one could say that the scientific theory which ended the cycle in the evolutionary dream cited in the last chapter, was the product of conscious reasoning, and that it was only accident which brought the latent thoughts of time intervals and embryological stages together in the first dreams. On this theory, reformulation of the symbols did not break up this chance relationship, although it did produce something which a fully awakened consciousness could grasp. According to this view, then, the conscious mind is the only one that reasons. When the unconscious throws two symbols together, the relationship of their latent meanings may be logical or illogical, and, on the theory of probability would usually be illogical and useless. Consciousness, then, could profit only by the rare accidents that brought together symbols, useful in combination, and the new idea formed by this combination would exist only when consciousness had grasped it as such.

The alternate view is as follows : If there be two objects or thoughts, known to consciousness as a and b, they would be represented in the unconscious language of symbols as x and y. According to the second view, x and y would be put into relationship in the dream in virtue of the relationship ab, which has never existed in consciousness and, moreover, never in the unconscious as ab but only as xy. In other words, the thought is ab for consciousness and xy for the unconscious and therefore has a functional value, which we might call ab apart from the formulation which it assumes. Whatever may be the philosophical implications of this conception, I think it must be adopted in dealing with dreams. No one can analyse dreams habitually and escape the conviction that the unconscious can reason. This, however, does not prove that it always does. Chance may determine the relationship established between symbols in many dreams. Indeed, it is possible that differences in intellectual fertility between different people may be reducible to relative capacities for unconscious fabrications of logical relationships.

But in adopting this second view we collide with an equivocation in nomenclature. Psychology began with introspective data and most of its terms refer, inevitably, to conscious phenomena. An idea or thought for psychology, *qua* psychology, is a subjective experience ; no matter whether there be entities having similar properties operating outside of awareness, either " idea " or " thought " is bound to suggest conscious experience. (This rationalizes much antagonism to psycho-analysis, by the way.) F. C. Bartlett has suggested a term for these unconscious processes which gets around the difficulty : he would call them " idea-functions ", which implies nothing as to their nature or their state of consciousness but merely states that they work. This term is worthy of adoption, I believe.

The following is a good example of unconscious reasoning as exhibited in dreams. Most of the examples coming to the daily attention of psychoanalysts are unsuitable for quotation as they represent judgments about personal matters that would be incomprehensible without tedious introduction. In this dream however, we have a simple example of medical reasoning presented, in true dream language. I should add that it was only a fragment from a long dream, the general trend of which was concerned with matters of purely personal significance.

One morning I read the following dispatch in " The Times " :

" A MAH JONG DANGER.

" New York, Feb. 11.

" Mah Jong, the Chinese game which has made great inroads on the popularity of auction bridge with Americans, has just been discovered to have unexpected perils.

" Most of the more elaborate sets of ' tiles ' with which the game is played are contained in red and black Chinese lacquer boxes. Recently physicians have been puzzled by the number of cases of dermatitis they have been called upon to treat in persons who were devotees of the new craze. Now it has been discovered that in the lacquer is the oil of rhus vernix, and rhus vernix is first cousin to rhus toxicodendron or poison ivy. The inflammation caused by the Mah Jong paraphernalia is so prevalent that it is the subject of two articles in the current issues of the *Journal of the American Medical Association* by New York and Chicago physicians."

That evening a companion mentioned this dispatch casually while we were playing bridge. But neither then, nor when I read it, did any thought come to me, consciously, about it, except the reflection, too cheap to utter, that it served defaulters from bridge right to be so afflicted. Of course I might have speculated consciously about this dermatitis and then repressed it, but I can see no possible reason for such repression. Presumably, then, the dream was the product of unconscious reasoning. On the other hand, there are excellent reasons for my being interested in poison ivy ; I am susceptible to it and have, on many painful occasions, had an opportunity to observe its mode of distribution on the skin.

Shortly before waking the next morning I had a complicated dream, one incident of which was the examination of some eruptions on the skin of my forearm and hand. Many fine vesicles were clustered on the back of my forearm, and the skin beneath them was slightly and evenly raised. On the back of my hand the vesicles were coalesced to form crossing bars. On looking at the forearm, I thought it might be either eczema or poison ivy. But when I examined the hand I thought, " These lesions are typical in shape and design [or something to that effect] of poison ivy. The whole disease is poison ivy."

On waking I thought of the curious crossing bars and was at

first reminded of the Tudor " portcullis " (this association belonged to the other part of the dream which I have not recounted).   Then my thoughts turned to poison ivy and the subtlety of its essential oil.   At this point I recalled the dispatch given above and suddenly realized that the figure on my hand was something in Chinese characters.   This, then, was the " Mah Jong Disease " of which I had been reading the day before.

The essence of this dream was visual images of lesions on the forearm and hand.   Associated with these were " thoughts " that more accurate introspection told me I had put into words only on waking.   They were much more " feelings " as to the meaning of the lesions, that could be represented for consciousness only in words.   What consciousness, that was intruding itself into the dream, saw was lesions of eczema or poison ivy.   These represent ideas associated with the two images, but they are not logical, for (to the fully awakened consciousness) the lesions on the forearm were characteristic of poison ivy, while those on the hand were fanciful.   However, if one looks for idea-functions expressed in symbols rather than in conscious language, logic is discernible.   In my experience poison ivy affects the forearms much oftener than the hands, although the " Mah Jong Disease " would certainly be on the hands.   While still in bed I realized that poison ivy eruption practically never appears on the palms or the thick skin on the inner side of the fingers.   When Mah Jong tiles touch the backs of the hands (or the fingers that have held them are rubbed on non-palmar surfaces) the toxic oil could reach sensitive skin.   The dream reflection, " This lesion is characteristic of poison ivy," is also nonsense from a conscious standpoint.   But, when the symbols are translated, it no longer is, for it says, " This is the characteristic thing," that is, " The Mah Jong disease will appear on the backs of the hands ".

If one considers this problem from the standpoint of ordinary introspection, the conclusion, that part of our minds, thinks in entirely different language from that with which we are familiar, seems so improbable as to be preposterous.   But a little attention to the mental operations of children and a little reflection on how thinking must begin, will show how the unconscious " language " can arise.   Children certainly begin to show discrimination—and definitely acquired discriminations—before they have any vocabulary beyond that of a few names.   If they discriminate, they must be using past experience in planning conduct, and this is thinking.   Abstract ideas, at bottom, are generalizations about qualities and relations of things.   Unless one is a thorough-going behaviourist and denies mind altogether, one must admit that discriminative planning implies some kind of mental representation.   Such a representation would be an image, and it is likely that a child has images long before he has words.   There are records, for instance, of children telling of incidents which occurred before they could talk ; this is inconceivable without images. We, as adults, still use images ; but for only simple elements or very simple combinations of them. For example, the visual image of a flash of lightning is more impressive to me than the word " lightning ", and I can think more readily of lightning striking a house in images than I can in words. But I cannot (consciously) think of lightning as an electric phenomenon in images.

But a child who has no form of mental representation but images must reason in these terms if at all. Their first recorded impressions are tactile sensations and visual or auditory contact with the environment comes later. Hence the environment is first grasped in terms of body sensations, that is, autoerotism is not merely a practice but a language as well.[1]

Similarly, after representations of the environment have become a vehicle for expression of idea-functions, they can persist as language into the period when words are also used. When images are totally supplanted by words in abstract thinking, the earlier language survives in symbols[1]. A boy I know was, at the age of six, a good draughtsman. He used to draw the objects with which he was most familiar, among them animals. He once drew a perfect outline of a duck but called it a chicken. There was no doubt as to his knowing the difference between ducks and chickens, and equally no doubt as to his knowledge of the names for them. But the image of duck was still all-important in his thinking, while the word for it was a matter to which he was relatively indifferent.

Only to-day a little girl of four and a half years put a question to me illustrating well the development of an abstract idea in terms of what is seen rather than in what is deduced. She sat beside me in a motor and suddenly asked : " Why do the people on bicycles start to go backwards quickly, when we catch up to them ? " She was wrestling with the problem of relative speeds, but she did not know those words, nor could think of any others, so she spoke of what she actually saw. Her brother, two years older, laughed at her from his eminence of sophistication ; but, then, *he* had not read the works of Mr. Einstein ! It is not impossible that the beginnings of relativity were first elaborated in a dream where people went backwards on bicycles or performed some similarly ridiculous act. But, if the unconscious can think logically, why does it disguise its ruminations in this cumbrous, outworn language. ?

Anything like an answer to this question would require a small volume for its exposition. (I hope it may appear before long !) Very sketchily, however, the reason may be indicated. It is the same problem as that underlying regression : why does consciousness ever lose its acuity or lapse altogether ? It is universally recognized that sleep is a resting or repair phase. When the

---

[1] I have elaborated this further in *Problems in Dynamic Psychology* in the chapters on " The Meaning of Autoerotism " and "The Origin of Symbols ".

organism is fatigued, waste products must be eliminated and tissues regenerated. The organism has, then, become insufficient for its most highly specialized functions. In the mental sphere, consciousness is the highest specialization : in demonstrable form it appears only in man and is best exhibited in the most specialized races and individuals. When the energy of the organism ebbs, consciousness is naturally the first function to weaken or lapse. Mental life must therefore cease, for the time being, or fall back to a less specialized type of function. It is a general rule in biology that specializations of functions are developed by the elaboration and integration of more primitive ones—more primitive both in evolution of the species and in the growth of the individual. For this reason, we should expect the mental functions of sleep to be those of the child before consciousness is developed, or else to be non-existent.

Consciousness, being bound up with awareness in general, is a function that is inevitably associated with recognition of the environment. Now our environment consists of things and people (as well as of intermediate groups of animals which need not be considered). Bodily behaviour is the medium for adaptation to things, while speech puts us in contact with our fellows. Consciousness, therefore, is inextricably intertwined with language. Thought-functions, which serve for adaptations to things in infants, anthropoids and deaf mutes, can exist quite inarticulate. A flux of images can serve the same purpose as a train of thought. It may, too, be just as logical. But it can never appear so to consciousness because words take on the function of labels for ideas rather than representations of objects. Images, in consciousness, are never labels ; they never refer to properties, or qualities, relationships. So when we are confronted with a series of images such as appear in the memory of a dream, we think only of the objects to which they refer. But language probably grew up as representations of objects and simple actions, as is shown in the etymology of many of our words. A simile begins to express the idea-function this turns to a metaphor, which is finally an abstraction. For instance : (1) The man is like an ass ; (2) the man is an ass ; (3) Assinity. In a dream the metaphor stage is reproduced (as it is in caricature), so that the man is given long ears or a donkey's body. All the abstract terms of common speech seem to have grown up in this way.

Supposing one were confronted with five detached hands, then a polished mallet lying on a plank across a stream, would that be comprehensible ? But let us translate it into words from images, that is to say, interpret it as Freud does a dream. " Hands " has a number of meanings ; it is a verb and also several nouns, a part of the body, the hand of a clock, a hand of cards. One is as good as another until a context is established. The mallet is on the plank, therefore they go together somehow. The actual mallet seen reminds us of an auctioneer's hammer ; but it might mean many different things. The plank could be timber, carpentry, etc., etc. In its situation, however, it is a bridge. Picking out the meanings that go together, we have the phrase " Five hands of auction bridge ". Playing bridge is a complicated process : could any reader name it (without words) in simpler metaphors than I have done ? The history of material civilization is epitomized in the metaphors, now becomes labels, that we use in describing it verbally. The metaphors, standing alone, as symbols, are meaningless for consciousness specialized in word thinking. But, as we must always remember, the dreamer is not conscious. The silliness of the dream may only appear when consciousness looks at it.

But, it may be objected, all dreams are not silly. Some appear highly rational, either duplicating actual experiences accurately, or producing new ideas logically expressed. This, however, is not at all at variance with my theory which assumes that waking up is a gradual process, consciousness and conscious thinking being gradually intruded into the action. The accuracy or bias of the introspectionist determines the point at which " dreaming " is said to end. If it be put late, the dreams will appear sensible. Unfortunately, there are other, although rare, phenomena that must be considered. What of the dreams in which we achieve what we cannot do when awake ? Such are compositions of poetry and music. As a general rule, if remembered, the composition is of an extremely inferior order. The idea of being a composer or poet has simply been dramatized in images that have not been reformulated to meet conscious standards. It is probably true that Coleridge composed Kubla Khan in a dream, but he was a poet, and therefore his conscious mind, when it made contact with the dream stuff, could transform it into excellent poetry. This, too, is the explanation of the work of Stevenson's " Brownies " the little elves, which, as he tells us, did all his work for him while he slept.

Occasionally, however, one hears of people who really do compose poetry in sleep, of which they are incapable when awake. I am inclined to think that this is always a product of dissociation of an hysterical type. That is, the capacity for metrical composition is dissociated from normal consciousness. It appears then in what is really a somnambulism, technically, although the subject speaks of it as sleep. I have been fortunate enough to observe one such case. The patient was full of grave hysterical symptoms, the nature of which is irrelevant. One only need be mentioned. At any time, day or night, she might go to sleep and then have the most extraordinary dreams. They appeared to awaken consciousness in excellent literary form and—to me—seemed to be the product of several different personalities. (None of them, however, had ever been awakened and so, to speak accurately, hers was not a case of multiple personality). There were also other dreams such as any person has, that were not garbed in any literary dignity. Stock figures appeared and re-appeared in her "dissociated" dreams, characters from history, romance and mythology : she lived (usually as some man) in many different ages and experienced a continuity in time that De Quincey might have envied. Consciously, she could only write the meanest doggerel, but many of her dissociated experiences came to returning consciousness as poetry of some merit. Occasionally long "dreams" would be entirely in blank verse. It is interesting that these memories vanished quickly, if her pen faltered for a moment in writing them down, the word or phrase would go. Her conscious substitutions I could always spot ; they lacked the ring which the composition had as a whole. I have in my notes hundreds of lines of this poetry. One is, perhaps, worth publishing as an example :

> Immortal One !
> Gentlest among the Gods :
> Stretch forth thy dusky wings,
> That under their vast shadow we may lie
> Who desire sleep, the weary who would die
> And know no more of life, no more of pain.
> (The lightning tracks the sky, the falling rain
> Gladdens the springing flowers,
> The wheeling stars circle and ring the void,
> And the quiet night brings rest to all that lives
> except mankind).
>
> Immortal One !
> Gentlest of all the Gods !
> Grant us the boon we crave : of life, surcease ;
> And in the shadow of thy great wings, peace !

Fifteen months later this "Invocation" was answered ! But the reply was too long to quote.

As I have had occasion to remark many times, dreams are only memories, but of what ? Obviously of imaginary experiences. But, if I interrupt my work to waft myself in fancy to the Alps, I do not call that expedition a dream ; and this is because I realize all the time that I really am at my desk. I never displace the environment totally with my imagination. There are two conditions under which imagination can assume such vividness, dreaming and insanity. In the former state an outside observer recognizes the immobility of sleep ; in the latter he does not. But to the subject himself the retrospect must often seem quite similar. Ordinarily, when after a lapse we recognize our environment, we find ourselves in bed or in a chair with sleepy eyes, we assume that we have been asleep. But if, when I was walking down the street, I suddenly remembered that a minute before I had been climbing an Alpine path, I would not know what to make of it—— or rather, *I* would, being a psychiatrist. My inevitable con-- clusion would not be comforting. We can understand, then,, how a patient, recovering from a psychosis with loss of orientation,. must feel. The natural tendency would be to call the remembered experiences dreams. Many of them do, of course, and that all do not so name them is probably owing to the fact that the return of normal consciousness is gradual and accompanied by many evidences of the patient being regarded as mentally ill.

The discussion of dreams may fittingly be closed with consideration of another of my own, because it illustrates almost every principle involved in the theories proposed. It is intricate, unfortunately, but every dream is, if one takes pains to pick up as many threads as possible immediately on waking. Complication was increased by there being a dream within the dream, the secondary one a product of the wish to awake that could not become effective short of a night-mare setting. Incidentally the nature of actual waking is prettily shown. The material may be conveniently divided into five parts.

1. *Actual experiences before going to bed.* In the evening I attended a concert in the rooms of a friend. I was much impressed by the singing of an undergraduate who had recently taken a leading rôle in a Greek play. During an intermission I criticized the furnish-ings of the room with another friend. This man left before the music was finished and I did not move up to take his place, as I might have done. When these incidents had been reflected in the dream I realized, consciously, for the first time, that my failure to take the next chair might have been interpreted as a slight on a third friend,, whom I made no effort to talk to. After the concert I returned to my rooms. First I relit my fire by covering a lighter with coals so completely that it was hidden from view and then set it going by throwing in a lighted match. It flared up almost explosively. (During the day I had had occasion to instruct a servant how to lay a fire with such lighters). I then sat down to read a novel for an hour. The heroine was a girl who reminded me of X, whom I had known many years ago, and also of Becky Sharp. When the hour was up I decided I ought to go to bed although I did not feel sleepy. I found my bed very cold and burrowed under the covers. My almost invariable custom is to lie on my left side till a change of position seems welcome ; I then turn on my right side and go to sleep at once. This time for no reason at all (consciously) I lay on my right side and have no further memories, except of the dreams. It would seem as if I had gone to sleep instantaneously but that was not so apparently.

2. *The main dream.* This was very long, although few details were remembered on waking. There was to be a Greek play and much discussion was in progress about who the actors were to be. One of them was a " Miss Steyne " (Becky Sharp) but the others were all undergraduates. [Later in the night, after recording these

dreams. I dreamed about X.] Next I was entering the theatre. I was late, a prologue was being said and in a half-light I looked about for my seat. I kept trying to find it on the left hand side but finally an usher took me to it. It was against the wall on the right. My companion at the concert was next to me and beyond him were other friends, possibly the others as at the concert. The seats were peculiar, reminiscent of furniture I had been criticizing that evening. Shortly after I took my place the curtain went up and light reflected from the stage illuminated the body of the theatre, which I inspected. The play went on, how long I do not know, for apparently I went to sleep and had another dream within the dream.

3. *The secondary dream.* I was lying in bed in my own bedroom, which was changed. My head was in a new position and a fire place had appeared. [It would be a boon at times !] The new arrangements I need not explain but can account for them by saying that it was as if I were sleeping in another bedroom in the College which I once occupied, the fire place of the dream occupying the position of a window in the second bedroom, through which coal gas used to come, much to my annoyance. I was awakened by the servant mentioned above whom I saw in the half light of the early morning trying to light the fire. Below the fire place there was, apparently, a gas pipe. She turned the gas on, threw in a lighted match, and a loud explosion followed. [Auditory images are rare in my dreams.] There was fire between me and the door but I could not see it for the smoke, although I knew it was there. The woman had run out of the door ; I called to her for help for I was ill and could not move. There was no answer and I yelled ; still no sound. The situation was desperate. Not only was I going to die but the College would be burned down. I must escape. I struggled to get out, beginning with throwing off the bed clothes. Over my eyes was a light cloth, which I first thought was a black sock I often put over my eyes on a bright morning when awakened early by a strong light, but I soon discovered that this was a sheet, while a heavy cover was over my mouth and nose. This I removed and at once got fresh air and thought I was awake. All fear had vanished abruptly and completely the moment my mouth was uncovered.[1]

4. *Waking dream.* I was back in the theatre, but it was pitch dark, apparently because the curtain was down. I asked my companions if I had been making a row and they answered, smiling, that perhaps I had made a slight sound. I felt vexed at admitting sleep, which they probably had not noticed, and to justify myself gave them a regular lecture on the inaudibility of sounds made by dreamers, illustrated with a long-winded reminiscence [a true one] of my personal experience with this phenomenon. While I was talking the lights were up in the theatre although I did not notice their being turned on. Perhaps it would be more correct to say that I was

---

[1] This is in contrast to ordinary nightmares of basically sexual origin when the panic is apt to persist for some time after waking.

visually aware of my companions, rather than that I was aware of light.

5. *Actual waking state.* I then awoke gradually realizing that I was in my own bed, that it was in its right place, and that I was on my left side ; I had no air hunger and was not panting.   I first examined my bed clothes.   I found that they were over my head but had been shifted enough to let air in.   Next I observed that the room was in total darkness and looked for the window in which there should have been a glow from a light in the Court.   It was not to be seen but I was so certain it was there that I pressed down the bedding, when it became visible.   I thought about my dreams for a quarter-of-an-hour and then looked at my watch.   I had been in bed for two hours.

Analysis.   I have no intention of giving any analysis of the first dream, beyond admitting that it is easily reducible to elements of deep unconscious significance.   Any experienced psychoanalyst could construct an interpretation that would not be far of the mark, except in so far as it involves matters of unique experience and Cambridge affairs that are of domestic interest.   It must be noted, however, that there is a steady dilution of these " unconscious " themes as the dreaming advances.   They include all the details of the first part of the dream, that is, the preparation for the play.   In the theatre itself lights going up and down begin to appear, otherwise there is no secondary interest intruded, although, of course, events prior to sleep are utilized in the dream structure.   In the secondary dream, there are no " unconscious " factors, a new element has effectually interrupted the trend.   In the waking dream, however, the latent theme appears again as my embarrassment.   To make this discrimination clear I should ennumerate the details belonging to the " unconscious " themes.   They are preparations for the play, including the choice of cast, all the events of finding my seat and identifying my companions and the action of the play itself.   Finally there is the embarrassment in the waking dream when the setting of the original dream is revived.

Of greater interest for our present purpose is the operation of the factor, foreign to all this, which was injected into the original dream. This seems pretty clearly to be a stimulus of a physiological order. I was suffering from lack of air.   Had I enjoyed waking consciousness a simple voluntary act would have abolished this somatic trouble without materially interrupting my train of thought.   But I was asleep, that is to say, my mind was not functioning in relation to the actual environment.   In sleep or reverie one can change the apparent environment by changing thoughts, hence problems can be solved in pure fantasy, their existence being merely fantastic. But a real, *i.e.*, physical stimulus, cannot be abolished in fancy ; it can only be disregarded.   If strong and persistent it will re-appear and eventually control the psychic situation.   This is what happened as a result of oxygen lack.

In order to understand the different reactions set up by this structure one should have clearly in mind the various ways in which idea-functions can be expressed. A mental process is most simply betrayed in bodily behaviour, that may or may not be accompanied by consciousness. Its other manifestations are those that affect consciousness, of which there are three. One is a subjective emotional reaction. A second is expression in images (symbols) that may be consciously illogical, although reasonable enough when the mental processes are identified and translated into abstract terms (*e.g.*, the Mah Jong dream). A third is abstract ideas which may be illogical in their conscious connections (as in many dreams) or logical (as in ordinary waking thought and in waking dreams).

Quite logical mental processes may be detected as resulting from the stimulus air hunger. They are : the obstruction to breathing must be removed ; but to do this I must awake ; I may be awakened by a light stimulus, a sound stimulus, or a violent emotional reaction (other possible stimuli such as touch, smell, taste or pain might appear but do not in this dream). Once a mental process is incorporated in an image or an idea the latter tends to wander into free associations. The connection between elements of free associations themselves are often unconscious mental processes (as in the ordinary dream), or they may be rather superficial and so lead to mere dramatization and secondary elaboration in a dream. Another result of superficial associations may be to side-track a useful mental process which, incorporated in an image or idea of clouded consciousness, does not lead to bodily behaviour. This last has its analogy in " absent-mindedness " of waking consciousness, where free associations lead a logical train of thought astray. Every one of all these mechanisms is represented in these dreams and we must see what was the fate of each imaginal or ideational presentation.

Since the image or idea of light is the first to appear we may begin with it. It was ineffective throughout in producing any expression sufficiently urgent to change the state of consciousness. The reason for this seems to have been that each time the light illuminated something to which attention could be given, and this something belonged to the existing dream. The first intrusion of light is in the theatre. When the curtain went up the audience became clearly visible and then I looked at the arrangements of the building and the people in it. In the bedroom scene the half-light of early morning probably represented the obtuseness of my consciousness. This may be the occasion as well for having the smoke obscure the view. I ought to have been awake and taking note of external realities but I could not achieve it. When I did succeed in actually getting at my bedclothes I first interpreted the sheet as a sock used to hide the light, an habitual remedy against being awakened by light. Throughout I was trying to see something that would orient me and always failed. Finally I became oriented by touch and had there been anything whatever to stimulate my sight I would probably have succeeded in waking up fully. But the room was dark. A clearer consciousness than I had had before, sought to establish itself more fully and found mere darkness. In this state free associational thinking is still dominant and its imagery can easily become hallucinatory if there are no external visual stimuli to correct the tendency. In other words, it is easy to drift back into dreaming, and this is what I did. The chief content was of waking but I staged an argument about it back in the theatre and with the companions of the original dream. When full consciousness was finally achieved I proved it by adopting an active, rather than a passive attitude towards the environment, that is, I did something which made actual visual perception possible, namely moving the bedclothes which were between my eyes and the window.

The stimulus which caused the secondary dreams and all their complications was a physiological one—need of air. This appeared in fairly direct form and then affected behaviour. First there was smoke in the room and at once, a fear of suffocation developed although this fear was even more of being burned, an irrelevant detail introduced by association from the explosion episode. The emotional reaction was sufficiently violent to rouse me from bodily inactivity, so that I was able to fumble with the bedclothes. An instinct to escape, always a well-trained and vigilant one, was utilized to effect movements fundamentally designed to improve breathing. This is theoretically of no small importance and goes right to the roof of the function of awakening dreams. The only usual bodily reaction to air hunger is panting, with its utilization of the accessory muscles of respiration. But forced inspirations do not help much if one's mouth and nose are covered. Had I been conscious I would have argued instantaneously " My mouth and nose are obstructed, I must remove the obstruction ". But I was not conscious, so my organism could only utilize the resources of unconscious mental processes. These are dependent for expression on the activation of pattern reactions. So a situation was fabricated which made escape from bed obligatory. The preliminary movements of escape relieved my air hunger and at once the whole secondary dream vanished[1]. But the interest in the obstruction

---

[1] The utilization of the fear reaction in the anxiety neurosis of sexual origin has probably just this mechanism. The sexual reactions are not integrated with the personality, and hence are not only unconscious but are also obstructive to the organism as constituted. Sex is kept from becoming conscious from affecting the behaviour of the subject by being symbolized as a danger. The danger reactions are then sufficiently prompt and effectual to prevent the appearance of sex in conscious thought or conduct, although the patient is uncomfortable. The mechanism of cure by psychoanalysis is the same as waking up. Sex is brought into consciousness, and can then be treated logically and directly. So long as it remains unconscious it can only be handled by the same means as are employed in dreams. In my secondary dream I had, in miniature, an anxiety state, the object of which—to speak teleologically—was the abolition of a disturbing condition, that did not appear in dream consciousness as such.

did not, for my first action on actually waking was to examine the bedclothes.

The problem or idea of waking as it appears in these dreams is of peculiar interest. It must be borne in mind that waking-up is a change in the level or capacity of consciousness. Consciousness is characterized by awareness of the environment and by a type of thinking. The latter is associated with use of abstract ideas or generalizations, logical connection between thoughts, and, above all, recognition by the subject that his mental content is mental, and not environmental in origin. More or less each one of these characteristics can appear in dreams, which become more like conscious thinking as the waking-up process advances, but the *sine qua non* of dreaming is the inability completely to discriminate between perceptual elements of inner and outer origin. To be conscious one must be sensorially aware of the environment. At least such are my views, and have been for many years, long enough for them to be grafted into my unconscious mental processes—and I was the dreamer of these dreams. Unconsciously, therefore, I seem to have reasoned as follows : Something must be done about my air hunger, that is I must externalize my activity, I must wake up. Waking can be accomplished by seeing bright lights, hearing sounds, making movements or concentrating consciousness on a logical train of thought. We practice all these methods in trying to keep awake when drowsy, and these devices appear in my dreams.

First came the light idea, which was ineffective, as we have seen. Next a loud sound was heard. It did not wake me, but it changed the dream from one of a passive spectator (of the fire-laying) to one of active planning. Up to this point there had been no feeling of willing anything in either of the dreams. Things had just happened. Now I wanted to do things, although consciousness was still so weak as to be represented in a paralyzed body. Also recognition of diurnal interests was strong enough to intrude concern over the safety of the College as well as my own security. Soon this higher type of thinking was effective in producing actual movements, which abolished the air hunger. Perhaps for an instant I was really awake. But, if so, the absence of an urgent need to maintain activity and the absence of visual stimuli made relapse easy. So I drifted back into a dream. But now the type of thinking was quite different, both in content and kind, from what had gone before. My theme was the abstract ideas of waking and sleeping, and my speech thereon, although socially *mal àpropos*, had no nonsense in it—that is from the standpoint of *my* diurnal judgment. Once launched on this topic I was thinking in a conscious way, my interest was aroused in a matter of day-time preoccupation, so naturally the audience, that is the dream, began to fade, and I really awoke. To prove that I was awake I looked for my window, and managed to find it. What kept me awake was the psychological interest that had appeared in the last dream. I now began to think of what I had been dreaming, and was soon sufficiently active to get out of bed and to write it all down.

Thus analysed, the dreams show a continuity of themes, which one would not expect from casual scrutiny of the manifest content. This continuity runs from actual experience, through dreams to actual conduct and conscious thoughts in the waking state. The thread can be followed in the theme of unconscious motivation as well. A social situation at the concert activated this theme. On going to bed I lie on my *wrong* side for no apparent reason at all, repress all memory of thoughts thereafter, and of turning over before going to sleep, then I dream of trying to sit on the wrong side of the theatre, and in the last dream am embarrassed at having fallen asleep at the play. But the continuity does not end there. The heroine in a novel I read before going to bed stirs a memory of a girl I once knew. She appears as a " Miss Steyne " in the first dream, and again, hours later on going back to bed, as herself, having a whole dream devoted to her.

The repression of memory for what happened between going to bed and falling asleep deserves comment. This period must have been of appreciable duration, for I did not feel sleepy on getting into bed, and, had I fallen suddenly asleep, I would not have turned over. This I do only when I have been long enough in one position for change to give a pleasurable relief. Since, on waking, my mind was an absolute blank for this time, cudgel it as I would, repression must have been operating. The object of this repression was presumably thoughts generated by events at the concert and what I had been reading, which appeared in the main dream and echoed on during the rest of the night. This is the simplest explanation for forgetting what I thought ; but another factor perhaps enters into the amnesia for what I did, namely, turn over. Not only had I no memory for this, but I succeeded in smothering myself in the process. For the latter there are two possible explanations. One is that this action was symbolic, was symptomatic behaviour like lying on the wrong side. If this were so the explosion dream, and all the trend connected therewith, would be the product of some unconscious death idea. This is conceivable, but hardly likely, since there was nothing in the other dreams nor the analysis of them to suggest it even remotely. Moreover there was absolutely nothing in any of the dreams to suggest that mouth or nose played any rôle in the unconscious drama. So the act could hardly have had any unconscious significance. On the other hand I did feel cold ; I was glad to get as much of me covered as possible. If consciousness with its accurate recognition of the environment was beginning to lapse when I turned over, clumsiness in covering my face would not be unnatural. This, I think, is the better explanation. One should give the devil his due, but repression should not be invoked to account for phenomena otherwise explicable. This, then, is like the forgetting in the waking-up state. It can largely be accounted for as the natural result of changed consciousness.

A corollary of this is the mechanism of remembering of past mental processes. In studying the recovery of dreams on awakening, it has been noted that free associations lead to more and more data coming into consciousness. One dates these as belonging to the past, and so calls them dreams. It would be difficult, in fact, impossible, to prove that these thoughts and images were not a product of the moment, and that the " dream " was an illusion. Indeed, we have seen that there is good reason for believing that many dreams are distorted in the remembering process. Naturally one is tempted to ask what the difference is between memory of such a thought process as is a dream, and the memory of a diurnal thought. If I recall that yesterday I was planning a holiday, how do I know, how can I convince myself that it was a " thought " and not a dream ? Apparently free associations bring the data to my mind in either case[1]. The difference between the two depends, apparently, on the nature of the circumstantial associations. If, when I think of the holiday plans, I can visualize the chair and room I was in, an interruption by the telephone, etc., then I call it a thought. If, on the other hand I imagine the thought taking place in an Alpine châlet with no detailed associations of journeys thither and return, then I conclude, instantaneously, that it was a dream. If the environmental associations are full of detail they seem " real " to me, and so the memory has validity. If there are few attendant thoughts, so that the memory seems to be suspended in space and time, so to speak, then I conclude that I am dealing with a fancy or a dream. Naturally all gradations are possible. One may be uncertain or make a wrong judgment either way. For instance, if a remembered dream have about it a large penumbra of rich associations, it seems real, and may constitute a delusion, or a false memory may be created. If I have such a firm intention of posting a letter that I visualize all the actions of finding a pillar box and dropping it in, the memory of this intention may seem to be of real events, or I may actually manufacture all these details and date them to the past. Again, if an automatic action be performed, memory of that is almost certain to be lacking. This is because the action is the product of a dissociated system of mental processes. Being dissociated they do not come into association

---

[1] I cannot recall anything by direct resuscitation : the best I can do is to think of something with which the required data are associated. For instance, if I be asked what I had for breakfast yesterday, I concentrate my attention on the idea (or image) " breakfast table " and imagine myself eating, at the same time I must think of the events of yesterday. The required data will then appear in consciousness, or they will not. The speed of different memories depends on the activity of the associational processes in question. The ideas associated in consciousness of five minutes ago are still fresh in my mind ; I can recall them quickly. Those of yesterday are not active unless they be related with habitual interests or experiences.

with the thoughts of consciousness. The latter are the ones concerned with the environment ; so, in effect, the automatic act has retrospectively, and for the conscious mind, no environment. No associations coming into consciousness will include the act in question. But, if the subject be hypnotized, the submerged consciousness that performed the act may be activated. In it associations will run toward the act. The hypnotized person will recall it.

PART XI

PSYCHOLOGICAL CONCLUSIONS

CHAPTER L

THE PSYCHOLOGY OF EMOTIONS

IN the Psychological Introduction, discussion of the theory of emotions (see Chapter XI) was left in abeyance till data could be secured as proof or disproof of the validity of the view put forward. It is now time to consider what conclusions may be reached. To avoid repetition I shall assume that the reader has in mind the hypothesis advanced. It will be recalled that there were three questions to which answer was sought : Are there such things as emotions existing as independent mental phenomena ? Is repression always demonstrable when emotion appears ? What are the psychological mechanisms by which an emotion comes into being ?

The first may be dealt with briefly. In the psychoses described, the weight of evidence was in favour of " pathological " emotions being reactions to pathological stimuli, rather than primary abnormalities. The study of dreams would tend to the same conviction, for it has been shown how dreams, although unremembered consciously, may produce moods after waking that last, sometimes, for many hours. The stimulus has become co-conscious, that is all. The apparently independent emotion is not demonstrable, provided, of course, that appropriate means of investigation are available.

The rôle of repression in production of emotion as revealed in the functional psychoses has already been reviewed in Chapter XLVII. We have still to consider what evidence dreams may furnish on this point. The data here have to do mainly with affect, rather than emotional expression, because the observations are almost entirely introspective. We must bear in mind that affect is a phenomenon

549

inevitably conscious, since it is discernible only to introspection. I have observed a sleeper moan and cry out without waking, who, in the morning, denied any but pleasant dreams. The sounds were instinctive responses to some situation that would have, presumably, been fearful or horrible, if consciousness had had an opportunity of knowing it. Other dreams displaced the ones of danger and with the latter the sleeper awoke. In this connection it might be mentioned that some good dream introspectionists report that they can, rarely, in the waking period, recover fragments of " deep " dreams, that have no affect although the content is melodramatic. These subjects have succeeded in getting an objective survey of their own dreams, that is, they have been able to see the dreamer, so to speak, rather than be the dreamer. But normally our striking dreams have an exaggerated personal reference, because in them, as De Quincey says, " . . . of necessity, we make ourselves central to every movement."

There are two conditions in which dream-produced affect appears : there are dreams recalled with strong feeling tone, and there is consciously inexplicable affect occurring in the waking state which can be traced to the influence of an unremembered dream. In the latter case the function of repression is clear : something keeps the dream from entering consciousness and its capacity to produce emotion may be annihilated by bringing the memory into awareness.

The other group demands more attention because the state is more like that of every day emotional experience. Dreams originate in the unconscious and exist, so it seems, as a flux of images. Remembered dreams, however, have suffered change in the process of becoming conscious, change in formulation and often change in the type of thinking exhibited in them. The conscious personality revolts at primitive dreams on both moral and intellectual grounds. Before they succeed in entering consciousness, therefore, resistance has to be overcome. When the dream has been absolutely repressed (that is, not merely put out of consciousness, but out of co-consciousness as well—rendered inactive in other words), or when it has been completely translated into conscious terms, there is no affect. In the latter case the awakened dreamer regards his nocturnal adventures with true objectivity. But where metamorphosis is incomplete an emotional aura does hang about them, and it may be intense. When full awakening banishes a painful experience or excludes us from some pleasure, it is because we have become real observers and not actors in the play. Often the dream images seem to show a stubborn tendency to enter consciousness as they are. Waking up is then difficult and charged with emotion. Or the subject may wake, have an objective view of his dream and still be troubled. In this case the unconscious mental processes have not been completely expressed in the remembered dream and the surplus has not been adequately repressed. The latter elements continue co-consciously and galvanize the conscious memories into life. Such, for instance is the usual nightmare. At bottom it is a sexual dream : a formulation of sexual outlet involving danger wakens the patient, but the sexual stirrings go on. The latter find their only outlet in the remembered dream and so activate this memory that a feeling of reality clings to it. When analysed, however, the sexual content is brought into consciousness and the anxiety disappears. In every case, then, when emotion is demonstrable, some unconscious mental processes are working against repression and reaching consciousness only in that form.

Essential to our theory of emotion is the operation of instinctive processes that, suffering some inhibition, reach expression in emotional behaviour and affect. The way in which this may occur can be discovered in the study of the mechanisms of unconscious thinking as revealed in dreams. All our evidence seems to point to unconscious mental functions being incorporated in images, succeeding one another as do free associations, that is, the bond between them is an idea-function. Dreams are remembered fragments of a riot of such imaginal free associations, which are brought into waking awareness as a result of consciousness being intruded into the dreaming. A continuity is thus established. We have seen that the " dream ", as something known to the diurnal personality, is really only a fragment. A psychoanalytic examination of this dream, conducted by free associations, can be regarded as a restitution of the nocturnal type of mentation. Theoretically, if one remembered enough of one's flow of images in sleep, the meaning of the symbols would be betrayed by comparisons of the different symbols expressing the various idea-functions. According to this view a successful psychoanalysis of a dream is a duplication, or reclaiming, of the dream " thoughts ". That is, by relaxation of ordinary conscious critique, the more primitive kind of thinking re-appears, and the same psychological state is established as exists in the terminal phase of sleep, that is, free-associational thinking coincident with enough awareness to have it registered. But these waking free associations, if they start from elements in the remembered dream, are found not to be guided by mere chance. They do incorporate definite idea-functions—at least, this is the claim made by all psychoanalysts.

Now this guidance must come from somewhere. The easiest assumption is that the flux of imagery going on in the night is not utterly abolished on waking but that it is latent during the day, ready to be activated by appropriate stimulus. Many phenomena cited in the last two chapters confirm the view that dream processes can live on during the day. And this is a crucial point in our theory of emotions. The study of dreams and dreaming demonstrates how connections exist between conscious and unconscious mentation, how they influence each other reciprocally. It makes it reasonable to suppose that a stimulus may be recognized by consciousness and at the same time set up a train of unconscious (co-conscious) imagery, which, in turn, will obtrude itself into consciousness as emotional expression or affect[1].

The mechanism whereby this may come about has also been illuminated. The unconscious formulation of an idea-function is meaningless for consciousness, *i.e.*, it is a symbol. But the reverse is not true. The conscious formulation is not meaningless for the unconscious (if one may speak so anthropomorphically of the unconscious). The metamorphoses of dreams show how the final formulation of the idea-function, accepted by consciousness, is still merely another symbol from the unconscious stand-point. This makes the basis of mind the unconscious flux and gives to consciousness a selective function. According to this view our mental operations are mainly unconscious and we are aware only of such fragments of them as appear in consciousness. The situation is comparable to that of the stage. A number of actors appear and attention is focussed on a small group of these picked out by a spot light. The observer watching them finds a *raison d'être* for the little group in the action performed. But beyond them are other actors who can with effort be made out (the fringes of consciousness) ; they too contribute to the significance of the spot light action. Further away and out of sight, are actors waiting to come on as well as a prompter (co-consciousness) ; and beyond that are the dressing rooms and the outside world (the deep unconscious). Now, from the view point of the audience, or of consciousness, the play is the thing. But the action on the stage may have quite different meanings to the actors—livelihood, self-display, romantic adventure, and so on. The actors are those who initiate activities, which, if they are performed on the stage, take on a special meaning. If the actor does not play his part on the stage but insists on being himself, the play is ruined. This is a psychopathic state.

Now when one examines the idea-functions latent in unconscious mental processes, they reveal what Freud has called a " wish ", or what I would call an " instinct motivation "[2]. This is the flux of symbols in an instinctive process (using " instinct " in a broad adjectival sense) in which images are substituted in the series both for stimulus and response. Thus instincts are the directing agencies in unconscious thinking. Broadly speaking one might say that the function of images is to prepare for bodily activity, the action being tried out in advance, so to speak. Whenever an instinct is activated a tendency to bodily expression is present. If this tendency is allowed full play the unconscious produces behaviour that is automatic—the ordinary instinctive action. If the first spontaneous activity be inhibited, the instinct leads to a train of images any one of which may be a stimulus for another reaction.

Now these other reactions may have two forms of expression :

---

[1] It must be borne in mind that Morton Prince has demonstrated this with his hypnotic technique.

[2] See Chapter VI and also *Problems in Dynamic Psychology*.

bodily behaviour or conscious thought. So long as neither takes place the inner activity is felt by the subject as affect. Observations based on introspection indicate this to be true, so far as it concerns overt conduct, as has been argued in the Psychological Introduction. Our dream material tends to confirm it for thoughts, for we have seen that when the idea-functions of the dream are presented to consciousness (either in the waking-up period or later) in a form that can be clearly grasped, there is either no detectable affect, or else it is exactly that which would appear were the fancied situation actually present. The most striking affects—analysis shows—are due to a failure of the idea-functions to be adequately formulated in terms suitable for acceptance by the waking personality. This leaves the train of unconscious, instinctive processes still active. It is not difficult to see why, on our theory, the incorporation of an idea-function in a form that consciousness can deal with should abolish emotional reaction. The latter is an expression of impeded activity. But, if a situation be presented to consciousness that is recognized by it as ridiculous or unreal, this judgment involves turning attention to other thoughts or to objective environmental stimuli ; that is, totally new reactions are substituted. Until the judgment of unreality is made, no complete substitution is possible. Indeed, this is one of the prime functions of consciousness. Again, if the first metamorphosis of the idea-function be one adaptive to the personality, activity pertinent to the waking thought or plan is initiated. In this case as well, there is no inhibition. Repressions and emotions are present only when idea-functions are active with which consciousness is incapable of dealing.

The matter may be put in other words. Instinctive mental processes have, for their emotional goal, bodily action. These processes are, then, a vehicle for expression of the energy of the whole organism, which they direct in somewhat the same way as an elaborate switch-board directs electrical energy. They are (except perhaps in deep sleep and in real physiological unconsciousness) continually active, continually responding to stimuli. There are two orders of stimuli, perceptions of the environment and images[1]. The effect of setting the instinct process into activity is to effect either overt behaviour (automatic) or images thereof. The latter, if unconscious, produce the stimulus for another instinct process, which may go on indefinitely (dreaming). But, if the image enters consciousness it can be used in planning, that is, consciousness can direct attention to the environment so as to make possible expression of the imaged movements in actual behaviour, or it can make possible perceptions (of environmental origin) that will stimulate totally new instinct processes. In either case the energy of the organism no longer flows through the original instinct channel. If it have no energy it cannot be active ; it is in abeyance till again stimulated

---

[1] For the purpose of this present argument I include abstract thoughts under " images."

and once more made a vehicle for energy. I am here using " energy " in its narrow physical sense, the kind that is measurable in calories or foot-pounds and not any metaphorical " mental energy ". It is therefore obvious that the energy used in the perpetuation of a flux of images is infinitesimal in comparison with that involved in muscular movement. That is why we can dream while still in the low state of vitality existing in sleep. In fact, we sleep (fundamentally) because the energy of the organism has been exhausted in diurnal activities. Psychologically, sleep is a condition in which consciousness ceases to operate. This is a protective mechanism. Consciousness involves direction of attention outward, and this implies reaction to environmental stimuli, be it only in the maintenance of posture. As a matter of actual energy output it is easier to dream of running a Marathon than to sit in a chair.

An emotional reaction is an exhibition of energy flowing through an instinct channel and not expressed—or not fully expressed—in planned or automatic behaviour. If this reaction include emotional expression it may use up a good deal of energy, but if it be merely affect, it may involve very little expenditure. Hence one may feel deeply in the waking up period without involving any material metabolic change. The energy expressed in emotion is deflected from the stream which produces behaviour by the free associational process, i.e., the activization of collateral instinct processes. If the flux of unconscious imagery flow in one stream only and that ends in muscle movements which abolish the stimulating perception, there can be no overflow and, therefore, no emotion. That is why the pure instinctive action is unaccompanied by emotion. It is not when I am saving myself from an actual danger that I am frightened but when I am saving myself, in imagination, from a danger that might happen.

At this point it may be well to consider some different types of unusual energy display in the psychoses. It must be borne in mind that the normal person, when awake, is preventing energy output in many ways, because, while conscious, he is keeping himself alert for the reception of a great variety of stimuli and, *ipso facto*, is not allowing any one instinctive process to monopolize all the energy of his body. Further, as consciousness has a discriminative function, behaviour is always adjusted to meet the demands of expedience, and this tends to inhibit wild and uncontrolled movement. We have seen, as well, that energy output is determined by outlet being directed into fantasy or into action. The interplay of these factors will account for the marked variations in motor activity observable in psychotic patients.

For instance, if consciousness exercise no inhibition, no discrimination, but the patient's attention is not withdrawn from the environment, instinctive processes tend to be excessive. This we see in the sudden wild actions of many dementia praecox patients, in stupor (impulsive suicidal efforts), and, not infrequently, in epileptic clouded states. It is further characteristic of all these that there is little, if any, evidence of emotion with the excitement. The patient may be assaultive, or self-destructive, with a blank facial expression. The reason for this is that there are not collateral instinct processes being activated. On the other hand, if some inhibition be maintained, as we have seen reason to believe it is in manic states, the muscular activity may be great, but it will be accompanied by emotion. The very fact that the patient is flighty in his talk shows that collateral paths are continually being opened up. But, if attention to the environment be displaced by intro-version of attention, outlet takes the form of imagery and ex-ternalized activity ceases.

Perhaps the most interesting problem is that of the stolid, deterior-ated dementia praecox patient. He is in contact with the environ-ment (i.e., he is at least oriented), but is nevertheless inert. The reason for this is that he does not sublimate his instinct motivations, they remain at an infantile level and therefore do not assume a form that has any reference to the actual environment ; they are indulged in fantasy. This is possible because the whole personality is changed and with it the function of consciousness, which has now different standards of reality. This altered consciousness does not dis-criminate between the real and the imaginary, so that outlet, adequate from a perverted standpoint, is obtainable in images for instinct processes that normally would imply action. Real behaviour and imaginal behaviour have become identical. So, as a rule, the outlet demanding least energy is chosen and the patient is stolid. But if, perchance, instinctive movements are initiated, they are explosive from lack of inhibition. Hence the incalculability of these patients.

One difficulty has probably occurred to the reader before this time. If emotion be the product of accessory mental processes that are essentially free associations, how can they appear in such brief time, in fact so quickly that it takes instruments of nice precision to demonstrate that they are not instantaneous ? A conscious train of thought we all know involves an appreciable passage of time and dreams seem to be actions enduring for long periods. This objection is not insuperable. Free associations that we *know*, *i.e.*, conscious ones, are translated into a cumbrous language of words or abstract thoughts which undoubtedly do move slowly in consciousness. But there is no reason to suppose that a flux of images would be so viscous. In fact we know that elaborate dreams can take place in incredibly short lapses of time, as has already been mentioned. It is when the action, there portrayed, has been put into words or conscious thoughts that the semblance of slowness appears. We judge, consciously, that many actions cannot take place consecu-tively, in no time at all. So in making the dream conscious we rationalize the activities by intruding a feeling of the action being prolonged. Roughly the dream seems to have lasted as long as the same actions would take for their performance in real life. This is one of the conclusions that Kriewiet de Jonge arrived at.

But, indeed, the phenomena of dreams need not be invoked to display rapidity of associations, for this is implicit in the popular phrase, " Practice makes perfect ". Instinct, in the sense used in this book, is a pattern reaction that operates, or tends to operate, when activated in an automatic way. It therefore includes habit reactions and, inevitably, acquired concepts and meanings. I was not born with an idea of " football match " in my consciousness. My conception of this event is a complex of experiences, which, it might be argued, have been so integrated as to form a mental unit that operates as a unit, although it is likely that these words really call up in my mind a series of memories that are generalized by consciousness, instantaneously, as " football match ". But, even regarding it as a unit, unconsciously as consciously, the fact remains that, as a stimulus, these words will produce different reactions in me at different times. I may be going to play in it, or watch it, or bet on it ; perhaps it may interfere with other plans I have, and so on. When the words " football match " are spoken my behaviour or my immediate conscious thought is not determined by a consciously elaborated train of images, which would consume appreciable time, but by unconscious associations that determine an almost instantaneous response. The very first time the reaction is elicited it is slow, but it becomes faster and faster until a certain end point is reached that is, from an introspective standpoint, instantaneity. If it were objected that the immediate response is the product of a new unit, functioning as a unit and not as an extremely rapid unconscious train of images, then how is one going to account for the gradual increase of speed in the reaction ? There must be, at some stage, a series of mental events that do operate with the facility that is demanded by my theory.

We must now consider the fate of unconscious mental processes. When some stimulus activates an unconscious train of thought, this appears in the form of co-conscious images. These can be demonstrated by hypnotic technique, as Morton Prince has done so effectively, or, rarely, they may penetrate into consciousness long enough for an introspectionist, interested in such phenomena, to grasp them. I may give an example of such an experience in myself. It occurred one morning following a night during which I had had little sleep and, therefore, was still tired. A state of fatigue facilitates the substitution of the conscious type of thinking by the dream type. (Exhaustion delirium is nothing but this). The events were these. A man passed me on a bicycle, who looked familiar. A quick scrutiny of his face convinced me that I did not really know him, but he reminded me of some one else. After several seconds I succeeded in summoning the memory of this other man. It was a friend S. whom I had not seen for a long time and was then on the other side of the Atlantic. Coincidentally with the resuscitation of this memory, so far as I could tell, I saw a Cambridge Undergraduate in cap and gown but carrying a golf bag slung over his shoulder.

An incongruous combination ! He was about fifty feet distant from me and at an angle of about thirty degrees from the axis of my eyes. At once I turned my eyes to get the spectacle in the centre of vision, and as soon as I had done so, the golf bag disappeared, although the undergraduate, cap and gown were there all right. The hallucination cannot have lasted more than a fraction of a second, although it was distinct and definite. I actually could describe the golf bag in detail. It took very little longer for me to discover the origin of the hallucination. I am very fond of golf and I played it frequently with S.

This is a good example of one of the functions of co-conscious images. Some detail of the bicyclist's face (probably his moustache) evoked an image of my friend S., that was latent in the unconscious. It became co-conscious and exhibited itself at first only in a feeling of familiarity. The next step should have been the immediate translation of the image " S " into the conscious thought " S ". But I was tired. Therefore it was easier to allow a more primitive type of thinking, a flux of images, to proceed co-consciously than to have the process elaborated from image to conscious thought. An habitual interest—golf—implies a low threshold for stimulation of the image processes connected with it. So, co-consciously, I associated from S to golf. This was a " dream ", and like a dream, entered consciousness only as one fragment that was rationalized at once by attaching it to something in the environment. But this something was not in the centre of vision and hence not in the focus of awareness. The moment I got it there, consciousness abolished the rationalization and turned the hallucination into an image.

From this the normal function of co-conscious images can be deduced. They are bound together as steps in instinct processes. When a given situation demands the presence of some thought in consciousness, attention is diverted from existing perceptions or thoughts in order that it may be given to something new. Some detail in the situation has set up a train of co-conscious imagery and the conscious thoughts into which these are translated are allowed into awareness long enough to be inspected for their relevance. The moment the right one comes attention is given to it, or, rather, the organism begins to react to the situation as modified by the addition of the required new element. This change of orientation, or of attention, prevents the entrance into consciousness of all the accessory images that may have been activated co-consciously.

This is plainly an adaptive process and it becomes ineffective only when consciousness fails in its task and allows attention to wander to the translation into thoughts of the ramifying co-conscious images. The path into consciousness is via utilization of conscious material as a medium for translation. There are, however, two general conditions in which it is difficult to effect a translation. One is where repression exists, i.e., the conscious thought, that would fittingly represent the co-conscious image, is repugnant to the personality.

The other is where co-consciousness is dealing with images of experiences so old that they are unfamiliar to consciousness, which means that the thought to be expressed is not habitual and so difficult to activate. Or, to put it in still other words, the co-conscious images incorporate an idea-function rather than an idea. (One of the difficulties of original thinking is to discover formulations in which really new idea-functions may be expressed).

When co-conscious images are active but do not succeed in penetrating consciousness, an affect results. A friend of mine has given me a pretty example of an affect betraying the presence of a memory that was very old and unhabitual, but was eventually brought into consciousness. He one day opened a thoroughly prosaic book and found himself experiencing a most peculiar affect. He felt himself—he could find no other words for it—to be in an atmosphere of romance. It was just a " romantic feeling ". The reaction was so inappropriate that he studied it closely and tried to trace it. Finally he succeeded : the pages of his book had precisely the same odour as that of a book of fairy-tales to which he was devoted as a little boy.

This illustrates a phenomenon of notorious frequence. Smells are particularly apt to be affectively toned. The reason for this is now plain. Our culture taboos the indulgence of smelling as a branch of æsthetics. Sounds and sights, as music and art, we extol, but smells never. The smells of food are of such inevitable biological importance that we cannot afford to neglect them utterly (although some dishonest folk pretend that delight in flavours is " low ".) But all other smells are either to be actively resisted (repressed) or treated with indifference. Consequently we have no vocabulary for them and, hence, little consciousness of them. But, nevertheless, our olfactory capacity is keen and, in some people, incredible. I have seen a woman who was utterly demented after scarlet fever at the age of five, who identified all her acquaintances by smell, although neither deaf nor blind. Under hypnosis this capacity is often capable of resuscitation. Sensory data connected with smell are, then, elaborated almost entirely outside of awareness. So they appear as emotional reactions. " Intuitive " likes or dislikes for strangers are sometimes traceable to distinctive personal odours.

One phenomenon should now be considered, which is a commonplace with every psychopathologist but has recently been elevated into a discovery in Baudouin's " Law of Reversed Effort ". It was well known to the moral theologians of the thirteenth century ! It is that, if an idea tend to be obsessive, a willed effort to dislodge it only increases the obsession. The theory of co-conscious trains of thought accounts for this adequately. An idea is originally obsessive when it is the conscious representation of something that is persistently active in the unconscious. For instance, obsessions about knives, or compulsions to use them assaultively, are frequently due to the knife being a phallic symbol. Now, as we have seen, any idea-function can, co-consciously, be expressed indifferently in a number of settings, each one of which is a symbol for it. Any one of these symbols will tend to call up the others on the free associational principle. In our example, for instance, " knife " is a symbol for the idea " phallus ". So, when the patient says to himself, " I will not think of ' knife,' " he is giving a stimulus to the co-conscious idea-function " phallus ". This, it happens, is a dominating instinct process. Hence " phallus " is re-activated co-consciously by the conscious thought " knife ". And, at once, it is retranslated into some conscious thought about a knife. Seven hundred years ago penitents were advised by their directors not to attempt to dislodge painful thoughts by direct effort !

A most important affect is the feeling of reality. In fact, it is, perhaps, the most important one in civilized life. Without it, religion, and philosophical or scientific endeavour, would be colourless and uninteresting. Perhaps one might go so far as to say that it is the feeling of reality which gives value to all thinking that is not adaptive to an immediate material situation. It must be borne in mind that the feeling of reality is quite a different thing from the sense of reality. The latter is an intellectual judgment, based, probably, on acceptance of conventional judgments, although the feeling of reality enters into it frequently. But the latter may be treated quite separately, and, indeed, the two may be dissociated. This is shown in depressions when the feeling of reality is lost. Such a patient may say : " I know the sun is the same as it always was and that you see it as bright as ever. But to me sunshine does not feel real any more. It feels artificial."

The mechanism of this invaluable affect may be explained as follows : Any stimulus sets up a train of co-conscious imagery, not specific enough, nor powerful enough to engender any of the usual affects but only a mild emotional reaction. This is projected in consciousness on to the content of consciousness, including, of course, the perception of the stimulus ; it is thus rationalized. It might be called spontaneous interest, perhaps. Attention is thus re-directed to the stimulus and it in turn initiates more co-conscious activity. And so the process goes on, being analogous to the obsessive thinking just discussed. The only—but vital—difference between this and obsession is that in the latter the co-conscious idea-functions are set and rigid, not fluid as in normal life. The greater the wealth of co-conscious activity set up by any stimulus, the greater will be the feeling of reality attaching to it. If consciousness be reduced to a narrow range of thoughts, as in the mystical experience, for instance, the affect aroused must be focussed on these thoughts exclusively. Hence they become " real " and, if dominating instincts are operating co-consciously, vividly real.

This formulation enables us to account with greater explicitness for the symptom of unreality than was possible when discussing the depressive conditions. The evidence in these states points, as we have seen, to the locking of unconscious processes in infantile, anti-social motivations. These must be repressed. So thorough is the repression that it inhibits interest in the environment. The affect engendered—that of sodden incapacity, heaviness, sluggishness—is rationalized mainly in projection on to the idea of self. In so far as it is projected on to the environment, the latter seems to be dull and inert. That is, it feels unreal.

This is the symptom of unreality as it appears among others in the course of an ordinary retarded depression. But there is also the so-called " Unreality Depression ". Patients suffering from this psychosis do not labour with the diffuse inhibition assailing the retarded cases. In fact, they may seem to be perfectly normal, from an objective standpoint, and even intimates may fail to observe their trouble. Yet they tell a sad story. All kinds of activity to which they force themselves fail to reward them with any emotional satisfaction. They can make themselves laugh in company with others, but the joke does not feel funny, they only know it is. They can recognize intellectually the beauty in any work of art, but there is no glow of pleasure in the sight. Above all in their human relationship they feel themselves lacking. Affection for others who ought to be dearest to them simply will not come. Consequently they sum up their subjective woes in the expression " unreality ".

Now this is a condition curiously like that seen in epileptics, with one great difference. The typical epileptic has never known the fine frenzy of love for either the good, the beautiful, or for a friend. Consequently he senses no defect. One epileptic, for instance, was a great collector of art treasures. His judgment of what was precious was almost unerring, but his intimates declared that the only satisfaction he had of his acquisitions was the pride of possession. A wealth of evidence shows that the anomaly in the instinctive equipment of epileptics is the weakness of social and sexual instincts as opposed to the egoistic ones of self-preservation, aggression or aggrandisement. The same disproportion probably exists in these unreality depressions. At bottom the dominant sexual motivations are of an infantile, anti-social order, and these are being repressed. The sexual is so intermingled with the social that instinct processes of the latter order are repressed with it. When the repression is truly wholesale all instincts are inhibited and a retarded depression results. The first group to escape are the ego instincts. These can motivate all kinds of adaptations that express expedience and can be achieved by intellectual effort. Hence the unreality depression patient can behave as normally as an epileptic can. But persuade either to sing and the wooden artificiality of the result will display the emotional poverty from which he suffers, or of which he is unaware. Theoretically the emotions associated with the ego instincts, which are chiefly fear and anger, ought to be present in the unreality cases as they are in epileptics. I have not seen anger in the former but I have witnessed attacks of panic in them. Anger may, perhaps, occur as well.

The reader has probably noted a discrepancy in my accounts of epilepsy. In Chapter XI I have spoken of the intense affect that these patients sometimes describe and now I claim that epileptics are apt to be deficient in emotional response except for such crude reactions as those of anger and fear. The paradox is heightened when I add that in cases of the kind mentioned in Chapter XI the affect may be described as a feeling of intense reality, just that which the epileptic, on theory, ought to lack. How may this be explained ? In the first place it should be noted that this affect is of episodic occurrence and is a definite symptom being an aura, or "warning", before an attack. Any one of us has, as a standard in guaging the intensity or quality of any subjective experience, nothing but his usual experience to go on. If then, an emotional state occurs which is different from the ordinary, its mere novelty will heighten the intensity of what is new. If I, "who have never turned a rhyme ", should suddenly find myself writing verse, I would feel myself, for the time being, the greatest poet living—that is, till I had got beyond this "first, fine, careless rapture ", and recovered my sanity sufficiently to look at the product critically. To the epileptic then, a feeling of reality must come as an illumination from on high.

The second point involves the whole story of reality feeling and of sense of self. The state of mind in an epileptic with an aura is interesting psychologically[1], because, for him, its very essence is its subjective aspect. The peculiar sensory experience which characterizes it for the physician is, to the patient, merely a signal for development of a fear of loss of consciousness. Against this he reacts, as a rule, by forcibly directing his attention to the environment, because he believes that, if he can keep from thinking about the aural symptom, consciousness will not lapse. He is a firm upholder of the view that consciousness means contact with the environment ! This is the ordinary method of aborting attacks and patients claim that it is often successful.

Now it should be noted that what he fears is not injury to body or life, but, merely, loss of self-awareness. That is, the instinct of self-preservation is operating to save the psychological, rather than the physiological organism, the former being represented by consciousness. But consciousness is awareness of two fields of experience, of one's own thoughts and of things. Therefore there are two ways in which consciousness may, presumably, be maintained—by maintaining contact with the world around (the customary method), or by heightening self-feeling. Normally, the more vividly we live with the world, the more do we feel ourselves to be alive. The epileptic, however, is relatively incapable of objectified interest :

[1] I read a paper on this subject to the New York Neurological Society about ten years ago, but have not yet published it.

he must seek direct satisfaction for his ego or perish. When therefore he fears that consciousness is ebbing away, he may try to
fabricate interest in the environment by an exercise of will, that is, he
may try to be " normal " by substituting intellectual for emotional
contact, or he may attempt to gain the desired goal by the reverse
means. He then follows his natural egoistic bent and stresses
consciousness of self, rather than consciousness of the environment.
So, with a God-like gesture, he makes the universe only part of
himself. For a brief moment the world and all that is therein
becomes himself.

The bearing of this on the reality feeling is instructive. When
we have emotional contact with anything—person, place or undertaking—we are identifying ourselves with it. When this identification takes place, the thing feels " real ", before that it is phantasmal,
shadowy. The most real experience in the lives of ordinary people
is love and, by the principle of paradox that haunts psychology,
the more objective love is, the greater is identification with the loved
one. The goal of devotion to another is a larger self. When therefore the quintessence of identification is achieved the maximum
feeling of reality is engendered. This explains—on its psychological
side—the mystical experience as it does the epileptic's glimpse of
Paradise. Both describe the experience as one of ineffable reality.
I have read no account of mystical experience in which the idea of
identification with the Divine is not put in the foreground, usually
with such plainness that no interpretation is necessary. It is
natural that the person who has vivid religious experience should
believe in God. The feeling of reality is something which tells us
that things about us are real : it is developed as an essential by-
product in normal adaptation. If, now, an excessive feeling of
reality developes in connection with thoughts or perceptions—no
matter how individual, how unobservable by others—are not
these experiences to be called " real ", and, moreover, real in
the very sense that the world around is real ? Ask the mystic
to abandon this belief and you ask him to abandon the subjective
criterion of reality which he and every normal person uses in
daily life.

But, one might ask at this point, are we therefore to conclude that
the more genuine religion is, the more is it a product of mental
disease ? Not at all. The mystical experience and the epileptic's
translation are equally unusual, and, in that sense, equally pathological. So then, is genius. Pedestrian creatures regard originality
and morbidity with equal distrust. Ordinary people have two ways
of judging reality, by sense and feeling. The sense of reality is,
essentially, the judgment of the group in which one lives, which is
exercised individually in a purely intellectual way. People say the
wind blows the tree, so, having been taught this, I say so too. That
the tree makes the wind I believe to be untrue, i.e., unreal. The man
of science belongs to a group with a more esoteric and modifiable

set of standards; but behaves, at bottom, in the same way. No matter how far science may advance it can never get further than this in its search for ultimate truth, because in the end it deals only with data secured through use of the special senses and of theories built thereon by minds that have grown up in the elaboration of stimulus and response to a material environment. If the universe consist only of the material, truth may, one day, be known; but daily the physicists are knocking out the props from under materialism. Sense of reality cannot give us the answer; the argument of the mystic would validate any sturdy delusion.

Under these circumstances, as psychologists, there seems to be only one way of gauging truth, and that is the pragmatic method. The mystical experience is, in itself, neither the mark of disease nor of genius; it is a proof neither of the reality nor unreality of the unseen. But, if it affect the subsequent life of the subject it has validity commensurate with the magnitude and quality of the change. This may be in the direction of insanity or of social usefulness. To a certain extent this direction may be predicted by the route followed in moving towards the goal of identification. "To travel hopefully is better than to arrive and the true success is to labour." One should note that, while the epileptic embraces the universe *within himself*, the mystic seeks to *melt himself* into the Divine. Both attain the same conviction, that of all-oneness; both, too, may enjoy the same affect of supreme reality. But one, in losing his life has found it; the other in saving his life is losing his only world.

A cognate problem has to do with the paradox that one may enjoy, or at least find satisfaction in, an emotionally painful situation. Conrad says of an heroic figure in one of his tales: " . . . . he had known remorse and power, and no man can demand more from life." How can the torture of remorse be regarded as a boon, even retrospectively? If the argument just made be sound, the answer is easily given. The conviction of reality comes from an emotional reaction. *Cogito ergo sum*, is probably wrong. It ought to be, *Sentio ergo sum*. That which is inviolably individual and personal is affect. Therefore the greater the feeling, the greater the conviction of personal individuality. No one can hurt my thoughts—they might belong to anybody—but, it is possible to hurt my feelings. Hurt them and it is I—only I—who am hurt. In other words we realize our identity in vivid emotional reaction. This may be of any kind, pleasant or unpleasant, but the derivation of the best adjective describing such affect—*poignant*—and its tendency to imply the painful, both exemplify the fact that the more vivid feelings are usually unpleasant. Moreover, as we view our lives and seek to find the agencies that have formed our characters, we tend to forget the gains and remember the losses. Egoists, as we are, we take our pleasant experiences as natural and give only to the unhappy ones a dramatic importance. So, in review, we mark the hazards through which we passed and our bravery as acquired in passing these without flinching. Our strength grew then, so we think, out of the fortitude *we* summoned, wherewith to meet the blow. It is probably largely for this reason that we value the tribulations we have suffered and count that man as never having lived, who has not known sorrow.

But this is retrospection. It is a rare creature who can summon such a philosophy in the day of trial. *That*, as a rule, is a time of agony. It is possible, however, to have one's cake and eat it, too—if one likes that kind of cake. Through the medium of the arts, chiefly the dramatic and literary, one may experience a dilute emotion vicariously and feel that one is " alive " in so doing. Hence the mawkish joy of crying in the theatre or over a novel. It is significant that the weaker one's personality is, the less one's " head is bloodied but unbowed ", the greater is the lust for vicarious woe. This is sentimentalism, a luxuriating in emotional response to artificial experience at the expense of real experience, *i.e.*, action. We distrust the sentimentalist because we realise, intuitively, that he shuns reality ; we suspect that in a crisis he will fail. The brave man or the good man does not need to talk of courage or of morals in order to enjoy the glow of virtue.

So far we have considered the manifestations of instincts that are plainly psychological in character, that is, the instinct motivations. But an instinct, at bottom, is a reaction of the whole organism. The body is a complicated machine and its simplest functions do not exist independently of others. I cannot bend my finger without involving not merely the muscles engaged and a large part of the central nervous system, but also including chemical reactions that reverberate off into all the vital organs and systems of organs. An instinct therefore, must be an integration involving both psychological and physiological elements. Darwin recognized this and James and Lange followed with their famous theory of emotions. This theory we have seen is untenable as originally stated but, with some modifications and additions still has great value. The chief emendation is the adoption of the suggestion of Lloyd Morgan and Sherrington that visceral events may have some kind of representation in the cerebral cortex. This is a cumbrous physiological expression for what is intended as a psychological process, because it means that part of the mental material may be representations of visceral sensations, when the viscera are not sending impulses through to the brain. Now if we apply the same terminology to sensory material derived from stimuli within the body as to those arising on its exterior, we must call these " representations " images. An ordinarily conceived image is a conscious reproduction of a perception when no stimulus activates the perception. For instance, I can have a visual image of a dog when no dog is visible.

I can see objections to this nomenclature but none that are insurmountable. The most obvious of these is that an image is, strictly speaking, a conscious phenomenon[1]. This is quite true, but then we know no mental datum directly unless it be conscious ; all unconscious elements are demonstrable by inference only ; not one is, by definition, open to inspection. So, whether there be unconscious images or not we cannot say with finality. We can only affirm that when a certain type of mental process reaches consciousness it takes the form of an image. If this proviso were added every time the word " unconscious " were used, our language would be very cumbrous. So we speak of unconscious images.

The second objection is that all the images we have been discussing represent duplications of experiences that at one time have been conscious and may become so again at any time, while a " visceral image " never has, and, presumably, never will be in awareness. Although this is true, it is not wholly so for internal stimuli may by mass effect succeed in presenting something to consciousness. If I feel nausea I am certainly not aware of the various changes in tension, circulation and secretion that are present in my alimentary canal, but the sum total I *do* know. I do feel sick. Or, again, I have never experienced tension in one tendon only, or pressure at one point only in a joint, quite isolated from any other perception. But I do have vividly conscious experience of an integration of such perceptions, whenever I am aware of the position of one of my limbs. Now in this second case we can have ample proof of sensory impulses from joints and tendons existing apart from specific stimuli because people who have lost arms or legs may feel them and feel them move. If " phantom limbs " be not images (or hallucinations) what are ? And it must be remembered that a phantom limb gives an experience so accurately like the earlier actual ones as to be embarrassing. Now it is true that such images are reproductions of complicated perceptions that once were fully conscious. But the elements that were integrated together to make the conscious complex were, many of them, not matters of conscious experience. Were they therefore non-mental ? I see no reason to suppose so. The experience of tension in one tendon could certainly, under proper conditions, enter into awareness ; in fact, the " queer sensations " that patients often complain of in various kinds of organic disease are probably the effects on consciousness of afferent impulses which have never been wittingly perceived before, because not occurring in isolation nor in sufficient strength. It is not unlikely that the whole story is one of threshold value, so that afferent impulses have to be more intense to enter consciousness than to affect the unconscious mind.

This is shown in experiments performed both by nature and artificially. If a man be blinded he can lower the threshold for touch and hearing stimuli to a marvellous degree. It is difficult to imagine this being a physiological change, or, at least, it is unaccom-

---

[1] So, too, is memory as ordinarily considered. Yet Sherrington goes so far as to speak of " Visceral and organic sensations and the *memories and associations* of them . . .", *Integrative Action*, p. 267.

panied by any alterations that can be detected with other than psychological tests. If not physiological, it is psychological and involves the bringing into consciousness of perceptions that previously were merely unconscious. In hypnotic experiments it has been shown innumerable times that consciousness can be so modified as to have an incredibly low threshold for sensory impressions.

At this point it is necessary to avoid misconceptions based on preconceptions as to nomenclature. So long as one has no category " The Unconscious ", it is easy to divide functions into psychological and physiological groups, because the former are only the ones revealed to introspection. If this division be selected a difficulty at once arises : there are a huge number of phenomena now " physiological " that can only be discussed in purely psychological terms. It is this embarrassment that has forced the adoption of the hypothesis of the unconscious. As this whole book has been written on the assumption that the mind can work outside of awareness, this is hardly the time to recant. But what are we to do with phenomena like visceral sensations that unquestionably enter into definitely mental complexes but also play a rôle in physiological processes ? I cannot see how, in theory, any line can be drawn, nor can I imagine what kind of new evidence could ever allow of a hard and fast discrimination. So I believe a procedure based on mere convenience should be adopted.

The one I propose is this : the simplest neurological processes—reflexes—are physiological. So are those more complicated ones that can be represented by a neurone (or analogous) diagram. But the moment an integration of reflexes of such complexity is reached as to make such a representation inadequate, let us call this function psychological. In practice this amounts to naming as a mental reaction any response that involves qualitative discrimination between stimuli. No qualitative discrimination can be *adequately* represented in a diagram. Of course, this extends the range of the psychic into fields that the physiologist can best investigate, but that is not so much of a crime as it would be to make the physiologist investigate, with his technique, all the phenomena we have been calling unconscious. Moreover, this is less an affront to the common meanings of terms than it is to speak—as some do—of the " consciousness " of the spinal cord or of an earthworm. After all, an animal that shows discrimination *looks* as if it thought.

If then, we adopt this grouping as a basis of pure expediency, it is obvious that there will be a large field—the unconscious mind—that slopes off on each side to another. These others are conscious functions on the one hand, and physiological ones on the other. This has an immediate bearing on our problem of emotions. There is now no theoretic reason why, if an instinct process be calling up others by association, purely physiological events as well as conscious ones should not occur. If the laws of psychology hold above the level where discriminative response begins, there may be perceptions that never reach consciousness, but may be nevertheless reproduced as images. Conscious images may be the stimuli for voluntary behaviour or for a train of thought. Unconscious images may similarly determine impulsive or automatic behaviour (Morton Prince has demonstrated this nicely), or may set up a flux of other images. These latter may initiate further behaviour (or thoughts) or set up definitely physiological reactions. *Emotional expression is the product of unconscious images which stimulate involuntary behaviour, either overt or visceral, accessory to purposeful actions. Affect is the impression made on consciousness by active unconscious imaginal processes, which do not gain any other outlet.*

The affect-producing images may be reproductions of environmental perceptions, of new combinations of these or of " perceptions " of bodily processes that never have been conscious. As we have seen, the energy flowing through any instinctive channel may be carried off or deflected by adequate expression in behaviour or conscious thought. If, however, an instinctive process be activated but denied these outlets, the energy is dammed up and flows into collateral channels. If these, in turn, fail to carry off the energy the backing-up goes on farther and farther till it ends in the production of somatic symptoms. The more damming up there is the stronger will the affect be until the point of physiological discharge is reached. If this actually drains off energy, the affect will then be reduced or, perhaps, abolished. This is why hysterical symptoms may be accompanied by no affect. For instance, comparing the two big groups of war neurosis, the anxiety states and the conversion hysterias, one saw fundamentally the same idea-functions producing violent affect on the one side, and physical symptoms with comparative or complete subjective comfort on the other. According to this view affect would be strongest when the damming up had reached the point of activization of images of internal bodily processes, but before the latter had actually led to physiological discharge.

An example may make this formulation clearer. Let us consider the probable train of events in the production of hysterical vomiting. Many cases of this disease have been investigated by psychoanalysts, and shown to be due to unconscious sexual disturbances. Without claiming that this is the only instinct that ever does produce such symptoms, a case with such etiology may serve as an example. Sexual tendencies are being repressed ; therefore, if once activated, damming up is bound to take place. This may lead to reformulation as sublimation or to further damming. *Qua* neurotic, the patient cannot sublimate adequately, hence overflow is going to take place. The sexual impulse is formulated, unconsciously, as an idea-function of pregnancy or impregnation. The images incorporating this are of the presence in the stomach of foreign substances. Associated with foreign substance images are those of poisons or indigestible material. These activate in turn the images of afferent stimuli set up in the digestive tract by the presence of such material in actuality. At this point there is a strong feeling of nausea, a feeling which is really an affect, according to our definition. Then these noxious-substance-images produce the complicated physiological response of vomitting. At once the nausea—the affect—disappears.

One advantage of this theory has probably occurred to the reader by now. It accounts equally well for emotional disturbances set up by stimuli that are originally purely psychological as for those of physical origin. Nausea is an excellent example of this. If I have indigestion, the afferent impulses from my digestive tract will evoke unconscious images that are felt as " nausea " before discharge takes place. And, with the exceptions of terror and deep depression, there is probably no affect as powerful as nausea. Or, if physiological disturbances excite my adrenal-sympathetic system, I may feel a vague anxiety without any psychogenic cause for it. Further, if the more complicated neurological functions follow psychological laws, and if our energy concept be sound, it is plain that associations from gastro-intestinal images will overflow into vasomotor channels until an adequate discharge of energy takes place one way or another. This explains why there may be such marked circulatory changes accompanying nausea, which disappear so soon as vomitting occurs.

The last matter to be discussed is the *raison d'être* of the various visceral changes that have been demonstrated by Cannon as accompaniments of emotion. Their biological purpose seems, plainly, to be the perpetuation rather than the initiation of violent muscular movements. Therefore one would expect them to appear after and not before exertion. It is probable that they do follow excessive work, where instincts are given free play, and come into operation when fatigue products produce stimuli specific for metabolic acceleration. But, according to our theory, these stimuli, as images, are associated with the images that stimulate strong and continuous muscular contractions. Or, to put it in Sherrington's terms, the accessory reactions are integrated with reactions of fighting, fleeing and so on. But when there is conflict (a matter of choice of reaction at the animal level, or intellectual and moral conflict as it may be in man) the primary instinct process is inhibited, so that overflow make take place into the associated, accessory outlets for energy. At the unconscious level voluntary and involuntary reactions are integrated together (associated). When the voluntary ones are impeded the involuntary ones will come into play. Hence the appearance of emotional expression, part of which is visceral changes, and of affect, or of both.

A final word should be added as to the elaboration and fate of affect once it has been aroused—a topic so far neglected except for some hints offered in the discussion above about the feeling of reality. According to my hypothesis affect is the effect produced in consciousness of the activization of unconscious image processes. Since these are unconscious, only a feeling penetrates into awareness, a feeling aroused by something of which the subject is quite ignorant. Self-conscious minds seem to have a repugnance for such isolated disembodied mental phenomena : they are felt to be morbid or eerie. Consequently a process of rationalization is undertaken at once. Whatever is in the focus of attention at the moment when the affect arises is held to be the direct cause of it. Consciousness is then focussed on two elements, on the object of external reference, which is a matter of pure cognition, and on to the affect. The two are thus combined to form a unit. Were the subject to report his introspection in the terms of everyday psychology, he would say that he was aware of a given perception that had a certain meaning. This meaning, I would claim, is the vital element, and is, in fact, the product of the affect. In the simplest case a preliminary perception activates a train of unconscious imagery which becomes conscious as an affect, and is given external reference by reflection on to the original stimulus. The latter is then re-perceived as having a special meaning. The second perception, the one that really gains serious attention is secondary to the affect. Striking perceptions are therefore liable to be secondary, rather than primary ones.

Several consequences flow from this. In the first place, since, when an affect is aroused, external reference offers to consciousness a perception as well, the latter must contribute to the quale of the emotional experience. The fear of a soldier before a stern officer may be due to unconscious images of escape. Similar images may be activated by the appearance of an enemy with a bomb. But the one is referred to a superior and the other to an enemy, and inevitably, the emotional experience is different.

How this comes about is not far to seek. The case I have mentioned of the initial stimulus reappearing as a secondary perception is too simple. Most of our perceptions are highly complicated ones ; it is some one detail that sets the affective process going. Attention, turned to the complicated situation, is liable to focus on some other detail, and this again sets up another train of unconscious imagery. Until some definite reaction—overt behaviour or conscious plan— is achieved, this echoing and re-echoing goes on from the perceived situation to affect and back again, and all the time the total affect is gaining a more complicated, and therefore more peculiar, quality. External reference therefore colours affect, and, in part, mediates it.

We are led then to the view that the quale of an affective experience may be determined by many trains of unconscious images. This may be put another way by saying that it is the product of the nature and proportions of the instinct processes unconsciously activated. This hypothesis allows—nay, it demands—the possibility of endless varieties of affects. It is plain that if more than one instinct process be involved, the proportions appearing in combination are capable of variation. But, according to our theory any single instinct process is itself liable to modification. That purely hypothetical entity a simple congenital instinct exists only as a tendency. Its actual exhibitions are the product of experience, the reactions slowly establishing new patterns. When images are incorporated into the structure, it becomes more plastic and takes on more of the modifiability of conscious mentation. We know, for instance, how behaviour in relation to some type of experience may be radically altered by one dramatic adventure. This means that the unconscious reaction patterns of no two people are alike, and further, that there is a slow unconscious evolution, parallelling the differentations of personality. It therefore follows that the affect of no two subjects, in the presence of the same stimulus are identical, and, further, that I may not produce the same emotional response to-morrow that I do to-day. In other words the variations of affect are like those of personality, which is natural enough since they are two exhibitions of the same underlying processes. I can never hope to know—except in the case of a crude emotion—what another feels ; to do so I would have to borrow his personality. Similarly I can never remember a refined or complicated affect except in such general terms as I would use to describe it to a second person. It can only be accurately reproduced by re-experience, and the latter would be possible only if I myself were absolutely unchanged. " The first free careless rapture " comes only once. Therefore the subject is a different person, be it only in having had that rapturous experience.

Another effect of the external reference of affect must be considered. As has been noted attention is turned to the environment in an effort of rationalization, as that another stimulus comes into play. The latter may activate processes of less dynamic, unconscious significance. The affect is thus diluted. This mechanism is of prime importance in psychopathology, because this is the one point where the stampede may be checked or turned. Sufficient exercise of will may keep attention fixed on some stimulus which activates less poignant affects. Thus a studied pre-occupation with everyday tasks may succeed in reducing depression. We have no control over affect directly, but we can put ourselves in or out of the way of what will excite emotions.

A corollary of this throws some light on the psychology of religious exercises. The more conscious any mental reaction is, the less emotionally toned is it. The greater then, is the attention given to the intellectual content of a ritual, the less religious feeling does it excite. No feeling, *qua* feeling, is rational, and religious emotion is not an exception. The psychology of religion owes much to Rudolf Otto[1] for his effective exposition of this principle, which, as he shows, is applicable to music as well. Music is a

---

[1] " The Idea of the Holy " translated by Harvey, Oxford University Press.

language that speaks to the unconscious or not at all. An attempt to translate it into terms of conscious ideas annihilates it. The real magic of religion is that an incomprehensible affect is produced by the utilization of means undertaken to that end. But the point of view of the worshipper must be similar to that of one expecting magic : he must not attempt to fathom the meaning of the words or ceremonies, except by feeling. Such, perhaps, is the meaning of entering the Kingdom of Heaven as a little child.

This, however, is too one-sided a statement. Were it wholly or exclusively true, the actual words or procedure in ritual would be a matter of indifference. Any mumbo-jumbo would do. So another factor has to be considered. When words are the effective stimulus in awakening affect, ideas are being used. Ideas gain a specific meaning from the comprehension of the subject. In other words an intellectual elaboration must be made before the idea can become effective as a stimulus. This, however, can be done unconsciously. A symbol can represent, and therefore evoke, an unconscious idea-function and still be senseless from a conscious point. But it is not any bit of nonsense whatever. Again, many of our aesthetic feelings depend on judgments that are intellectual. For instance, diction is surely an intellectual affair, but a particular grouping of words will excite a stylist pleasantly or unpleasantly. If, in ritual, the words do not flow in a stream that seems beautiful, all those sensitized for language will find the performance exciting affects far from harmonious with religious atmosphere. On the other hand, words, sounds, colours or odours that satisfy aesthetically, all contribute to the quale of the desired affect.

CHAPTER LI

FUTURE PROBLEMS

The Imagination is one of the highest prerogatives of man. By this faculty he unites former images and ideas, *independently of the will*, and thus creates brilliant and novel results.

The Descent of Man, Darwin.

IN order to explain emotions I have fabricated an hypothesis·of unconscious mental processes which, in continuous operation, not merely parallel consciousness but actually support and nourish it. These unconscious processes issue, I have claimed, in behaviour, (both voluntary and involuntary), in emotions, and in conscious thinking. Plainly, if this be sound theory, it must be possible to explain all psychological phenomena in these terms. In fact, if it be not universally applicable, it would fail even in its initial task of accounting for emotions, because the emotional is thoroughly intermingled with the intellectual in all mental life. This is an ambitious task, so ambitious that I would not undertake to achieve it. For, like every proper *Kerl der spekuliert*, I have a greater respect for my theories than I have for myself as their expositor. Moreover, this is a study of emotions, not a treatise on psychology. It has already extended itself far past its projected length. The book is finished, so, perhaps, a post-script may be allowed in which I point out how our cognate problems may, perhaps, be solved.

For the purposes of the study of emotions the fundamental process has been termed " free association ". The reader has, perhaps, suspected before this that free associations are but one form assumed by some more fundamental process. Something that extends down to the physiological level cannot be accurately labelled in a terminology derived from conscious mental experience. Yet I have retained the term here, because it is applicable to the major portion of the phenomena discussed. Eventually, however, if the theory is to be given wider application, it will have to be abandoned, and have its place taken by some word that can be used indifferently in the description of conscious, unconscious and neurological events.

How free associations may explain a number of general psychological problems has already appeared in accounting for various symptoms observed in manic-depressive insanity. Since it is along these lines that I believe further researches may extend, it may be well to mention some of them again.

Vagaries of *attention* appear in the manic symptom of distracti-bility. In this psychosis we saw that attention may be directed to a conscious perception which is a suitable vehicle for expression of a co-conscious idea-function. All attention may be of this nature and inevitably dependent on the dominance in the co-conscious of some group of idea-functions. A change of attention would then result from the introduction of a stimulus strong enough to activate another train of idea-functions.

Recognition receives a good deal of illumination from the observa-tion of patients who are subjectively perplexed. In studying such cases the conclusion was reached that a feeling of familiarity grows around any perception when it leads to activization, co-consciously, of images that duplicate, or closely resemble, the percept in con-sciousness. When the co-conscious image come into conscious-ness there is memory of an event or object that is identical with or different from the perception. The process of recognition is complete. One then knows that the present is not providing a new experience or that it is. In either event the affect of familiarity disappears with the entrance of the image into con-sciousness. It has served its function of arresting conscious attention till the memory image can be inspected by awareness.

It is possible that all the phenomena of *memory* may be ex-pressible in terms of free associations. That any explanation beyond that of *recall* can issue from such a translation is yet to be proved. But, at least, in studying dreams it seemed that free associations were the vehicle by which past mental experience travelled into consciousness again. The magnitude and importance of this problem is obvious.

Meaning, seems as well to depend, somehow, on free associations or on the nature of free associations. In ordinary, introspective psychology the study of this problem is rendered difficult by the fact that in normal life the definition meaning and the behaviour meaning of a word, percept or concept, may be closely allied. When we deal with symbols, that are regarded as symbols by the subject, such differences as may exist between the two meanings are still perhaps explainable by specious argument. But when we examine psychopathological material, the two can by no verbal agility be put side by side. When behaviour is determined solely by the symbolic meaning, and not by the obvious significance, and when attendant conscious judgments are similarly formed, one has to discard the dictionary altogether, and realize that symbols—images —form a language of their own, the meaning of which is to be found in what is, broadly, behaviour. And at this point one may perhaps be able to use free associations in deciding which gauge of meaning is to be used. There is a vast difference in the nature of the successive elements of the associations of one who is merely dis-cursive, mildly flighty, in full manic flight, given to scattered speech, suffering from distraction of thought or dreaming. There is a parallel change in meaning.

No psychology that pretends to be biological can fail to be genetic. Beginning with some relatively simple principles it must construct mind out of these. There are then, two great problems at the two extremes of mental life. That physiological functions are developed into mental ones, and how do these culminate in consciousness ? To the last we have no satisfactory answer as yet, and none, it seems to me, that is even promising. The behaviourists cut the Gordian knot by denying there is any such thing. To characterize this solution I can find no epithet but " silly ". Not only is it an affront to universal experience, but, as we have seen repeatedly, consciousness is a term for a variety of functions, working together, that would have to be accounted for were there no such experience as subjective awareness. To reconstruct consciousness, is, I believe, the most ambitious task in psychology, but I also believe that it may be possible to fabricate a hypothesis as to how it might arise, even if no finality be achieved.

Then there is the physiological end of this spectrum, the infra-red, that warms us, nourishes us, although we do not sense it directly. One cannot explain emotions without entering the domain of physiology. If, then, the explanation be valid for these physiological processes, why not for others ? In other words, if the physiology of emotions be sound physiology, it must be applicable elsewhere. One begins to suspect that any principle, which can be evoked to account for the varied phenomena mentioned so far, is likely to be useful in studying any integration of functions whatever. At least it may give us a language in which to discuss all psycho-pathological phenomena without being forever guilty of tautology, of " neurologizing psychology ".

What these problems will include is for the future to reveal, but one of them must be mentioned now. This is *pain*. In the Psychological Introduction I argued that pain must be an affect on any definition of affect that includes phenomena normally spoken of as affective. To this topic I have not recurred as yet, because its discussion would involve the introduction of physiological data irrelevant to the general purpose of this book. But, now that I am indulging in what may fairly be called fantasy, I may mention my view, which, without evidence, I would expect neither physiologist nor psychologist to accept.

Sherrington says, " Pain is the psychical adjunct of a protective reflex "[1]. Abolish consciousness (as, for instance, by severing the conduction paths to the brain), and what is seen is the protective reflex, appearing, perhaps, in exaggerated form. When one feels pain, then, it may be that one feels not merely the stimulus but the response as well. If one felt merely the stimulus he would be experiencing a pure " sensation ", that is, a psychologist's myth. Only perceptions (that is sensations qualified by experience, by

---

[1] *Integrative Action of the Nervous System*, p. 252.

meaning) ever enter consciousness. The interpretative quality which the word " pain " implies may be the response, represented in consciousness as pain. But, it will be objected, the subject may feel pain when motionless. Yes, and he may feel pain when there is no stimulus, as many patients do, " Imaginary pains " as the non-psychological doctor calls them. (As if pain, *qua* pain, had any existence except as a subjective experience ! If a pain were imaginary, it would cease to be a pain.) The something which gives the specific quality we call " pain " may, therefore, be produced psychologically. At this point the hypothesis of images of physiological processes may solve the problem. If the withdrawal reaction be represented as an image, this may be evoked by the process of association. It will be associated both with noxious stimuli at one end, and with images of a conscious order at the other. The image of a withdrawal movement may, then, be elicited from either end of the chain. If I am pricked with a pin I will feel as pain the tendency to withdraw, whether I do move or not. Similarly, if I incorporate some co-conscious idea-function in the image of a pin-prick, that will incite either withdrawal or an image of withdrawal, and I shall feel pain again. In broad outlines, therefore, the same kind of processes—in so far as they affect consciousness, explain the affect of pain, or the affect of nausea, or the affect of fear.

All these problems I am planning to discuss in a small book, which, I hope, may appear soon, under the title of *The Basis and Development of Mental Life.*

GLOSSARY

Note. *Technical terms not included here are probably defined in the text, and should be sought out in the Index.*

ACHILLES REFLEX : *See* REFLEX.

ACHILLES TENDON : The big tendon running from the calf muscles to the back of the heel bone.

ACIDOSIS : A disturbance of balance in body chemistry between acid and alkali products, the former tending to predominate.

AFFERENT : A physiological term for nervous impulses conducted from the point of stimulus toward the central nervous system, and, inside the central nervous system for impulses travelling towards the brain. (The central nervous system comprises the brain and spinal cord.)

AMNESIA : Forgetting. A term usually not employed so much in cases where there is a general defect of memory, but rather for failure to recall specific data that one would expect the subject to be able to remember.

ANLAGE : An embryological term, meaning a nest of cells from which some organ will develop, which is now given a wider reference as a metaphor.

ANTHROPOMORPHISM : Assigning human qualities (consciousness and personality) to organisms or functions, although there is no direct evidence therefor.

APPERCEPTION : Conscious recognition of mental processes.

ARCUS SENILIS : A whitish opaque ring at the periphery of the cornea.

ARTERIOSCLEROSIS : " Hardening of the arteries ". A disease incidental to advancing age, but apt to appear before other evidences of senility. It often affects particularly the vessels of the brain. This leads to apoplexy, with destruction of part of the brain, or it may simply lead to interference with the nutrition of the brain tissue, and hence its gradual diffuse decay. The mental symptoms are a reduction in the speed and accuracy of mental processes, which may go on to severe dementia.

AURA : In epilepsy a " warning " which the patient has of an approaching seizure. It usually takes the form of an unusual bodily perception, but may be an hallucination or peculiar affective state.

AUTISTIC : A term coined by Bleuler to denote that the mental experience so characterized is a product of imagination. Autistic thinking includes dreams, delusions, hallucinations, but also the creative productions of poetry, art, invention and theoretic speculation.

BEHAVIOURISM : A doctrine which claims that mental processes can be adequately and best studied by purely objective observation, eliminating introspection. It denies the usefulness of the concept of consciousness, and attempts to formulate mind in terms of physiological processes.

CATALEPSY : A maintenance of positions or postures in which a patient's body or limbs have been artificially placed. Associated with it is *flexibilitas cerea*, in which condition joints bend when manipulated, but do so with a steady resistance as if made of wax.

CATATONIA : *See* DEMENTIA PRAECOX.

CLONUS : Continuous oscillatory movements, usually of the foot or lower leg, produced on sudden passive bending of a joint. The muscles, which are thus stretched, contract ; this stretches the muscles on the opposite side, which contract in turn, and so the process goes on indefinitely. It bespeaks a loss of voluntary control, which is usually the result of disease in the central nervous system, but may be a purely neurotic phenomenon.

CLOUDING (of consciousness) : A dulling of perception which results in confusion about the environment, although mental processes of internal origin may be quite active. A dream-like state.

CO-CONSCIOUS : Unconscious mental processes in a state of activity.

COMPLEX : A group of ideas constellated by an instinctive process. The ideas are linked together because they form a chain in some potential instinctive reaction. A complex is always unconscious, or at least, owes its importance to elements in it which remain unconscious.

CONATION : That part of a psychological reaction which moves toward expression, towards behaviour, or to the initiation of other content. It is equivalent to, or rather includes, impulse and striving ; in the sphere of conscious mental processes it may be represented by desire.

CONJUNCTIVAE : The mucous membranes covering the front of the eye-balls and lining the lids.

CONSCIOUSNESS : (1) Simple awareness—awareness of self and awareness of environment. (2) The totality of mental processes associated with and involving awareness.

CONTENT, MENTAL CONTENT, OR IDEATIONAL CONTENT : That which a subject is consciously thinking of, as judged by his speech and actions.

CONTRACTURE : A permanent shortening of a muscle or of one muscle group.

CORNEA : A transparent membrane in the centre of the front of the eye-ball. The iris, or coloured part of the eye, is visible through it.

CYANOSIS : A dusky blue colouration due to stagnation of the blood, or to lack of oxygen in the blood of the part of the body where the change is observed.

DELUSION : A false idea, held to be true by the subject.

DEMENTIA : Chronic, and often progressive, mental disease.

DEMENTIA PRAECOX : A constitutional, chronic, mental disease characterized by delusions, hallucinations and scattered speech, as well as reduction, or dissociation, of emotional reaction. Only one of these may be prominent, but all are always potentially present. Dementia praecox is often divided into three types : hebephrenia, in which scattered speech and dissociation of emotional reaction are prominent, giving an impression to the observer of extreme silliness ; catatonia, characterized by sullenness, negativism, silence (often actual stupor), punctuated by wildly irrational, impulsive acts ; and a paranoid form. In the last, false ideas may be the only obvious symptom, so that the patient may make quite a normal impression except in so far as his delusions induce odd behaviour.

DISORIENTATION : A disturbance or loss of orientation (*q.v.*) in any of its spheres.

DISSOCIATION : (As a psychopathological term) the segregation of a group of mental processes, separated off from consciousness, but functioning as a unitary whole, *as if* they belonged to another person. This, when greatly elaborated, may lead to a double personality, but only if the dissociated complexes displace the normal consciousness, becoming themselves conscious.

DISSOCIATION OF AFFECT : A loose term used in psychiatry to cover both the appearance of only one element in a complicated emotional reaction (e.g., tears without other evidence of woe), and also exhibition of a kind of emotional response inappropriate to the situation. The former alone ought to be called " Dissociation of Affect " or, better still, " Dissociation of Emotion".

EFFERENT : A physiological term for nervous impulses proceeding from the brain and towards the muscles or glands.

EMOTION : *See* Chapter VI.

ENDOCRINE (glands) : Glands of internal secretion. These are often spoken of as a separate system, for instance, one speaks of endocrine functions.

ETIOLOGY : Causation ; but etiology is a little wider in its reference than causation because under the former term are grouped all possible factors that might operate as contributary, if not as direct, causes.

EUPHORIA : An abnormal feeling of well-being.

EXTROVERSION : Turning of interest and attention to the world around.

FEMUR : The bone of the thigh.

FLEXIBILITAS CEREA : *See* CATALEPSY.

FLIGHT (of ideas) : A wandering train of thought rendered inconsequent and often incomprehensible by the interruption of sound associations (often rhyming) and of comments on the environment, and the occurrence of associations of purely personal origin.

FORECONSCIOUS : A term used by Freud to cover mental processes, not in awareness, but capable of appearing there under appropriate stimulation from without, or in response to studied conscious effort toward that end.

FUGUE : A state of dissociated (*q. v.*) mental activity which exhibits itself in conduct over which the subject has no control, and of which he is not, as a rule, aware so far as his normal consciousness is concerned.

GONADS : The sexual glands.

HALLUCINATION : A false sensory experience. A mild type of this is " illusion ", which is a distorted perception of some actual environmental event. A completely developed hallucination occurs independently of any demonstrable environmental stimulus.

HYDROCOELE : A cyst containing watery fluid, usually in the testicle.

HYPNOGOGIC : Referring to the period of time and the mental state during the induction of sleep, that is between normal waking thought and dreaming.

HYPNOPOMPIC : A term equivalent to hypnogogic, but referring to the time between sleeping and waking up.

HYPNOSIS : An artificially induced condition in which the functions of consciousness are directed by the hypnotist instead of by the subject and in which the range of this vicarious control is much wider than that of the subject's normal consciousness. Hence there results an activation of bodily processes or of ideas which is normally impossible, while there is also a recognition of afferent stimuli and a production of memories such as cannot be brought into consciousness voluntarily.

HYSTERECTOMY : An operation for removal of the womb and usually of the ovaries as well.

HYSTERIA : A psychoneurosis (some forms reckoned as a psychosis), the symptoms of which are, rather exclusively, the product of dissociation (q.v.). If the dissociation affect conscious control of bodily processes, " Conversion " Hysteria (Freud) results, that is a condition in which there appears to be physical disease. For instance, there may be loss of functions : blindness, deafness, mutism, absence of voiced sounds so that the patient can only whisper, almost any kind of paralysis or loss of sensation ; or functions may be disturbed, so that there are automatic movements, or some simple habitual movements are distorted (e.g., gait disturbances). If, on the other hand, obviously mental processes are affected, there are losses of memory or any of the symptoms which may result from the irruption into consciousness of dissociated material. Thus there are attacks of clouding or consciousness, deliria, fugues and even multiple personality. Many so-called occult phenomena, such as automatic writing, are really hysterical phenomena.

ILLUSION : *See* HALLUCINATION.

IMAGE : The reproduction of a perception in the absence of environmenta stimulus, but recognized by consciousness as being a purely mental product, being thus differentiated from hallucination.

IMAGO : The object existing only in unconscious fantasy of an unconscious affection or repulsion.

INSTINCT : *See* Chapter VI.

INSTINCT MOTIVATION : *See* Chapter VI.

INTROVERSION : The turning of interest and attention to the world within, i.e., to oneself as body and as personality, to the products of one's mind.

INVOLUNTARY NERVOUS SYSTEM : A system of ganglia (groups of nerve cells) which lie outside the central nervous system and are connected together, and with the organs they supply, and with the central nervous system, by separate nerves. The involuntary nervous system controls immediately the contraction or dilation of blood vessels, the secretions of all glands, both internal and external, and all muscles which are not under direct voluntary control, as, for example, the muscles in the walls of the stomach and intestines, the muscles that move the hairs on the surface of the body, and so on. It is called the involuntary nervous system because consciousness has no direct control over it. Correlated with this is the fact that all afferent impulses arising in the involuntary nervous system do not reach consciousness, or, if they do, do not lead to accurate or accurately localised perceptions.

INVOLUTION : The opposite of evolution—regressive rather than progressive development. Specifically it refers to the period of life after a mature vigour is achieved, when strength is beginning to go, but before actual senility is demonstrable.

ISCHAEMIA : Insufficient blood supply.

LEUCOCYTOSIS : The increase of white blood cells in the circulating blood. It often occurs in conjunction with some infections and fevers, but may be caused by other factors as well.

LIBIDO : A psycho-analytic term for sexual appetite ; it stands to sexual instinct in the same relation as hunger does to nutritional instinct. It refers mainly to unconscious strivings of a sexual nature. According to psycho-analytic theory, however, through symbolisations and sublimations, this sexual factor comes to be the driving force back of most interests. I do not use the term in the cosmic sense which Jung gives it.

MENTATION : A purposely vague term covering any kind of mental activity. It is roughly equivalent to " mental processes ".

NEGATIVISM : A perversity in behaviour. Sometimes it is exhibited merely in refusal to speak, but often consists in the patient's doing opposite of what commanded to do or expected to do.

NEURONE : The unit element, anatomically, in the nervous system. It consists of the nerve cell, which has a central cell body from which run long processes, that, although of microscopic diameter, may be several feet long. The processes are of two types, dendrites and axones. The former carry nervous impulses towards the cell body, while the latter carry them away. The present-day physiology of the nervous system is based on the neurone doctrine. According to this hypothesis, impulses pass from the axone of one nerve cell to the dendrites of another or to more than one other. The second pass the impulses along to the dendrites of a third group, and so on. Eventually the axone of some cell connects with a gland or muscle, which then secretes or contracts. Thus a stimulus from one part of the body may effect an action in a far-distant part of the body. A " reflex " is of this order. Theoretically, a reflex is constituted of three simple elements. A nerve end organ in the skin transmits an impulse along a sensory nerve to a ganglion lying next the spinal cord (that is, along the dendrite of a cell, the body of which is in the ganglion) ; an axone from the ganglion runs into the spinal cord, and there transmits the impulse to a second, or connector, neurone, this links up with a third neurone which sends out an axone to a muscle or gland through an efferent nerve. Since the afferent cell may connect with many connectors and the latter with many efferent neurones or even with still other connectors, a great complexity of reaction is possible on this theory.

NOSOLOGY : Classification of diseases.

ONANISM : Masturbation.

OPISTHOTONOUS : A condition of muscle spasm in which the muscles of the neck, back and legs are so contracted as to make an arch, the body resting on head and heels.

ORIENTATION : Knowledge of one's whereabouts, including recognition of the people about (or at least of their status, in a hospital as doctors, nurses and patients), and of day, date and year and of approximate time of day. We therefore speak of orientation for time, place and persons.

PARANOIA (Paranoid state) : Mental disease characterized by "ideas of reference", i e., misinterpretation of the actions of other people, and ascription to them of motives which they do not possess, such as enmity towards the patient, and so on.

PARESIS : (1) As a general term meaning simply weakness. (2) Specifically, as a psychiatric term, a dementia due to the late effects of syphilis. It is also called general paralysis of the insane, and is known to the layman frequently as " softening of the brain ".

PARTURITION : The process of childbirth.

PATHOGNOMIC : Giving conclusive evidence of a specific pathological process or of a specific disease.

PERCEPTION : An effect produced on the mind by some stimulus originating in the environment or in some physiological change within the body, but outside of the nervous system. Before this effect can be called a perception it must be given some meaning, that is it involves the utilization of past experiences in the interpretation of the present one.

PERSEVERATION : Useless and inappropriate maintenance of any reaction. It always implies an incapacity of consciousness to change the direction of attention or to control a response that has been elicited, so that the latter goes on autonomously.

PHALANX (Phalangeal) : One of the bones of the fingers or toes.

PHARYNX (Pharyngeal) : The throat.

PHOBIA : A fear regarded by the subject as irrational and inexplicable, of some innocuous object or situation.

PRE-CONSCIOUSNESS : The period of mental life in an infant prior to the development of consciousness.

PRE-MENSTRUUM : A period just before menstrual flow begins marked by a feeling of tension and often by nervous symptoms. It may last for only a few hours or for several days.

PSYCHIATRY : The study of mental disease from a medical standpoint.

PSYCHOLEPTIC CRISIS : An abrupt appearance of dramatic mental symptoms. It is often associated with the delusion of the world coming to an end, or of its being radically altered in the twinkling of an eye. Or, on the other hand, the change seems to be in the patient himself ; then something " gives way ", in his head as a rule.

PSYCHONEUROSIS : See PSYCHOSIS.

PSYCHOPATHOLOGY : The study and science of mental disease, particularly from the psychological standpoint.

PSYCHOPATHY : A vague term for mental disorder, but of wider reference than the term mental disease because it includes all that is ordinarily called mental disease, and, in addition, alcoholism, crime, social maladjustment, epilepsy, and so on.

PSYCHOSIS : Mental disease. It is roughly equivalent to insanity, but the latter is, strictly speaking, a legal term referring to the condition of one who is certified through legal procedure as being mentally incompetent. This implies serious disability, whereas psychosis being a medical term implies only the existence of mental derangement, no matter in how slight a degree. A psycho-neurosis is a state of ill-health, the symptoms of which are produced psychologically, but it is differentiated from a psychosis by the retention, in the case of a psycho-neurosis, of insight; that is, the patient regards the symptoms of a psycho-neurosis as being something abnormal, as representing disease in some form, no matter whether he regards the cause of it as being physical or mental. A patient with a psychosis, on the other hand, regards the environment as being really changed, or that he himself (either in body or in mind) is altered. The change in himself he may regard as being the product of disease, but in this case the symptoms are palpably ridiculous. Amongst psychoses are also included marked abnormalities in emotional reaction to be pathological. For instance, a normal person may feel anxious or distressed and regard his mood as abnormal. A psychotically anxious or distressed patient will consider that circumstances justified his emotional state.

REACTION FORMATION : The development, in the conscious personality, of traits representing a tendency directly opposed to a strong unconscious trend, e.g., a sympathetic nature in one who is unconsciously cruel.

REACTION TYPE : See Chapter IV.

REFLEXES (Deep) : Contractions produced by sudden passive stretching of muscles. The ones usually elicited are known as the knee-kick and ankle-jerk (Achilles reflex), which are produced by tapping the tendon below the knee-cap or the Achilles tendon. These reflexes are normally present, but when greatly exaggerated or absent, they are suggestive or significant of a disease in the central nervous system. A considerable increase may, however, be present in a purely psycho-neurotic state.

SCATTERED SPEECH (Scattering) : See pages 422, 466.

SCHIZOPHRENIA : A term roughly equivalent to dementia praecox, but having wider reference inasmuch as most authors who use it include therewith some cases of manic-depressive insanity, particularly those in which delusions are prominent.

SENSATION : A purely hypothetical element in psychology representing the effect on the mind of a single simple afferent stimulus. It is assumed by many psychologists that perceptions are built up by the correlation of sensations, but others insist that a sensation, as properly defined, would be too primitive an element to have any mental existence whatever, and that the simplest possible mental unit would be already a perception.

SENTIMENT : The union of an idea or a group of ideas with an emotion to form a unit in mental reactions. The idea activated will arouse the emotion, while the special significance of the idea for the subject is due to the emotion.

SKOTOMATA : Spots in the field of vision in which nothing is seen. Blind spots.

SMEARING : Of faeces on body, clothes or furniture.

SOMATIC : Having to do with the body as opposed to the mind, or, physiologically, with the functions of the body rather than with those of the central nervous system.

SOMNAMBULISM : A state in which the normal consciousness is abrogated so that all physical and mental activity is no longer " willed " except for the fact that the subject may move, speak and even answer questions. It may occur spontaneously (in hysteria) or be produced by suggestion.

SPHINCTER : A ring shaped muscle that when contracted closes the opening of a hollow organ. The only ones mentioned in this book are those of the bladder and rectum which may keep urine and faeces from escaping.

SUB-CONSCIOUS : A term used only in quotations from other authors. Essentially, it is synonymous with " unconscious " as I use that term.

SUGGESTION : The process which produces the kind of modification of consciousness, which in its extreme form is known as hypnosis ((q.v.).

SYNDROME : A group of symptoms occurring together with such frequence as to justify the view that they are causally connected. Often the term is equivalent to the " symptom picture " of a disease.

TAXONOMY : Classification.

THERIOMORPHISM : The ascription to conscious mental life of an infra-human or purely physiological nature.

TIC : An habitual, more or less involuntary contraction of some muscle or of a group of associated muscles.

TREND (Trend of Ideas) : A term which has grown up at Ward's Island to denote the delusional and autistic ideas of a patient as opposed to his adaptive thoughts. The trend may include thoughts about actualities, but these are then distorted and imaginary attributes assigned to the reality.

TROPISM : A term in physiology for reactions produced by simple physical or chemical stimuli, e.g., turning to or away from heat or cold, light, positive electricity, a specific chemical substance, etc. Much of the behaviour of animals, extremely low in the evolutionary scale, can be expressed in terms of tropisms.

" UNCONSCIOUS " : Part of the mind not in normal awareness. Its mental processes reach consciousness only in abnormal mental states, dreams, and as a result of special psychological technique. (This is Rivers's definition).

" UNTIDY " : A psychiatric euphemism for wetting and soiling with urine and faeces.

VASOMOTOR SYSTEM : That part of the involuntary nervous system that presides over the contraction and dilatation of blood vessels. Blushing and pallor, for instance, are vasomotor phenomena being due to a contraction of small blood vessels which squeeze the blood out of the vessels in the part that turns pale, or the dilatation of vessels which allows engorgement of blood locally and so produces a red colour.

(IN) VITRO (literally " in glass ") : A state of artificial isolation like that of an organ taken out of the body and put into a jar.

WISH : See Chapter VI.

INDEX